Nursing Approach to the Evaluation of Child Maltreatment

SECOND EDITION

STM **Learning**, Inc.

Leading Publisher of Scientific, Technical, and Medical Educational Resources

Saint Louis

www.stmlearning.com

Our Mission

To become the world leader in publishing and information services on child abuse, maltreatment, diseases, and domestic violence. We seek to heighten awareness of these issues, and provide relevant information to professionals and consumers.

A portion of our profits is contributed to nonprofit organizations dedicated to the prevention of child abuse and the care of victims of abuse and other children and family charities.

This book is dedicated to:

To Jamie Ferrell, BSN, RN, CA/CP-SANE, DABFN, Forensic Nursing Clinical Manager at the Memorial Hermann Healthcare System who over the years stands out as a trusted colleague to many, a highly regarded expert, and an inspiring advocate for the vulnerable in need of care.

—APG and ERG

To my husband Jerry and my children Karl, Patrick, and Alice, who I am thankful to have in my life and are the heart of my inspiration.

—TFH

Nursing Approach to the Evaluation of Child Maltreatment

Second Edition

Paul Thomas Clements, PhD, RN
Associate Clinical Professor
Coordinator - Contemporary Trends in Forensic Health Care Certificate Online
Drexel University
College of Nursing and Health Professions
Philadelphia, Pennsylvania

Ann W. Burgess, DNS, APRN, FAAN
Professor, William F. Connell School of Nursing
Boston College, Chestnut Hill, Massachusetts

Theresa M. Fay-Hillier, MSN, PMHCNS-BC
Drexel University College of Nursing and Health Professions
Assistant Clinical Professor
Philadelphia, Pennsylvania

Eileen R. Giardino, PhD, RN, APRN, ANP-BC, NP-C
Associate Professor of Nursing
School of Nursing
University of Texas Health Science Center
Houston, Texas

Angelo P. Giardino, MD, PhD
Professor and Section Chief
Academic General Pediatrics
Baylor College of Medicine
Senior Vice President/Chief Quality Officer
Texas Children's Hospital
Houston, Texas

STM **Learning**, Inc.

Leading Publisher of Scientific, Technical, and Medical Educational Resources
Saint Louis
www.stmlearning.com

Publishers: Glenn E. Whaley and Marianne V. Whaley

Graphic Design Director: Glenn E. Whaley

Managing Editor: Paul K. Goode, III

Associate Editors: Lindsay Westbrook and Caoimhe Ní Dhónaill

Editorial Intern: Mia Garchitorena

Book Design/Page Layout: Jennifer M. Jones

Print/Production Coordinator: Jennifer M. Jones and G.W. Graphics

Cover Design: Jennifer M. Jones and G.W. Graphics

Color Prepress Specialist: Kevin Tucker

Acquisition Editor: Glenn E. Whaley

Developmental Editor: Kristen Prysmiki

Copy Editor: Kristen Prysmiki

Proofreader: Paul K. Goode, III

Printed in the United States.

Publisher:

STM Learning, Inc.

55 Westport Plaza, Suite 455, Saint Louis, Missouri 63146 USA

Phone: (314) 434-2424 Fax: (314) 434-2425 Toll Free: (800) 600-0330

http://www.stmlearning.com

Library of Congress Cataloging-in-Publication Data

Nursing approach to child maltreatment / [edited by] Paul T. Clements, Ann W. Burgess, Angelo P. Giardino, Eileen R. Giardino, Theresa Fay-Hillier. -- Second edition.

p. ; cm.

Preceded by Nursing approach to the evaluation of child maltreatment / Eileen R. Giardino, Angelo P. Giardino. c2003.

Includes bibliographical references and index.

ISBN 978-1-878060-17-4 (pbk. : alk. paper)

I. Clements, Paul T. (Paul Thomas), 1962- editor. II. Burgess, Ann Wolbert, editor. III. Giardino, Angelo P., editor. IV. Giardino, Eileen R., editor. V. Fay-Hillier, Theresa, editor.

[DNLM: 1. Child Abuse--diagnosis. 2. Mandatory Reporting. 3. Nurse's Role. 4. Nursing Assessment--methods. 5. Physical Examination--methods. 6. Social Responsibility. WA 325]

RJ375

616.85'8223--dc23

2014011220

Contributors

Marisa V. Atendido, CRNP, MSN
OB/GYN Nurse Practitioner
Adolescent Care Center
Children's Hospital of Philadelphia
Philadelphia, Pennsylvania

Kathy Bell, MS, RN, SANE-A, SANE-P
Tulsa Police Department
Forensic Nursing Administrator
Tulsa, Oklahoma

Kathleen M. Benasutti, MCAT, ATR-BC, LPC
Treatment Research Institute
Registered and Board Certified Art Therapist
Trauma Consultant
Philadelphia, Pennsylvania

Melanie D. Bragg, JD
Bragg Law PC
Houston, Texas
President, Legal Insight, Inc.
Houston, Texas

Kathleen Brown, PhD, RN, NP
University of Pennsylvania
School of Nursing
Associate Practice Professor
Philadelphia, Pennsylvania

Michelle Clayton, MD, MPH
Assistant Professor of Pediatrics
Eastern Virginia Medical School
Children's Hospital of The King's Daughters Child Abuse Program
Child Abuse Pediatrician
Department of Pediatrics
Norfolk, Virginia

Lisa Creamer, BSN, RN
Assistant Director
Texas Children's Hospital
Child Abuse Pediatrics
Houston, Texas

Marcella M. Donaruma-Kwoh, MD
Baylor College of Medicine
Assistant Professor
Program Director
Child Abuse Pediatrics Fellowship
Department of Pediatrics
Houston, Texas

Elizabeth Burgess Dowdell, PhD, RN, FAAN
Professor
Villanova University College of Nursing
Villanova, Pennsylvania

Sandra L. Elvik, MS, RN, CPNP
Harbor-UCLA Medical Center
Associate Professor of Pediatrics
UCLA School of Medicine
Assistant Medical Director
Child Crisis Center
Harbor-UCLA Medical Center
Torrance, California

Erin Endom, MD
Co-director, Texas Children's Emergency Center Disaster Preparedness and Response
Texas Children's Hospital
Houston, Texas

Tracy A. Evanson, PhD, PHCNS-BC
University of North Dakota
Associate Professor
College of Nursing and Professional Disciplines, Nursing Department
Grand Forks, North Dakota

Diana Faugno, MSN, RN, CPN, SANE-A, SANE-P, FAAFS, DF-IAFN
Barbara Sinatra Children's Center
Eisenhower Medical Center
Forensic Nurse Examiner
Emergency Room
Rancho Mirage, California

Beverly L. Fortson, PhD
Centers for Disease Control and Prevention
Behavioral Scientist
Division of Violence Prevention, National
Center for Injury Prevention and Control
Atlanta, Georgia

Rebecca Girardet, MD
Associate Professor of Pediatrics
University of Texas—Houston Medical School
Houston, Texas

Karen C. Harpold
Children at Risk
Staff Attorney
Houston, Texas

Tomika S. Harris, DNP, RN, CPNP
UT Health Medical School at Houston
Center for Evidenced Based Research
Houston, Texas

Elizabeth Henderson,
RN, MSN, MS, SANE-A, AFN-BC
Massachusetts General Hospital
Clinical Nurse Specialist
Boston, Massachusetts

Tanya Hinds, MD, FAAP
Children's National Medical Center
Child Abuse Pediatrician
Child and Adolescent Protection Center
Washington, DC
The George Washington University
Assistant Professor Pediatrics
Department of Pediatrics
Washington, DC

Karyn E. Holt, CNM, PhD
Director of Online Quality
Associate Clinical Professor
Division of Nursing
College of Nursing and Health Professions
Drexel University
Philadelphia, Pennsylvania

Reena Isaac, MD
Assistant Professor of Pediatrics
Baylor College of Medicine
Department of Pediatrics
Child Protection Section of
Pediatric Emergency Medicine Services
Texas Children's Hospital
Houston, Texas

Annie Lewis-O'Connor,
NP-BC, PhD, MPH
Brigham and Women's Hospital
Nursing Scientist and Founder and
Director of the Women's CARE Clinic
Center for Community
Health and Health Equity
Harvard Medical School
Instructor in Obstetrics, Gynecology
and Reproductive Biology
Boston, Massachusetts

Colby Lokey, MS
Centers for Disease Control and Prevention
Health Scientist
Division of Violence Prevention
National Center for Injury
Prevention and Control
Atlanta, Georgia

Joanne B. Martin, DrPH, RN, FAAN
Indiana University School of Nursing
Assistant Professor, Emerita
Department of Environments for Health
Goodwill Industries of Central Indiana, Inc
Consultant, Program Development,
Evaluation and Research
Community & Workplace
Initiatives Department
Indianapolis, Indiana

Stacey A. Mitchell,
DNP, MBA, RN, SANE-A, SANE-P
Harris Health System
Director
Forensic Nursing Services
Houston, Texas

Hillary Mowbray, MD
Pediatric Hospitalist
St. Mary's Pediatric Hospital
Evansville, IL

Mary Muscari,
PhD, MSCr, CPNP, PMHCNS-CS
Associate Professor
Decker School of Nursing
Binghamton University
Binghamton, New York

Frances M. Nadel, MD, MSCE
Children's Hospital of Philadelphia
Attending Physician
Division of Emergency Medicine
Professor of Clinical Pediatrics
Affiliate Faculty
Perelman School of Medicine at the
University of Pennsylvania
Philadelphia, Pennsylvania

Julie A. Nadkarni, MS, ARNP, CPNP
USF Child Protection Team,
Suncoast Center Child Protection Team,
Pasco Kids First Child Protection Team
Pediatric Advanced Registered Nurse Practitioner
Department of Pediatrics, College of Medicine,
University of South Florida
Tampa, Florida

Sandra W. Shulman, BSN, ARNP, CPNP
Senior Nurse Practitioner
Child Protection Team
Department of Pediatrics,
University of South Florida
College of Medicine
Tampa, Florida

Ann L. O'Sullivan, PhD, FAAN, CRNP
Professor
Pediatric Primary Care Nursing
University of Pennsylvania
School of Nursing and Medicine
Director Pediatric Nurse Practitioner Program
School of Nursing
The Children's Hospital of Philadelphia
Philadelphia, Pennsylvania

Julie Pape, CPNP
Director of Programs
National Children's Alliance
Washington, DC

Jennifer Pierce-Weeks, RN, SANE-P, SANE-A
Project Director
International Association of Forensic Nurses
Elkridge, MD
Forensic Nurse Examiner
Emergency Department
Memorial Hospital
University of Colorado Health
Colorado Springs, Colorado

Judith A. Rosenberg, PhD, MPH, CPNP-PC
University of Tampa
Assistant Professor
Department of Nursing
Tampa, Florida

Teresa Scalzo, JD
Former Prosecutor
Easton, Pennsylvania

Sandra W. Shulman, BSN, ARNP, CPNP
Senior Nurse Practitioner
Child Protection Team
Department of Pediatrics,
University of South Florida
College of Medicine
Tampa, Florida

Barbara Speller-Brown, RN, MSN, CPNP
Department of Pediatrics
Walter Reed Army Medical Center

Suzanne Starling, MD, FAAP
Eastern Virginia Medical School
Professor of Pediatrics
Department of Pediatrics
Division of Child Abuse Pediatrics
Children's Hospital of The King's Daughters
Medical Director
Child Abuse Program
Norfolk, Virginia

Foreword

As is true for every professional who interacts with children, nurses are mandated reporters and, therefore, must notify appropriate authorities when they encounter cases of child maltreatment. They are responsible for understanding what constitutes abuse or neglect, what signs and symptoms are indicative of child maltreatment, what identifies families at risk for developing a pattern of child maltreatment, and how to intervene effectively. The nurse's focus must be on the safety and well-being of the child.

Nurses interact with other health care providers in rendering care for families and children, playing a major role in the health care team. Nurses may be considered the eyes and ears as they are often the first health care professionals who notice signs and symptoms suspicious for maltreatment. Therefore, it is essential that they be well prepared to identify problems and make accurate assessments. Their ability to obtain a complete history and perform a thorough physical examination may be crucial in exposing abuse or neglect. This is particularly true when they are functioning as clinical nurse specialists or nurse practitioners and in independent nursing centers. They also need to be sensitive to the various verbal, physical, and behavioral cues that alert one to the possibility of maltreatment. Suspicions that are raised must be thoroughly evaluated and the possibility that abuse or neglect is present must be considered along with other diagnoses.

This book offers nurses the tools required to fulfill these roles. We begin with the basics: a definition of the problem of child abuse and neglect, the presenting signs and symptoms of child maltreatment, obtaining a complete history, and conducting an appropriate interview and physical examination. Then, we move through the various aspects that must be considered in greater depth, such as laboratory findings and obtaining proper forensic specimens, dealing with sexually transmitted infections, considering suitable differential diagnoses, documentation, and mental health problems. The rare but fascinating medical child abuse, formerly known as Munchausen syndrome by proxy, is outlined along with information pertinent to sexual abuse of adolescents. How the nurse can effectively interact with other professionals is addressed, with full chapters on child protective services and legal issues that occur in child maltreatment cases. The special risks that children face on the Internet are also explored. These chapters should equip the nurse to be a well-informed and effective guardian of children's health.

The practical information that nurses require is often outlined in special sections focused on nursing interventions. These discussions detail the hands-on actions that nurses can take in specific situations.

Health care professionals can only function well when they are given adequate, accurate information. This textbook offers in-depth, well-documented information that should help guide nurses to be exceptional providers of health care to the families they encounter each day. The editors are to be thanked for assembling a dedicated team of authors who offer their expertise in the important area of child maltreatment education for nurses.

Diana K. Faugno, MSN, RN, CPN, SANE-A, SANE-P, FAAFS, DF-IAFN
Barbara Sinatra Children's Center
Eisenhower Medical Center
Forensic Nurse Examiner
Emergency Room
Rancho Mirage, CA

FOREWORD

Child maltreatment (CM) is a significant health problem in the United States and across the globe. According to child protective services, more than 676 000 children in the US are victims of maltreatment each year with substantial emotional and economic consequences. A recent study by the Centers for Disease Control indicates that the total lifetime estimated financial cost associated with just one year of confirmed cases of child maltreatment is approximately $124 billion.

Given its wide-spread prevalence, nurses practicing in a variety of clinical settings, including emergency departments, schools, inpatient, and outpatient settings, are highly likely to encounter children who have experienced one or more forms of child maltreatment. It is critical, therefore, that nurses be well versed in the latest science on the prevention, identification, and treatment of various forms of child maltreatment. *Nursing Approach to Child Maltreatment*, 2nd edition is an excellent resource for all nurses who work with children and families as well as adult survivors of child maltreatment. It is highly relevant for nurses in advanced practice roles, such as NPs and CNSs, as well other registered nurses and health professionals.

A number of nursing experts in the area of child maltreatment edited and contributed to this second edition of *Nursing Approach to Child Maltreatment*; they include Paul Clements, Ann Burgess, Elizabeth Dowdell, Sandra Elvik, and Eileen Giardino, as well as many others. Angelo Giardino, a leading pediatrics expert in the field of child abuse and neglect, is also an editor and major contributor to *Nursing Approach to Child Maltreatment*, 2nd edition.

This book begins with a comprehensive overview of the evaluation of suspected cases of child maltreatment, followed by detailed chapters on the role of history taking, physical examination, and diagnostic testing. Other chapters cover a range of critical topics, including sexually transmitted infections; conditions that mimic CM; medical child abuse (also known as Munchausen's syndrome by proxy); as well as neglect, the most prevalent form of CM. Given the risks associated with child and adolescent internet use, the chapter "Risks to Children in the Digital Age of the Internet and Social Networking" is particularly timely. The chapters on child abuse prevention and forensic nursing emphasize the important role of nurses in the protection and safety of children. Throughout the book, an interdisciplinary approach to child maltreatment is emphasized, with particular attention to the contribution of nurses.

The second edition builds upon the strong foundations of the original edition, providing up-to-date, detailed information that nurses and other health care professionals will find beneficial in clinical practice and in research. Chapters are comprehensive and well organized and provide systematic approaches to treatment associated with the particular form of child maltreatment being addressed. A detailed reference list is included with each chapter that directs readers to additional up-to-date, evidence-based knowledge.

In summary, our knowledge related to the various aspects of child maltreatment has grown exponentially over the past several decades; thus, it is critical that nurses possess the most advanced level of knowledge available in order to provide optimal nursing care to children and families. *Nursing Approach to Child Maltreatment,* 2nd ed. is an outstanding resource for nurses and other health care professionals. The editors and contributors are to be commended for providing readers with such an inclusive, state-of-the art approach to the nursing care of maltreated children.

Susan J. Kelley, RN, PhD, FAAN
Professor
Byrdine F. Lewis School of Nursing and Health Professions
Director, Project Healthy Grandparents
Georgia State University
Atlanta, GA

Foreword

Care is the core of the nursing profession. For nurses, caring for children is a responsibility greater than other acts because they are a uniquely vulnerable population.

As nurses, we belong to one of several professions that are required by law to be knowledgeable of child abuse and neglect and legally mandated to report suspected maltreatment. This is true in every state. Nurses bear witness to such acts in a variety of settings, making the responsibility of knowledge even greater.

This text provides an overview of the multiple settings in which child maltreatment can be identified. Of note is the wonderful and enlightening section on prevention. The review of successful evidence-based programs, such the as the *Period of Purple Crying and the Adults and Children Together Against Violence Parents Raising Safe Kids Program (ACT Program)*, gives nurses and other health care professionals the tools they need to educate parents and caregivers.

The nurse's role in prevention is pivotal. This text helps frontline health care professionals identify high-risk populations for child maltreatment and equips nurses with the tools they need to do something about it before it happens.

Lori Armstrong MSN, RN, NEA-BC
Senior Vice President
Chief Nursing Officer
Texas Children's Hospital
Houston, TX

PREFACE

Abused and neglected children need a voice. These often invisible victims frequently suffer in silence, confusion, and in fear of repercussion for revealing the secret. The abused child frequently wonders, "Why would someone who is supposed to love me do things to hurt me?"

The history of childhood is replete with suffering. Prior to the sixteenth century, children were frequently maltreated, murdered, and sold into slavery. It was not until the end of the nineteenth century that attitudes toward the treatment of children began to change with the landmark Mary Ellen Wilson case of 1874. Mary Ellen, age 8, lived with her adoptive parents in New York City; she was kept in chains, starved, and beaten. Although her screams brought complaints, the police responded that it was a family matter and the adults had rights, not the child. Finally a social worker contacted Henry Berg for help. Berg was able to extricate Mary Ellen from her family torture chamber through skill and guile. Who was Henry Berg and why was he called? Henry Berg had founded a protective group the preceding year, The Society for the Prevention of Cruelty to Animals. It is thought-provoking to realize that during that era, animals had more protection from abuse than children.

The Honorable Charles D. Gill, judge in Superior Court Litchfield, Connecticut, presents a provocative exercise in role-playing. He asks that you pretend you are the chairperson of a commission for the city of New York. Presume also that the stork delivers babies. Today, the stork delivers 3 babies and it is your task to distribute them to families. Being a professional, you will interview applicants for the positions as parents.

Couple number one is married. Husband and wife are in their mid-thirties. Dad is an alcoholic who physically abuses Mom and the children. Mom is an alcoholic abuser herself and unable to defend the children from Dad's physical and verbal abuse. Dad has been arrested several times and hospitalized twice with alcohol-related illnesses. He has an erratic work history and relates poorly to work associates. There are 3 children in the family already. The oldest is in sixth grade and in special education. He has brain damage of unknown etiology. The middle child is in second grade and receives medication for hyperactivity and lack of concentration. The youngest is in preschool, and little is known about her at this time.

The second pair of applicants is an unmarried couple who are both in their twenties. They have been living together off and on for 2 years. They are cocaine abusers. The female has had 3 medical interventions and is she willing to enter another program so she can "get this kid." The man works sporadically as a house painter. They have had 3 different addresses in the past year and done some traveling with friends.

The third applicant is a single, 15-year-old female who lives at home with her mother, who is 32, and her mother's current boyfriend. The applicant is "madly in love" with 19-year-old Lenny. She and Lenny do not do heavy drugs. They only partake of alcohol and marijuana recreationally on weekends. At present, Lenny is in jail for some minor larcenies, but when he gets out, he is going to get 2 good jobs, a super apartment, a new car, and toys for the child.

Now, let us start distributing the 3 babies. What is this? You hesitate? Stop looking through the eyes of these babies. This is only pretend. In the real world, distribution is automatic. Whoever begets them, gets them.

One baby, perhaps with fetal alcohol syndrome, goes to couple number one. The second baby, perhaps with the relentless wailing characteristic of cocaine withdrawal, goes to couple number 2. The third baby, perhaps with low birth weight and problems associated herewith, goes to the 15-year-old female and Lenny.

These 3 examples are just a sample of the situations that threaten children at birth and thereafter. They are by no means the most graphic. We see these children as they develop in hospitals, the courts, the schools, the prisons, and television programming, and we wonder why.

The contributing authors of this book have years of clinical practice with maltreated children. They provide clinical skill and wisdom regarding various problems associated with child maltreatment. The text is designed as a handbook for professionals working with children as well as for students studying the problems of maltreated children.

Chapters cover the problems of child abuse and neglect, evaluation of child maltreatment, the health care interview and physical examination, laboratory findings, sexually transmitted infections, differential diagnosis, photodocumentation, mental health aspects of child survivors, sexual abuse of adolescents, medical child abuse (Munchausen Syndrome by proxy), Child Protective Services, legal issues, intimate partner violence and child maltreatment, media risks, prevention, human trafficking, substance abuse, and forensic nursing. Chapters include key points and case studies. Tables, figures, and photographs emphasize key aspects of each chapter.

Ann W. Burgess, DNS, APRN, FAAN
Paul Thomas Clements, PhD, RN

Reviews

Nursing Approach to Child Maltreatment, *2e is a well-articulated, comprehensive overview of violence perpetrated against children. It underscores the indispensable role of nurses in the assessment, evaluation, and treatment of vulnerable children seen on the "frontline" of health care and emphasizes adverse consequences of child abuse, including those affecting the physical, emotional, cognitive, and social well-being of the family. The risk of early trauma reaching beyond childhood into adolescence and adulthood is also explored. Nurses practicing in diverse specialties will benefit from the clinical and theoretical applications proposed in the text. This insightful composition of scholarly work is a welcome addition to the science of nursing.*

Marie E. Mugavin, PhD, FNP-BC, SAFE-A
Adjunct Assistant Professor
University of New Mexico
School of Medicine
Department of Emergency Medicine
Family Nurse Practitioner
Sexual Assault Forensic Examiner
First Choice Community Healthcare
Albuquerque, NM

This new edition of Nursing Approach to Child Maltreatment, *2e offers essential, updated information about the evaluation procedures and techniques necessary for a comprehensive assessment of a child with potential physical and sexual abuse and other forms of maltreatment. There have been major advances in our understanding and approach over the 10 years since the first edition, and this revised text provides a broad knowledge base to understand key aspects of medical history, examination, and laboratory evaluation while recognizing additional critical steps needed within the multidisciplinary team to promote emotional healing and prevent further injury. Frontline nurses and advanced practice nurses play a vital role in the safety net for children, and the nursing approach in this text builds upon our evolving science to extend these contributions to children in a variety of settings in the hospital, office, and community.*

Vincent J. Palusci, MD, MS, FAAP
New York University
School of Medicine
New York, NY

This text, written by experts in the field of child maltreatment, is set to become the most widely used reference for those in practice today. It is comprehensive in its approach to the care of child maltreatment victims. Experts in various fields share their knowledge, from understanding the scope of the problem to assessment and treatment, while including a thorough review of legal implications. Our knowledge in all areas affecting maltreated children has grown exponentially over the past several years, and research supports changes in assessment techniques and treatment. These authors came together to produce a text that, while written for the nurse clinician, has the potential to serve various collaborating professionals as well. It is set to become a standard reference in the library of the many clinicians who work to make life better for children and to prevent maltreatment in the future.

L. Kathleen Sekula, PhD, APRN, FAAN
Professor
Director, Forensic Graduate Programs
School of Nursing
Duquesne University
Pittsburgh, PA

Geared to the specialized needs of the nursing community, Nursing Approach to Child Maltreatment, *2e succeeds in covering the field of child maltreatment admirably. It moves from the global view of child abuse and neglect in all of its manifestations to the specifics of evaluation, diagnosis, and management of the child who has suffered maltreatment. The importance of ruling out conditions that could be mistaken for abuse and neglect are considered fully in one chapter, and in another chapter, the necessity for precise documentation is stressed. In a particularly important chapter, the intersection of domestic violence and child abuse is explored. Outcomes are addressed, particularly those that involve life-long mental health harms, and the need for working with child protective services is highlighted in another chapter. The inevitable Legal issues are discussed fully and rounding out the book are chapters devoted to the pitfalls of social networking for children and adolescents, human trafficking, and the close relationship of substance abuse and maltreatment. Taken together, this book should find high usage among nurses confronted with this blend of medical, nursing, social, and legal problems.*

Robert M. Reece, MD
Editor, The Quarterly Update

Contents in Brief

Contents in Detail

Nursing Approach to the Evaluation of Child Maltreatment

Second Edition

STM **Learning**, Inc.

Leading Publisher of Scientific, Technical, and Medical Educational Resources

Saint Louis

www.stmlearning.com

Chapter 1

The Problem of Child Abuse and Neglect

Mary Muscari, PhD, MSCr, CPNP, PMHCNS-CS
Eileen R. Giardino, PhD, MSN, FNP, ANP

Key Points

1. Nurses should have an understanding of the comprehensive meaning of child maltreatment.
   a. Nurses should be able to identify risk factors associated with child maltreatment and provide competent and comprehensive interventions to children who have experienced child abuse and neglect.
2. Physical, sexual, emotional and psychological abuse, and neglect are the broad categories of child maltreatment.
3. Both the National Association of Pediatric Nurse Practitioners (NAPNAP) and the American Association of Colleges of Nursing (AACN) have position statements that address child maltreatment.
   a. To limit trauma to the child, NAPA believes that it is essential for all nurses to practice the quick prevention and identification of child maltreatment. Pediatric nurse practitioners (PNPs) are in an ideal situation to assess for the presence of risk factors of child maltreatment and provide primary prevention interventions. PNPs can also screen for maltreatment, provide anticipatory guidance related to potential maltreatment, and assist children and families who are engaged in maltreatment by making a referral to the local child protection agency.[1]
   b. AACN believes that nurses should be "aware of assessment methods and nursing interventions that will interrupt and prevent the cycle of violence," particularly intimate partner violence (IPV). They also believe that all baccalaureate and higher degree programs should contain curricula with opportunities for all students to gain knowledge and clinical experience regarding IPV that should at least include: assessment, interventions, cultural competence in dealing with violence, legal and ethical issues, and activities to prevent IPV.[2]
4. Multidisciplinary child fatality review (CFR) teams are a coordinated approach to understanding child deaths. A 1992 amendment to the Child Abuse Prevention and Treatment Act (CAPTA) requires states to include information obtained through CDR teams in their program plans. The purpose of CFR teams is to conduct a comprehensive, multidisciplinary review of child death, better understand how and why children die, and use the findings to take action to prevent other deaths and improve the health and safety of children.

5. It is helpful for health care providers to be able to place abuse into a framework in order to develop a greater sociological perspective. The 4 different frameworks used to further understand the dynamics associated with child maltreatment are: (1) the epidemiological framework, (2) the ecological framework, (3) longitudinal progression model for child sexual abuse, and (4) the traumagenic dynamics model for child sexual abuse.

Introduction

Violence touches the lives of children with alarming frequency, and the problem of child abuse and neglect, collectively known as child maltreatment, impacts the nation and the world through its profound and far reaching effects. Victims of child abuse and neglect may suffer physical, psychological, social, and even financial trauma (eg, parents using the child's social security number to get around their own bad credit). The social and occupational implications of child maltreatment have the potential to ultimately slow a country's economic and social development.[3]

Health care professionals have made great progress in the recognition and treatment of child maltreatment since Kempe[4] and associates first published their description of battered child syndrome in 1962. Child maltreatment is now recognized as part of the continuum of family violence that also includes IPV, elder abuse, and animal cruelty.[5] However, this progress still appears minimal, considering that the statics of child maltreatment remain staggering.

Nurses interact with children and their families and caregivers at all levels of health care. They educate people, intervene in primary care and institutional settings, and provide services to help children and families heal. It is important for nurses to have a clear understanding of child maltreatment, how to identify risk factors, how to intervene to provide competent and comprehensive health care for children who have experienced child abuse and neglect, and when prevention strategies may be employed. This chapter discusses the problem of child maltreatment, offers a conceptual framework to help explain how and why specific types of child abuse and neglect occur, and identifies the role of nurses in evaluating and treating child sexual abuse.

Defining the Problem

Child maltreatment encompasses various situations in which a parent or caregiver fails to provide for the health and well-being of a child. Abusive caregiver acts are those of commission or omission that have an injurious effect on the physical, psychosocial, or developmental well-being of the child. CAPTA, as amended by the Keeping Children and Families Safe Act of 2003, defines child abuse and neglect at a minimum as "any recent act or failure to act on the part of a parent or caretaker which results in death, serious physical or emotional harm, sexual abuse or exploitation; or an act or failure to act, which presents an imminent risk of serious harm."[6]

Categories of Maltreatment

Federal legislation provides broad categories of maltreatment, including physical, sexual, emotional and psychological abuse, and neglect. Each category contains definitions for further clarification. Federal legislation also provides a basis for state definitions of maltreatment by identifying a minimum set of acts or behaviors that characterizes maltreatment and defines specific acts that are considered physical abuse, neglect, and sexual abuse.[6] While not specifically listed in federal legislation, the following section also touches on parental financial abuse of children by way of identity theft.

Physical Abuse

Physical abuse is defined as the infliction of physical injury resulting from acts that may or may not have intended to hurt the child. Physical abuse is usually defined as nonaccidental or intentional physical injury to the child. Injuries range from minor bruises to severe fractures to death as a result of punching, beating, kicking, biting, shaking, throwing, stabbing, choking, hitting with a hand or object, burning, or otherwise harming a child. The injury is considered to be abuse regardless of whether the caregiver intended to hurt the child.[7] Medical child abuse (MCA)—formerly known as Munchausen syndrome by proxy (MSBP)—and abusive head trauma (AHT)—formerly known as shaken baby syndrome—are also characterized as physical child maltreatment. However, physical discipline, such as spanking or paddling, is not considered abuse provided that it is reasonable and causes no bodily injury to the child. Additionally, the following folk healing practices, which can mimic abuse, are not characterized as such:

— Cao gio: also referred to as coin rolling or coining; rubbing a coin on the skin until a red mark is produced

— Cupping: applying a cup to the skin until pressure is created, also causing a mark

— Moxibustion: applying heat from burning herbs, causing burn marks

Sexual Abuse

Sexual abuse is defined by CAPTA as:

> (T)he employment, use, persuasion, inducement, enticement, or coercion of any child to engage in, or assist any other person to engage in, any sexually explicit conduct or simulation of such conduct for the purpose of producing a visual depiction of such conduct; or the rape, and in cases of caretaker or inter-familial relationships, statutory rape, molestation, prostitution, or other form of sexual exploitation of children, or incest with children.[7]

A central component of sexual abuse is the misuse of an adult's power relationship with a child and betrayal of the child's trust by the older adult.[8] Specific activities noted as sexual abuse include any sexual activities by an older person that involve a dependent, developmentally immature child or adolescent and that are for the sexual stimulation or gratification of that person or of other persons, such as in child pornography or prostitution. Specific activities include sexualized kissing; fondling; exhibitionism; masturbation; digital or object penetration of the vagina or anus; and oral-genital, genital-genital, and anal-genital contact.[8]

Emotional and Psychological Abuse

Emotional abuse, or ***psychological abuse***, is a pattern of abusive behavior that impairs a child's emotional development or sense of self-worth. It is almost always present when there is another form of child abuse. Emotional abuse may include constant criticism, name-calling, or threats as well as withholding love, support, or guidance. One example is the use of extreme forms of punishment such as confining a child in a dark closet. Emotional abuse can be difficult to prove; therefore, child protective services (CPS) may not be able to intervene without evidence of harm to the child.[7]

Child Neglect

Neglect is the failure of a caregiver to provide for a child's basic needs. Neglect can be:

— Physical: failure to provide adequate food, clothing, or shelter

— Medical: failure to provide necessary medical treatment

— Educational: failure to educate a child

— Emotional: permitting the child to use alcohol or other drugs

These circumstances are not always related to neglect, as evidenced by certain cultural practices or impoverished conditions; however, when a family fails to use information and resources and the child's health or safety is at risk, intervention is required.

Many states now define abandonment as a form of neglect. A child is usually considered to be abandoned when his or her parent's identity or whereabouts are unknown, the child has been left alone in circumstances where the child suffers serious harm, or the parent has failed to maintain contact with the child or provide reasonable support. Many states also consider substance abuse as a form of child abuse or neglect. Circumstances in which substance abuse is considered abuse or neglect include prenatal exposure to harm due to the parents' use of substances; manufacturing of drugs in the presence of a child; selling, distributing, or giving alcohol or illegal drugs to a child; and the use of a controlled substance by a caregiver that impairs the caregiver's ability to adequately care for the child.[7] Individual statutes define issues of child neglect and abandonment for each state. Health care providers can access information specific to the state within which they practice through the federal Child Welfare Web site at www.childwelfare.gov/systemwide/laws_policies/state/.

Financial Abuse

Financial abuse or exploitation, a long-time problem in elder maltreatment, is now becoming an issue for children. Criminals steal children's identities by fraudulently using their social security number (SSN) and birth date to open credit accounts, take out loans, apply for jobs, receive government benefits, access medical care, and even commit crimes. Perpetrators may be strangers; however, they may also be the child's parents.[9] Research regarding this problem is practically nonexistent at this point. Many anecdotal cases involve a close family member as the perpetrator, often a parent or relative, who has damaged his or her own credit or other personal records. These individuals often have the easiest access to the child's information.[10] Child victims of financial abuse face very serious consequences, including inheriting significant debt, carrying a tarnished credit history, or suffering emotional impacts, especially when the offender is a parent.[9]

Children's Exposure to Violence

Children are more likely to be exposed to violence than are adults. Millions of children and adolescents in the United States are exposed to violence in their homes, schools, and communities as both victims and witnesses. A recent comprehensive national survey on children's exposure to violence confirms that most of the children in the United States are exposed to violence on a daily basis. More than 60% of the children surveyed were exposed to violence within the past year, either directly or indirectly, 46.3% were assaulted at least once in the past year, while a little more than 25% witnessed a violent act, and 9.8% saw one family member assault another.[11]

Exposure to violence can have a significant impact on a child's developmental processes and the formation of intimate relationships throughout childhood adulthood. Some children experience chronic community violence and are exposed to guns, knives, drugs, and random violence in their neighborhoods; some witness IPV on a regular basis; and some are exposed to a plethora of violent acts through television programming, computer and video games, and other media. Still, many children are exposed to all of these instances of violence. Risk factors are cumulative; therefore, the risk of negative outcomes multiplies for children who are in double jeopardy, such as those who are exposed to IPV and community violence. Children who are direct victims of assault and who witness repeated violence are more likely to have significant negative outcomes than children who are exposed to a single instance.[11]

The Child Abuse Prevention and Treatment Act

Child maltreatment is defined by federal and state laws. As previously mentioned, CAPTA provides the minimum standards that must be incorporated into state statutory definitions of child abuse and neglect. CAPTA, which was reauthorized and amended by the Keeping Children and Families Safe Act of 2003, supports individual state efforts to develop, run, expand, and increase community-based, prevention-focused efforts and family resource and support programs. CAPTA was enacted by Congress to ensure that child victims of abuse and neglect receive a comprehensive approach to care through the integration of multiple state agencies, such as social services and legal, mental health, education, and substance abuse agencies.[6] Health care providers can access information specific to the state within which they practice through the federal Child Welfare Web site at www.childwelfare.gov/systemwide/laws_policies/state/.

Nursing Organization Position Statements Related to Child Abuse

Nursing is the largest group of health care providers in the United States, and as such, nurses care for both victims and perpetrators of violence, including child abuse, on a regular basis. Not all nursing organizations have position statements; however, of those organizations that do, NAPNAP and AACN have position statements relevant to child maltreatment.

National Association of Pediatric Nurse Practitioners Position Statement on Child Maltreatment

One of the goals of the NAPNAP[1] is to enhance the quality of health care for infants, children, and adolescents; therefore, NAPNAP believes that a strenuous effort should be made to prevent child maltreatment and to identify and manage maltreatment as soon as possible to cause the least amount of trauma to the child.

> Pediatric nurse practitioners (PNPs) are in a strategic position to assess for the presence of risk and protective factors [and to] provide primary prevention interventions...PNPs can screen for maltreatment, provide anticipatory guidance regarding potential maltreatment, and assist children [and] families already engaged in maltreatment by referring them to a local child protection team.[1]

While these actions are aimed at PNPs, all nurses play a role in the prevention, identification, management, and referral of child maltreatment.

American Association of Colleges of Nursing Position Statement on Violence as a Public Health Problem

AACN states that nurses should be aware of assessment methods and nursing interventions that will interrupt and prevent the cycle of violence, particularly domestic violence.[2] AACN defines IPV as physical, sexual, or emotional-psychological violence directed toward men, women, children, or elders that occurs in current or past familial or intimate relationships, whether the individuals are cohabiting or not. The AACN recommends that educational programs that prepare nurses in baccalaureate and higher degree programs contain curricula with opportunities for all students to gain knowledge and clinical experience regarding domestic violence to include, at a minimum, acknowledgment of the scope of the problem; assessment skills related to the identification and documentation of abuse and its health effects; interventions to reduce vulnerability and increase safety especially of women, children, and elders; cultural competence in dealing with violence as a health care problem; legal and ethical issues in treating and reporting; and activities to prevent domestic violence.

Incidence

The United States Department of Health and Human Services (USDHHS) collects and analyzes data annually from reports filed by state CPS agencies in an effort to track the data on child abuse and neglect. The 2009 report shows that an estimated 3.3 million referrals involving the alleged maltreatment of approximately 6.0 million children were received by CPS agencies, and 61.0% of these referrals were escalated for a response by CPS.[12] The incidence of child maltreatment declined from a rate of 10.9 in 2005 to a rate of 9.3 in 2009 (**Table 1-1**).

As with previous years, most children included in the CPS report suffered from neglect; however, report findings indicated that some children may have suffered from multiple forms of maltreatment and, as a result, were counted once for each applicable maltreatment type (**Figure 1-1**). According to the 2009 report,[12] children aged 1 year and younger had the highest rate of victimization at 20.6 per 1000 children in the population of the same age, while children aged 1, 2, and 3 years had victimization rates of 11.9, 11.3, and 10.6 victims per 1000 children, respectively. Children aged 8 through 11 years had victimization rates of 18.8 per 1000 children; children aged 12 to 15 had victimization rates of 17.8 per 1000 children; children aged 16 through 17 had victimization rates

Table 1-1. Rate of Child Maltreatment From 2005 Through 2009

Reporting Year	Number of States Reporting	Child Population of Reporting States	Number of Reported (Unique Count) Victims	Child Victimization Rate
2005	49	72 751 837	793 558	10.9
2006	49	72 647 455	793 558	11.0
2007	49	71 886 504	690 482	9.6
2008	50	74 398 024	704 429	9.5
2009	50	74 495 280	693 174	9.3

Adapted from United States Department of Health and Human Services, Administration for Children and Families, Administration on Children, Youth and Families, Children's Bureau. Child maltreatment 2009. Administration of Children and Families Web site. http://www.acf.hhs.gov/programs/cb/stats_research/index.htm#can. Accessed May 25, 2013.

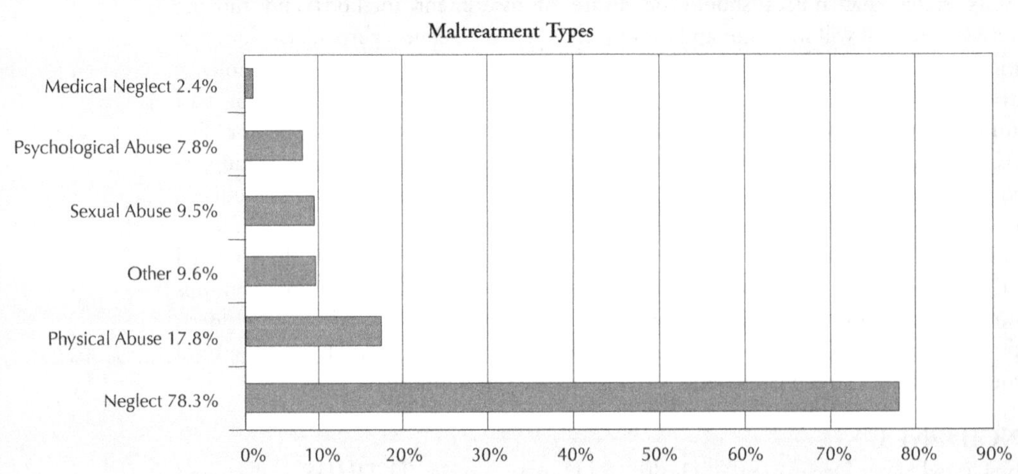

Figure 1-1

Figure 1-1. *Maltreatment Types. Adapted from United States Department of Health and Human Services, Administration for Children and Families, Administration on Children, Youth and Families, Children's Bureau. Child maltreatment 2009. Administration of Children and Families Web site. http://www.acf.hhs.gov/programs/cb/stats_research/index.htm#can. Accessed May 25, 2013.*

of 6.3 per 1000 children. Victimization was fairly equal between the sexes with boys at 48.2% and girls at 51.1%. The majority of victims (87%) was composed of 3 races or ethnicities: African American (22.3%), Hispanic (20.7%), and white (44.0%).

Fatalities

Filicide is the killing of a child by his or her parents; subcategories include neonaticide in which the victim does not survive the first 24 hours of life and infanticide in which the child is less than 1 years old at the time of death. Filicide may also occur within the context of filicide-suicide, the offending parent also kills himself or herself, or in the context of familicide, the entire family is killed. The United States has the highest rate of child homicide among developed countries, and many child abuse specialists believe child fatalities due to abuse and neglect are still underreported.

Even with underreporting, the number of child fatalities has been increasing since 2006. An estimated 1770 children died from abuse and neglect in 2009, compared with 1720 children in 2008. Of the children who died in 2009, 66.7% suffered neglect either exclusively or in combination with another type of maltreatment type and 44.8% suffered physical abuse either exclusively or in combination. The youngest children are more vulnerable to fatal child maltreatment as four-fifths (80.8%) of all child fatalities were under the age of 4 years. Boys (2.36 boys per 100 000) had a slightly higher child fatality rate than girls (2.12 per 100 000), and more than 80% of child fatalities were comprised of African American, Hispanic, and white victims. Three-quarters (75.8%) of child fatalities were caused by 1 or both parents, with more than one-quarter (27.3%) of fatalities perpetrated by the child's mother acting alone.[12]

The response to child abuse and neglect fatalities is often hampered by inconsistencies, including underreporting of the number of children who die each year as a result of abuse and neglect; lack of consistent standards for child death investigations or autopsies; varying roles of CPS agencies in investigations; uncoordinated, single discipline investigations; and medical examiners or coroners who do not have specific child abuse and neglect training.

To address some of these inconsistencies, multidisciplinary CFR teams have emerged to provide a coordinated approach to understanding child deaths. An amendment to the 1992 reauthorization of CAPTA supports the development of CFR teams by requiring states to include information regarding their CFR teams in their annual program plans. Such program plans are frequently attached to a state's receipt of government funding.[12] According to the National Maternal Child Health (MCH) Center for Child Death Review, the purpose of CFR teams is to conduct a comprehensive, multidisciplinary review of child deaths, better understand how and why children die, and use the findings to take action to prevent other deaths and improve the health and safety of children. The objectives of the review process are complex and meet the needs of many different agencies, ranging from the investigation of child deaths to prevention. Nurses can provide expertise on both child death investigation and prevention and, as a result, should become involved in their local CFR. **Table 1-2** provides contact information for national CFR resources.

Children with Disabilities

The numbers of children who survive disabling medical conditions as a result of technologic advances and children who have disabilities are increasing. The rates of child maltreatment have been found to be high in children with blindness, deafness, chronic illness, developmental delays, behavioral or emotional disorders, and multiple disorders.[13] The 2009 report[12] detailed 11.1% of maltreatment victims as having a disability. Of those victims with a disability, 2.9% were recorded as having behavior problems, 2.1% emotional disturbances, and 3.8% other medical conditions

Table 1-2. Child Death and Fatality Review Resources

Organization	Contact Information	Mission Statement
National MCH Center for Child Death Review	Phone: 800-656-2434 Web site: www.childdeathreview.org	"The National Center for Child Death Review is a resource center for state and local CDR programs, funded by the Maternal and Child Health Bureau. The center promotes, supports, and enhances child death review methodology and activities at the state, community, and national levels."[14]
National Center on Child Fatality Review (NCFR)	Phone: 626-455-4585 Web site: www.ican-ncfr.org	"The Mission of NCFR is to develop and promote a nationwide system of Child Fatality Review Teams to improve the health, safety and well-being of children and reduce preventable child fatalities and severe injuries."[15]

(**Figure 1-2**). Victims could have been reported as having more than one type of disability, and children with risk factors may have been undercounted since not every child receives a clinical diagnostic assessment from CPS agency staff.

The causes of abuse and neglect of children with disabilities are the same as those for all children; however, additional factors may increase their risk for maltreatment. Children with chronic illnesses or disabilities frequently place higher emotional, physical, economic, and social demands on their families. Parents with limited support may be at an especially high-risk for maltreating their children with disabilities if they feel overwhelmed and unable to cope with the required responsibilities with regard to care and supervision. A lack of breaks in child care responsibilities can contribute to an increased risk of maltreatment as well. Finally, the added requirements of special health care and educational needs can result in neglect when the parent fails to provide the child with needed medications, adequate medical care, or appropriate educational placements.[15]

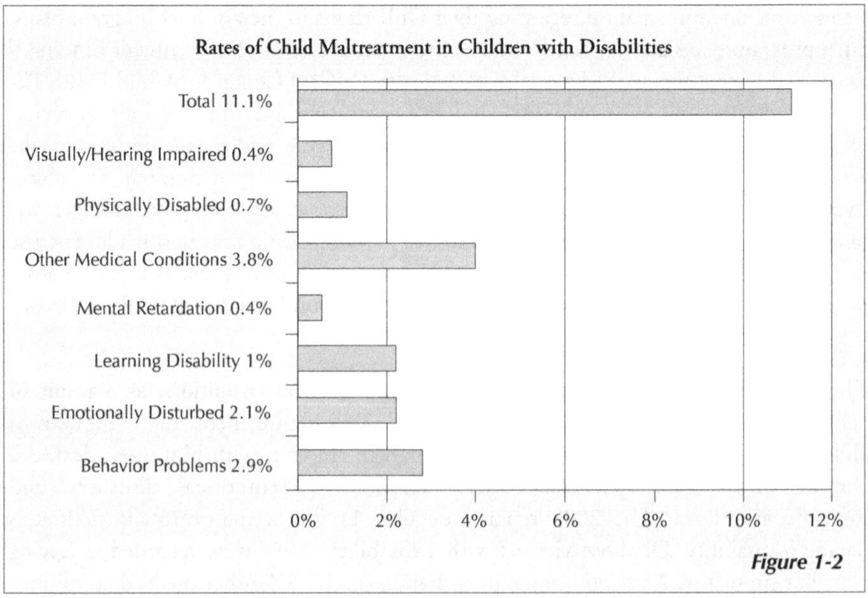

Figure 1-2. *Rates of Child Maltreatment in Children with Disabilities. Adapted from United States Department of Health and Human Services, Administration for Children and Families, Administration on Children, Youth and Families, Children's Bureau. Child maltreatment 2009. Administration of Children and Families Web site. http://www.acf.hhs.gov/programs/cb/stats_research/index.htm#can. Accessed May 25, 2013.*

Costs of Maltreatment

Not all costs are monetary. Children who have been abused or neglected are more likely to experience adverse outcomes throughout their life span in a number of areas such as poor physical health, poor emotional health, social difficulties, cognitive difficulties, high-risk health behaviors, and behavioral problems. The costs of responding to the consequences of child maltreatment are borne by the victims, their families, and society. In 2007, the estimated annual cost of child maltreatment was $103.8 billion, which equates to an estimated $258 million per day.[16]

The Impact of Physical Abuse and Neglect

Child maltreatment can result in both short- and long-term negative outcomes, even if the abuse itself is short lived. The impact on each child depends upon a number of factors, including age of the child when abuse began, severity of the abuse, frequency of the abuse, the child's relationship to the abuser, availability of support systems, and the child's ability to cope. The negative outcomes can be compounded when children are exposed to more than one type of maltreatment, including exposure to IPV and community violence. Children who are exposed to one type of maltreatment are frequently exposed to other types on several occasions or continuously. A review of the impact of physical abuse and neglect on children by Turnera et al[17] revealed multiple effects of child maltreatment to persist even after accounting for family characteristics and individual risk factors, including strong associations between child maltreatment and obesity and an association between child sexual abuse and eating disorders, such as bulimia and anorexia nervosa. Turnera et al[17] also revealed relationships between child physical abuse and neglect and multiple child adversities and between child maltreatment and a range of health outcomes in adulthood, including ischemic heart disease, cancer, chronic lung disease, skeletal fractures, and liver disease.

Child maltreatment may cause important regions of the brain to fail to form or fail to grow properly, resulting in impaired development. These changes in brain maturation have long-term consequences for cognitive, language, and academic abilities. Child maltreatment is associated with long-term deficits in educational achievement. Studies, such as one conducted by Boden et al,[18] have shown that abused children have lower educational achievement than do their peers and are more likely to receive special education. The educational deficits caused by abuse can, in turn, have long-term economic consequences since abused children are more likely to end up in menial and semiskilled jobs than will their peers who have not experienced abuse.[18-20]

Studies that have examined the relationship between child maltreatment and sexual behavior in adolescence and adulthood have focused on outcomes for sexual abuse. In one prospective study, Wilson and Widom[21] reported a significant association between physical or sexual abuse or neglect and arrest for prostitution or being paid for sex (13% of cases compared to 4% of controls for girls), but no significant associations with promiscuity or teenage pregnancy. Abused children are more likely to smoke cigarettes, abuse alcohol, or take illicit drugs during their lifetime than are non-abused children. A report from the National Institute on Drug Abuse (NIDA) notes that as many as two-thirds of people in drug treatment programs reported being abused as children.

Abused children are more likely to be arrested for criminal behavior as a juvenile, more likely to be arrested for violent and criminal behavior as an adult, and more likely to be arrested for one of many forms of violent crime as a juvenile or adult. Abused and neglected children were 11 times more likely to be arrested for criminal behavior as a juvenile, 2.7 times more likely to be arrested for violent and criminal behavior as an adult, and 3.1 times more likely to be arrested for one of many forms of violent crime as either a juvenile or an adult.[22]

Conceptual Frameworks

Conceptual frameworks can put aspects of child physical abuse, neglect, and sexual abuse into the greater perspective of overall family and social systems. These theories, as noted in the following paragraphs, address abuse as part of dysfunctional family or societal systems. Theoretical frameworks that explain the complex causes of abuse are helpful to the practitioner who may be the one to identify abusive situations or treat the individual child or family members.

The following sections describe the 4 different frameworks— epidemiological, ecological, longitudinal progression model for child sexual abuse, and traumagenic dynamics model for child sexual abuse—that put abuse into a greater sociological perspective. Although it is sometimes the case that a child who is sexually abused may also experience physical abuse in addition to neglect and vice versa, there seem to be certain individual and family dynamics that lead a person to abuse in a specific manner. Dynamics of the phenomena suggest that physical and sexual abuse represent separate phenomena with unique patterns of abuser behavior, etiology, and treatment modalities.[23,24]

The Epidemiological Framework

The epidemiological approach to child abuse and neglect builds an understanding for the short- and long-term effects of abusive processes on normal child development.[25] Children raised in abusive situations may have sensory system modifications that make it difficult for them to process their environment in a healthy way. Therefore, a child who struggles with difficult family situations and unrealistic expectations learns inappropriate and maladaptive ways to meet his or her needs from adults, a process that continues throughout his or her lifespan.[25] In essence, abusive situations may continue because the child-turned-adult learned few healthy interaction skills and developed poor decision-making abilities.

Helfer[25] describes 4 categories that help to make up the potential for abuse: (1) how parents were raised, (2) ability of caregivers (families) to use other people to help them when they are stressed, (3) quality of relationship between parents, and (4) how parents view the child.[26] The epidemiological approach accounts for how a person who develops an abusive caregiving style begins to feel out of control through the negative interactions of unmet needs, muted senses, and limited choices. This combination of factors leads to poor self-esteem, an inability to trust others, and a possible series of unhealthy decisions about friends and partners.[25]

The Ecological Framework

Child physical maltreatment occurs when there is dysfunction between the adult and child. The incidence of child maltreatment seems to increase as stressors outweigh the supports that people have within their environment.[27] The ecological approach to the study of abuse and neglect identifies the multifaceted causes of child abuse and then works to integrate divergent viewpoints of the role of the child, patterns of family interaction, and cultural values and social stress in the etiology of child maltreatment.[28,29] The model recognizes that although abusing parents and caregivers may have developmental histories that predispose them to possible maltreatment of children, there are then stress-producing forces from within the family (microsystem) and the outside environment (exosystem) that may increase the likelihood of conflict between parents and child.[28] The response of the parent or caregiver to such conflicts results in maltreatment.

The ecological model can serve as a guide for both the prevention of child abuse and neglect and the identification of at-risk families. This model can help nurses understand factors and forces within a family system that may predispose a person to acting on abusive tendencies. Health care providers who understand the dynamics of individuals with their microsystems and exosystems are better prepared to intervene with support.

Longitudinal Progression Model for Child Sexual Abuse

The phenomenon of child sexual abuse occurs when there is a breakdown of protective mechanisms within the child's sociological system. The failure of protective mechanisms in some cases of sexual abuse occurs in a relatively systematic manner.[30] The actual sexual encounters between adults and children often occur within predictable patterns. The patterns are described by 5 separate phases[31] known as engagement, sexual interaction, secrecy, disclosure, and retraction. A practitioner's understanding of the dynamics of child sexual abuse enables more appropriate interventions.

Engagement

In child sexual abuse, the opportunity for a perpetrator to engage in inappropriate behaviors is made possible because he or she has entrée to private interactions with the child. Often the abuser is someone within the child's family circle or an adult who has access to the child through age-appropriate group activities.[8] The perpetrator typically engages the child in sexual behaviors by first proposing interactions and activities that are acceptable and interesting to the child, such as going for ice cream or becoming a friend who meets psychological needs or provides material rewards.[8]

Sexual Interaction Phase

In the sexual interaction phase the perpetrator engages in sexually inappropriate behavior through activities such as undressing, exposing his or her genitals, and touching. These activities may progress in the level of sexual interactions suggested and encouraged by the perpetrator. Fondling, masturbation, and penetration of the child's body in a variety of ways may be realized at this phase.[8] The mouth and anus are areas for possible penetration for both boys and girls. Penetration of the vagina may progress from digital penetration. In general, the sexual interaction phase involves a series of inappropriate sexual expectations and activities required of the child. Successful perpetrators may be subtle in their coerciveness to persuade compliance; however, there are also many situations, often in family relationships, in which the child is threatened into compliance through force or threat of force.[8]

Secrecy Phase

A perpetrator's desire is to keep the age-inappropriate sexual activity a secret to the rest of the world. Secrecy allows repetition of the behaviors, maintains a lack of accountability and responsibility, and avoids the interference of and judgment by society[8]; therefore, the perpetrator must persuade the child to keep the secret through direct or indirect coercion. Perpetrators encourage secrecy in many ways, often by offering rewards or bribes or using threats. A subtle threat may involve the perpetrator indicating disapproval of the child if the child does not comply, whereas an explicit threat is one by which the perpetrator may indicate harm to the child or loved ones if secrecy is broken. The secrecy phase may last for weeks, months, or years and only ends when the maltreatment comes to light.[8]

Disclosure Phase

A child's disclosure of sexual abuse occurs in either an accidental or purposeful manner.[8] Accidental disclosure occurs when external circumstances come into play that reveal a perpetrator's inappropriate sexual behaviors. The following are usual scenarios that occur in accidental disclosures:

— A third party observes the child and perpetrator in inappropriate activity and tells someone else.

— Physical injury occurs to the child and is noted by an outside observer.

— Signs of a sexually transmitted infection (STI) are noted through evaluation of a new onset of symptoms in the child, such as penile or vaginal irritation or discharge.

— The child becomes pregnant.

— The child engages in age-inappropriate sexual activity in other settings, such as in school or with playmates, that indicates his or her exposure to developmentally inappropriate behaviors.

Accidental disclosure may precipitate a crisis within the family system because the child did not purposely set out to disclose the situation; therefore, health care providers should be prepared to anticipate problems and foresee the need for crisis intervention when disclosure occurs.[8]

Purposeful disclosure occurs when the child decides to tell another person about the sexual abuse. The reasons for sharing the secret with others are numerous and vary with the child's developmental level. A young child may want to share the experience, whereas an older child may want to end the abuse and escape family or individual pressure or release personal anger or frustration with the abusive situation.[8] Disclosure often brings the child mixed emotions of relief, guilt, and disloyalty because the circumstances surrounding the abuse are complex and family relationships are likely to be affected and potentially disrupted.

Retraction Phase

After a child discloses sexual abuse and the events surrounding it, it is not uncommon for the child to recant the story. Family members are often overwhelmed by the situation and may want to forget about it.[8] The perpetrator may exert direct or indirect pressure on the family as well as the child to induce guilt or fear that the family will be disrupted or destroyed as a result of legal actions taken against the perpetrator. This may be especially true if the perpetrator is the breadwinner of the family, because incarceration will inevitably lead to financial loss. Additional pressure may result as family members attempt to persuade the child to retract the story and details of the abusive events. Family members may also assert that the child fabricated the accounts of abuse and, therefore, his or her story should be dismissed as a flight of the imagination.

Traumagenic Dynamics Model for Child Sexual Abuse

Models that explain the dynamics of how child abuse and neglect come to be in a family system are important because they help practitioners understand and then identify risk factors during the course of health care visits with children and their caregivers. Models provide frameworks that help to characterize the kinds of psychological injury that happen to a child who has been sexually abused. The traumagenic dynamics model developed by Finkelhor and Browne[32] describes how specific dynamics come together in a child to alter the child's cognitive and emotional being and distort aspects of worldview, self-concept, and the child's ability to receive and give affection. This model describes 4 trauma-causing dynamics that come together in the circumstance of sexual abuse and are responsible for the child's psychological alterations:

(1) traumatic sexualization, (2) betrayal, (3) powerlessness, and (4) stigmatization. These dynamics are used to assess child sexual abuse victims and then anticipate potential problems to which the child may be vulnerable.[32] While there may be common types of trauma to a person's psyche caused by physical, sexual, and emotional abuse and neglect, Finkelhor and Browne[32] postulate that the trauma caused by sexual abuse is unique.

Traumatic Sexualization

Traumatic sexualization caused by sexual abuse is a process that shapes a child's sexual feelings and attitudes in a way that is developmentally inappropriate and interpersonally dysfunctional.[32] It is a complex process that occurs when a child is rewarded by a perpetrator for sexual behavior that is developmentally inappropriate or given attention or privileges for inappropriate behavior. Traumatic sexualization also occurs through the perpetrator's distortion of the importance and meaning of a child's sexual anatomy and through the child's resulting misconceptions of sexual behavior and sexual morality. Furthermore, the child's mind begins to associate frightening memories and events with sexual activity.[32] A traumatically sexualized child may demonstrate age-inappropriate sexual behaviors along with a myriad of confusion surrounding his or her own sexual self-concept, and may experience difficult emotional associations with sexual activity.[32]

Betrayal

Betrayal occurs when an individual who should be a trusted person or one on whom a child is vitally dependent causes the child harm. The child may experience different levels of adult betrayal, one involving the person who actually molests the child and others involving family members who should have protected the child but perhaps failed to believe the story or take the child out of an abusive situation. The degree of betrayal experienced is affected by the child's relationship to the perpetrator, how much trust there was in the beginning between the two, and the possible disbelief of others when the child does disclose the abuse.[32] All of the situations experienced throughout abusive activities contribute to betrayal dynamics. One aspect of emotional trauma resulting from betrayal is the impairment the child may have in future relationships with adults and others to be able or willing to form trusting relationships.

Powerlessness

Powerlessness is a process whereby the child attempts to halt the abuse or have it halted by others but is unable to do so. Over time, the child learns to feel disempowered or powerless to change situations.[32] There are resultant feelings of powerlessness loss and a loss of self-efficacy over his or her life. Child sexual abuse involves the invasion of a child's body space and territory as well as coercion and manipulation that tend to cause feelings of entrapment and an inability to change situations. Powerlessness is a process that occurs to the psyche, inner being, and will of a child. Impaired coping strategies may result from this phenomena and manifest in symptoms such as phobias, nightmares, depression, clinging behavior, and running away.[32]

Stigmatization

A child experiences *stigmatization* when negative connotations of the abusive behavior become incorporated into the child's psyche. These connotations include feelings of shame, badness, or guilt.[32] It is often the abuser who helps instill such thoughts and inferences through activities such as blaming or demeaning the child for the abusive behavior or conveying shame concerning the nature of the activity. Stigmatization comes from the child knowing that family and community consider a certain sexual activity taboo. The term "damaged goods" has been applied to how a child victim of sexual abuse often feels that he or she is less than whole or is damaged in some way.[8]

Children experience a myriad of emotional and psychological reactions to child sexual abuse, and factors such as how well or poorly the abuser treats the child or the burden of keeping a difficult secret reinforce the stigma of the abuse. The stigmatization phenomena may manifest as feelings of isolation or a gravitation toward others who feel the same, self-destructive behavior, depression, and attempted suicide. Victims of child sexual abuse often carry a great amount of shame and guilt for a long time and experience a low sense of self-esteem.[32]

The organizing framework of traumagenic dynamics helps health care providers understand possible outcomes in the emotional and physical development of survivors of child sexual abuse. Manifestations may be seen at all stages of development and include age-inappropriate sexual behaviors, such as masturbation or sexualized play with other children. The list of problems that adult survivors of child sexual abuse experience is lengthy. Survivors report flashbacks, an inability to form intimate relationships with others, and a higher incidence of sexual victimization.[32] The more a nurse knows about the dynamics of child sexual abuse and the manifestations of abuse, the better able he or she is to deal with the problems that patients may have.

The Role of the Nurse in Child Abuse and Neglect

Mandated Reporting

All 50 states as well as the District of Columbia, American Samoa, Guam, the Northern Mariana Islands, Puerto Rico, and the United States Virgin Islands have statutes identifying persons who are required to report child maltreatment. As health care providers, nurses are mandated reporters. The circumstances under which a mandatory reporter must make a report vary from state to state, but, typically, a report must be made when the nurse suspects or has reasons to believe that a child has been abused or neglected. Another common standard requires the nurse who has knowledge of or has observed a child being subjected to conditions that would reasonably result in harm to the child to make a report to his or her local CPS agency or authorities.[33] Therefore, it is important nurses understand reporting laws in their specific state, the circumstances under which one reports abuse, and to whom reports are made.

Managing Child Maltreatment

According to the American Nurses Association (ANA) code of ethics,[34] nurses promote, advocate for, and strive to protect the health, safety, and rights of patients. These nursing general functions as well as those of assessment, intervention, prevention, and collaboration with the multidisciplinary team functions apply to victims of child maltreatment. The application of specific nursing functions is based on whether the nurse is a generalist or advanced practice nurse (APN) and the nurse's occupational setting. Forensically trained nurses who have successfully completed a pediatric sexual assault nurse examiner (P-SANE) course or a pediatric sexual assault forensic examiner (P-SAFE) course conduct sexual assault exams, collect evidence, and provide expert witness testimony.

Nursing assessment of child maltreatment requires a comprehensive history and physical examination. The history can be stressful for the nurse, parent, and child, warranting the use of nonjudgmental, therapeutic communication skills, and a quiet, unhurried environment. Successful assessment also requires understanding of the developmental level and abilities of the child to determine if the parent or caregiver history provides a plausible explanation for the child's injury or condition. The nurse should ascertain the child's general health status, past illness and trauma history, sources of health care, and developmental and psychosocial history. Data collected during the history is critical for comparison with the physical examination findings, particularly when discrepancies exist. Careful and objective documentation is critical, and child maltreatment typically warrants narrative, diagrammatic, and photographic documentation.[35]

The application of nursing interventions, like assessment, depends upon the nurse's role but include preventing further injury, providing supportive care, and reinforcing the importance of follow up. Interacting with parents suspected of abusing their child can be difficult. Nurses should debrief after managing child maltreatment cases by talking with colleagues about the events and their feelings. Team meetings can also better enable nurses and other professionals to work with abused children and their parents.[35]

Research and Evidence-Based Practice on Child Abuse and Neglect

Ongoing research in child abuse and neglect is important because of the many problems that abuse is known to cause for both individuals and society. Specific problems such as poor academic performance, delayed development, depression, delinquency, and substance abuse are known outcomes for some victims, while others demonstrate criminal and domestic violence and inappropriate sexual behaviors[33] in response to childhood traumas.

As with other health care issues, child maltreatment is an area of focus for nursing research (**Box 1-1**). Nursing research provides the scientific basis for nursing practice and is more important than ever given the changes in nursing roles and health care. Research is not a typical responsibility of an entry-level nurse; however, these nurses can still participate in the process by assisting with literature reviews or data collection and, even more importantly, by utilizing both evidence-based practice for child maltreatment and

Box 1-1. Recent Nursing Research on Child Maltreatment

— Sutherland MA. Examining mediators of child sexual abuse and sexually transmitted infections. *Nurs Res.* 2011;60(2):139-147.

— Pabi M, Wroska I, Lusarska B, Cuber T. Paediatric nurses' identification of violence against children. *J Adv Nurs.* 2011;67(2):384-393.

— Hornor G, Scribano P, Curran S, Stevens J. Emotional response to the ano-genital examination of suspected sexual abuse. *J Forensic Nurs.* 2009;5(3):124-130.

— Francisco MA, Hicks K, Powell J, Styles K, Tabor JL, Hulton LJ. The effect of childhood sexual abuse on adolescent pregnancy: an integrative research review. *J Specialists Pediatr Nurs.* 2008;13(4):237-248.

— Tingberg B, Bredlov B, Ygge B. Nurses' experience in clinical encounters with children experiencing abuse and their parents. *J Clin Nurs.* 2008;17(20):2718-2724.

— Gabriel LS. Patterns of injury in nonaccidental childhood fatalities. *J Forensic Nurs.* 2009;5(1):18-25.

— Bowman K, Rew L, Murphey C. Childhood maltreatment among community dwelling adult Latinas. *Issues Ment Health Nurs.* 2009;30(7):443-450.

— Holm AL, Bégat I, Severinsson E. Emotional pain: surviving mental health problems related to childhood experiences. *J Psychiatr Mental Health Nurs.* 2009;16(7):636-645.

— Weber S. Treatment of trauma- and abuse-related dissociative symptom disorders in children and adolescents. *J Child Adolesc Psychiatr Nurs.* 2009;22(1):2-6.

creating research questions based on their own nursing practice. APNs, particularly now with the advent of the doctor of nursing practice (DNP), can also be leaders in developing evidence-based nursing assessment and intervention for child maltreatment.

Conclusion

The pervasive nature of child abuse and neglect in society is immense, and the effects of abuse and neglect are great on those children and adults who survive the trauma. Nurses have a critical responsibility to understand the issues involved in maltreatment and to be an advocate for children by providing direct clinical care to the child and family. As nurses grow in their knowledge of the types of maltreatment and the underlying causes, opportunities for better identification of the problem, intervention, and prevention efforts are made possible.

Later chapters outline the major aspects of the health care approach to the care of children suspected of having been abused or neglected and detail the nurse's role in meeting the needs of these children and their families.

References

1. National Association of Pediatric Nurse Practitioners (NAPNAP). NAPNAP position statement on child maltreatment. National Association of Pediatric Nurse Practitioners Web site. http://www.napnap.org/Files/NAPNAP_PS_Child_Maltreatment_2011_FINAL.pdf. Published March 21, 2011. Accessed May 25, 2013.

2. American Association of Colleges of Nursing (AACN). Violence as a public health problem. American Association of Colleges of Nursing Web site. http://www.aacn.nche.edu/publications/position/violence-problem. Published March 15, 1999. Accessed May 25, 2013.

3. World Health Organization. Child maltreatment. World Health Organization Web site. http://www.who.int/mediacentre/factsheets/fs150/en/index.html. Published August 2010. Accessed May 27, 2013.

4. Kempe C, Silverman F, Steele B, Droegmuller W, Silver H. The battered-child syndrome. *JAMA*. 1962;181(1):17-24.

5. Flaherty E, Stirling J; the American Academy of Pediatrics Committee on Child Abuse and Neglect. Clinical report—the pediatrician's role in child maltreatment prevention. *Pediatrics*. 2010;126(4):833-841.

6. Child Abuse Prevention and Treatment Act, as amended, 42 USC 5101 et seq; 42 USC 5116 et seq (2003).

7. Child Welfare Information Gateway. What is child abuse and neglect? Child Welfare Information Gateway Web site. http://www.childwelfare.gov/pubs/factsheets/whatiscan.pdf. Published April 2008. Accessed May 25, 2013.

8. Sgroi SM. *Handbook of Clinical Intervention on Child Sexual Abuse*. New York, NY: DC Heath and Co; 1982.

9. Napp J, Case B. Stolen futures: a snapshot on child identity theft. *Office for victims of crime—Issue article*. Office of Justice Programs Web site. http://www.ojp.usdoj.gov./ovc/pdftxt/Article_ChildIDTheftSnapshot.pdf. Published July 2011. Accessed May 25, 2013.

10. Javelin Strategy & Research. Child identity theft study. Debix Web site. http://www.debix.com./docs/Child_ID_Theft_Study_2008.10.pdf. Published October 2008. Accessed 2012.

11. Finkelhor D, Turner H, Ormrod R, Hamby S, Kracke K. Children's exposure to violence: a comprehensive national survey. *National Survey of Children's Exposure to Violence*. National Criminal Justice Reference Service Web site. https://www.ncjrs.gov/pdffiles1/ojjdp/227744.pdf. Published October 2009. Accessed May 25, 2013.

12. United States Department of Health and Human Services, Administration for Children and Families, Administration on Children, Youth and Families, Children's Bureau. Child maltreatment 2009. http://www.acf.hhs.gov/programs/cb/stats_research/index.htm#can. Accessed May 25, 2013.

13. Hibbard RA, Desch LW; American Academy of Pediatrics Committee on Child Abuse and Neglect; American Academy of Pediatrics Council on Children with Disabilities. Maltreatment of children with disabilities. *Pediatrics*. 2007;119(5):1018-1025.

14. National MCH Center for Child Death Review. http://www.childdeathreview.org/home.htm. Accessed May 25, 2013.

15. ICAN/NCFR and ICAN Associates. The National Center on Child Fatality Review (NCFR). http://www.ican-ncfr.org/. Accessed 2012.

16. Wang C, Holton J. Economic impact study: total estimated cost of child abuse and neglect in the United States. Prevent Child Abuse America, a report funded by The Pew Charitable Trusts. Prevent Child Abuse America Web site. http://member.preventchildabuse.org/site/DocServer/cost_analysis.pdf?docID=144. Published 2007. Accessed 2012.

17. Turnera H, Finkelhor D, Ormrod R. The effect of lifetime victimization on the mental health of children and adolescents. *Soc Sci Med*. 2006;62(1):13-27.

18. Boden J, Horwood L, Fergusson D. Exposure to childhood sexual and physical abuse and subsequent educational achievement outcomes. *Child Abuse Negl*. 2007;31(10):1101-1114.

19. Gilbert R, Spatz Widom C, Browne K, Fergusson D, Webb E, Janson J. Burden and consequences of child maltreatment in high-income countries. *Lancet*. 2009;373(9657):68-81.

20. Mills C. Problems at home, problems at school: the effects of maltreatment in the home on children's functioning at school: an overview of recent research. London, UK: National Society for the Prevention of Cruelty to Children Web site. http://www.nspcc.org.uk/Inform/publications/Downloads/problemsathome_wdf48202.pdf. Published 2004. Accessed 2012.

21. Wilson H, Widom C. An examination of risky sexual behavior and HIV in victims of child abuse and neglect: a 30-year follow-up. *Health Psychol*. 2008;27:149-58.

22. English DJ, Widom CS, Brandford C. Another look at the effects of child abuse. *NIJ J*. 2004;251:23-24.

23. Finkelhor D. *A Sourcebook on Child Sexual Abuse*. Beverly Hills, CA: Sage Publications; 1986.

24. Jason J, Williams S, Burton A, Rochat R. Epidemiological differences between sexual and physical child abuse. *JAMA*. 1982;247:3344-3348.

25. Helfer R. The developmental basis of child abuse and neglect: an epidemiological approach. In: Helfer R, Kempe R, eds. *Battered Child*. 4th ed. Chicago, IL: The University of Chicago Press; 1987:60-80.

26. Helfer R. The etiology of child abuse. *Pediatrics*. 1973;51(4):777-779.

27. Belsky J. Etiology of child maltreatment: a developmental-ecological analysis. *Psychol Bull.* 1993;114(3):413-434.

28. Belsky J. Child maltreatment: an ecological integration. *Am Psychol.* 1980;35(4):320-335.

29. Justice B, Calvert A, Justice R. Factors mediating child abuse as a response to stress. *Child Abuse Negl.* 1985;9(3):359-363.

30. Hibbard RA, Desch LW; American Academy of Pediatrics Committee on Child Abuse and Neglect; American Academy of Pediatrics Council on Children with Disabilities. Maltreatment of children with disabilities. *Pediatrics.* 2007;119(5):1018-1025.

31. Sgroi SM, Blick L, Porter F. A conceptual framework for child sexual abuse. In: Sgroi SM, ed. *Handbook of Clinical Intervention on Child Sexual Abuse*. New York, NY: DC Heath and Co; 1982:9-37.

32. Finkelhor D, Browne A. The traumatic impact of child sexual abuse: a conceptualization. *Am J Orthopsychiatry*. 1985;55:530-541.

33. Child Welfare Information Gateway. Mandatory reporters of child abuse and neglect: summary of state laws. Child Welfare Information Gateway Web site. http://www.childwelfare.gov/systemwide/laws_policies/statutes/manda.cfm. Published 2010. Accessed 2012.

34. American Nurses Association (ANA). Code of ethics with interpretive statements. American Nurses Association Web site. http://nursingworld.org/codeofethics. Published 2001. Accessed May 25, 2013.

35. Giardino A. Physical child abuse. Emedicine Web site. http://emedicine.medscape.com/article/915664-overview. Updated April 1, 2013. Accessed May 25, 2013.

Chapter 2

Presentation and Overview of the Evaluation of Child Maltreatment

Sandra L. Elvik, MS, RN, CPNP
Eileen R. Giardino, PhD, MSN, FNP, ANP
Angelo P. Giardino, MD, PhD

Key Points

1. Child maltreatment, in any form, is a crime. All 50 states have mandatory reporting laws that define the steps that professionals must take when a child presents with findings that suggest abuse or neglect.
2. As the child's injuries are examined, the health care provider should pay close attention to the location of the injury, injury pattern, mechanisms that could plausibly explain the injury as opposed to the one that was provided by the caregiver on presentation, and the developmental level and capabilities of the child.
3. Inflicted trauma may at times cause bruising in protected, clothed areas of the body that would be viewed as uncommon in accidental trauma. Injuries seen in hidden or protected body areas are of significant concern and may be easily overlooked during an examination. Hidden areas include the neck, axillae, abdomen, back, and inner thighs, which are more difficult to reach.
4. Immersion burns are among the most serious burns seen in children and carry a high rate of morbidity and mortality. Often, sharp lines of demarcation between burned and unburned skin form in a stocking-and-glove type of pattern when different parts of the child are forcefully held in the scalding water. These sharp lines of demarcation are not expected findings in cases of accidental immersion for a couple of reasons: (1) Force is not used to hold the child in place. (2) The child normally splashes around to try and get out of the water.
5. The differential diagnoses for subdural hematoma (SDH) in an infant with no witnessed injury are limited, so abuse is usually at the top of the list. Children with his injury have sustained a serious, life-threatening injury and require appropriate medical evaluation and treatment as well as child protective services (CPS) reporting and investigation.
6. Sudden infant death syndrome (SIDS) is diagnosed when no other explanation fits the unexpected death of an infant aged 1 year and younger once a complete investigation has been conducted, including autopsy, death scene investigation, and review of clinical history.
7. The most important component of the sexual abuse evaluation has proved to be the information collected from the child and caregivers during the medical interview or

history-taking process. It is during the history taking process that the child is likely to disclose the inappropriate activity that has been occurring while in the care of the perpetrator.

8. Health care providers should familiarize themselves with normal anatomical changes that occur throughout the child's life by routinely examining the anogenital area and documenting findings from these specific areas during each health care visit.

Introduction

Child maltreatment, in any form, is a crime. All 50 states have mandatory reporting laws that define the steps that professionals must take when a child presents with findings that suggest abuse or neglect.[1] These laws clearly define mandated reporters as those who, by virtue of their work with children, are obligated to alert appropriate authorities of suspicions concerning abuse and neglect. Nurses are mandated reporters in all 50 states. Such laws and regulations vary from state to state in terms of the time parameters for reporting, the format for the report, and how law enforcement is involved and at what point. It is important for nurses and other health care providers to familiarize themselves with laws of the state within which they practice as well as the policies and procedures of their place of employment (see *Chapter 14, Legal Issues*).

There are many presentations for child abuse and neglect, ranging from obvious pathognomonic situations to subtle occult injuries. Additionally, there are high-risk situations that are only uncovered as a result of a high index of suspicion and meticulous medical evaluations. Some forms of maltreatment related to sexual abuse and exploitation may only present with nonspecific behavioral concerns that might also be seen in children experiencing other serious situations, such as parental divorce or moving to a new location, and are not necessarily specific to maltreatment. Often, the nurse is among the first health care professionals to have contact with the child who is being maltreated; therefore, nurses involved in all areas of practice must not only be able to recognize the signs and symptoms that may suggest maltreatment, but also be familiar with situations in which child maltreatment is seen. Nurses, and all health care providers, must be attuned to the many faces of child maltreatment and be sensitive to verbal, physical, and behavioral cues that alert to the possibility of maltreatment. The health care professionals involved in the care of the child who is being maltreated must then work to evaluate these suspicions and findings in light of the following child- and family-specific information:

— Historical details

— Physical signs

— Laboratory and diagnostic testing data

— Family background and cultural practices

— Expected developmental level and abilities of the child

To serve the best interests of the child and family, a health care provider must have a low index of suspicion for the possibility of child maltreatment while generating a broad differential diagnoses that considers child abuse and neglect and its various forms as a possible explanation for what is before him or her. In the early years of professional study of child maltreatment, Sgroi[1] recognized that a prerequisite for health care providers diagnosing sexual abuse is a willingness to consider that it exists. When abuse or neglect is not part of a differential diagnosis, a health care provider is not likely to rule in or out that diagnosis.

The health care evaluation of child maltreatment is best carried out in a multidisciplinary manner with each discipline contributing its expertise in the process.[2] The role of nurses in evaluating abuse and neglect is far-reaching and requires intervention in all aspects of care, including prevention, evaluation, and treatment. The advanced practice nurse (APN) has assumed major areas of responsibility in collaboration with physician colleagues around the following areas of child abuse evaluation:

— Interviewing the child for the medical history

— Examining the child for physical findings and collecting forensic evidence when appropriate

— Ordering and interpreting appropriate laboratory and diagnostic tests

— Observing interactions between child and family

— Generating differential diagnoses

— Carefully documenting the findings of a complete health care evaluation

The diagnostic approach to caring for a child suspected to have been abused or neglected relies on the clinical process of taking a history; performing a physical examination; obtaining laboratory findings to allow the development of a differential diagnosis composed of a wide variety of conditions; and, ultimately, a diagnostic impression and treatment plan. This chapter provides an overview of the health care evaluation process related to physical abuse, sexual abuse, and neglect.

Presentation and Evaluation

Physical Abuse

Eighteen percent of the nearly 1 million annual substantiated reports of child maltreatment can be categorized as physical abuse.[3] A diagnosis of physical abuse is made when a child sustains an injury inflicted by a parent, caregiver, or anyone else in a position of authority over the child. Injuries from physical abuse may present in various ways and may be obvious or occult and only discovered later in the comprehensive evaluation.

Ludwig describes a "building block" approach to the evaluation of a child suspected of physical abuse in which each block represents a component of the health care evaluation and the blocks build on each other[4] (**Figure 2-1**). As suspicion for abuse increases with findings from the history and physical examination, the blocks are stacked and the evidence in the growing tower may rise to the *concern threshold* requiring further consideration of the possibility of child maltreatment. Consequently, the concern for abuse may increase where the block tower then exceeds the concern threshold and crosses into the *reporting threshold*. Such concern requires the health care provider to make a report to the state CPS agency.

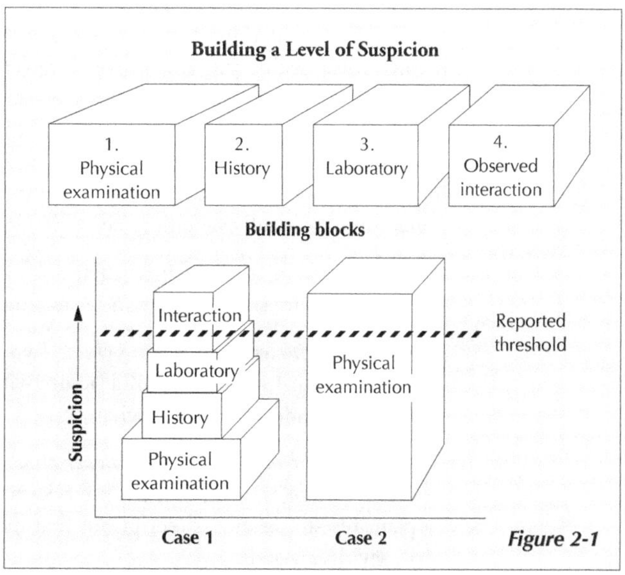

Figure 2-1. *Building a level of suspicion. Reprinted with permission from Ludwig S. Child abuse. In: Fleisher GR, Ludwig S, eds.* Textbook of Pediatric Emergency Medicine. *4th ed. Philadelphia, PA: Lippincott Williams & Wilkins; 1999:1669-1704.*

The physical examination during a well-child evaluation or an acute illness visit may uncover physical injuries indicative of child abuse. Additionally, a child may exhibit a pattern of injuries that suggests repeated abuse over a time period. In some cases, injuries may be such that the child is brought to the hospital moribund and in need of emergency medical care and resuscitation, while some children are brought to the hospital with fatal injuries and cannot be saved. Physical abuse is considered a medical emergency. It is imperative that children brought to a health care provider for evaluation of possible physical abuse be evaluated immediately. The goal of the evaluation is to accurately assess injuries, treat inflicted injury, and ensure that the child will be safe and protected from risk of subsequent injury.

Once a child is brought to a health care facility to receive treatment for an injury, the health care provider should complete a thorough health care evaluation to accurately diagnose the extent of injury and the mechanism by which it resulted. A complete health care evaluation in the face of possible maltreatment includes the following components:

— History from child and caregiver, including the periods before, during, and after the injury occurred

— Physical examination to evaluate obvious injury as well as possible hidden injuries

— Laboratory and diagnostic testing as appropriate for possible findings

— Observation of the child and caregiver interaction throughout the health care episode, noting caregiver-child communication and caregiver responses to the child's needs

— Meticulous documentation of the entire evaluation, beginning with the initial presentation for care and concluding with a diagnostic impression

Obtaining a history for an injury can begin with simply asking the question in an open-ended, nonthreatening manner, such as "What happened here?" or "How did the injury happen?" An open-ended approach gives the verbal child or the caregiver the opportunity needed to provide details of how the injury occurred. Other questions related to the injury may be asked. All answers should be documented.[5] As any information given in a health history may have varying degrees of accuracy, the health care provider must consider the history in light of physical examination findings and determine the plausibility of the mechanism of injury offered. The level of suspicion is raised to the point of reporting the information to CPS when reasons for the injury are not in agreement with the physical findings or the details of the story do not make sense.

Careful documentation of the caregiver's account at the time of presentation is essential, because it is possible that an abusive caregiver's initial report will change over time as the seriousness of the situation becomes clearer.[6] It is important for the health care professional to carefully document the time and content of statements made by the parent or caregiver in the medical record so that it can then be shared with other professionals involved in the case. Discrepancies noted during the evaluation are an important component in the overall evaluation (see *Chapter 3, History and the Health Care Interview*).

Presentations and subsequent evaluations of injuries with the following characteristics are among the most worrisome in regard to possible child maltreatment:

— ***Magical injuries in the young child:*** Two-month-old is brought to a hospital with a femur fracture or skull fracture without any witnesses to any trauma that would provide an injury mechanism.

— ***Changing history of the injury over time:*** Initial mechanism of injury that was offered changes in subsequent interviews to, what are thought to be, more plausible stories or to descriptions that may account for injuries that have been newly discovered.

— ***History incongruous with injury seen on physical examination:*** History of minor trauma provided despite evidence of massive injury.

— ***History implausible for injury:*** Mechanism of injury does not explain the injury found on examination.

— ***Developmentally incompatible history:*** Child is not developmentally capable of doing what caregiver said he or she did to sustain observed injury.

— ***Self-inflicted trauma history:*** Child threw himself into bathtub of scalding hot water.

— ***Young sibling or playmate blamed for serious injury:*** Eighteen-month-old sibling blamed for massive intracranial injury found in 6-week-old brother.

— ***Delayed presentation or late medical care:*** Caregiver brings child for care of injury long after a reasonable caregiver would have sought health care assistance.

Differentiating Between Accidental and Inflicted Injuries

As the child's injuries are examined, the health care provider should pay special attention to the location of the injury, the injury pattern, the mechanisms that could plausibly explain the injury as opposed to the one that was provided by the caregiver on presentation, and the developmental level and capabilities of the child. Children and adults can be injured accidentally despite reasonable precautions taken in the environment, and careful evaluation of the injury is necessary to accurately determine if the mechanism of injury was accidental (noninflicted) or inflicted. In the context of a case in which the injury sustained is suspected to be the result of physical abuse, several types of injuries are discussed, including bruises, burns, skeletal fractures, and central nervous system injury.

Bruises

Bruising is the most common soft tissue injury seen in childhood and is nearly a universal finding on the routine well-child examination. However, certain characteristics invoke more concern for possible inflicted trauma. These characteristics are related to the location, shape, amount, and extent of the bruising.

In active children, accidental bruises are generally seen over areas with a bony prominence, such as the knees and shins. The forehead and chin are other sites of accidental trauma, especially in toddlers who are learning to walk and run. Inflicted trauma may at times cause bruising in protected, clothed areas of the body that would be viewed as uncommon in accidental trauma (**Table 2-1**). Injuries seen in hidden or protected body areas are of significant concern and may be easily overlooked during an examination. Hidden areas include the neck, axillae, abdomen, back, and inner thighs, which are more difficult to reach. The use of objects as well as one's hands are among the countless ways in which bruising injuries can be inflicted on a child's skin. Pinches and slaps by the caregiver may or may not leave patterned markings while some objects have characteristic shapes that, when forcefully applied against the child's skin, leave characteristic geometric markings (**Figure 2-2**). Patterned bruising on the child's skin makes the identification of the implement possible. The nurse should describe in detail the pattern of the injury, including shape, dimensions, pattern, and coloring variability, such as areas of normal skin interspersed with reddish-blue linear markings. **Figure 2-3** illustrates shapes of commonly used objects that may be employed in bruising children.

Child abuse typically occurs longitudinally and represents a pattern of caregiving behaviors over time that results in the child's injury. Indication of ongoing battering of the child raises the concern of physical maltreatment. The child may have a large

Table 2-1. Typically Accidental Versus Possibly Nonaccidental Injury Sites

Typically Accidental	Possibly Nonaccidental	
— Forehead	— Scalp	— Head and face
— Elbows	— Behind ears	— Chest
— Knees	— Neck	— Upper back
— Shins	— Axillae and arms	— Lumbar region
— Iliac crest	— Inner thighs	— Thighs and buttocks
	— Webs of fingers and toes	— Fracture(s) and burn(s)
	— Genitalia	

Adapted from Roberton DM, Barbor P, Hull D. Unusual injury? recent injury in normal children and children with suspected non-accidental injury. Br Med J (Clin Res Ed). *1982;285(6352):1399-1401.*

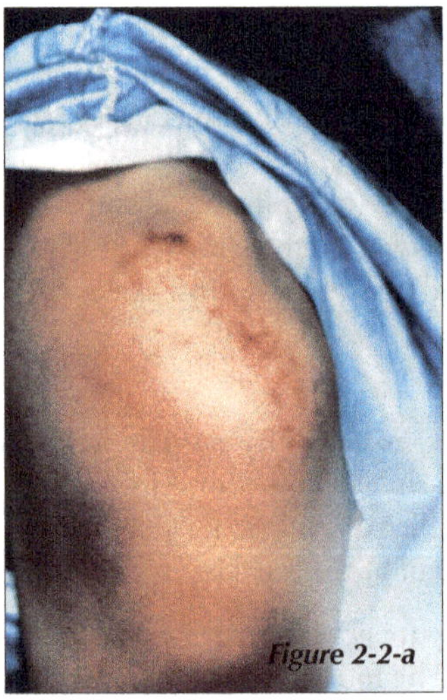

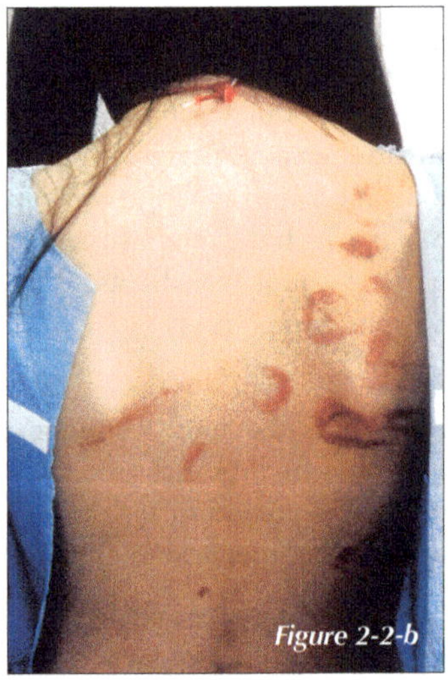

Figure 2-2-a. *Shoulder and upper arm bruises of a 9-year-old female. Historical details indicated that the child's biological father became angry with the child for getting a bad grade on a test. The grade was a B, and the father wanted the child to get straight A's. The father began punching the child with his fist, but soon tired and grabbed a hanger.*

Figure 2-2-b. *Bruises on the back of aforementioned child. Note the fixed loop marks, which are consistent with the child's history of being hit with a hanger. No court case was conducted; the father confessed to the beating and was imprisoned.*

Figure 2-3. *Shapes of commonly used objects that may be employed in bruising children. Reprinted with permission from Johnson CF. Inflicted injury versus accidental injury.* Ped Clin North Am. *1990;37(4)791-814.*

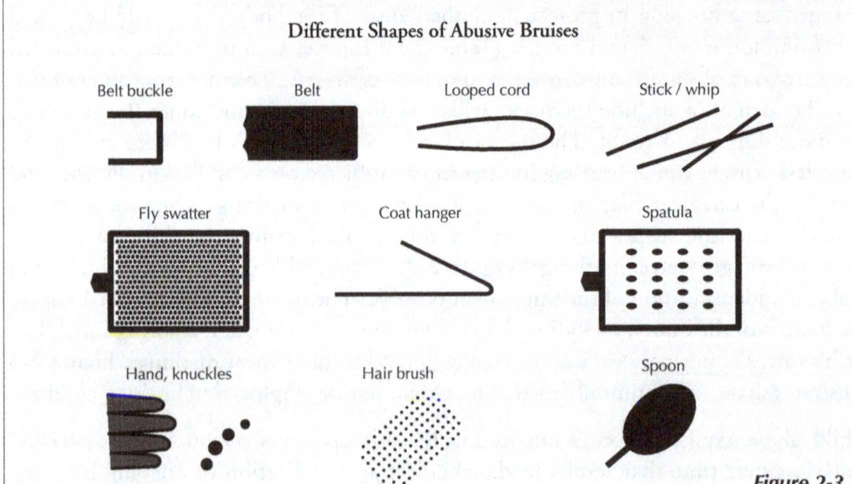

Figure 2-3

amount of bruising or the bruising may be composed of crops of bruises at different stages of healing. Caution is needed when attempting to specifically date bruises based on their color.[8] In general, bruises undergo a series of color changes from the reddish-blue seen in the immediate phase following injury to the yellowish-brown seen during final stages of resolution.[9] As a result of the variant nature of bruises, it is difficult to determine the exact time at which a bruise should change colors. Additionally, the literature does not support certainty in actual dating[8]; therefore, color changes in bruises should not be used as a universal rule of thumb to date bruises in children. However, health care providers can evaluate the color and stages of bruising on a specific child and, by comparison, determine the age of the injury based on color changes. When evaluating and then documenting the bruises of a specific child, health care providers should state only broad ranges of how old different bruises are suspected to be in comparison to other bruises on the child (see *Chapter 4, The Physical Examination in the Evaluation of Suspected Child Maltreatment: Physical Abuse and Sexual Abuse Examinations*).

Cultural Considerations in Suspected Abuse

When evaluating the child with bruising, cultural factors must be taken into consideration. Families who have emigrated from other parts of the world bring with them certain traditions. Besides foods and celebrations of particular holidays, there are customary forms of health and healing that may differ from those of traditional Western practices. The health care provider should consider the child's cultural background because the folk healing practices common to some cultures may leave characteristic marks on a child's skin.[10] Some Asian families practice *cao gaio*, or coining, in which a coin is rubbed over an area of pain or illness. The friction results in petechiae and bruising, usually over the ribs and chest. *Cupping*, practiced in some parts of China since the third century BC, involves lighting a match into a small round cup made of glass, bamboo, ceramic, or metal. Once heated, the cup is quickly applied to the skin. The heating and cooling creates a partial vacuum as the cup sticks tightly to the skin, and this suction-like action creates a bruise that resembles a circular burn. Several cups may be applied at any one time to a particular part of the body for the purpose of increasing blood circulation and promoting healing.[10]

Some additional findings may raise concern for possible abuse but on evaluation are found to have a nonabusive cause. For example, a Mongolian spot is a finding commonly mistaken for abuse (**Figure 2-4**). This blue-black macule is seen on the skin, most often over the sacrum, of many dark-skinned children. Other youngsters have small circular spots scattered over the skin. A nurse concerned about the identification of this birthmark can review birth records, previous histories, and prior examinations. If the assessment for abuse is benign and the child is felt to be safe, the nurse can schedule a 2-week follow-up visit to re-examine the skin. A bruise would be expected to fade in the time between the initial visit and the follow-up visit, whereas the Mongolian spot would remain constant. Mongolian spots usually lighten after the first few years of life.

Figure 2-4. *Mongolian spots. This is a 4- to 5-month-old child who was seen in the failure-to-thrive clinic. The lesions, though commonly thought to be bruises as a result of their extensive nature, are Mongolian spots.*

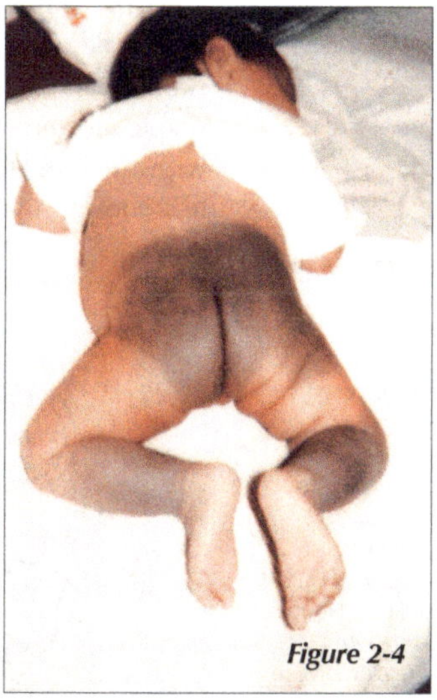

Figure 2-4

When assessing bruising, the nurse examiner considers a broad differential diagnosis that includes organic disorders that can cause the child to bruise or injure easily (see *Chapter 7, Differential Diagnosis: Conditions That Mimic Child Maltreatment*). A number of hematological conditions can cause easy bruising, and appropriate laboratory tests may reveal the presence of such conditions and explain certain bruises (**Table 2-2**).

Table 2-2. Medical Conditions Presenting With Skin Lesions That May Be Confused with Child Maltreatment

CONDITION	POTENTIAL MIMICS
Connective Tissue	— Ehlers-Danlos syndrome
Genetic	— Osteogenesis imperfect (bruises with fractures)
Hematological	— Leukemia — von Willebrand's disease — Idiopathic thrombocytopenic purpura (ITP)
Infectious	— Meningococcemia
Pediatric	— Physical abuse

After completing a history, physical examination, and review of laboratory and diagnostic testing, the nurse and other collaborating health care professionals should weigh the possibility that the bruising is likely to have occurred in the way the caregiver described. They may draw on knowledge of the general mechanism of injuries, the developmental level of the child, and the consistencies of the history provided, and then compare these impressions with observations of the child's actual injuries to reach a diagnosis.

Burns

Burns are a common soft tissue injury seen in children and have significant public health implications related to prevention efforts. Burns may be minor, severe, and at times fatal, with significant potential to disfigure the child's appearance. When examining the child with a burn injury, the health care provider must consider several important factors, including the location, shape and pattern, and extent of the burn, and has an essential responsibility to then compare the findings against the history offered by the caregiver.

Various kinds of burns are possible based on the mechanism of injury. For example, hot liquids may come in contact with the child's skin causing scalding burns. Scalding burns are further subdivided into splash burns, in which the liquid spills or pours onto the skin, and immersion burns, in which the child's skin is submerged in the hot liquid. Contact burns are seen when a hot object comes in contact with the child's skin. Characteristic shapes or patterns may be left on the child's skin depending on the shape and temperature of the object and the amount of time the object is in contact with the child's skin. Open fire flame burns and electrical burns are also possible but less commonly seen in the context of physical abuse. **Figure 2-5** demonstrates the

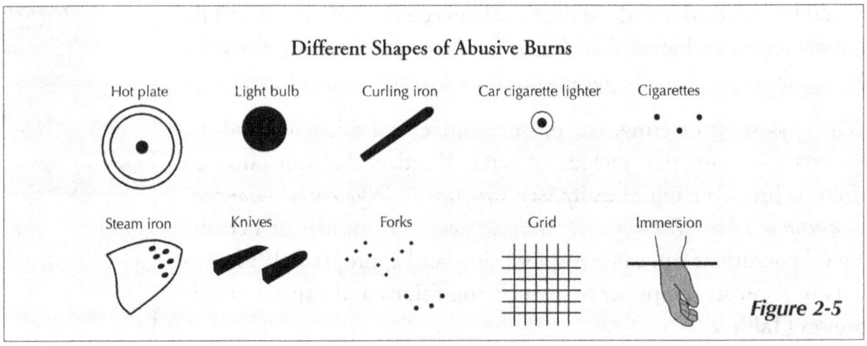

Figure 2-5. *Shapes of commonly used objects that may be employed in burning children. Reprinted with permission from Johnson CF. Inflicted injury versus accidental injury.* Ped Clin North Am. *1990;37(4) 791-814.*

shapes of commonly used objects that may be employed in burning children. Certain presentations of a burned child raise particular concern for possible abuse, as follows:

— Implausible history based on child's development, age of the burn, and appearance of the burn

— Magical injury with no history offered for burn; child just found to have a burn

— Caregiver who was watching the child is not present during the health care evaluation

— Sibling or playmate blamed for child's burn

— Pattern that suggests the child was restrained during injury

— Delay in seeking health care

— Presence of other injuries

— Signs and symptoms of neglectful caregiving, including poor hygiene, malnutrition

— History of previous injury

Given the history and physical examination of a child with a scald burn, the health care provider must consider what would be reasonable to expect on examination given the caregiver's report about how the burn occurred. Children are naturally curious and explore their environment in a developmentally appropriate manner. As a result, they may attempt to pull objects that contain hot liquids off of stoves, tables, and countertops. If a 2-year-old boy is brought to a facility for care with a history of having walked over to the stove and pulled a pot of boiling water onto himself, the expected burn from such a mechanism would have a characteristic shape created by falling liquid. One could expect the liquid to hit the child's face, neck, and shoulder as he looked up and reached to pull the pot off the stove. The hot liquid would then be expected to pour down the child's skin, most likely involving the outstretched arm, chest, and back, cooling as it spread across the skin and resulting with the most distal area of skin being the least severely burned. The initial point of contact is the hottest and would have the most serious burn. An examination that reveals a circular burn on the child's back is not consistent with the mechanism described in the history. The finding of a spreading burn would be more consistent with a hot liquid being thrown at the child rather than a spill or pouring of liquid onto the child. Such a discrepancy should raise concerns about physical abuse using a hot liquid and requires reporting to CPS (**Figure 2-6**).

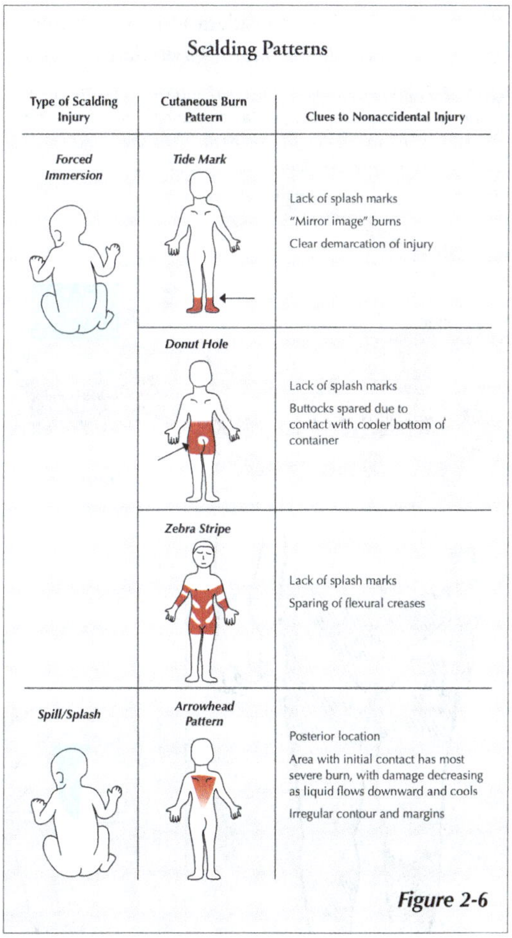

Figure 2-6. *Illustrations of characteristic patterns of scald abuse. Reprinted with permission from SLACK Incorporated: Mahindra P, Guillen C, Glick S. A 5-year-old girl with scarring.* Pediatric Annals. *2009;38(7):362-364.*

Immersion burns resulting from abuse are among the most serious burns in children and carry a high rate of morbidity and mortality. Forced immersion burns often have a characteristic pattern that is formed as the caregiver uses physical strength to hold the child in contact with the hot liquid, as in hot bath water. As the child is plunged into the hot liquid, he or she typically tries to recoil from the hot liquid but cannot overcome the larger, more powerful caregiver. If the caregiver were to hold the child by arms and plunge him or her into the scalding hot liquid buttocks or feet first, the child would instinctively attempt to pull his or her legs up in an attempt to escape. In the classic abusive immersion burn, the buttocks are submerged and pressed against the container holding the hot liquid. In such a case, the skin of the child's anterior thigh comes in close approximation with the skin of the femoral area as the child struggles against the attack and effectively seals out the hot water, sparing that skin. This scenario also leads to a central area of protected skin on the buttocks resulting in a "hole-in-doughnut" pattern. In forced immersion burns, there are often sharp lines of demarcation between burned and unburned skin in a stocking-and-glove type of pattern that forms as different parts of the child are forcefully held in the scalding water. These sharp lines of demarcation are not expected in an accidental immersion, because the child, if not forcefully held in place, would splash around, trying to get out of the water (**Figure 2-7** and **Figures 2-8-a, b,** and **c**). In evaluating scald burns, the health care provider must consider a broad list of differential diagnoses that takes into consideration conditions that may initially appear similar to burns (see *Chapter 7, Differential Diagnosis: Conditions That Mimic Child Maltreatment*).

Figure 2-7. *Immersion burn. The child appears to be 10 to 12 months old. Of interest are the areas of sparing where the body was "folded" up to protect the skin as much as she could. (Contributed by James Williams, MD; Stockton, CA.)*

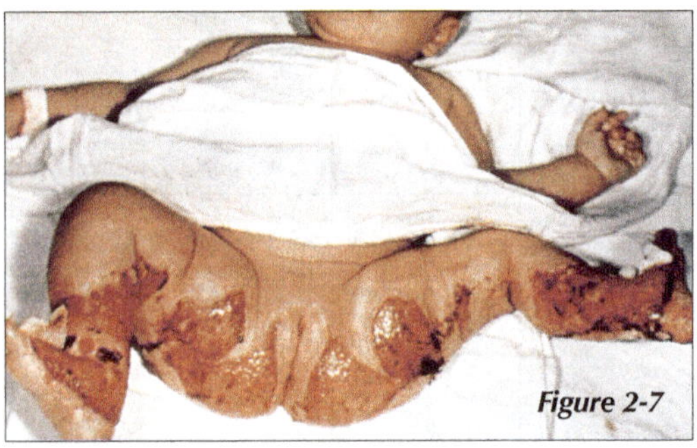

Figure 2-7

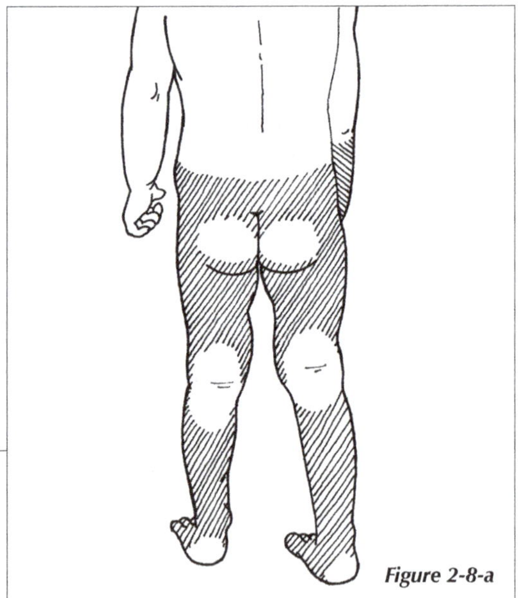

Figure 2-8-a

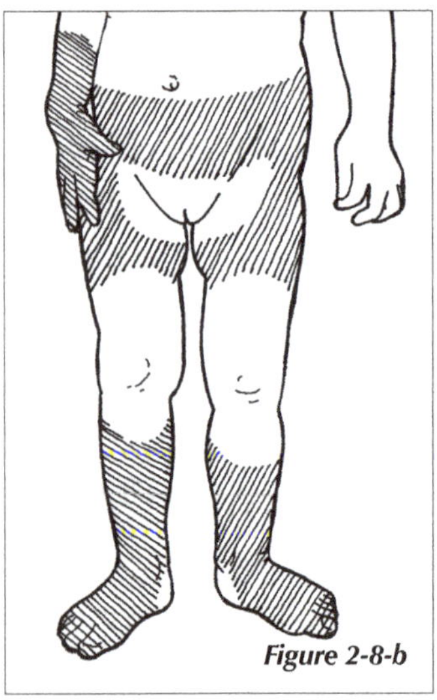

Figure 2-8-b

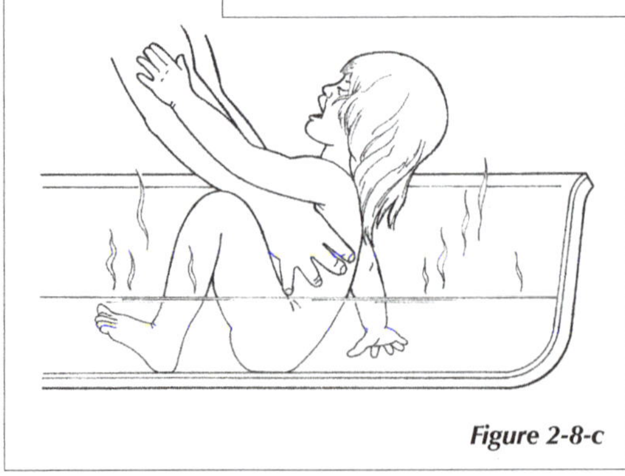

Figure 2-8-c

Figure 2-8-a. *Hole-in-doughnut burn pattern of immersion burns seen from behind.*

Figure 2-8-b. *Hole-in-doughnut burn pattern of immersion seen from the front.*

Figure 2-8-c. *How hole-in-doughnut pattern is produced.*

Fractures

Fractures in the long bones are common injuries found in children, especially as they grow older and become involved in sporting activities; however, skeletal injuries are also frequently seen in physically abused children. Other than clavicle fractures that occur during birth, skeletal fractures in infants and young children should raise concerns about possible maltreatment. Healthy bones are strong; a fair amount of force is required to break even a child's bone, especially the relatively large femur. Histories for injury containing inconsistencies already described in this chapter are of concern with abusive fractures as well. The presence of long bone fractures and histories of minor trauma or unwitnessed falls in the non-walking infant should be considered highly suspicious. The child's developmental abilities must always be taken into consideration when evaluating the plausibility of mechanism of injury leading to a skeletal fracture. Other bones besides the long bones may be fractured during maltreatment, with the most worrisome fractures being those of the rib and skull. Because of the amount of force required to generate long bone fractures and the risk of other associated injuries, infants who have such fractures without a reasonable, witnessed mechanism of injury are considered at risk for potentially life-threatening injury. Therefore CPS should be notified for an immediate evaluation to prevent re-injury to the child.

Skeletal fractures in young children are not always obvious initially and may be uncovered only during a thorough health care evaluation. Because of this, the American Academy of Pediatrics (AAP) recommends a skeletal survey, a complete set of radiographs with examination of each bone for possible fracture, be done for children aged 2 years and under who are being evaluated for possible physical abuse.[11] The specific radiographic views contained in a skeletal survey include the following:

- Anteroposterior views of the appendicular skeleton
  - Humeri
  - Forearms
  - Femurs
  - Lower legs
  - Feet
- Oblique and posteroanterior views of the hands
- Lateral views of the axial skeleton, along with the additional views contained in parentheses
  - Cervical spine
  - Lumbar spine (lateral)
  - Thorax (anteroposterior)
  - Pelvis (anteroposterior, including mid- and lower lumbar spine)
- Frontal and lateral views of the skull bones

Many different types of fractures are defined by the location of the break on the bone. All fracture types have been seen in child maltreatment-related injuries, although some patterns are more commonly associated with child maltreatment than are others[12] (see *Chapter 4, The Physical Examination in the Evaluation of Suspected Child Maltreatment: Physical Abuse and Sexual Abuse Examinations*). The skills of knowledgeable pediatric radiologists are invaluable in identifying fractures and in assessing potential mechanisms and risk of abuse-related trauma.

Health care providers may be asked to help investigators determine when a fracture may have occurred. It is possible to date skeletal injuries within a relatively certain time frame based on a combination of factors related to tissue formation and bone healing,[13,14] including soft tissue changes, visibility of fracture line, callus calcification, and ossification of new periosteal bone.[12] Additionally, it is important to recognize that the younger the bones, the more rapidly the fracture may heal. Each of the 4 phases of healing indicates specific aspects of healing that can be viewed via radiography. For example, periosteal bone formation occurs in the second phase of healing and begins to occur after injury, approximately 7 to 10 days in infants and 10 to 14 days in older children. In general, more precise dating can occur when there is a shorter time period between injury and the dating process[13] (see *Chapter 4, The Physical Examination in the Evaluation of Suspected Child Maltreatment: Physical Abuse and Sexual Abuse Examinations*).

A broad list of differential diagnoses should be assessed, including all relevant medical conditions, whenever a health care provider is considering child maltreatment in the context of skeletal fractures. A common differential diagnosis when considering skeletal fracture is osteogenesis imperfecta (OI), a genetic disorder affecting the formation of collagen that has various characteristic manifestations that might be confused with child maltreatment. The presence of these manifestations should be explored during the health care evaluation (see *Chapter 7, Differential Diagnosis: Conditions That Mimic Child Maltreatment*).

Central Nervous System Injury

Among the most serious patterns of injuries identified in maltreated children are the inflicted brain injuries and subsequent central nervous system (CNS) impairment seen with abusive head trauma (AHT), formerly known as the shaken baby syndrome (SBS) or shaking impact syndrome (SIS). Brain injuries seen in AHT are a result of the application of rotational forces to the child's head and neck. These forces were initially described as "whiplash shaken baby syndrome" to capture the "to and fro" movement of the child's head as the child is violently shaken.[15] Rotational forces are distinct from the low-velocity translational forces seen in common household falls. Infants, with their relatively large heads, weak neck muscles, and relatively strong spinal ligaments, may sustain serious injuries to the brain and its associated vascular and neural connections and significant impairment.

The presence of a subdural hematoma (SDH) is a classic manifestation of AHT and may be of different ages, appearing radiographically as both chronic and acute. SDHs are often associated with retinal hemorrhages and may occasionally occur with other injuries, including various other intracranial findings. Whether the injuries to the brain in AHT require a mechanism of injury that includes impacting of the child's head against a fixed surface remains a debate in the professional literature. From a clinical evaluation and overall investigation perspective, the child is violently attacked by shaking alone or shaking plus the impacting of his or her head against a fixed surface. Regardless of the ultimate outcome of this scientific inquiry, the fact remains that the injury is inflicted and not accidental.

Children who sustain AHT injury are typically young, almost always aged 2 years and younger, with many aged 6 months and younger.[16,17] Less severe cases of AHT include symptoms of irritability, lethargy, and poor feeding, while more severe cases include symptoms of apnea, seizures, and unresponsiveness.[18] Histories offered by abusive caregivers are often misleading and inaccurate. Physical examination typically finds neurological impairment referable to the brain injury; approximately 50% present with severe impairment.[15]

Other physical findings may be present, with retinal hemorrhages present in 65% to 95% of infants with AHT.[17,19] A smaller percentage have skull, rib, or long bone fractures. The absence of extracranial injuries is not uncommon and should not be viewed as evidence for nonabusive injury. Laboratory and diagnostic imaging demonstrates that a child with CNS injury often has bloody cerebrospinal fluid (CSF) and imaging studies demonstrating SDH. The differential diagnoses for SDH in an infant with no witnessed injury are limited, so abuse is usually at the top of the list. Children with this injury have sustained a serious, life-threatening injury and require appropriate medical evaluation and treatment as well as CPS reporting and investigation (see *Chapter 13, Child Protective Services and Child Abuse*).

Minor household falls are frequently offered as reasons for AHT. The consensus among experts in the field is that severe, life-threatening injuries from common household falls are uncommon.[18,20] The more suspicious the history initially offered, the more classic the findings for AHT; the more severe the injuries, the higher is the suspicion for inflicted trauma.

Dating the age of a head injury has strong implications for the medical evaluation and an ensuing investigation of the injury by CPS and possibly law enforcement. Magnetic resonance imaging (MRI) can distinguish between fresh blood in an acute SDH and older blood that is undergoing resorption in subacute and chronic SDH. The significance of finding both acute and chronic SDHs is the subject of current debate. The analysis of these debates requires an extensive literature review; however, several key clinical points may be made on the presentation of a child who has sustained AHT and have been summarized here. It can be said with a high degree of certainty that traumatic acute SDH associated with brain swelling and severe neurological impairment, including death, is associated with the following[15]:

- Injury from major mechanical forces
- Presentation of rapidly progressing symptoms that progress with no long lucid period between injury and onset of symptoms, as contrasted with a slowly evolving epidural hemorrhage
- No occult subclinical injury occurring unexpectedly and without any explanation in an otherwise healthy infant

Child Fatality

Each year approximately 2000 children, or 5 children per day, die as a result of child maltreatment.[21,22] Some children are brought to the emergency medical services system with catastrophic, life-threatening central nervous system (CNS) and thoracoabdominal injuries. The more obvious battering cases are typically identified as inflicted injuries. More commonly, however, children die from subtle forms of neglectful caregiving. For the year 2000, neglect and abuse was determined to be the cause of death in 1.7 of every 100 000 child fatalities. Of those maltreatment-related fatalities, 34.9% resulted from abuse and 27.8% resulted from neglect.[23]

Correct identification of child fatalities associated with maltreatment may be difficult, depending on the circumstances surrounding their presentation and a number of associated community-specific factors. Health care providers may have an impact on the accuracy of maltreatment-related child fatality statistics and should be aware of how to ensure an appropriate response in such cases. The following broad systemic issues are identified as underlying the ambiguity in maltreatment-related child fatalities:

— Variation in the way child deaths are reported, leading to inaccurate reporting of the number of children who die from child maltreatment

— Lack of national standards for child death investigations and child autopsies

— Variation in the manner in which CPS, law enforcement, and medical examiners handle the investigative process

— In many states, use of elected coroners who are not required to have medical training or child maltreatment training rather than physician medical examiners

In response to these concerns, state and local governments have impaneled multidisciplinary child fatality review (CFR) teams that review all cases of child death in a given locality. The teams seek to correctly identify causes of death and support the need for systemic reforms to prevent similar deaths. CFRs also facilitate system improvements to enhance future investigations and attempt to build broad coalitions between the disciplines and agencies involved.[24]

Perhaps one of the more difficult areas to understand when making a determination of nonaccidental or accidental cause of natural death is that of sudden infant death syndrome (SIDS). SIDS is diagnosed when no other explanation fits the unexpected death of an infant aged 1 year or younger once a complete investigation, including autopsy, death scene investigation, and review of clinical history, has been conducted.[25] To assist in distinguishing SIDS from fatal child abuse, the AAP has issued a policy statement to clarify several key points.[25] SIDS is more common than infanticide and is the most common cause of death in child aged 6 months through 1 year. Approximately 90% of SIDS deaths occur by age 6 months, with the peak incidence between age 2 and 4 months. The etiology of SIDS is not understood and has been associated with various factors:

— Prone sleeping position

— Sleeping on a soft surface

— Maternal smoking, antepartum and postpartum

— Bundling and overheating of the child

— Delayed or absent prenatal care

— Young maternal age

— Prematurity

— Low birth weight

— Male gender

Since 1992, the AAP has recommended that infants be placed on their back to sleep.[26] Campaigns to decrease infants sleeping in a prone position (eg, "Back to Sleep") have been associated with an approximately 50% decrease in prone sleeping and an approximately 40% decrease in SIDS deaths. The AAP is clear that, despite some of the uncertainty around SIDS, it is a diagnosis of exclusion and should only be made after thorough investigation and medical admission that the death is completely unexplained.[25] Specifically, the following criteria must be met to diagnose an infant death as SIDS:

— Complete autopsy, including cranium and cranial contents; findings compatible with SIDS

— No gross or microscopic evidence of trauma or significant disease process

— No evidence of trauma on skeletal survey

— Other possible causes of death are adequately ruled out, including meningitis, sepsis, aspiration, pneumonia, myocarditis, abdominal trauma, dehydration, fluid and electrolyte imbalance, significant congenital lesions, inborn metabolic disorders, carbon monoxide asphyxia, drowning, or burns.

— No evidence of current alcohol, drug, or toxic exposure

— Negative findings in thorough death scene investigation and review of clinical history

Further, the AAP Committee on SIDS offers recommendations for health care providers with regard to the evaluation of sudden unexplained infant deaths.[25] The AAP encourages health care providers to rigorously pursue the medical evaluation, contribute to the investigation, and maintain a supportive approach to the parents because of the uncertainty surrounding the case and their stress and bewilderment at the loss of the child.[26] The AAP policy statement on SIDS and other sleep-related infant deaths addresses risk factors for infant deaths and recommends approaches to child care that decreases the occurrence of sleep-related deaths.[27]

Sexual Abuse

Sexual abuse accounts for approximately 9.1% of child maltreatment cases annually[28] and is recognized as a significant health problem affecting the well-being of a relatively large number of children (approximately 61 000 children in 2011).[28] The following are some of the ways in which sexual abuse presents to the health care provider:

— Purposeful disclosure by the child that inappropriate sexual activity is occurring[29]

— Accidental discovery in which a third party, other than the child or perpetrator, observes or suspects inappropriate sexual activity and reports it or when another child victim discloses the perpetrator's behavior

— During medical evaluation for genital signs or nonspecific physical symptoms leading to the discovery of genital trauma, sexually transmitted infection (STI), or other findings suggestive of sexual abuse. (As a result of heightened recognition of sexual abuse, parents are more attuned to genital complaints, especially from their daughters.) **Table 2-3** identifies specific and nonspecific physical and behavioral complaints of sexual abuse.

— During medical and mental health evaluation for nonspecific behavioral complaints leading to the discovery of sexual abuse

Sexual abuse is a unique form of child maltreatment separate from physical abuse. Sexual abuse of the child typically occurs over time by a perpetrator with whom the child or family is acquainted. The most important component of the sexual abuse evaluation has proved to be the information collected from the child and caregivers during the medical interview or history-taking process. It is during the history-taking process that the child is likely to disclose inappropriate activity. The physical examination in cases of child sexual abuse is often without specific findings of either acute or chronic trauma[30-33] (see *Chapter 4, The Physical Examination in the Evaluation of Suspected Child Maltreatment: Physical Abuse and Sexual Abuse Examinations*). Many families and some relatively uninformed professionals mistakenly think that the physical examination will provide evidence to confirm the child's allegation and inappropriately place too much

Table 2-3. Identification of Sexual Abuse

Physical Complaints		Behavioral Complaints	
Specific	— Genital injury: bruises and lacerations — Rectal laceration, fissures — STI — Pregnancy	**Specific**	— Explicit descriptions of sexual contact — Inappropriate knowledge of adult sexual behavior — Compulsive masturbation — Excessive sexual curiosity, sexual acting out
Non-specific	— Anorexia — Abdominal pain — Enuresis — Dysuria — Encopresis — Evidence of physical abuse in genital area — Vaginal discharge — Urethral discharge — Rectal pain	**Non-specific**	— Excessive fears, phobias — Refusal to sleep alone, nightmares — Runaway behavior — Aggressive behavior — Attempted suicide — Any abrupt change in behavior

Reprinted with permission from Ludwig S. In: Fleisher GR, Ludwig S, eds. Textbook of Pediatric Emergency Medicine. *4th ed. Philadelphia, PA: Lippincott Williams & Wilkins: 1999;1669-1704.*

emphasis on the presence or absence of findings. However, laboratory findings positive for STIs or forensic evidence indicating the presence of sperm or seminal products in the prepubertal child are usually indicative of sexual abuse.[34]

How a child discloses inappropriate activity may be problematic. In nearly all cases of sexual abuse, the perpetrator forces the child to keep the abuse secret. Coercion may be implicit, as in subtle threats that if the secret is disclosed then the child may be left alone without friends, or explicit, by direct threats to the safety of the child or family.[29] Even after disclosure, the child may be ill-prepared for the maelstrom of activity and emotions that ensue from the people involved and may be overwhelmed by the events that occur in the course of investigating the situation. Such events include the involvement of CPS and law enforcement, the need for a medical examination that may be perceived as stressful, and the potential arrest of someone known and potentially valued by the family.

Children often feel helpless when in the midst of a sexually abusive situation. The sense of helplessness arises from the child's realization that the people and environment that were supposed to protect him or her have failed. As a result, the child may lose faith that disclosure of sexual abuse would serve to make things better. Additionally, after disclosure occurs, the child may be subjected to pressure from family members and other caregivers to recant and retract the disclosure in an effort to return life to the way it was before the abuse came to light.[29] These circumstances place the child in a very difficult position and account for the observed cycle in which the child discloses abuse, recants, and then discloses again through the course of the investigation and aftermath.

Nonspecific Behavioral Complaints

Presenting symptoms that suggest the need for a sexual abuse evaluation are often nonspecific behavioral complaints that span the entire continuum of emotional and behavioral symptomatology. Symptoms vary from externally oriented symptoms, such as various forms of acting out, to include aggression and delinquent-type behaviors, to internally focused symptoms, such as appearing withdrawn, feeling depressed, and becoming suicidal. The behavioral and emotional manifestations are nonspecific in that they can also result from other stressful situations that the child may experience, such as the loss of a parent, parental divorce, or diagnosis of a serious illness. Therefore, no specific behavioral symptom automatically implies that a child has been sexually maltreated. The following behaviors are examples of nonspecific complaints:

— Extremes of activity, ranging from hyperactivity to withdrawal

— Poor peer relationships

— Regressing to behaviors from an earlier developmental stage

— Enuresis and encopresis

— Fear of adults who were formerly liked

— Poor school performance

— Sexualized play and promiscuity

— Excessive and compulsive masturbation

— Sexual aggression toward playmates or younger children

— Running away

— High-risk and delinquent behaviors

— Suicidal gestures and suicide attempts

Nonspecific Genital Complaints

Presenting symptoms of child sexual abuse may include nonspecific genital complaints. These signs and symptoms may be directly related to the genital manipulation that occurred during the abuse, or the signs and symptoms could be related to the child's increased

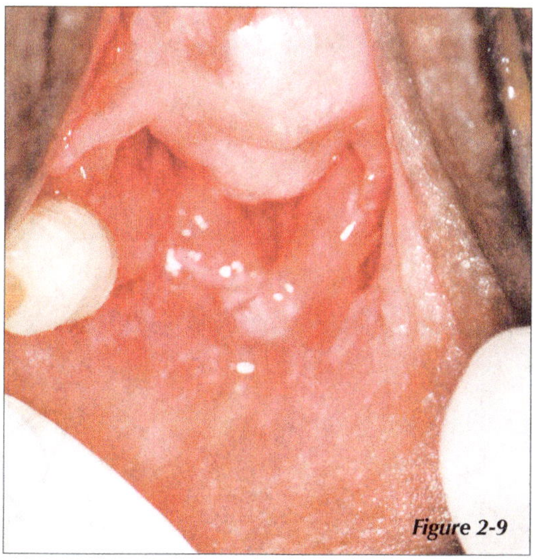

__Figure 2-9.__ Adolescent with abnormal genital examination demonstrating chronic abuse. This 17-year-old girl lived with her mother and stepfather in another state, but regularly visited her biological father and stepmother. On visits to the father, the girl complained of a chronic vaginal discharge. The stepmother took her to several clinics, all of which told the girl the discharges were normal at her age; no cultures were done. During a visit to her father the girl finally disclosed years of sexual abuse by both her stepfather and her stepbrother, which included ongoing vaginal and anal penetration. On examination, there was a minimal amount of hymenal tissue. The applicator demonstrated a hymenal defect that ran through the hymen to its base, a finding consistent with a healed tear. Her vaginal culture was positive for trichomonal and chlamydial organisms. Her serological test results were positive for syphilis and human immunodeficiency virus (HIV). She was referred to a specialty clinic for HIV-positive patients, where she was noncompliant with medications. She was reportedly having sex with her current boyfriend without barrier protection. It was unclear whether she had shared her immune status with her partner. Soon after that she turned age 18 years old and was lost to follow-up.

focus on the anogenital area as a result of the age-inappropriate sexual contact imposed on him or her by the perpetrator (**Figure 2-9**). The evaluation of genital complaints may present unique challenges for both the child and the health care provider. Health care providers commonly overlook genital and anal areas in a well-child examination, even though sound clinical practice would promote assessing the genital area at every visit.[33,34] Health care providers should familiarize themselves with normal anatomical changes that occur throughout a child's life by routinely examining the anogenital area and documenting findings from these specific areas during each health care visit.

Some nonspecific complaints can be confused with sexual abuse. For example, vulvovaginitis is the most common pediatric gynecological diagnosis seen in a primary care setting.[33] Presenting problems generally fall into 1 of 3 categories: erythema, discharge, and spotting or blood in the diaper or underwear.

Genital erythema is a common finding in the prepubertal female. Most often the redness is associated with nonsexual etiologies. The health care provider must ask the caregiver about the hygiene habits practiced by the child and family. Chemical irritation can result from harsh soaps used for bathing or laundry detergents that leave a residue in the child's underwear. Frequent bubble baths or the use of a harsh product in the water, such as dishwashing soap, can also be a culprit and cause a chemical irritation and subsequent signs and symptoms.[6] Mechanical irritation may be characterized by maceration of the skin, as in diaper dermatitis, and can be caused by tight-fitting clothing and nylon underpants. Girls who spend a great deal of time in wet bathing suits for swimming or in leotards and tights for ballet are prone to mechanical irritation.[34]

There are 2 times in a young girl's life when a vaginal discharge may be viewed as normal. The first is the newborn period, when white or blood-tinged exudates may be noted around the vaginal opening. This occurs in response to the systemic withdrawal of the mother's estrogen from the baby. The second time a vaginal discharge would be expected is approximately 6 to 12 months before the onset of menses.[35] At this time, some girls may experience a white discharge called physiological leukorrhea (**Figure 2-10**). This occurrence may continue for several years. Once the young pubertal woman's menstrual cycle is well established, she may notice a cyclical change of secretions from clear or mucoid to white.[36]

Figure 2-10. *Adolescent with normal redundant hymen. This 13-year-old, Tanner-stage-3 girl has a normal hymen reflecting increased estrogen effect. Note the white substance in the labia minora, which is normal physiological leukorrhea.*

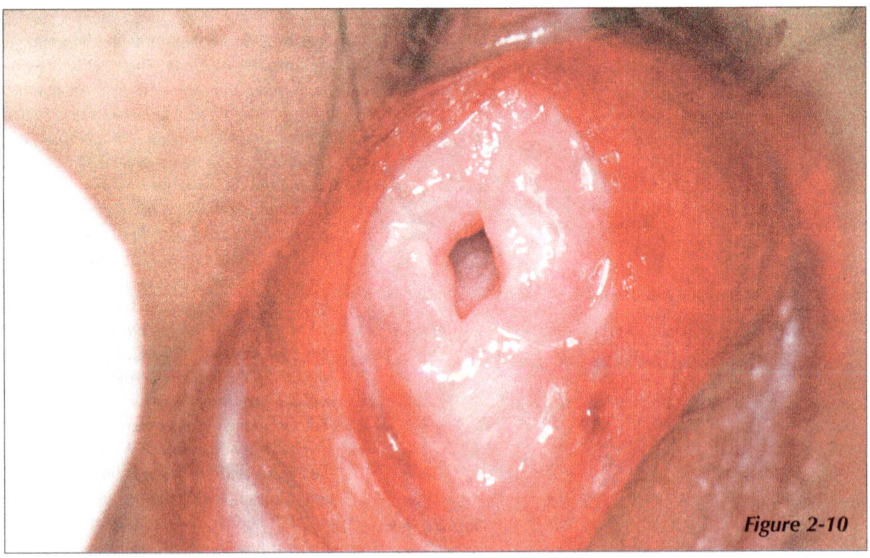

Table 2-4. Causes for Vaginal Discharge

CONSISTENCY	COLOR	CAUSE
Thin	White or yellow	Chemical irritation, *Chlamydia trachomatis*
Thin	Clear or white	Physiological
Cheesy	White	*Candida* sp
Thick, profuse	Green or yellow, purulent	*Trichomonas* sp *Neisseria gonorrhea*
Moderate	Brown, bloody	Foreign body, *Shigella* sp

There are other nonabuse-related causes of vaginal discharge that the clinician should consider, among which are poor hygiene, autoinoculation, and pinworms (**Table 2-4**). Poor hygiene, wiping from the perianal area toward the genitalia after a bowel movement, may lead to a vaginal whitish-yellow discharge. Autoinoculation of pathogenic bacteria, especially with organisms from the respiratory tract during an illness, is another possible cause of vaginal discharge. Additionally, pinworms (*Enterobius vermicularis*), with a symptom pattern composed of vaginal discharge, erythema, and anal pruritus, are another possible nonabuse-related cause of vaginal discharge.

Any vaginal discharge in a prepubertal girl, from scant to copious or clear to purulent, warrants cultures for infectious agents, including STIs. Gonorrhea notoriously presents as a purulent discharge in the prepubertal girl[36] while the discharge associated with chlamydial organisms is usually less impressive (see *Chapter 6, Sexually Transmitted Infection in the Setting of Maltreatment*).

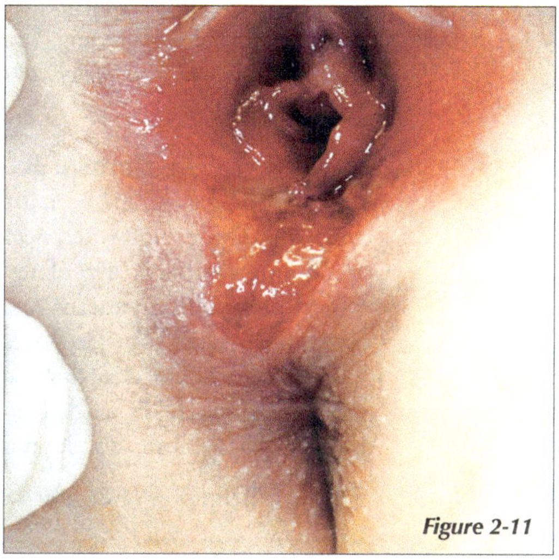

Figure 2-11

Figure 2-11. *Prepubertal child with evidence of acute sexual assault. A 2½-year-old girl had blood in her diaper. The history given by the mother and aunt was that the child had sustained a straddle type injury on the padded arm of an overstuffed chair. The laceration transected the hymen completely at the 6 o'clock position and ran through the vaginal floor, then through the perineum and into the anus. This injury required surgical intervention. It was later discovered that the uncle had vaginally penetrated her; both the aunt and the child's mother tried to protect him. He was eventually convicted, and because of the mother's actions, the child was placed into a loving foster home. The child was later relinquished by the mother and adopted by the foster mother.*

Blood in the diaper or underwear is cause for alarm in both parent and health care provider (**Figure 2-11**). The nurse's primary objective is to locate the source of the bleeding and determine whether it is vaginal, urethral, or anal. Frank vaginal bleeding in a prepubertal child calls for an expedient gynecological referral, although several nonabuse-related causes are possible. For example, urethral prolapse may present as a beefy-red mass of varying size and can cover the vaginal opening, giving the appearance of a traumatized hymen. It is often accompanied by mucosal ulceration and bleeding and is most common in African-American girls.[37] Small masses of prolapsed mucosa may resolve with simple symptomatic treatment, such as warm sitz baths and attention to proper hygiene. Large masses of prolapsed mucosa, on the other hand, may be difficult to manage. Those that do not resolve after 3 days of sitz baths should be referred to a pediatric urologist for further evaluation and management.

Occasionally, presenting symptoms of brown, blood-tinged, foul-smelling vaginal discharge may be seen in the prepubertal girl. Although this may be a sign of shigellosis, the most common etiology for these symptoms is a retained vaginal foreign body primarily caused by overzealous wiping, resulting in small pieces of toilet tissue to be deposited in the vagina. The foreign body acts as a direct irritant and also plays host to a myriad of bacteria that make the genital mucosa friable and prone to bleeding. Careful examination of the area is necessary, and lavage of the area is a mainstay of diagnosis and treatment.[36,38] One of the authors of this chapter has experience with removing pieces of carpet fiber from the vagina of a very young child who presented with genital erythema, edema, and a bloody, foul-smelling discharge. The child responded well when the fibers were gently lavaged from the vaginal vault using warm saline solution and an infant feeding tube.

Genital bruising and external lacerations may result from straddle injuries that can occur when a female child falls onto an object such as the crossbar of a bicycle or the bar of the jungle gym. The hard, fixed object forcefully sandwiches the tissues of the genitalia between the object and the pubic bone, causing bruising of the labia majora and minora and lacerations with bleeding. Straddle injuries rarely cause trauma to the vagina and hymen[39] (see *Chapter 7, Differential Diagnosis: Conditions That Mimic Child Maltreatment*).

Neglect

Neglect, defined as a pattern of caregiving that does not adequately meet the needs of the developing child, has been under-recognized in the past when compared to physical and sexual abuse.[40] However, neglect is the single most common type of maltreatment, accounting for over 78% of reported and substantiated cases of abuse.[41] There are typical presentation patterns for the various types of neglect, although the signs and symptoms related to neglect are often more subtle than those seen in physical abuse and, to some extent, sexual abuse. Neglect often presents in an insidious manner, over time, with the child's needs being inconsistently met in various dimensions, such as nutrition, health care, development, and supervision.

The legal definition of neglect varies from state to state. From a presentation perspective, however, the health care provider may identify neglect using the following 3-part categorization system[42] (**Table 2-5**):

— ***Provisional neglect:*** Caregivers are not able to give the child basic necessities such as food, clothing, shelter, and health care.

— ***Developmental neglect:*** Caregivers do not provide the child with an appropriately stimulating environment.

Table 2-5. Presentation of Neglect

Provisional	Developmental	Supervision
Failure to provide basic needs: — Shelter — Food — Clothing — Education — Immunizations — Health care	— Preventing normal growth and development by curbing normal exploration — Having unrealistic expectations of a child's ability — Keeping a child restrained	— Placing a child in a situation that may result in serious injury or death — Leaving a very young child in the care of a sibling who is too young or immature to provide adequate care

— ***Supervisional neglect:*** Caregivers do not adequately protect the child from environmental hazards, thus risking injury and placing the child at times in imminent danger and risk.

When evaluating a child for possible neglect, the health care provider must pay careful attention to all the components of the health care process, including history over time, physical examination, appropriate laboratory and diagnostic studies, and observation of parent-child interactions (see *Chapter 8, Clinical Aspects of Child Neglect*). The health care record should reflect meticulous documentation of what is heard and seen during each encounter with the parent and child as well as attempted efforts to address problems and the results of such efforts. The evaluation should be focused on the child's present needs and how the caregivers attempt to meet those basic needs. In the primary care setting, neglect often presents over time and is more clearly identified as a pattern of caregiving emerges that inconsistently meets the child's needs. Nurses have close contact with the child and caregivers and are, therefore, ideally suited to participate in the evaluation of neglectful caregiving (see *Chapter 8, Clinical Aspects of Child Neglect* and *Chapter 7, Differential Diagnosis: Conditions That Mimic Child Maltreatment*).

Provisional Neglect

Parents are expected to provide for the basic needs of their children, such as food, shelter, clothing, nurturance, schooling, and health and dental care. Caregivers may intentionally deprive a child of these things or be so distracted by their own problems that they become inattentive to the child and the child's needs. Caregivers may also be unable to understand the child's needs based on their own cognitive level or learning style or may be unable to marshal community or personal resources to meet their child's needs. Regardless of the underlying reason, the outcome is that the child's needs are not met satisfactorily.

One of the most common presentations of provisional neglect is failure to thrive (FTT). Children with FTT fall below the third to fifth percentile for height or weight respectively, or show a drop in 2 percentiles between health visits.[43] In FTT that results from neglect, there is often no organic cause that can be associated with the small stature and weight of the child. Several medical conditions can predispose a child to be at low percentiles for height and weight; however, nurses can monitor a child's growth during each encounter and plot the increments on a standardized growth curve to evaluate for positive gains in growth at regular intervals. Additionally, observing how the caregiver responds to the child's cues about hunger and the manner in which the caregiver provides the child with food can be very informative when evaluating FTT (see *Chapter 7, Differential Diagnosis: Conditions That Mimic Child Maltreatment*).

Immunizations have become a controversial topic of concern in recent years because some parents oppose vaccines and are afraid of potential complications. The parent who has researched the pros and cons of vaccines and makes a decision based on the information obtained contrasts dramatically with parents whose inattention to the child's preventive health care needs causes them to "forget" to immunize their child (see *Chapter 8, Clinical Aspects of Child Neglect*).

Developmental Neglect

Children must be exposed to a large spectrum of activities and events to progress developmentally. From the earliest days, an infant learns about his or her environment by being held, looking into an expressive face, and hearing verbalizations from caregivers. Physical examinations provide an opportunity to assess children for developmental neglect. Babies and children who have no other developmental complications or illness will interact with the examiner on some level. A child who experiences developmental neglect may demonstrate certain behaviors, including an inability to make eye contact, a resistance to being held, and an inability to relate to the nurse at all during the evaluation. In such cases, it is critical to discuss such findings with the child's caregiver. The health care provider should be aware of parents who complain that the child is hyper or into everything, especially when the child's behavior represents developmentally appropriate exploration of his or her surroundings. Such statements indicate that the parent may have unreal expectations of the child's capabilities, such as expecting an 18-month-old child to sit quietly in front of a television set for hours.

Supervisional Neglect

The ongoing development of a young child's new skills may present a challenge for the parent in terms of supervision and protection. The most conscientious parent can turn away for just a minute, and the child can get into a deadly situation. When this happens and the child presents with injuries, the bruises and burns will have plausible explanations. Although such injuries may not constitute physical abuse, they are reportable as neglect in some states. The following case study is an example of supervisional neglect:

Case Study 2-1.

An 18-month-old female was brought to a small community emergency room with a deep, fresh, circularly patterned burn to her left mandible. The hospital staff reported the injury as suspicious, and CPS escorted the family to a suspected child abuse and neglect (SCAN) team at another hospital.

The parents were in their late teens. When they arrived at the second hospital, they were tearful and visibly shaken. The child was crying as well.

It was found that the family had attended a barbecue earlier that day with some friends. Out of concern for their child's safety, the parents had placed her in her car seat and employed the safety restraints. Unfortunately, the car seat was close to a small hibachi-type barbecue grill that was on the ground and still hot from the afternoon meal. To free herself, the girl started rocking back and forth in the seat and flipped it on its side, landing the child on the barbecue grill. This incident was witnessed by a number of people at the party. The child was immediately taken to the community hospital.

Although the injuries to the child were consistent with the mechanism described by the parents and were deemed to have not been inflicted, it was suggested that the social worker visit the home of the child and instruct the parents on diligent supervision and safety issues when dealing with a young child.

Supervision problems also arise when parents allow older siblings to watch younger ones while playing or bathing. A number of tragic situations have developed when an older, but still immature, child is left to care for an infant. A child who repeatedly presents with signs of neglect in provisional, developmental, or supervisory areas should be reported to the proper authorities, as should the child aged 2 years and younger who is alleged to be accident-prone. The nurse who regularly addresses the issues of safety, supervision, and normal development may protect a child from long-term disability or death.

Conclusion

Although it may be difficult to believe that an adult is capable of injuring a small child, a nurse who cares for children must keep this possibility in mind whenever a young patient presents with an unusual injury. As with any presenting complaint, it is important to obtain a complete history and physical examination while considering the differential diagnoses for the signs and symptoms. The nurse must then decide whether or not findings are suspicious based on knowledge of abuse and experience in identifying signs and symptoms associated with child abuse and neglect. Although abuse and neglect cases are challenging and cause conflicting emotions in all parties involved, to ignore child maltreatment or to deny its existence places a vulnerable child at risk for further abuse or death. Although nurses have legal mandates to report child maltreatment, the care and safety of children should serve as an even greater motivation to become involved in the life of a child who is abused in any way.

References

1. Sgroi SM. Sexual molestation of children. the last frontier in child abuse. *Child Today*. 1975;4(3):18-21,44.

2. Giardino A, Ludwig S. Interdisciplinary approaches to child maltreatment: accessing community resources. In: Finkel M, Giardino A, eds. *Medical Evaluation of Child Sexual Abuse: A Practical Guide*. 2nd ed. Thousand Oaks, CA: Sage Publications, Inc; 2002:215-231.

3. Peddle N, Wang CT. *Current Trends in Child Abuse Prevention, Reporting, and Fatalities: The 1999 Fifty State Survey.* Chicago, IL: National Center of Child Abuse Prevention Research, Prevent Child Abuse America; 2001.

4. Ludwig S. Child abuse. In: Fleisher GR, Ludwig S, eds. *Textbook of Pediatric Emergency Medicine*. 4th ed. Philadelphia, PA: Lippincott Williams & Wilkins: 1999;1669-1704.

5. Farley R, Reece R. *Recognizing When a Child's Injury or Illness is Caused by Abuse. Portable Guides to Investigating Child Abuse.* Washington, DC: United States Department of Justice, Office of Justice Programs, Office of Juvenile Justice and Delinquency Prevention. NCJ 214125; 2006.

6. Elvik S. Child maltreatment. In: Soud T, Rogers J, eds. *Manual of Pediatric Emergency Nursing*. St. Louis, MO: Mosby; 1998:586-605.

7. Roberton DM, Barbor P, Hull D. Unusual injury? recent injury in normal children and children with suspected non-accidental injury. *Br Med J (Clin Res Ed)*. 1982;285(6352):1399-1401.

8. Schwartz A, Ricci L. How accurately can bruises be aged in abused children? literature review and synthesis. *Pediatrics*. 1996;97(2):254-256.

9. Wilson E. Estimation of the age of cutaneous contusions in child abuse. *Pediatrics*. 1977;60(5):750-752.

10. Feldman K. Evaluation of physical abuse. In: Helfer M, Kempe R, Krugman R, eds. *The Battered Child.* 5th ed. Chicago, IL: The University of Chicago Press; 1997:175-220.

11. American Academy of Pediatrics (AAP). Diagnostic imaging of child abuse. *Pediatrics*. 2000;105(6):1345-1348.

12. Launius G, Silberstein M, Luisiri A, Graviss E. Radiology of child abuse. In: Monteleone J, ed. *Child Maltreatment*. 2nd ed. St. Louis, MO: GW Medical Publishing, Inc; 1998:31-58.

13. Cooperman D, Merten D. Skeletal manifestations of child abuse. In: Reece R, Ludwig S, eds. *Child Abuse: Medical Diagnosis and Management*. 2nd ed. Phildelphia, PA: Lippincott Williams & Wilkins; 2001: 123-156.

14. Islam O, Soboleski D, Symons S, Davidson LK, Ashworth MA, Babyn P. Development and duration of radiographic signs of bone healing in children. *Am J Roentgenol.* 2000;175(1):75-78.

15. Duhaime AC, Christian CW, Rorke LB, Zimmerman RA. Nonaccidental head injury in infants: the "shaken-baby syndrome." *N Engl J Med.* 1998;338:1822-1829.

16. Berkowitz CD. Pediatric abuse: new patterns of injury. *Emerg Med Clin North Am.* 1995;13(2):321-341.

17. Duhaime A, Partington M. Overview and clinical presentation of inflicted head injury in infants. *Neurosurg Clin N Am.* 2002;13:149-154.

18. Monteleone J, Brodeur A. Identifying, interpreting, and reporting injuries. In: Monteleone J, ed. *Child Maltreatment.* 2nd ed. St. Louis, MO: GW Medical Publishing, Inc; 1998:1-29.

19. Reece R, Sege R. Childhood head injuries: accidental or inflicted? *Arch Pediatr Adolesc Med.* 2000;154(1):11-15.

20. Chadwick DL, Chin S, Salerno C, Landsverk J, Kitchen L. Deaths from falls in children: how far is fatal? *J Trauma.* 1991;31(10):1353-1355.

21. National Clearinghouse on Child Abuse and Neglect Information. *Child Fatalities Fact Sheet.* Washington, DC: United States Department of Health and Human Services; 2001.

22. National Clearinghouse on Child Abuse and Neglect Information. *What is Child Maltreatment?* Washington, DC: United States Department of Health and Human Services; 2001.

23. Administration for Children and Families, Department of Health and Human Services. Child Maltreatment 2000. Administration for Children and Families Web site. http://www.acf.hhs.gov/programs/cb/pubs/cm00/table5_6.htm. Accessed December 17, 2002.

24. Kolilis DM. Child fatality review teams. In: Monteleone JA, ed. *Child Maltreatment.* St. Louis, MO: GW Medical Publishing Inc; 1998.

25. Kairys SW. Distinguishing sudden infant death syndrome from child abuse fatalities. *Pediatrics.* 2001;107(2):437-441.

26. Kattwinkel J. Changing concepts of sudden infant death syndrome: implications for infant sleeping environment and sleep position. *Pediatrics.* 2000;105(3):650-656.

27. American Academy of Pediatrics (AAP). SIDS and other sleep-related infant deaths: expansion of recommendations for a safe infant sleeping environment. *Pediatrics.* 2011;128(5):1030-1039.

28. Sedlak AJ, Mettenburg J, Basena M, et al. *Fourth National Incidence Study of Child Abuse and Neglect (NIS-4): Report to Congress.* Washington, DC: United States Department of Health and Human Services, Administration for Children and Families; 2010.

29. Sgroi SM, Blick L, Porter F. A conceptual framework for child sexual abuse. In: Sgroi SM, ed. *Handbook of Clinical Intervention on Child Sexual Abuse.* New York, NY: DC Heath and Company; 1982:9-37.

30. Adams J, Harper K, Knudson S, Revilla J. Examination findings in legally confirmed child sexual abuse: it's normal to be normal. *Pediatrics.* 1994;94(3): 310-317.

31. Bowen K, Aldous M. Medical evaluation of sexual abuse in children without disclosed or witnessed abuse. *Arch Pediatr Adolesc Med.* 1999;153:1160-1164.

32. American Academy of Pediatrics (AAP) Committee on Child Abuse and Neglect. Guidelines for the evaluation of sexual abuse of children: subject review. *Pediatrics.* 1999;103(1):186-191.

33. Reichert S. Medical evaluation of the sexually abused child. In: Helfer M, Kempe R, Krugman R, eds. *The Battered Child.* 5th ed. Chicago, IL: The University of Chicago Press; 1997:313-328.

34. Christian C, Lavelle J, DeJong A, Loiselle J, Brenner L, Joffe M. Forensic evidence findings in prepubertal victims of sexual assault. *Pediatrics.* 2000;106(1):100-104.

35. Emans SJ, Laufer MR, Goldstein DP. *Pediatric and Adolescent Gynecology.* 4th ed. Philadelphia, PA: Lippincott-Raven; 1998.

36. Ingram D, Everett D, Flick L, et al. Vaginal gonococcal cultures in sexual abuse evaluations: evaluation of selective criteria for preteenaged girls. *Pediatrics.* 1997;99:1-4.

37. Abrams M, Lewis KH. Prolapse of the female urethra in young girls. *J Urol.* 1954;72:222-225.

38. Giardino AP, Christian CW. Vaginal foreign bodies. In: Henretig F, King C, eds. *Textbook of Pediatric Emergency Procedures and Techniques.* Baltimore, MD: Williams & Wilkins; 1997:971-974.

39. Berkowitz CD. Child sexual abuse. In: Berkowitz CD, ed. *Pediatrics: A Primary Care Approach.* Philadelphia, PA: WB Saunders; 1996:411-415

40. Dubowitz H, Giardino A, Gustavson E. Child neglect: guidance for pediatricians. *Pediatr Rev.* 2000;21(4):111-116.

41. United States Department of Health and Human Services (USDHHS), Administration for Children and Families, Administration on Children, Youth and Families, Children's Bureau. Child maltreatment 2011. Administration for Children and Families Web site. http://www.acf.hhs.gov/programs/cb/research-data-technology/statistics-research/child-maltreatment. Published December 2012. Accessed May 30, 2013.

42. Cantwell H. The neglect of child neglect. In: Helfer M, Kempe R, Krugman R, eds. *The Battered Child.* 5th ed. Chicago, IL: The University of Chicago Press; 1997:347-373.

43. Berkowitz CD. Failure to thrive. In: Berkowitz CD, ed. *Pediatrics: A Primary Care Approach.* Philadelphia, PA: WB Saunders; 1996:415-420.

Chapter 3

History and the Health Care Interview

Kathleen Brown, PhD, RN, NP

Key Points

1. The focus of an investigation varies based on the type of child abuse encountered by the victim.
2. The circumstances surrounding an injury are central to the history in physical abuse cases, whereas a child's description about inappropriate sexual activity is the focus in sexual abuse cases. In neglect cases, the pattern of care described by the caregivers is the focus of the health care interview.
3. Basic research on interviewing children coupled with theory on child development demonstrates that children can clearly remember incidents they have experienced; however, the relationship between age and memory is complex and a variety of factors influence the quality of the information. Valuable information can be obtained from child victims, but obtaining this information requires careful investigative procedure and interviewers with an awareness of children's capacities and developmental levels. The most important factors related to interviews in cases of suspected abuse and neglect are the interviewers ability to elicit information and the child's willingness and ability to express it.
4. The interviewer should minimize the size difference between himself or herself and the child by getting on the same physical level. At the beginning of the history-taking process, the health care provider should start by establishing a dialogue with the child. Introductions should be made, and a simple explanation of the role of the health care provider as interviewer should be given to the child. During the interview, it is essential that the health care provider assure the child he or she is not in any trouble.
5. During the interview process, the child should be told that it is okay to answer that they do not know or understand rather than to guess a response. It is important to ask questions that encourage the child to give more than a yes or no answer and to avoid leading questions that start with did or does. The health care provider should be aware of the child's nonverbal communication, be patient, and allow the child ample time to respond to any question asked. The health care interviewer must encourage the child to be comfortable and must remain neutral in responding to the child's responses so as not to influence answers.
6. Behaviors of and interactions with caregivers that demonstrate indifference to the child's injuries, lack of support for the child, or lack of awareness of the seriousness of the injuries raise concerns for the stability of the relationship between the adult and child.[1] Also concerning is a child who does not look to the caregiver for emotional support or a caregiver who belittles the child.

7. The history-taking effort often does not hinge on one episode but, instead, on multiple histories elicited over time during well-child and sick visits. The histories are usually linked together to form a comprehensive picture of how caregivers meet the child's physical and emotional needs.
8. The direction of the specific assessment depends on information uncovered during the generic screening and on the form of suspected neglect. In the health care setting, the provider can focus on physical neglect, medical neglect, and ***failure to thrive (FTT).***
9. In assessing for ***physical neglect,*** exploring protection from avoidable environmental hazards is essential and specific questions should include anything from poisonous or hazardous material in easy reach of children to appropriateness of clothing for environmental conditions.
10. In assessing ***medical neglect,*** compliance with or adherence to health care recommendations and whether noncompliance has resulted in potential or actual harm to the child is the focus. Questions should focus on the existence of barriers to care, such as insurance or transportation, whether past recommendations were clear and followed, and the relevance between the child's current condition and noncompliance.
11. In assessing for FTT, nutritional intake and patterns of the child's growth and development is the focus. The questions should focus on a detailed dietary history, barriers to acquiring food, perceptions of feeding and meal times, and an understanding of caloric intake and appropriate food selections.
12. There are rarely witnesses to a child's molestation, offenders infrequently admit to an offense, and there is often no medical evidence to prove that sexual abuse has occurred. The words spoken by children and adolescents about their experiences of victimization are often the most significant pieces of evidence in cases of sexual abuse. Case studies demonstrate that less than 5% of sexually abused children have physical findings that, on their own, are diagnostic of sexual abuse.
13. Pediatric health care providers are in an important position to obtain information from children by virtue of the relationship with their patients and the helping role they embody. As a result, children will reveal more information with medical professionals about sexual abuse when issues of their health may be at stake than they would share with caregivers or investigators. Additionally, and as with cases of suspected physical abuse, the statements about potential abuse made by the child to the health care provider in the course of medical diagnosis and treatment may be admissible in court and as such are dependent on the health care provider's skillful and developmentally sensitive interviews as well as the preservation of the information through accurate and thorough documentation.
14. In all circumstances, health care providers should strive to maintain an objective, nonjudgmental stance and be careful not to take a position of blame. This approach encourages an open exchange of information with the caregiver and establishes a productive working relationship that may lead to needed services for the child and family.

Introduction

Review of literature and clinical experience indicates that child abuse or neglect cannot be ruled in or out during the course of a single episodic visit to a health care provider. A history and physical examination are the necessary components of a child's visit with a health care provider when abuse or neglect is suspected (see *Chapter 2, Presentation and Overview of the Evaluation of Child Maltreatment*). Every health care provider should be aware that well-trained teams of professionals that diagnose and treat chronic victims of child abuse and neglect are available to all providers of medical and nursing care. This child abuse team is usually composed of physicians, health care providers, social workers, and members of the law enforcement community. The team closest to the child geographically is an invaluable resource for the child, his or her family, and health care providers. Every health care provider who works with children should be familiar with the location, telephone number, and Web site of the closest child abuse team. This chapter discusses the interview of a child and the child's caregiver when abuse or neglect is suspected.

Nonurgent and Urgent Cases

Determining whether or not the child is a victim of abuse of neglect may not be possible during a onetime visit to an emergency room (ER), clinic, or an office.[2] When during the course of an episodic health care visit the health care provider suspects child abuse or neglect, the first goal of the provider is to determine and ensure the health and safety of the child. Follow-up may be necessary by way of a child abuse team or individual services represented within a team. Pediatric cases that may be related to child abuse and neglect can be categorized as urgent and nonurgent. In nonurgent situations in which child abuse or neglect is suspected, but the child lacks physical complaints and evidence collection is not needed, the interview portion of the visit can be brief. Still, a physical examination should be performed and safety of the child assured. At the conclusion of the visit, a referral may be made to the child abuse team. Every effort should be made to ensure that the follow-up visit to the child abuse team is completed. At the follow-up appointment with the child abuse team, a forensic interviewer can conduct a more extensive interview than is possible in an episodic visit to an ER, clinic, or office. The most important goals in nonurgent episodic cases are to ensure the child is safe, the family is supported, and the immediate concerns are fully addressed.

If the child is in need of medical and nursing care urgently, an in-depth interview can be conducted at a later time. The child must be diagnosed, treated, and perhaps admitted to the hospital. While in hospital, the child and the child's family can be interviewed at length and in detail. If hospitalization is not required, appropriate referrals can and should be made by social worker(s).

Unfortunately the simple recipe described above is not always possible to follow. All health care providers know that cookbook strategies for complex problems are often ineffective. This chapter discusses how the provider who does not have special forensic training might conduct an interview of a child in a non-forensic setting. This chapter is valuable in cases in which disclosure from the child, caregivers, or both takes place in a health care setting. Disclosure of information related to abuse and neglect can occur while the health care provider is asking questions related to the nature of the current visit.

Caregivers seek health care due to concerns about the health and safety of a child. Medical and nursing providers are trusted professionals. As Dr. Finkel stated in 2008, individuals often share information with health care professionals that they would not otherwise share.[3] While telling the health care provider about the signs and symptoms that brought the child to the health care setting, the child, caregivers, or both may give the provider information related to abuse or neglect. Nurses and physicians are comfortable with discussing very personal and, usually, private information with families. Families believe the health care providers can be trusted with personal information. In that context, providers need guidelines for conducting an interview of children and parents in cases of possible abuse or neglect. The information derived from the health care provider's interview will be utilized for treatment of any physical injury, and it may be used by law enforcement in the form of charges against the caregivers of the affected child. The following 3 case studies are examples of the importance of the interview in urgent and nonurgent pediatric cases.

Case Study 3-1. MA, a 3-year-old female, was brought to the ER by her young mother. During the health care interview, MA's mother explained that she had just picked up MA from a visit with her father, who has visitation rights with MA every other weekend, and her father's girlfriend. The mother verbalized concern that MA was being sexually abused, a concern the mother based on a conversation she had with MA in the car on the way home from a visit with the girl's father. At first glance, the mother appeared to be in psychological distress, as she sobbed and wrung her hands. MA appeared to be tired, as she closed her eyes, leaned back, and verbally expressed a need to "go home."

Case Study 3-2. TK, a 10-year-old male in an unconscious state, was brought to the ER early in the evening by his mother. During the health care interview, the mother explained that TK fell down the stairs after awakening from his afternoon nap. When TK did not regain consciousness, she decided to bring him in to the ER for evaluation.

Case Study 3-3. BW, a 4-year-old male, was brought to the clinic by his mother for a well-child check-up required for enrollment in all-day kindergarten. During the health care interview, the mother provided a dietary history that indicated that BW was underfed. The health care provider noted that BW had been underweight since birth and that he was missing vaccinations. It was also noted that BW was wearing dirty and torn clothing, had dark circles under his eyes, and was pale in appearance. Additionally, developmental testing indicated that he was functioning at a level much lower than that of a typical 4-year-old. BW's last health care visit was at 12 months of age.

The health care interview, or history-taking process, is an important component of any medical evaluation. A child's caregiver and the communicating child provide the history through verbal or written means or sign language as necessary. When carefully documented, the history provides a record of what was described and explained during the interview and accomplishes the following goals for the overall evaluation:

- Lays the groundwork that frames the entire evaluation
- Suggests areas for detailed examination
- Assists in targeting laboratory and diagnostic testing
- Provides clues to possible diagnoses

The history component of the health care evaluation has become somewhat standardized and is traditionally composed of individual sections that contain specific information related to the presenting problem. The following sections are each explained in the context of a complete history and physical examination:

- ***History of the present illness (HPI):*** Provides an account of the problem(s) for which the child or caregiver is seeking care. It includes information to describe the reason the child is being evaluated. The HPI elaborates on the details of the problem or symptom(s), such as the timing of the complaint, the location and setting in which the problem occurred, factors that aggravated or alleviated the problem, and other relevant information such as the patient's response to the problem and the effect of the problem on the child's life.[4]
- ***Past medical history (PMH):*** Includes childhood illnesses, such as measles and chickenpox, or chronic conditions with which the child has been diagnosed and for which he or she has been treated, if necessary.
- ***Birth history:*** Includes relevant information concerning the mother's health during pregnancy; complications before or during delivery; birth order if a multiple birth; and birth weight of the child. Also included may be problems the child encountered with breathing, feeding, infections, or parent-child interactions, such as bonding or early caregiving. The birth history also includes neurological or developmental problems the child may have experienced after birth.

— ***Social history:*** Aids in determining lifestyle issues relevant to the health and well-being of the family and risk factors for health and health maintenance issues of the family.[4]

— ***Family history:*** Explores disease patterns in the family and factors that may influence health risks for particular diseases. The family usually includes the child's parents, siblings, and grandparents; aunts and uncles are of secondary importance. The amount of information gathered usually depends on the child's specific problem(s) and the relevance of family disease patterns to the particular problem(s).[5] For example, a family history of alcoholism or drug abuse may be more important to maltreatment and neglect than diabetes or heart disease.

— ***Review of symptoms (ROS):*** Generally documents relevant subjective information related to each of the major body systems. The purpose of the ROS is to ensure that other important symptoms the child may be experiencing have not been missed.[4] Each system review can be introduced with questions such as— "Has the child ever experienced any problems with hearing or ear infections?" or "Does Jane have any problems with breathing or allergies?"

Guidelines for Interviewing Children when Maltreatment is Suspected

In the setting of suspected child maltreatment, the history provided by the caregiver(s) and the communicating child is a very important part of the overall evaluation process and may supply information for legal investigation. In alleged physical abuse, the circumstances surrounding the injury are central to the history, whereas the child's description about inappropriate sexual activity is the focus in sexual abuse cases. When neglect is suspected, the pattern of care described by the caregivers is the focus of the health care interview (**Table 3-1**).

Interviewing children about abuse and neglect is not an intuitive process.[6] The victims are often the only source of investigative information; therefore, the interview must be conducted with great care. Basic research on interviewing children coupled with theory on child development demonstrate that children can clearly remember incidents they have experienced; however, the relationship between age and memory is complex with

Table 3-1. The Health Care Interview

Development of guidelines	Every department that works with children and adolescents should develop a flow chart appropriate for the diagnosis and treatment of children suspected of abuse or neglect. The flow chart should include guidelines for reporting in the department's geographical area. The flow chart should also include the location, phone number, and Web site of the closet child abuse team.
Roles and responsibilities	The role of physicians, health care providers, and social workers should be clearly defined in protocol for cases of suspected child abuse or neglect.
Referral process	Indications for referral to child abuse teams, child protective services, mental health professionals, and social workers should be clearly defined in a written protocol.
Follow-up procedures	Outpatient and inpatient follow-up in cases of suspected abuse should be clearly defined and described in protocol.

a variety of factors influencing the quality of the information. Valuable information can be obtained from child victims, but obtaining this information requires careful investigative procedure and interviewers with an awareness of children capacities and developmental levels. The most important factors related to interviews in cases of suspected abuse and neglect are the interviewers ability to elicit information and the child's willingness to and ability to express it.[7] Since 1990, highly publicized cases in the United States and United Kingdom have drawn attention to inappropriate interview techniques through which alleged victims' interviews were compromised and contaminated.[8]

The American Professional Society on the Abuse of Children (APSAC) has published recommendations for forensic interviewing of children.[9,10] Additionally, several articles and books have been written detailing effective techniques for interviewing children of suspected abuse and neglect.[11-17] Professional groups agree that the child should be interviewed as soon as possible after the alleged offense(s).

Interviewers should introduce as little information as possible while encouraging the child to provide information.[7] The use of open-ended prompts is recommended to allow the child to recall information from memory instead of forcing him or her to recognize one or more focused choices suggested by the interviewer. Responses to individual open-ended, or free-recall, prompts are 3 to 5 times more informative than responses to focused prompts.[18-20]

The National Institute of Child Health and Human Development (NICHD) investigative interview published by the National Institute of Health (NIH) is a structured interview protocol designed for forensic interviewers. The concepts presented in this protocol can be very helpful to health care providers when interviewing children in a clinical setting. The protocol is divided into 3 phases:

1. ***Introductory:*** The interviewer introduces him or herself, clarifies the child's task, and explains ground rules. Ground rules permit the child to say that he or she does not remember, know, or understand.
2. ***Rapport building:*** A relaxed and supportive environment is created and the child can be asked to describe a recent neutral event. In this phase, the child should be introduced to the concept of open-ended questions or prompts.
3. ***Interview:*** Prompts are used to identify what the health care provider wishes to talk about. If the child makes an allegation, the free-recall phase begins when the health care provider might prompt the child to share more information by saying, "Tell me everything." Alternatively, the health care provider may say, "Tell me what happened." Exhaustive free-recall prompting is recommended for health care providers in cases of possible abuse or neglect.

Interviewing Children when Physical Abuse is Suspected

In pediatric practice, the child's caregiver typically provides the health care interviewer with the details of the history. This is especially true with infants, young children, children who are extremely frightened or fearful, and children who are severely injured or unconscious. However, older children who have mastery of some form of language are able to complement the caregiver history. When interviewing a child, the health care provider must remember both the developmental level and communicative abilities of the child and the circumstances surrounding the interview.[4,21] In dealing with children, attention should be paid to both the physical environment and the tone in which the history and interview are conducted.

Preparing the Environment

In cases of physical abuse in which the child presents to the ER with needs for immediate care, the urgency of the child's medical condition determine how much attention can be paid to modifying the setting. When possible, it is best to make the physical environment as quiet and private as possible. It is advisable to interview children when they are not hungry, sleepy, or otherwise physically uncomfortable. In less urgent circumstances, measures can be taken to accommodate the child to some extent, but that may not be possible in situations where critical care and life-saving interventions are necessary.

Setting the Tone

Establishing rapport with the child before beginning to discuss the incident in question provides a good foundation for open dialogue. Various techniques can be employed to avoid both intimidation on the part of the health care provider. The interviewer should minimize the size difference between himself or herself and the child by getting on the same physical level. If possible, the interviewer should sit on a chair by the side of the bed or stretcher and position himself or herself in a comfortable spot that will allow for eye contact to be made with the child. Standing over and looking down on the child is the least favorable position for the interview. At the beginning of the history-taking process, the health care provider should establish a dialogue with the child. Introductions should be made, and a simple explanation of the role of the health care provider as interviewer should be given to the child. At this time, it is essential that the health care provider assure the child that he or she is not in any trouble. Depending on the child's developmental and maturity level, it is ideal to speak with the child without the caregiver present.

In this instance, the role of the health care provider is to ask potentially difficult questions of the child while respecting the child's feelings. The health care provider's job is to develop rapport with the child and put the child at ease while asking questions about difficult issues. The health care provider should explain one important rule: the child has the right to ask the health care provider to stop at any time during the evaluation and examination, and the health care provider will stop. If the interviewer fails to follow the rule, any trust established with the child will be forfeited.

It is important to keep questions and sentences simple when speaking with the child and to use words familiar to the child's vocabulary and understanding. For example, the interviewer should use the child's words for body parts, such as "belly" rather than stomach. Interviewers must not assume that their meaning of a word is the same as the child's or that pronunciation is consistent. Care must be taken when using pronouns like "he" or "she" and words like "there" and "that" because the child may be unable to follow the meaning of the scenario; therefore, it may be clearer to use the names or titles of the people involved rather than pronouns.

While it may be difficult, it is preferred that interviewers use open-ended, nonleading questions with the child. The interviewer should first start with general or neutral questions to allow for the narrative and then move slowly to more specific prompts to determine the information needed for a medical evaluation with appropriate evidence collection.

Typical questions that might help to establish rapport with the child include the following:

— What is your name? How old are you?

— Where do you live? Who lives with you? Who visits you?

— What is your mother's and father's name?

— What school do you go to? What grade are you in?

— What is your favorite subject? Your least favorite subject?

— What is your teacher's name? Who was your teacher last year?

— What makes you happy? Sad? Mad? Scared?

— What do you like best about the people you live with? Least?

— Why are you here today?

The child's developmental level should be assessed quickly and considered throughout the evaluation. The developmental history is used to determine when the child reached developmental milestones and if the child has any special needs. The child's developmental level is often a guideline for determining if the stated cause of the injury is consistent with the child's physical and psychological development. The child who is a slow developer may be a source of frustration to a caregiver and increase the risk for abuse.[1]

In suspected physical abuse, the history is important and conducted by asking open-ended questions about what happened. Asking the child, "Why are you here today?" may help the child open up and relate his or her story. When a child is developmentally able to interact with the health care provider, it is ideal to interview both the child and the caregiver separately and then compare the answers.[21]

Interview of the Child

With cases of suspected child physical abuse, the child has sustained some sort of injury and may be upset and in discomfort; therefore, the health care interviewer should try to ask as few direct questions as possible and instead attempt to obtain the what, who, how, where, and when of the events surrounding the time that the injury occurred using open-ended prompts. This history taker should avoid why questions, because they may imply blame to the child.[22] The child requires ongoing reassurance that the interviewer believes him or her and that he or she is not at fault for what happened.

Along with obtaining specific history about the child and the injury, the interviewer also observes the child's interactions with his or her caregiver(s). Behaviors and interactions that demonstrate indifference to the child's injuries, lack of support for the child, or lack of awareness of the seriousness of the injuries raise concerns for the stability of the relationship between adult and child.[1] Other concerning signs are a child who does not look to the caregiver for emotional support or a caregiver who belittles the child. Although these are not definitively indicative of abuse, they raise the level of suspicion.[1]

Interview of the Caregiver(s)

The interviewer should question the caregiver about the child's past medical history, birth history, social history, and family history, and conduct a complete ROS. The data collected are then explored for findings or patterns that might suggest child maltreatment. Information from all of these sections of the history is important, particularly if there were prior incidents of injury, because it is essential to determine how the caregiver(s) responded. The interviewer may ask several questions of the caregiver:

— When did the injury occur (date and time)?

— Where did the injury occur (eg, child's home, other caregiver's home, school)?

— Who had caregiving responsibility for the child at the time of the injury?

— Were you watching the child?

— Had you left the child in someone else's care?

— Did you witness the injury?

— What was happening during the time before the injury occurred?

— What was the response to the injury?

— What was the child's response?

— What was the caregiver's response?

— If someone else was watching the child, what was been his or her response? Is that person here with the child?

— What happened after the injury?

Concluding the Interview

At the end of the history-taking process, the interviewer should ask the child and caregiver if they have any questions. It is appropriate to comfort the child, but the health care provider should not make promises about what will happen to the alleged perpetrator in the case. Also, it is out of the health care provider's realm to know or discuss with the child to whom he or she will be discharged after the health care encounter, because these decisions are not under the health care provider's complete control.

Interviewing Children When Neglect Is Suspected

In cases of possible neglect, the focus of the evaluation is on the patterns of care the child receives. As such, the history-taking effort often does not hinge on one episode but, instead, on multiple histories elicited over time during well-child and sick visits. The histories are usually linked together to form a comprehensive picture of how the caregiver(s) meets the child's physical and emotional needs (see *Chapter 8, Clinical Aspects of Child Neglect*).

The history-taking process for cases where neglect is suspected is best viewed in terms of both generic and specific assessments. The generic assessment screens for patterns of care or symptoms that might suggest the need for further exploration. The specific assessment screens then builds on the findings of the generic assessment and focus on particular forms of neglect that may be suspected. A generic assessment should evaluate the following:

— Circumstances related to the child's basic needs being met; whether actual or potential harm exists

— Patterns of neglect observed in the past or present; whether child protective services (CPS) has been involved

— Possible contributing factors at the child, caregiver, family, and community levels

— Strengths and challenges for the child, family, and community

— Information regarding previous interventions and the results

— Prognostic information related to motivation to change and availability of formal and informative resources[23]

The direction of the specific assessment then depends on what was uncovered during the generic screening and the form of suspected neglect. In the health care setting, the provider can focus on physical neglect, medical neglect, and FTT. In looking at physical neglect, protection from avoidable environmental hazards is paramount and specific questions should explore the following:

— Poisonous or hazardous materials in easy reach of children

— Tobacco smoke around children with respiratory conditions

— Presence of intimate partner violence (IPV)

— Failure to use automobile restraints, smoke detectors, bicycle helmets; access to firearms

— Appropriateness of clothing for environmental conditions

— Perceptions of caregiver and child regarding clothing being worn

— Whether others have made comments about clothing or have teased the child

In considering medical neglect, the specific assessment focuses most heavily on whether there is compliance with or adherence to health care recommendations and whether noncompliance has resulted in potential or actual harm to the child. Questions should revolve around the following:

— The child's condition and the relevance of the noncompliance

— Existence of barriers to care (eg, insurance, transportation, skills)

— Whether past recommendations were clear and suggestions followed

Finally, when looking specifically at FTT, the history should focus on nutritional intake and patterns of the child's growth. Questions should address the following:

— Dietary history

— Perceptions of feeding and meal times

— Barriers to acquiring food

— Understanding of caloric intake and appropriate food selections

Interviewing Children When Sexual Abuse Is Suspected

There are rarely witnesses to a child's molestation, offenders infrequently admit to an offense, and there is often no medical evidence to prove that sexual abuse has occurred. The words spoken by children and adolescents about their experiences of victimization are often the most significant pieces of evidence in cases of sexual abuse. Case studies demonstrate that less than 5% of sexually abused children have physical findings that, on their own, are diagnostic of sexual abuse.[3] Health care providers encounter various situations that may raise suspicion about sexual abuse. Physical symptoms, behavioral difficulties, or comments from a child may warrant questioning about possible sexual victimization to determine whether maltreatment has occurred and what type of medical, mental health, or legal intervention is needed.

Health care professionals may gather information from children and adolescents about their health and well-being and whether or not they have been sexually abused. Paluski et al[24] "(examined) the relationship of behavioral symptoms, interview disclosures, and physical examination findings with changing legal outcomes in child sexual abuse." It was found that children who disclosed child sexual abuse or assault were 4 times more likely to have a positive examination finding, and cases with a positive examination finding were 2.5 times more likely to result in finding a perpetrator guilty.[24] Pediatric health care providers are in an important position to obtain information from children by virtue of the relationship with their patients and the helping role they embody. As a result, children reveal more information to medical professionals about sexual abuse when issues of their health may be at stake than they would to caregivers or investigators. Additionally, and as with cases of suspected physical abuse, the statements about potential abuse made by a child to the health care provider in the course of medical diagnosis and treatment may be admissible in court and, as such, are dependent on the health care provider's skillful and developmentally sensitive interviews as well as the preservation of the information through accurate and thorough documentation.[25]

Interview of the Caregiver(s)

An important first step in exploring concerns that a child may be the victim of sexual abuse is to gather information from the child's caregiver. It is most appropriate that this conversation take place privately, without the child present, so that the caregiver can speak freely and openly about his or her concerns and the caregiver's statements do not influence or contaminate what the child subsequently reports. Talking first with caregivers informs the health care provider about the basis for the sexual abuse concerns and provides information about the child's physical, developmental, and mental health status. This information provides the framework for conducting a productive medical history with the child. A detailed caregiver history may also guide diagnosis and treatment decisions.

The medical interview with the caregiver should include several elements pertaining to both sexual abuse concerns and the child's general physical, developmental, and mental health status. Questioning specific to sexual abuse should address the caregiver's cause for concern. When a child has made statements suggesting sexual abuse, it is helpful to know how the child's disclosure came about, whom the child has told, and the extent to which others have questioned the child. Eliciting information from the caregiver regarding his or her knowledge of the child's statements and types of sexual contact the child may have experienced may be critical to determining the child's need for medical evaluation, as well as safety. The caregiver's knowledge of the perpetrator, including name, relationship to the child, age, and high-risk behaviors or conditions specific to the perpetrator, such as drug use, sexual promiscuity, and known sexually transmitted infections (STIs), is also important. In situations involving acute assaults, such information may guide medical decisions about providing prophylaxis to the child for infections or, in non-acute cases, may help determine the need to test for STIs.

The health care provider should also explore the caregiver's knowledge of the child or adolescent's sexual history, including prior incidents of consensual and nonconsensual sexual activity, exhibition of sexualized behaviors, and exposure to sexual information and sexually explicit media. Inquiring about the child's sexual knowledge and the child's terminology for male and female private parts provides information that may be critical to understanding the history the child provides. This will also help guide the health care provider's language and ensure that he or she asks questions of the child using terms the child understands.

In regard to a child's general health status, it is helpful to discuss with the caregiver the child's past medical history, as well as current problems or symptoms. A report of past anogenital injuries, bladder or kidney infections, or episodes of unexplained vaginal or rectal bleeding may be of particular importance. A developmental history, including the age at which the child reached motor and language milestones, is also useful. Knowledge of the child's cognitive, speech, or language difficulties should also be obtained at this time.

Finally, eliciting information about patterns in the child's academic, social, behavioral, and emotional functioning may identify the existence of problems that may warrant mental health intervention and may yield data to help clarify the diagnostic picture.

Hearing caregivers talk about their children's suspected sexual abuse may evoke feelings in the health care provider, ranging from sadness to shock to anger. Particularly difficult are situations in which it appears that the caregiver may have contributed to the circumstances that enabled the abuse, such as exposing the child to a known perpetrator, ignoring signs that abuse was occurring, or failing to believe the child's disclosure of molestation. In all circumstances, health care providers should strive to maintain an objective, nonjudgmental stance and be careful not to take a position of blame. This approach encourages an open exchange of information with the caregiver and establishes a productive working relationship that may lead to needed services for the child and family.

Caregivers should be told that information obtained during the interview process may be shared with CPS when there is reasonable cause to suspect that the child has been abused. Explaining to caregivers the dictates of state child abuse reporting laws and the importance of complying with the law may help caregivers understand and accept why reporting is necessary. Health care providers should also be knowledgeable about state statutes related to the issue of consent for the medical examinations of children for whom abuse is suspected. In all jurisdictions, examinations of children for suspected abuse can be conducted without the consent of the child's parent or legal guardian. Whenever possible, it is important to inform caregivers of the nature and purpose of the medical evaluation and seek their assent and cooperation.

Discussing the Examination

Caregivers concerned that their child may have been molested often have many questions and look to health care providers for information, guidance, and support. One of their immediate concerns may be the nature of an anogenital examination. Caregivers often fear that a forensic medical evaluation will be painful and invasive and mistakenly believe the examination will determine conclusively whether or not their child has been molested. Correcting such misconceptions and sharing accurate information is important in allaying caregivers' anxieties and creating realistic expectations regarding the outcome of their child's examination.

If an anogenital exam is required at the health care visit, many caregivers request that they be present during the examination. Whereas preschool-age children often want and need their caregiver present during the examination for support and assistance, school-age children and adolescents may prefer be on their own. Allowing school-age children and adolescents to decide who is present during their examination can give the child a measure of control over the situation and demonstrates respect for their needs and preferences.

Interview of the Child

Obtaining medical history from a child or adolescent, particularly when there is concern about sexual abuse, is a challenging task that requires careful attention to both the content and the process of the interaction. In regard to the content, the health care provider's questions should focus on information relevant to medical diagnosis and treatment. It is not the place of medical professionals to conduct exhaustive investigative interviews that detail the dates, circumstances, and contexts of each reported episode of sexual abuse. Such interviews are best left to specially trained CPS workers, forensic interviewers, and law enforcement investigators.

Preparing the Environment

Whenever possible, health care providers should conduct the questioning in a room that is quiet, private, and child friendly. Providers should talk with the child or adolescent alone, without caregivers present. Maintaining a position at eye level; sustaining a calm, accepting demeanor; and respecting the child's pace for providing information will set the stage for a productive exchange of information.

Establishing rapport with a child or an adolescent is a critical precursor to eliciting sensitive information about a child's experience of maltreatment. An important first step is to establish for the child what will occur during interaction with the health care provider. Supplying this information will help allay the child's anxieties or fears. The health care provider should introduce him or herself and describe the evaluation process. Children should be told the rationale for questioning what will happen to the information provided. Specifically, children should be told in simple terms that the interview is for the purpose of medical diagnosis and treatment. For example, the health care provider may say, "I want to know about problems you've been having with your body and about things that have happened to your body, so I can check to see if you're okay or need any medicine." Once the health care provider establishes the purpose of the evaluation, he or she may ask the child or adolescent about general topics, such as school, extracurricular activities, or hobbies. Inquiring about topics that are nonthreatening and of interest to the child helps to put the child at ease, promote verbal exchange, and build a relationship between the child and interviewer. A child's conversation regarding general topics also provides the health care professional with important information about the child's cognitive, language, and speech skills, so that subsequent questioning can be adjusted accordingly.

Confidentiality

It is necessary to inform children about the limits of confidentiality during the initial phase of the interview. Children and adolescents should never be told or led to believe that the information they provide will remain private, because a disclosure of abuse necessitates reporting. Explaining to the child or adolescent that his or her statements may be shared with others to ensure their safety and protection is critical for honest, informed communication with a child.

Once adequate rapport is achieved and guidelines for clear communication are established, the health care provider may question the child or adolescent about significant past medical history and recent health problems or concerns. Such questioning should focus the child on issues related to his or her body. This is a good time for the health care provider to learn the child's terms for various body parts, including the genital and rectal areas. The health care provider should inquire about any physical problems the child or adolescent is experiencing as well as the presence of mental health difficulties. Symptoms such as sleep disturbances, behavioral regression, somatic complaints, anxiety, depression, fearfulness, irritability, aggressive conduct, and drug and alcohol use are not uncommon in children who have been abused.[26] When health care providers discuss general health concerns with a child or an adolescent, they may uncover stressful or traumatic events the child has experienced, including molestation. If not, then it is appropriate to proceed to the next phase of questioning, which is inquiring specifically about sexual abuse.

Setting the Tone

Health care providers must be sensitive to the process of gathering information about molestation from children. Many children have difficulty acknowledging or talking about their sexual victimization for fear of social and legal repercussions, shame or embarrassment, or retaliation by the perpetrator. Approaching children and adolescents in an empathic and supportive manner and being sensitive to changes in a child's affect or behavior during questioning may increase the likelihood that a child will divulge information to the health care provider.

Inquiring about Sexual Abuse

When questioning a child about sexual abuse, it is best to use open-ended questions that invite the child to provide a narrative account of his or her experiences. Such questions typically elicit the most accurate reports and are least likely to be misleading.[7] Open-ended questions will sometimes yield a disclosure from a child about abuse. Examples of questions that may be used include "Do you know why you're here today?" and "What happened?"

If a child indicates that he or she has recently been involved in inappropriate sexual contact, there are pieces of information that the health care provider should try to obtain for the purpose of medical diagnosis and treatment, namely who perpetrated the act, what occurred, and when the abuse transpired. Identifying who molested the child is critical for the protection of the child, helps guide decisions about the type of examination that may be needed, and determines whether testing for STIs is indicated. For example, a 4-year-old girl who experienced penile-genital contact with an adult male may have different medical needs than a 4-year-old girl experiencing the same act by a 9-year-old boy. After a child has indicated that a particular person molested him or her, it is important to remember to ask the child if anyone else has engaged him or her in sexual activity, because some children and adolescents will have been molested by more than one individual and some will have engaged in consensual sexual contact.

Questions asked to determine what happened to the child should focus on the types and extent of sexual contact the child experienced. Specific information regarding the parts of the perpetrator's body that made contact with the child's body is essential for guiding decisions regarding examination of the child and interpretation of medical findings. Questions about whether the child experienced pain or bleeding after sexual contact are important as well.

It is important to establish when the incident(s) of sexual abuse occurred, as reported by the child. Of particular relevance is the time and date of the child's most recent sexual contact. A child or adolescent who has been sexually assaulted within the previous 24 to 72 hours may require forensic evidence collection and may be eligible to receive prophylaxis for pregnancy and disease (see *Chapter 6, Sexually Transmitted Infection in the Setting of Maltreatment*). The answers collected as to the who, what, and when of the events determine if, what, and from where evidence should be collected.

Concluding the Interview

The final step in the interview process is to provide the child with some closure. After responding to multiple questions and perhaps revealing sensitive and emotion-laden information, the child may need an opportunity to express his or her feelings and seek information from the health care provider. The experience of sexual abuse evokes many questions and issues for children and adolescents, including concerns about the intactness and health of their bodies, fear of human immunodeficiency virus (HIV) and other diseases, uncertainty about virginity, and confusion about sexual orientation. An open and honest discussion of these issues with a health care provider can often be enlightening and reassuring to children.

Development Considerations in Interviewing Children When Maltreatment Is Suspected

It is essential that health care providers tailor their questioning to meet the developmental needs of the child they are interviewing. Studies suggest that the quality of a child's report depends on the competence of the interviewer to ask questions using language the child can comprehend about concepts they can understand. Following are some guidelines for questioning children of different ages about their experiences of abuse.

Preschool-Age Children

Obtaining reliable and understandable information from children aged 3 through 5 years is a formidable task. Although many preschoolers can provide accurate accounts of personally significant events, they may not be able to give an organized or consistent description of incidents of maltreatment and may have a limited capacity to describe events in detail.[27] Preschool-age children exhibit thinking that is egocentric and concrete. They focus on their own experiences and have difficulty understanding the viewpoints of others. Additionally, their language is simple and often very literal.

Most children aged 3 years and older can label body parts, although their terms for the genital and rectal areas may be idiosyncratic, and they may be unfamiliar with anatomically correct labels. A useful strategy for questioning preschoolers about sexual abuse is to have them label body parts using a picture of a person or their own body. This strategy establishes the child's knowledge of and terms for various body parts, including private areas. The interviewer can then ask about contact to the body using anatomical terms the child understands. Many interviewers use anatomical drawings to help identify a child's labels for private parts and provide the child with another means of indicating what type of sexual contact they experienced by allowing the child to point to areas on the image. Drawings, whether formal or informal, may be useful aides in communicating with young children.

Between ages 3 and 5 years, most children can respond accurately to questions regarding the who, what, and when of a situation. Therefore, questions about who touched their bodies, where on their bodies they were touched, and what the perpetrator did to their bodies are appropriate and generally within the developmental capacity of preschoolers. Preschoolers cannot reliably answer questions about when an event occurred or how many incidences of abuse occurred, because they have not yet mastered the concepts of time and enumeration.[28] As a result, providing details about when an abusive incident occurred, the timing of the most recent abuse or assault, or the number of abusive episodes is beyond the capabilities of children aged 6 years and younger.

Although preschoolers are able to recall salient experiences accurately, they tend to recall only that information about which they are asked. Consequently, open-ended questions may yield little information. Concomitantly, preschoolers may be particularly susceptible to the effects of leading and suggestive questions, which can contaminate children's reports and undermine their credibility.

Keeping language simple and questions contained to one idea at a time is key to eliciting information from preschoolers. For example, the health care provider should avoid asking the preschool child, "What did Johnny do after you left his house and drove to the farm?" Instead, he or she should ask, "Where did you go with Johnny? What did you do there?" Preschoolers may be reluctant to admit when they do not understand a question or do not know an answer. The health care provider may help the preschooler to overcome this reluctance by asking the child for clarification and giving the child permission to say that they do not know when unsure of an answer. Given the inherent difficulties and pitfalls of obtaining information from young children, questioning of preschoolers, if possible, should be kept to a minimum.

School-Age Children

Between ages 6 and 12 years, children's thinking becomes more logical and their vocabulary expands rapidly. Consequently, school-age children may seem to understand adult questions and provide responses that seem to reflect an adult-like understanding of concepts. However, an adult-like use of language does not necessarily reflect adult-like linguistic or cognitive capabilities.[29] Children may use words before they really understand them; therefore, it is important for health care providers to clarify statements made by school-age children. For example, the health care provider may restate what the child said using different terms in order to remove any doubt as to the meaning of the information conveyed by the child.

Compared with preschoolers, school-age children have a better-developed sense of time. They can use words to describe clock and calendar time and duration in seemingly appropriate ways. Still, an adult-like concept of time may not be fully developed until they reach their mid-teens.[30] When questioning a school-age child about when an event occurred, it may be more useful to help the child place the event in relation to a concrete event in the child's life, such as the school year, summer vacation, Christmas, daytime, or nighttime, and establish a time frame based on whether the abuse occurred before, during, or after the concrete event.

School-age children are able to respond to open-ended questions and to provide a narrative account of their experience. Because school-age children can think about the consequences of revealing a history of abuse, they may be more reluctant than preschool-age children to share such information. It is helpful, therefore, to attend to a child's nonverbal signals during questioning, particularly when inquiring about abuse. A child's change in behavior, voice level, or emotional expression or attempts to avoid or divert the interviewer when questions about abuse are broached may signal a problem, even if the child does not admit to victimization.

Adolescents

Developmentally, adolescents have adult-like cognitive and language skills and can accurately relate details of abusive experiences, including when contact occurred and the circumstances surrounding any type of abuse. Still, it is important to assess whether the adolescent understands terms being used by the provider and vice versa. The health care provider should clarify the use of terms and definitions with the adolescent since, at times, terms have a different meaning for the adolescent than they do for the provider. For example, "hooking up" can mean something very different to the health care provider than it does to an adolescent.

Although they are capable of providing a narrative account of their victimization, they may be reluctant to do so out of shame, concern for the perpetrator, fear or mistrust of the legal system, concern about social embarrassment, or anxiety regarding parental response. Adolescents may be particularly concerned with issues of privacy and confidentiality and want to know what the health care provider will do with the information obtained during the medical encounter.

The general medical history obtained from the adolescent should include menstrual history and use of contraception and consensual sexual activity. Genital complaints, which may be symptomatic of an STI, should be addressed in a detailed ROS. A report of drug or alcohol abuse, depression, anxiety, eating disorders, self-injury, poor academic achievement, or problematic peer relationships may indicate a need for mental health services.

When questioning an adolescent about suspected abuse, the health care provider should determine:

— Identity of the perpetrator

— All forms of contact that occurred

— Date of most recent incident

— Regularity of abuse (eg, onetime or repeated)

— Associated pain or bleeding

Documentation in Cases of Suspected Maltreatment

Although careful documentation of the findings of a physical examination is essential for quality patient care in cases of suspected maltreatment, documentation of observations and statements pertaining to alleged child abuse has forensic significance as well. Details regarding the questioning and examination of the child may provide critical information to CPS, law enforcement, and legal systems and is consequently scrutinized by all involved agencies. A timely, accurate, and comprehensive written recording of conversations conducted with the child and his or her caregiver(s) about abuse is essential to not only preserve evidence, but also protect health care providers who may be called on to testify in court about his or her evaluations.

Most states allow medical professionals who have gathered information in the course of diagnosing and treating a child to testify in court as to what the child reported to him or her. This exception to the hearsay rule, commonly referred to as the medical diagnosis and treatment exception, means that statements from the child about abuse, when made in the course of diagnosis and treatment, may be admissible in court; however, statements made to other individuals are considered hearsay and are typically not admissible.

The child's medical record should include several elements to increase the likelihood that the information obtained will meet the medical diagnosis and treatment exception to the hearsay rule. Health care providers should document, whenever possible, that the child was informed that the purpose of questioning was for medical diagnosis and treatment and that the child was told of the importance of providing accurate information. In addition, the information elicited and documented from the medical history of the child should be pertinent to effective diagnosis and treatment.

Health care professionals should take particular care in recording information obtained during their inquiry about abuse. Documentation should include the question or context that led to a particular response from the child, and statements by the child about abuse should be recorded verbatim.[31] It is important, as well, to record the child's affect and demeanor during questioning, because they may be useful in assessing the credibility of the child's history and the child's response to the abuse. Dubowitz and Bross[31] summarize information that should be included when documenting interviews with children about abuse. When written in a thorough, objective, legible manner and when using terms that are easily understood by nonmedical professionals, the medical record should be useful to investigators, caseworkers, and attorneys. This provides an accurate record of the child's statements and how they were obtained. A detailed record of such conversations will also be useful should the health care provider be called to testify several months or years from the time the information was gathered, when memory about the details of such conversations has long since faded. Careful documentation, therefore, has important implications for both the disposition of the child and the credibility and integrity of the health care provider.

Conclusion

Health care providers are often the gatekeepers to specialized medical, social, and mental health interventions for children and families. Obtaining a health history and an interview of a child when there are concerns about abuse may be the critical first step in stopping the child's victimization and connecting the child and his or her caregivers with the services needed to effectively deal with their situation. The health care provider is an important link in the safety net created to identify and treat victims of abuse. It is the responsibility of health care providers to make sure this link is a strong one.

References

1. Giardino A, Christian C, Giardino E. Evaluation of abuse and neglect. In: Giardino A, Christian C, Giardino E, eds. *A Practical Guide to the Evaluation of Child Physical Abuse and Neglect*. Thousand Oaks, CA: Sage Publications, Inc; 1997:23-59.
2. Faller KC, Cordisco-Steele L, Nelson-Gardell D. Allegations of sexual abuse of a child: what to do when a single forensic interview isn't enough. *J Child Sex Abuse*. 2010;19(5):572-589.
3. Finkle M. "I can tell you because you're a doctor." *Pediatrics*. 2008;122(2):440-441.
4. Bickley L, Szilagyi P. *Bates' Guide to Physical Examination & History Taking*. 8th ed. Philadelphia, PA: JB Lippincott Co; 2003.
5. Coulehan JL, Block MR. *The Medical Interview: Mastering Skills for Clinical Practice*. 4th ed. Philadelphia, PA: FA Davis Co; 2001.
6. Fivush R. Developmental perspectives on autobiographical recall. In: Goodman G, Bottoms B, eds. *Child Victims, Child Witnesses: Understanding and Improving Testimony*. New York, NY: Guilford Press; 1993:1-24.
7. Lamb, ME, Hershkowitz I, Orbach Y, Esplin, PW. *Tell Me What Happened: Structured Investigative Interviews of Child Victims and Witnesses*. Hoboken, NJ: Wiley; 2008.
8. Bruck M, Ceci S. The suggestibility of children's memory. *Annu Rev Psychol*. 1999;50:419-439.
9. American Society on the Abuse of Children. *Guidelines for Pyschosocial Evaluation of Suspected Sexual Abuse*. Elmhurst, IL: American Professional Society on the Abuse of Children; 1990.
10. American Society on the Abuse of Children. *Practice Guidelines: Psychosocial Evaluation of Suspected Sexual Abuse in Children*. Chicago, IL: American Professional Society on the Abuse of Children; 1997.
11. Jones DPH. Oregon interviewing guidelines. http://www.doj.state.or.us/victims/pdf/oregon_interviewing_guidelines.pdf. Updated 2012. Accessed January 2014, 2014.
12. Lamb ME. The investigation of child sexual abuse: an interdisciplinary consensus statement. *Child Abuse Negl*. 1994;18(12):1021-1028.
13. Lamb ME, Sternberg KJ, Esplin PW. Effects of age and delay on the amount of information provided by alleged sex abuse victims in investigative interviews. *Child Dev*. 2000;71(6):1586-1596.
14. Lamb ME, Orbach Y, Hershkowitz I, Esplin PW, Horowtiz D. A structured forensic interview protocol improves the quality and informativeness of investigative interviews with children: a review of research using the NICHD investigative interview protocol. *Child Abuse Negl*. 2007;31(11-12):1201-1231.

15. Poole DA, Lamb ME. *Investigative Interviews of Children: A Guide for Helping Professionals*. Washington, DC: American Psychological Association; 1999.

16. Sattler JM. *Clinical and Forensic Interviewing of Children and Families: Guidelines for the Mental Health, Education, Pediatric and Child Maltreatment Fields*. La Mesa, CA: Jerome M Sattler; 2008.

17. Warren AR, McGough LS. Research on children's suggestibility: implications for the investigative interview. *Criminal Justice Behav*. 1996;23(2):269-303.

18. Lamb ME, Hershkowitz I, Sternberg KJ, Boat B, Everson MD. Investigative interviews of alleged sexual abuse victims with and without anatomical dolls. *Child Abuse Negl*. 1996;20(12):1251-1259.

19. Sternberg KJ, Lamb ME, Orbach Y, Esplin PW, Mitchell S. Use of a structured investigative protocol enhances young children's responses to free recall prompts in the course of forensic interviews. *J Appl Psychol*. 2001;86(5):997-1005.

20. Dunne MP, Zolotar AJ, Runyan DK. ISPCAN child abuse screening tool retrospective version. *Child Abuse Negl*. 2009;33(11):815-825.

21. Ludwig S. Child abuse. In: Fleisher GR, Ludwig S, Henretig FM, Ruddy RM, Silverman BK, eds. *Textbook of Pediatric Emergency Medicine*. 4th ed. Philadelphia, PA: Lippincott Williams & Wilkins; 2000:1669-1704.

22. Feiring C, Cleland C. Childhood sexual abuse and abuse-specific attributions of blame over six years following discovery. *Child Abuse Negl*. 2007;31(11-12):1169-1186.

23. Dubowitz H, Giardino A, Gustavson E. Child neglect: guidance for pediatricians. *Pediatr Rev*. 2000;21(4):111-116.

24. Palusci VJ, Cox EO, Cyrus TA, Heartwell SW, Vandervort FE, Pott ES. Medical assessment and legal outcome in child sexual abuse. *Arch Pediatr Adolesc Med*. 1999;153(4):388-392.

25. American Academy of Pediatrics Committee on Child Abuse and Neglect. Guidelines for the evaluation of sexual abuse of children: subject review. *Pediatrics*. 1999;103(1):186-199.

26. Kendall-Tackett KA, Williams LM, Finkelhor D. Impact of sexual abuse on children: a review and synthesis of recent empirical studies. *Psychol Bull*. 1993;113(1):164-180.

27. Sattler JM. *Clinical and Forensic Interviewing of Children and Families*. San Diego, CA: Jerome M. Sattler, Publisher, Inc; 1998.

28. Hewitt S. *Assessing Allegations of Sexual Abuse in Preschool Children*. Thousand Oaks, CA: Sage Publications, Inc; 1999.

29. Saywitz K, Compero L. Interviewing child witnesses: a developmental perspective. *Child Abuse Negl*. 1998;22(8):825-843.

30. Graffam Walker A. *Handbook on Questioning Children: A Linguistic Perspective*. Chicago, IL: American Bar Association Committee; 1994.

31. Dubowitz H, Bross DC. The pediatrician's documentation of child maltreatment. *Am J Dis Child*. 1992;146(5):596-599.

Chapter 4

The Physical Examination in the Evaluation of Suspected Child Maltreatment: Physical Abuse and Sexual Abuse Examinations

Eileen R. Giardino, PhD, MSN, FNP, ANP
Tomika S. Harris, DNP, RN, CPNP
Angelo P. Giardino, MD, PhD

Key Points

1. An examination that reveals no abnormal physical findings is common in children who have been sexually abused and does not rule out the possibility of sexual abuse.[1]
2. Routine pediatric visits should include an assessment of the genitourinary system in the context of the Tanner stages.
3. A thorough examination of the genital and anal areas is necessary in a sexual abuse evaluation.
4. Health care providers cannot provide an estimated age range for bruising because the exact age can rarely be determined.
5. Every child suspected of being the victim of physical abuse should be evaluated for bone fractures because the child may have an occult fracture without any specific sign and symptoms.
6. Inflicted head injury may result from a variety of mechanisms, including the rotational forces associated with shaking and the translational forces associated with impact injuries resulting from being slapped, hit, or punched.
7. Intentional poisoning, seen more commonly in children aged 2 years and younger, may be used as a type of discipline or punishment and is a form of child physical abuse.
8. One of the best predictors of discovering abnormal findings in the female genital examination is the time frame between the actual assault and the examination. The closer the examination is to the actual assault, the better the possibility of finding physical evidence of the assault.
9. A health care provider who is not familiar with the abuse evaluation should refer the victim of child abuse to an expert health care provider. Ideally, a child should undergo only one physical examination because the examination experience can be emotionally upsetting.

10. The appearance of the normal hymen in prepubertal and postpubertal children varies. The range of normal variants is wide, and examination techniques and positioning of the child can affect what the health care provider sees.

Introduction

The health care provider plays an important role in the evaluation of the child suspected of being the victim of maltreatment. Advanced practice nurses (APNs) or sexual assault nurse examiners (SANEs) with enhanced pediatric training complete all aspects of the medical evaluation, including gathering the comprehensive history, conducting the physical examination, and collecting samples for appropriate laboratory tests. The health care provider also coordinates diagnostic studies and documents observations of child and caregiver interactions.

The 3 major categories of child maltreatment are physical abuse, sexual abuse, and neglect, the latter of which is the most prevalent form of child maltreatment. Each maltreatment category has a specific evaluation focus and presents unique challenges to the health care provider. The evaluation of a child who may have been physically abused focuses on determining if physical injuries are consistent with the inflicted injuries of child physical abuse. The physical examination of a suspected victim of child sexual abuse focuses on physical and forensic findings that are consistent with inappropriate sexual contact in light of the fact that sexual abuse may not leave any physical evidence at all. The evaluation of the suspected child victim of neglect can be challenging. Typical signs of neglect with very specific findings may be obvious to the health care provider, while other signs may appear in a more insidious manner.

This chapter focuses on techniques for conducting a comprehensive physical examination in cases of suspected physical and sexual abuse. The chapter emphasizes ways to approach the child that are sensitive to the developmental needs of the child and caregivers. Because the physical examination may be stressful for the child and caregivers, it is important that the health care provider exhibit patience, kindness, and support during the examination process. The issues surrounding the comprehensive evaluation and physical examination for suspected neglect are discussed in greater detail in *Chapter 8, Clinical Aspects of Child Neglect.*

Evaluation Versus Investigation

The evaluation and investigation of suspected child maltreatment is a multidisciplinary process[2] that includes a health care evaluation as well as a broader assessment of the child's home environment and the people and situations to which the child is exposed. A home and environment evaluation is initiated as a result of a report to child protective services (CPS) personnel or law enforcement officers by health care providers who suspect maltreatment after having completed an evaluation. Mandated reporters and other individuals might also trigger an investigation that may in turn lead to the request for a health care evaluation.

Evaluation

The health care provider who conducts the physical examination portion of the investigation is part of the team that evaluates the suspected victim of physical or sexual child maltreatment. The primary role of the health care provider is to evaluate the child's health care needs. The health care evaluation is well defined and includes a history, a physical examination, laboratory assessments, and observations of both child-caregiver interactions and individual child and caregiver behaviors. The information gathered should lead to a differential diagnosis and diagnostic impression of the possibility that the findings indicate abuse. The health care evaluation is oriented first toward assessing the child's health status and then toward intervening to restore health to the child and family.

The health care provider who evaluates child maltreatment should have specialized training in the medical evaluation of physical and sexual abuse. One aspect of the health care evaluation is to help the child and family understand the goals of the evaluation. The clinician is called upon to answer difficult questions asked during the evaluation and provide an age-appropriate approach to ease the child's fears during the potentially uncomfortable or embarrassing physical examination and specimen collection process. The health care provider cooperates with investigators and reports findings and information collected during the medical evaluation. The child and family should see the health care provider as someone working with them to identify medical conditions, provide treatment modalities, and address health and wellness issues stemming from the abuse.

Investigation

There is a distinction between the health care evaluation and the investigation completed by CPS or law enforcement.[3] Investigators are individuals from disciplines and agencies, such as law enforcement and CPS personnel, mandated by laws and regulations to explore allegations of suspected maltreatment. Law enforcement officers determine whether or not a crime has been committed and begin appropriate legal action toward holding the abuser responsible for his or her actions. CPS agencies and CPS workers, often social workers, operate hand-in-hand with law enforcement agencies and police officers to protect children. CPS focuses on the functioning of the child's family and the family's ability to protect the child. CPS agencies provide necessary social support services to families in need and may ultimately remove the child from an environment determined to be unsafe.

The health care evaluation generates information concerning physical findings that support the diagnosis of child maltreatment. In addition, the health care provider collects and preserves forensic evidence that is key to the investigation of alleged child abuse. At this point in the evaluation process, the health care provider participates with law enforcement, social services, CPS, and the courts to obtain evidence for the forensic investigation team. The health care provider interacts with other members of the investigation team to share medical evaluation information with other team members, such as prosecutors. The prosecutor seeks evidence to support the prosecution of an alleged perpetrator and is responsible for pursuing court-related processes that hold offenders accountable for illegal activities. Prosecutors as well as victim service agencies provide support to the child and family. A victim service agency is a general rating to an organization that provides service from trained forensic interviewers and counselors. Various disciplines come together through the victim service agency to make the whole experience better for the child, help the child prepare for testifying in court, and provide support persons to accompany the child to court.

The Physical Examination of the Suspected Victim of Child Maltreatment

Accurate physical examination findings of a suspected victim of child maltreatment are important to the health care evaluation and related investigation. The health care provider must be comfortable working with team members of other disciplines whose perspectives about the information uncovered during physical examination may differ from their own. The medical evaluation of child maltreatment focuses on evaluating the child's health, supporting and reassuring the child and caregivers, and, ultimately, restoring the health of the child. The forensic aspect of the medical evaluation is focused on preserving and documenting evidence that will withstand scrutiny in court. Each aspect requires training and experience to understand how team members work together to ensure that both the evaluation and investigation proceed in a way that best serves the overall goals of each team member. The health care provider must know which team member to consult for assistance with medical or forensic concerns related to the evaluation before, during, and after the physical examination. The health care team may provide consultations regarding medical and nursing concerns, while those with more forensic expertise may address concerns regarding the preservation of photographs and evidence.

Clinical findings that suggest a diagnosis of sexual abuse can have far-reaching consequences for those suspected or accused of the crime, especially if incorrect findings and conclusions are reached.[4] Also, investigators must understand that a normal examination, or one without abnormal physical findings, is common in children who have been sexually abused and does not rule out the possibility of sexual abuse.[1]

Comprehensive Medical Examination for Suspected Child Abuse

The goal of the comprehensive medical examination where maltreatment is suspected is to assess for findings that support abuse while providing reassurance to the child and family.[5] Examining a child who has been physically or sexually abused is both a science and an art. The science involves the theory and details related to what to examine and what the findings may signify. The art of examination is learned through experience and involves the knowledge of how to work with a child to gain cooperation for an exam that is possibly uncomfortable and threatening to that child.

The health care evaluation of a suspected victim of child maltreatment necessarily includes a complete physical examination during which each body system and structure is examined in a systematic manner. In cases of sexual abuse, special attention is given to areas of suspected injury, such as the anogenital area. It is recommended that routine pediatric visits in primary care settings include a Tanner assessment of the genitourinary system to determine development of secondary sexual characteristics. However, anogenital assessment is not always completed[6]; therefore, primary care providers may not be skilled in identifying the specific structures that are comprised in the external genital examination of prepubertal children.[7-10] Skill in the accurate evaluation of the anogenital structures to determine normal versus abnormal is particularly important for the evaluation of the child suspected of sexual abuse.[6]

The physical examination of suspected victims of child maltreatment is an essential element of the comprehensive health care evaluation and an important component of the overall maltreatment investigation. **Table 4-1** shows what the health care provider accomplishes through the health care evaluation. Physical examination findings are combined with findings from other components of the health care evaluation, such as the history, laboratory and diagnostic data, and observations of caregiver and child interactions, to determine whether the child was abused. The investigative team uses the history, examination findings, and diagnostic impression to guide other aspects of the maltreatment investigation.

The physical examination of a child suspected of having been sexually abused is a unique situation that requires specific techniques for examining the child and collecting forensic evidence. Because the examination has forensic implications, clinicians who perform these examinations must have additional training in examining the genitalia and collecting evidence.

Table 4-1. Clinical Accomplishments of the Health Care Evaluation

Considerations for the Health Care Provider	— Identify physical injuries or conditions that require treatment. — Document physical findings at the time of the examination using notes, drawings, and photographs. — Obtain necessary laboratory specimens and diagnostic studies. — Collect and preserve forensic evidence. — Provide appropriate treatments directed at restoring health when findings or conditions are present. — Reassure child and family of ways to attain or restore health and well-being.

General Issues

Evaluating Stress and Distress

The health care setting in general can be a source of stress for children who may fear the thought of painful procedures and separation from their family.[11] A child with physical injuries may be distressed about having painful body parts physically manipulated and examined. In cases of sexual abuse, the child may experience stress from the thought of having a genital examination.[12-14]

Health care providers have learned a great deal about how to help children cope with the stress they may feel when visiting the health care setting. Studies determining the degree of a child's fear and feelings of distress toward medical procedures have offered ways to enhance the child's coping strategies.[5] Efforts to decrease the child's anxiety include establishing familiarity with the setting and communicating in a child-friendly way about what to expect of the process. **Table 4-2** shows stressors associated with a physical examination for suspected child maltreatment while **Table 4-3** offers coping strategies for the child.

Table 4-2. Clinical Stressors Related to the Child's Physical Examination

Health Care Provider Considerations	— Age and developmental level — Previous interactions with the health care system — Circumstances of the alleged maltreatment — Potential concern about future safety — Perceived potential for further inflicted injury

General Appearance

The first step in the physical examination in cases of suspected physical or sexual abuse is to assess the overall appearance of the child. The health care provider should look for signs indicative of caregiving practices that meet or fail to meet the child's basic needs. The overall appearance of the child may be reflective of the general treatment of the child. Caregiving that does not adequately deal with the child's physical condition

Table 4-3. Strategies to Help the Child Cope During the Health Care Evaluation

— Explain the examination to the child before performing the examination.

— Allow a nonabusing caregiver to be present during the examination.

— Allow time to relieve the child's anxiety.[15]

— Take the history from the adult who is accompanying the child.

— Provide the child distance from the process by encouraging play in another part of the room.

— Offer child choices during the physical examination (eg, what robe to wear, what position to use, what ear to examine first, what instrument to use first).

— Use distraction techniques during the examination with conversation about topics of interest.

— Use words that are less threatening to the child; for example, a little bump or scratch versus tears or scarring.

and health needs may indicate neglect. Often, the legal community defines insufficient caregiving practices that result in harm as neglect; however, health care professionals often expand the definition of neglect to include those instances in which the caregiving practices allow for a potential for harm. Based on this expanded definition, health care professionals should make every effort to make appropriate referrals to meet the needs of the child (see *Chapter 14, Legal Issues*). **Table 4-4** shows parameters to consider when evaluating the general appearance of a child suspected of physical or sexual abuse.

Specific Examination Issues Related to Cases of Suspected Physical Abuse

Accidental Versus Inflicted Injury

The health care provider must determine whether the injuries seen on physical examination appear to be accidental or inflicted. Law enforcement officials can help differentiate between accidental and inflicted injury by retrieving, when possible, the exact object used to inflict injury. The health care provider may use the following general guidelines to differentiate between accidental and inflicted injuries.[16]

— Injuries to the prominent areas of the child's body, such as the forehead and shins, are consistent with accidental injuries.

— Injuries to padded areas (eg, buttocks) and well-protected areas such as neck, trunk, and genitalia are highly suspicious of abuse.

— Inconsistencies between physical findings and the history raise suspicion for abuse.

When formulating a diagnostic impression, the health care provider should consider the following:

— Is the injury location consistent with the given history of events?

— Are injuries consistent or inconsistent with the developmental level of the child?

— Is it developmentally possible for the child to have performed the task described and become injured as a result?

Additionally, injury characteristics that support suspicion for an inflicted injury and raise concern for physical abuse include an examination or review of the medical record that suggests repetitive or cumulative injuries over time; the appearance of an injury pattern

Table 4-4. Evaluation of the Child's Appearance in Cases of Suspected Maltreatment

— Height and weight	— Scars
— Age-appropriate growth parameters	— Insect bites
— Evidence of nutritional deficiencies (eg, subcutaneous fat deposits)	— Physical evidence of neglect
— Evidence of diaper rash; if present, severity	— Nourishment
— Signs of skin infection	— Overall cleanliness of child
	— Appropriate dress for weather and climate

that reflects cigarette burns, belt marks, or bite marks; an examination that reveals a severe central nervous system (CNS) injury that seems inconsistent with the history provided; and the presence of defensive injuries on the arms. The following situations should raise suspicion about physical abuse and prompt a complete health care evaluation:

— No explanation or a vague explanation is given for the injury, especially a significant injury.

— Suspicious history given for injury changes over time.

— Injury observed is not congruent with history given.

— Injury observed is incompatible with the child's developmental stage and abilities.[17]

— Caregivers demonstrate untimely delay in seeking medical attention for an injury that a reasonable caregiver would have brought to the attention of a health care provider.

Skin Injuries

The skin is the largest organ in the body and the one most commonly injured in cases of physical abuse.[18] The physical examination of suspected victims of child abuse involves a careful search for findings suggestive of inflicted injury to the skin. The health care provider must inspect the child's skin from head to toe, looking for injuries requiring treatment and injuries supportive of the diagnosis of inflicted injury.

Bruises

A bruise injury generally results from blunt force trauma to the skin that disrupts capillaries and causes leaking and the collection of blood beneath the skin.[19] Relatively deep bruises may not appear for hours or days. Bruise injuries can develop on body areas where a child was struck or in areas where the child was held down or restrained (**Figures 4-1** to **4-6**).

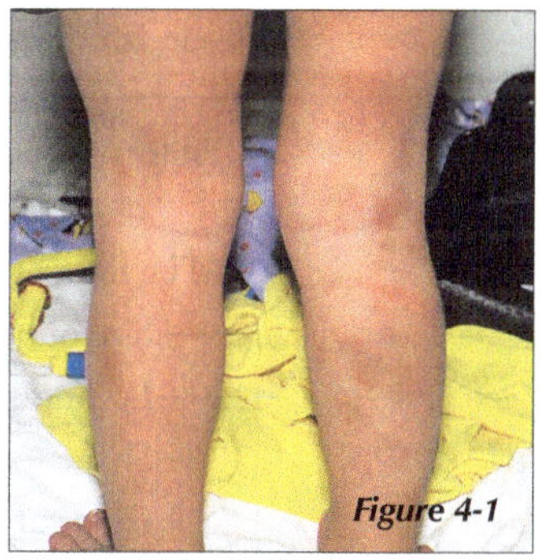

Figure 4-1. *Bruises inflicted with a belt. (Contributed by Lawrence R. Ricci, MD; Portland, ME.)*

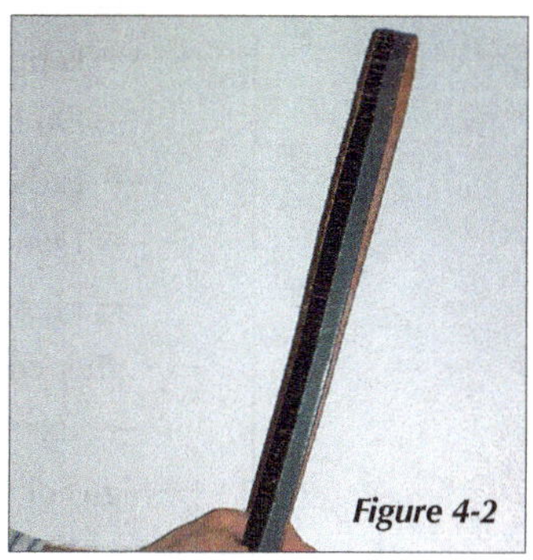

Figure 4-2. *Belt used on child in Figure 4-1. (Contributed by Lawrence R. Ricci, MD; Portland, ME.)*

Physical Examination of Bruises

Assessment of skin injuries includes the examination of all areas of the body where injuries are expected, such as bony prominences of the forehead, chin, and shins, as well as the atypical areas, such as the trunk, bottoms of the feet, and inside of the mouth. It is important that the health care provider carefully document the location and

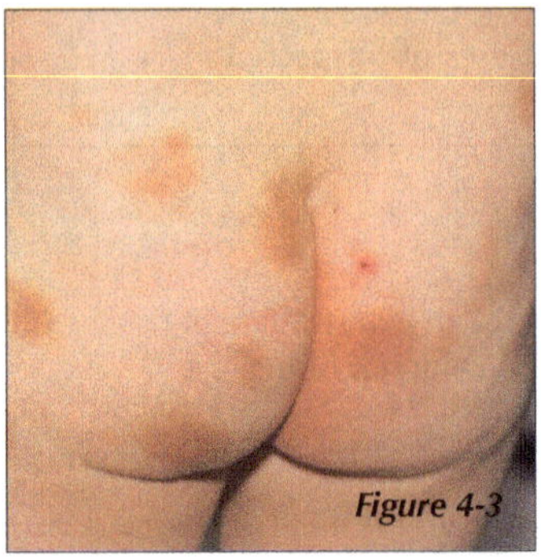

Figure 4-3. *Bruises inflicted with a wooden spoon. (Contributed by Lawrence R. Ricci, MD; Portland, ME.)*

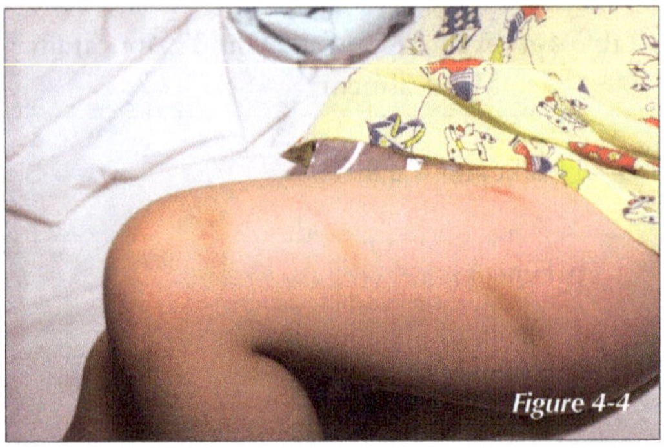

Figure 4-4. *Bruises inflicted with a switch. (Contributed by Lawrence R. Ricci, MD; Portland, ME.)*

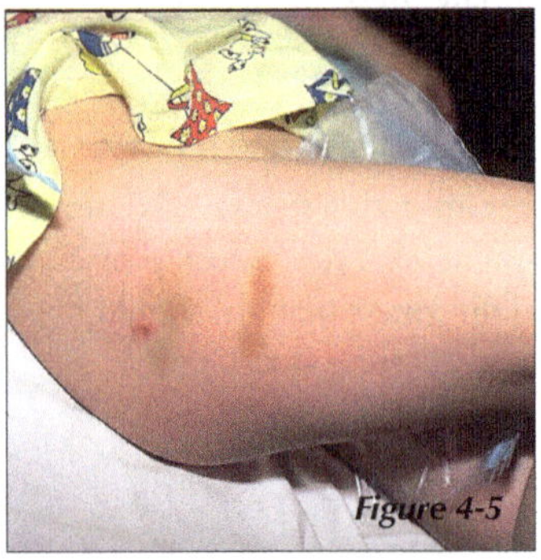

Figure 4-5. *Same child as Figure 4-4. (Contributed by Lawrence R. Ricci, MD; Portland, ME.)*

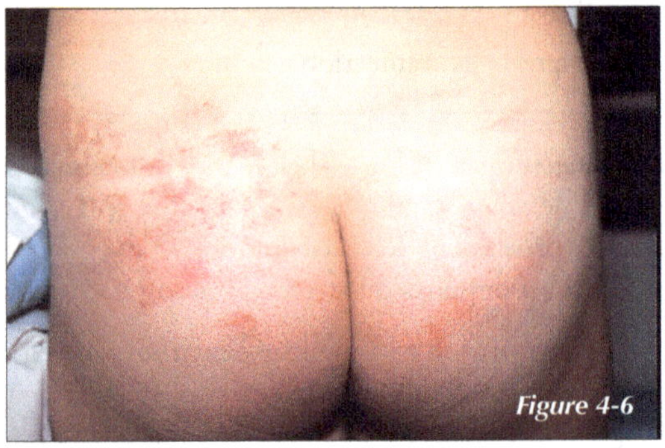

Figure 4-6. *Bruises inflicted with a belt. (Contributed by Lawrence R. Ricci, MD; Portland, ME.)*

description of each injury. The health care provider should document each identified injury in the medical record, noting the size, specific location using anatomical landmarks, and appearance. The health care provider should note whether the injury appears to be acute, in a healing phase, or totally healed. Ideally, each injury should be described in written form, with a hand-drawn diagram and a photograph indicating the location of the injury (see *Chapter 9, Documenting the Evaluation of Suspected Child Maltreatment Cases*). A standard form may be used to document examination findings (**Table 4-5**).

Table 4-5. Documentation of Bruising

The following should be documented for each bruise:

—Size of bruise
—Location (on what body part[s])
—Shape (object used)
—Color of injured area
—Characteristics and pattern of bruise(s)
  — Is bruise centrally located or in a protected area?
  — Do multiple bruises have different colors or different ages?
  — Is there a consistency of bruise pattern with history given?
  — Does the pattern indicate a specific mechanism of infliction?
  — How many body surfaces are injured (single or multiple episodes of trauma)?
—Other considerations of injury
  — Examine for other signs of organ or bone injury
—Signs of physical neglect

Patterned Injuries

Patterned injuries have geometric shapes that resemble the object used to physically injure the child (see **Figure 4-3**) (see *Chapter 2, Presentation and Overview of the Evaluation of Child Maltreatment*). Patterned marks may be obvious or subtle in appearance. Generally, patterned injuries indicate that the child was struck with something that created an impression of the object used, of which common implements include the hand, belts, cords, and shoes.[19] Grab or pinch marks are often indicators of inflicted skin injury. Bruising in the shape of an outline of fingers or grasp marks indicates forceful holding of the child. The outline of the perpetrator's fingers may appear on the child's skin at the point of holding and show up as linear bruises surrounding a clear center.[20] The violent holding is the identified mechanism of injury; the circulation in the child's skin is forced beyond the area where the force is applied, creating a bruise around it. Other objects, when administered with force, can create a similar pattern (**Figures 4-7** to **4-10**).

Dating of Bruise Injuries

The ability to determine the approximate time that a bruise was inflicted is based on the progression of color changes that occur in a bruise as the skin and underlying tissues undergo the healing process. The dating of skin bruises has received a great deal of attention over the past several decades.[21,22] Bruise dating is not an exact science, and the health care provider must be careful to speak in typical age ranges for various bruises rather than pronounce the specific age for a given bruise. In many cases, the health care provider can evaluate the approximate age range of a bruise based on the color of the skin and underlying tissues as the bruise goes through the healing phase and document whether the given time frame between the suspected time of injury and the date of the examination is consistent or inconsistent with the estimated age. It is best to document that a bruise is consistent with a given estimated age range because the exact age can rarely be determined.[19,21,22] When examining a child, it is reasonable to compare bruises that seem newer or older; however, it is not accurate to compare the color of one

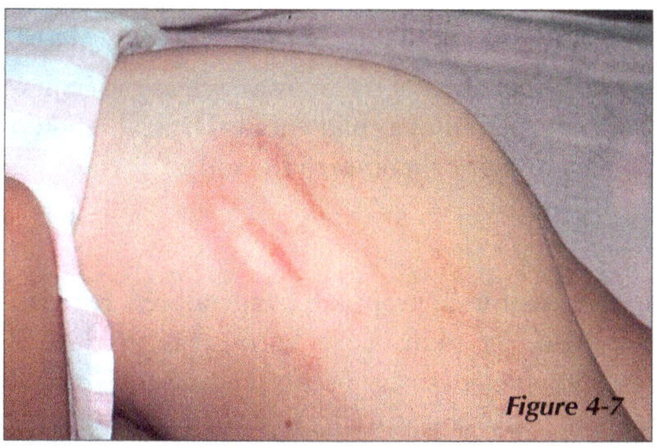

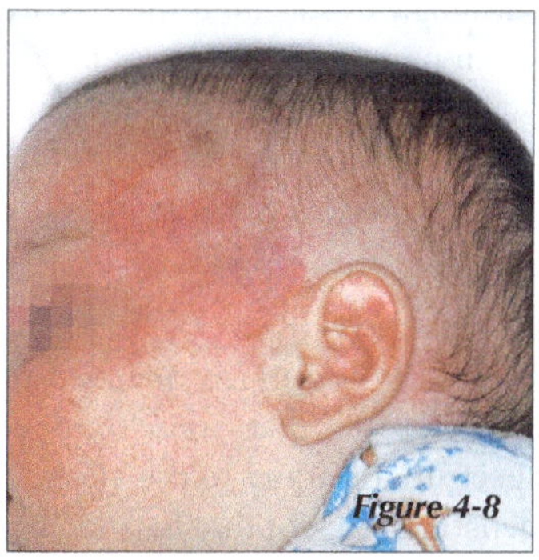

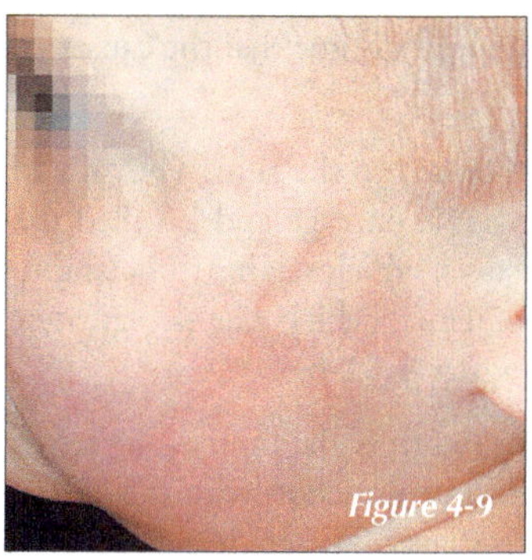

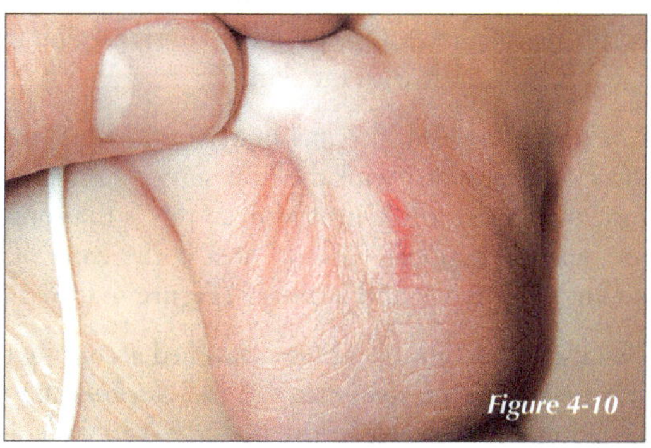

Figure 4-7. Handprint on leg. (Contributed by Lawrence R. Ricci, MD; Portland, ME.)

Figure 4-8. Handprint on face. (Contributed by Lawrence R. Ricci, MD; Portland, ME.)

Figure 4-9. Slap mark. (Contributed by Lawrence R. Ricci, MD; Portland, ME.)

Figure 4-10. Fingernail scratch. (Contributed by Lawrence R. Ricci, MD; Portland, ME.)

child's bruise to the same color of a bruise in another child and say that the age of both bruises is the same. Serial or follow-up examinations for bruises are suggested, so that the progression of the healing process can be documented in cases of suspected physical abuse. **Table 4-6** details the color progression and associated age ranges of bruising.

Table 4-6. Progression of Bruising

Approximate Age of Bruise	Color Range
—Fresh injury	—Red coloration
—First day or 2	—Red, swollen, tender
—1 to 5 days	—Red, purple
—5 to 7 days	—Green
—7 to 10 days	—Yellow
—10 or more days	—Brown
—14 to 28 days	—Gone

Adapted from Farley RH, Reece RM; United States Department of Justice. Recognizing When a Child's Injury or Illness Is Caused by Abuse. *Washington, DC: United States Department of Justice; 2002.*

Other Related Injuries

Bite marks and traumatic alopecia are other skin injuries that can be identified during the physical examination. A bite mark, especially a full bite mark, can help reveal the identity of the perpetrator because of its size and identifiable dental characteristics.[24-26] Identifying the specific characteristics of a bite mark is an area where forensic experts can assist the health care provider in completing documentation and preserving evidence. Although extragenital injuries are not often a common finding in child sexual abuse, when present such injuries may manifest as contusions, erythema, tearing, bite marks, scratch marks, and finger pressure marks in other areas of the body as well as the genitalia. Traumatic alopecia occurs when hair is pulled out of a child's head. The scalp should be inspected for findings indicating the loss of hair or trauma to the scalp.[27]

Burns

Pathophysiology

The skin is an organ designed to function within appropriate temperatures. Extreme temperatures that come into contact with the skin cause burns that produce a spectrum of injury to the affected cells. Permanent damage occurs when there is a total denaturation of proteins and enzymes and a resultant inability of cellular mechanisms to function.[28] Each of the 3 layers of skin can be affected in varying degrees, depending on the temperature of the causative substance and the amount of time that the causative agent is in contact with the skin.

Concentric zones of thermal injury result after heat is applied to the skin. The area in most direct contact with the heat source sustains irreparable damage and is called the zone of coagulation. Outward from this is the zone of stasis, which retains some ability for repair. The most outward area is the zone of hyperemia, which has the greatest potential for repair and healing[28] (**Figure 4-11-a** and **Figure 4-11-b**)).

There are 4 categories of burns classified according to the depth of the injury. The terms ***superficial, partial-thickness***, and ***full-thickness*** are used in conjunction with the 4 classifications. First-degree burns are limited to the epidermis layer. The epidermis consists

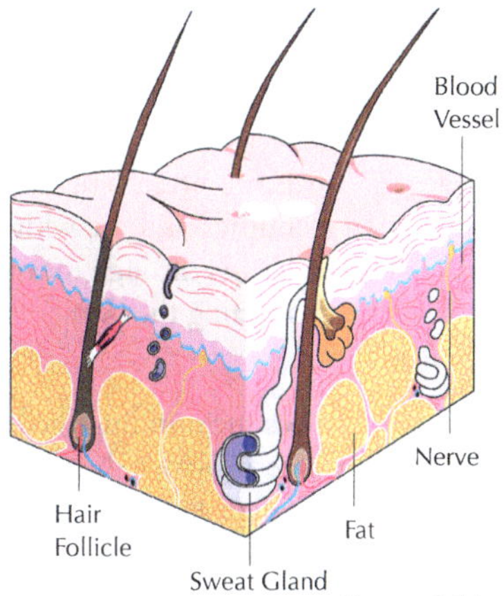

Figure 4-11-a

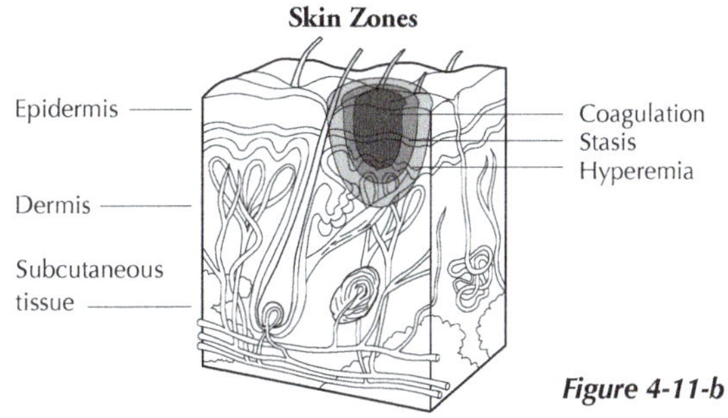

Figure 4-11-b

Figure 4-11-a. *Skin consists of 3 layers, making up a dynamic network of cells, nerves, and blood vessels.*

Figure 4-11-b. *Diagram showing the 3 layers of skin with concentric zones of thermal injury. Adapted from Robson M, Heggers J. Pathophysiology of the burn wound. In: Carvajal HF, Parks DH, eds.* Burns in Children: Pediatric Burn Management. *St. Louis, MO: Year Book Medical Pub; 1988:27-32.*

of an outer layer of anucleated cornified cells, called the stratum corneum, and an inner layer of cells that mature and differentiate into cornified cells of the stratum corneum. The stratum corneum acts as a barrier to the entrance of microorganisms and the loss of water and electrolytes. Although painful, the superficial burn is self-limiting and rarely leads to scarring. Within a few days, the injured skin sloughs and heals as the healthy cells regenerate from the underlying skin cells. Treatment usually involves local wound care.[29]

Second-degree burns involve injury that extends into the dermis with some viable dermis remaining. The dermis is composed of a dense fibroelastic connective tissue that contains collagen, elastic fibers, and an extracellular gel, also called the ground substance. The dermis has an extensive nerve and vascular network, which includes glands and appendages that communicate with the epidermis. A second-degree burn usually causes blistering of the skin, vessel disruption, and a resultant beefy, red appearance of the

Table 4-7. Evaluating a Burn Injury

Burn Injury Evaluation Questions:

— How did the burn occur?

— How did the child come into contact with the burning agent?

— For how long was the burning agent in contact with the child?

— Was the skin covered with clothes or was the skin uncovered?

— Who was supervising the child?

— In what timeframe was the child taken for medical care?

— If there was any delay in seeking treatment, what is the reason for the delay?

— Who brought the child to medical care?

— Did anyone other than the child witness the burn incident?

— What was the child's immediate response to the burn situation (eg, cry, run)?

Adapted from Giardino AP, Christian CW, Giardino E. Evaluation of abuse and neglect. In: Giardino AP, Christian CW, Giardino E, eds. A Practical Guide to the Evaluation of Child Physical Abuse and Neglect. *Thousand Oaks, CA: Sage Publications; 1997:23-59.*

affected area.[30] Exposed nerve endings cause greater pain and discomfort during the injury and healing process. Partial-thickness burns heal in approximately 2 weeks, though deep partial-thickness burns may take 3 to 4 weeks.[31]

Third- and fourth-degree burns, also called full-thickness burns, involve destruction of the entire epidermis and dermis to the subcutaneous tissue (third-degree), or the muscle, fascia, and bone (fourth-degree). Fourth-degree burns are often lethal. Full-thickness burns completely destroy blood vessels and nerve endings and are white in appearance as a result of exposed subcutaneous tissue. Healing occurs through means of surgical grafting or by inward growth of skin from tissues surrounding the skin.

History-Taking for the Evaluation of Burns

The caregiver's history describing the cause of and circumstances surrounding the burn is an important part of the overall evaluation. The health care provider should note the responses of both the child, when possible, and the caregiver because responses provide clues as to whether the injury was accidental or inflicted. All answers should be carefully documented in the medical record. **Table 4-7** identifies questions that should be asked when completing a history for a burn injury. The following specific points can help determine whether the history provided by the caregiver correlates with physical findings and should be taken into consideration by the health care provider:

— What is the time of occurrence, nature, extent, and location of the burn?

— Does the burn pattern correlate with the history of the accident?

— Is the history from the caregiver plausible or implausible?

— When more than one family member is involved and questioned separately, is each story consistent with the other and with what has been observed?

— Is the history consistent with what the health care provider has heard from the child?

— Is the child's developmental level consistent with the actions described as having caused the burn injury?

— Does the child have any medical conditions that mimic burning?

— Are there any other signs of abuse?

Physical Examination of Burns

The physical examination may reveal burn patterns characteristic of inflicted injury that raise suspicions about the possibility of abuse. The findings of the physical examination may give clues that the caregiver's history or the given mechanism of injury may be implausible based on the child's developmental level and the depth and distribution of the burn[32] (**Table 4-8**).

The health care provider should note all aspects of a burn injury, including:

— Location

— Size

— Appearance or severity (first-, second-, or third-degree; percentage of body surface) (see **Figure 4-12**)

Characteristics of the Accidental and Inflicted Burn

Evaluating the shape of a burn is important because the pattern may indicate the object used, such as an iron, radiator, or cigarette lighter (**Figure 4-13**). Burns by forced immersion can cause sharply demarcated, circular-type injuries to the lower and upper extremities causing a stocking-and-glove pattern. In forced immersion burns, characteristic patterns involving the buttocks and genitalia may result. If a child falls

Table 4-8. Burn Examination Guidelines

Description of the Burn(s)	— Type and degree of burn(s) (superficial, partial thickness [superficial or deep], full thickness) — Amount of body surface area (BSA) involved (see Figure 4-12)
Characteristics and Pattern of Burn(s)	— Apparent age of burn (Does it appear older than given history?) — Consistency of burn distribution with history provided — Burn incompatible with described events in history — Note signs of restraint — Signs of immersion in hot fluid — Stocking-and-glove demarcation on extremities — Sparing of flexure areas — Presence or lack of splash marks — Hole-in-doughnut pattern
Identification of Other Signs of Inflicted Injury	— Presence of other injuries (eg, bruises, fractures, burns of different ages) — Maltreatment evidence (eg, scars, malnourishment) — Restraint-related injuries (eg, multiple bruises resembling fingers and hands on upper extremities)

Adapted from Giardino AP, Christian CW, Giardino E. Evaluation of abuse and neglect. In: Giardino AP, Christian CW, Giardino E, eds. A Practical Guide to the Evaluation of Child Physical Abuse and Neglect. *Thousand Oaks, CA: Sage Publications; 1997:23-59.*

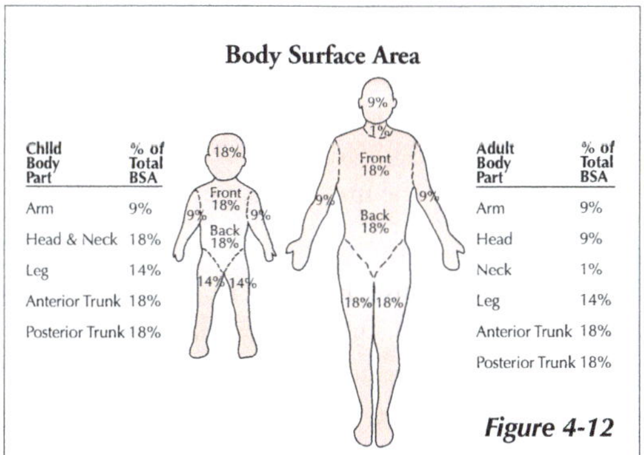

Figure 4-12

Figure 4-12. Rule of nines. Image reprinted with permission from eMedicine.com, 2010. Available at: http://reference.medscape.com/article/934173-overview. Besner GE, Otabar IA. Surgical treatment of burns. eMedicine Web site. http://emedicine.medscape.com/article/934173-media. Updated March 10, 2009. Accessed December 10, 2010.

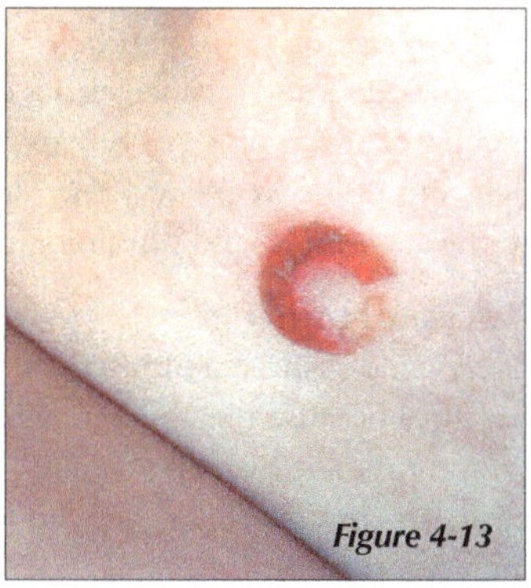

Figure 4-13

Figure 4-13. Inflicted burn from cigarette lighter. (Contributed by Lawrence R. Ricci, MD; Portland, ME.)

into a tub, the health care provider would expect to find an irregular burn pattern with burns on the skin areas hit by the hot liquid. Sharp lines of demarcation would typically be absent because the child would splash around in the struggle to escape from the hot liquid. However, if a child is forcefully immersed in hot liquid in a sitting position, the health care provider would expect to find burns on the buttocks and the legs with the skin on the knees, hands, and arms spared.

The unique hole-in-doughnut pattern occurs when a child is forcefully held against the surface of a container holding hot liquid, such as a bathtub. The central part of the child's buttocks is spared from burns because the container is relatively cooler than the hot liquid it contains; therefore, the point at which the skin touches the tub may be less burned or affected than the skin surface that came in contact with the hot liquid. The

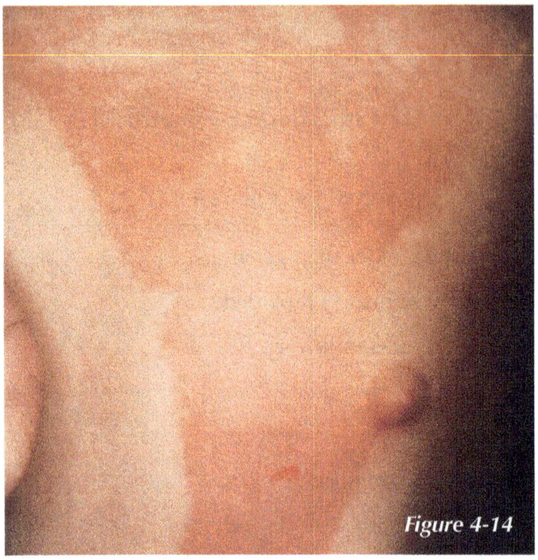

Figure 4-14. *Accidental spill burn pattern.*

hole-in-doughnut pattern is highly associated with forced immersion burns.[32]

Most accidental burns are related to splash or spill injuries; however, splash and spill burns can be inflicted, and an overlap exists in the physical findings between the 2 mechanisms of action. The severity of the burn is related to the temperature of the burning agent, amount of time the hot liquid is in contact with the skin, and thickness of the skin where the burn occurred. Clothing tends to keep the burning agent in contact with the skin for a longer amount of time and, therefore, causes a more severe burn.

Accidental scalds occur in situations in which the child reaches for a container holding hot liquid and then pours the liquid down onto him or herself. A child who pulls down a cup of hot coffee onto himself from a table would manifest a burn pattern consistent with hot liquid falling onto the body from above. Splash marks may also appear in body areas separate from the most severely burned areas (**Figure 4-14**). In an inflicted burn, the perpetrator may pour a hot liquid onto or throw a liquid at a child. A burn on the back may indicate liquid was thrown. The history given by the caregiver is important and should be evaluated in relation to the pattern of the injury (**Table 4-9**).

Skeletal Injuries

Fractures are the second most common manifestation of physical abuse after skin injuries[33] and are found in approximately 30% of physically abused children.[34,35] Fractures usually result from traumatic injury to bone that causes the continuity of bone tissues or bony cartilage to be disrupted or broken. **Table 4-10** outlines the classifications and characteristics of fractures. Common physical signs of skeletal injury include reduced range of motion (ROM), swelling, tenderness, ecchymosis, and limb deformity. The frequency, type, location, and healing of pediatric fractures are related to the anatomical and physiological characteristics of the immature, porous skeleton.[36]

Relevant History

Every child suspected of being the victim of physical abuse should be evaluated for bone fractures because the child may have an occult fracture without any specific signs and symptoms. The history of a child who is brought to a health care facility for treatment of skeletal trauma or a child who is suspected to have experienced physical abuse should include the following details[37]:

— Developmental stage of the child

— Supervision given by caregivers

— Child's behavior that signaled pain

— Prior history of injuries or fractures

— In cases of falls, questions regarding the height from which the child fell

— Contact surface

— Witnesses to the event

— Description of possible injury mechanisms, such as twisting, compression, traction

Table 4-9. Distinguishing Accidental From Inflicted Burns

Indications That Burns May Not Have Been Accidental	
History	— The burns are attributed to siblings. — An unrelated adult brings the child in for medical care. — Accounts of the injury differ. — Treatment is delayed for more than 24 hours. — There is evidence of prior accidents or absence of parental concern. — The lesions are incompatible with the history.
Location	— The burns are more likely to be found on the buttocks; in the anogenital region (the area between the legs, encompassing the genitals and anus); and on the ankles, wrists, palms, and soles.
Pattern	— The burns have sharply defined edges. For example, in immersion burns, the line of immersion gives the appearance of a glove or stocking on the child's hand or foot. — The burns are full thickness (all of the skin, and possibly muscle and bone is destroyed). — The burns are symmetrical. — The burns are older than the reported history indicates. — The burns have been neglected or are infected. — There are numerous lesions of various ages. — The burn patterns conform to the shape of the implement used. — The degree of the burns is uniform (usually indicating forced contact with a hot, dry object), and they cover a large area.
Indications that Burns are More Likely to be Accidental	
History	— The history of the mechanism of the burns is compatible with the observed injury.
Location	— The burns are usually found on the front of the body. They occur in locations reflecting the child's motor activity, level of development, and the exposure of the child's body to the burning agent.
Pattern	— The burns are of multiple depths interspersed with unburned areas and are usually less severe, such as splash burns. — The burns are of partial thickness; that is, only part of the skin has been damaged or destroyed. — The burns are asymmetrical. — Apparently only one traumatic event has occurred because the skin injuries are all of the same age.

Reprinted from Farley RH, Reece RM; United States Department of Justice. Recognizing When a Child's Injury or Illness Is Caused by Abuse. *Washington, DC: United States Department of Justice; 2002.*

Table 4-10. Classification of Fractures

FRACTURE CLASSIFICATIONS

Fracture	Characteristics
Simple (closed fracture)	—Surface of skin intact and not ruptured; bone broken in one place.
Compound (open)	—Fracture ruptures skin, exposing bone and causing soft tissue injury and possible infection.
Greenstick (incomplete)	—Bone is partly broken and partly bent; fracture occurs partly across a bone shaft, often resulting from bending or crushing mechanisms on the bone.
Complete	—Break is completely through the bone.

CLASSIFICATION BY FRACTURE LINE

Fracture	Classifications
Hairline	—Fracture appears as a narrow crack along surface of a bone.
Linear	—Fracture runs parallel to the bone's axis or direction of the bone's shaft.
Oblique	—Angled fracture crosses bone at approximately a 45-degree angle to the bone's axis.
Transverse	—Fracture at a right angle to the bone's axis, at a 90-degree angle.
Stellate	—Fracture lines radiate from a central point.
Spiral	—Oblique fracture line encircles a portion of bone, crosses the bone at an oblique angle, creating a spiral pattern.

CLASSIFICATION BY FRACTURE LINE

Fracture	Characteristics
Comminuted	— More than 1 fracture line and more than 2 bone fragments; usually produced by high forces in a very fragile bone.
Nondisplaced	— Fragments of bone maintain their normal alignment after fracture.
Impacted	— Compression fracture, involves entire bone.
Overriding	— Bony fragments overlap and shorten the total length of the bone.
Angulated	— Fragments result in pieces of bone being at angles to each other.
Displaced	— Bony fragment occurs from disruption of normal bone alignment; deformity of segments separate from one another.
Avulsed	— Bone fragments pulled from normal position by forceful muscle contractions or resistance from ligaments.
Segmental	— Segmental alignment occurs when fractures in 2 adjacent areas happen with an isolated central segment, for example, when arm bone fractures in 2 separate places with displacement of the midsection of bone.

(continued)

Table 4-10. Classification of Fractures *(continued)*

Torus (buckle)	—Impact injury specific to children; bone buckles, usually at or near the metaphysis.
Depressed	—Skull fracture with inward displacement of a part of the roof of the skull.
Diastatic	—Significant separation of bone fragments.

FRACTURE CLASSIFICATIONS

Fracture	**Characteristics**
Distal	Fracture located away from center of body, usually in hands or feet.
Occult	Clinical, but not radiographic evidence of fracture; may also indicate a fracture seen radiographically but without manifestations of actual fracture.
Pathological	Fracture occurs in area of disease-weakened bone.
Proximal	Fracture located more near trunk or center of body.
Supracondylar	Fracture area is above condyle, is typically of the humerus.

Patterns of Fractures in Abuse

There is no single fracture pattern that can determine abuse beyond any doubt in an infant or child; however, there are a few fracture patterns that should raise suspicions as to the possibility of abuse, especially when considered in light of several other pieces of historical data. When evaluating fractures, it is important to consider the pattern of fracture as well as the following:

— The child's age: most fractures related to abuse are found in infants younger than 1 year of age.[38]

— Stated mechanism of injury: fractures can occur from blunt force or torsion.[37,38]

— Overall injury pattern: fractures are commonly seen in the extremities in abuse and may include occult fractures. It is also important to consider associated head and visceral trauma.[38]

— Pertinent psychosocial factors[38]

The location of a fracture may be a clue in diagnosing child abuse. Accidental fractures that occur in the active child are often the result of falls and commonly include injuries to the clavicle, distal forearm, and hand.[34,39] However, the presence of certain types of metaphyseal lesions in young children, multiple fractures in various stages of healing, fractures to the posterior ribs, and long bone fractures in children younger than 2 years of age suggest inflicted injury[38] (**Figures 4-15** to **4-20**). For example, fractures of the femur or ribs in a young child should increase the suspicion for child abuse. Rib and metaphyseal fractures in infants should also raise concern for abuse in the absence of a significant history. Fractures of the distal femur in the infant are a strong indicator of abuse and should be carefully evaluated with high-detail skeletal radiographs in all cases.[36] Other uncommon and, therefore, suspicious fractures include fractures of the vertebrae, sternum, or pelvis.

Radiographic Evaluation

The use of radiographic imaging in child abuse cases helps to identify the extent of physical injury and is the method of choice for global skeletal imaging in cases of suspected abuse.[40] A full skeletal survey is a series of radiographic images of the entire

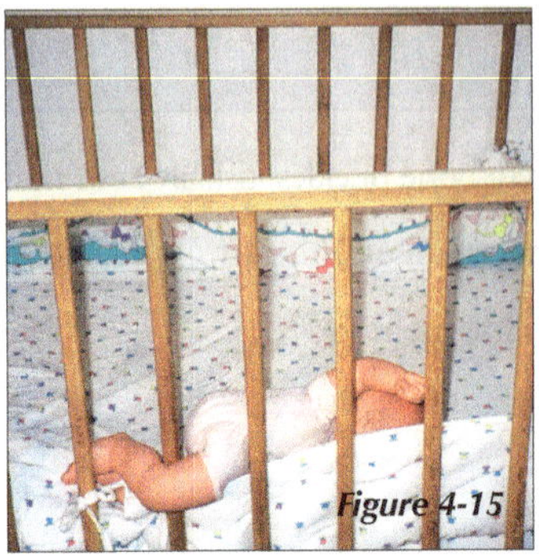
Figure 4-15

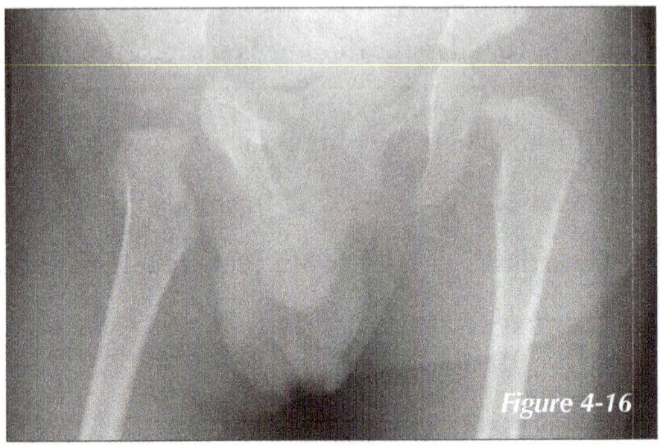
Figure 4-16

Figure 4-15. Model for Figure 4-16. (Contributed by Lawrence R. Ricci, MD; Portland, ME.)

Figure 4-16. Femoral neck fracture from being yanked from crib in Figure 4-15. (Contributed by Lawrence R. Ricci, MD; Portland, ME.)

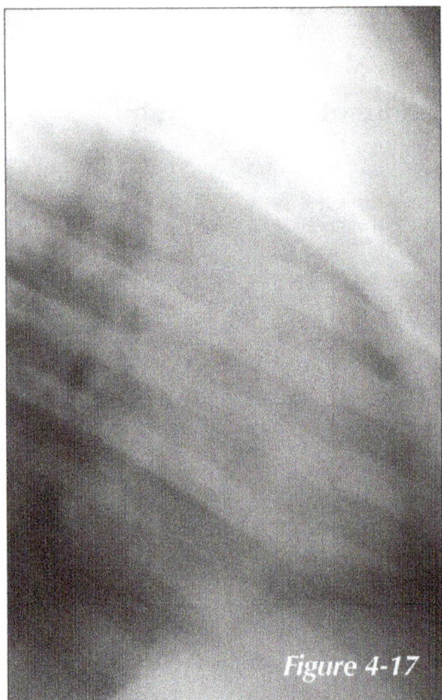
Figure 4-17

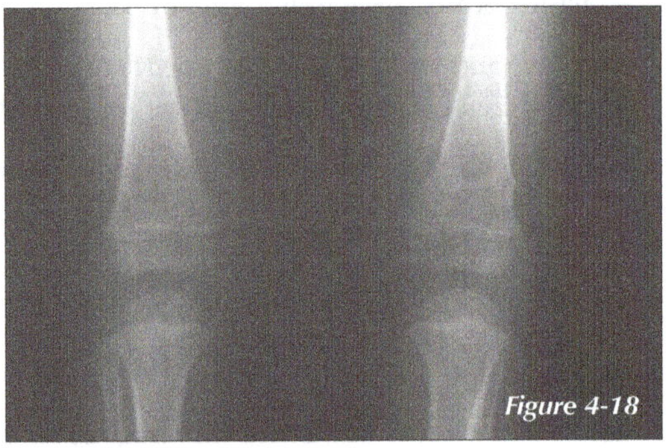
Figure 4-18

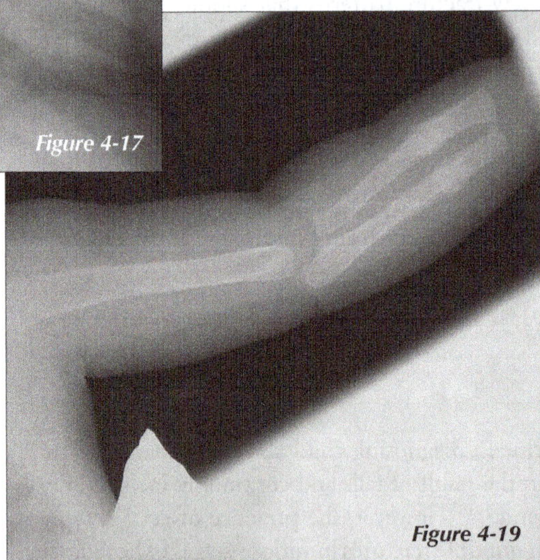
Figure 4-19

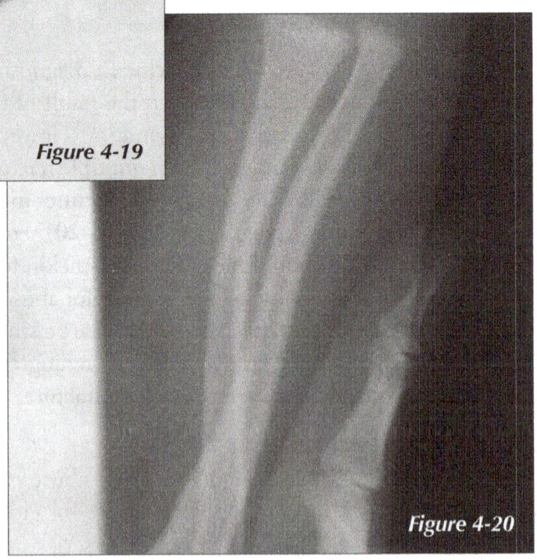
Figure 4-20

Figure 4-17. Child with multiple rib fractures. (Contributed by Lawrence R. Ricci, MD; Portland, ME.)

Figure 4-18. Buckle fracture distal femur shaft inflicted. (Contributed by Lawrence R. Ricci, MD; Portland, ME.)

Figure 4-19. Same child as Figure 4-9 with old radius and ulna fracture. (Contributed by Lawrence R. Ricci, MD; Portland, ME.)

Figure 4-20. Old and new radius fracture. (Contributed by Lawrence R. Ricci, MD; Portland, ME.)

skeleton, or those anatomic regions appropriate for the clinical indications,[41] that helps identify both old and new injuries and determine the presence of metabolic or genetic conditions that mimic abuse. A full skeletal survey is a useful screening tool for children aged 2 years or younger for whom child maltreatment is being considered[40] and in cases involving head or visceral trauma. The patient's age and type of suspicious injury can guide the health care provider as to the appropriateness of obtaining a skeletal survey.[42] For those aged 2 through 5 years, the health care provider must use clinical judgment when deciding whether a skeletal survey is warranted. However, no matter what the child's age, the clinician should follow the customary radiographic protocol whenever clinical findings point to a specific site of injury.[40]

Radiographs can reveal spiral fractures resulting from the twisting of the long bones as well as old and healing fractures. The skeletal survey includes lateral spine views to assess vertebral fractures and dislocations and hands and feet views to identify subtle digital injuries (**Table 4-11**). Mandatory anteroposterior and lateral views of the skull are taken even when cranial computed tomography (CT) has been performed because a CT scan can miss certain skull fractures.[43]

Table 4-11. The Standard Skeletal Survey

Appendicular Skeleton	— Humeri (AP)
	— Forearms (AP)
	— Hands (AP)
	— Femurs (AP)
	— Lower legs (AP)
	— Feet (AP)
Axial Skeleton	— Thorax (AP, lateral, right and left obliques), to include ribs thoracic and upper lumbar spine
	— Pelvis (AP), to include ribs, thoracic and upper lumbar spine
	— Lumbosacral spine (lateral)
	— Cervical spine (lateral)
	— Skull (frontal and lateral)

Adapted from American Academy of Pediatrics. Diagnostic imaging of child abuse. Pediatrics. *2000; 105:1345-1348.*

Thoracic and Abdominal Injuries

Abdominal injuries in cases of child physical abuse are relatively uncommon, but often serious, and represent the second most common cause of mortality in cases of child physical abuse.[43] When a child sustains serious abdominal or chest injury without a known or observed mechanism, an investigation for potential child abuse must be conducted. Internal injuries usually result from blunt trauma, such as a direct blow to the abdomen. Blows to the anterior abdomen may cause epigastric injury, mesenteric tears, or pancreatic injury, whereas blows to the side of the abdomen may cause splenic, hepatic, or renal injury. It is important to inspect the abdomen carefully and examine the child for external bruises and internal injuries of underlying organs. Abdominal injuries that heighten the suspicion of child abuse include blunt thoracoabdominal injury, duodenal hematomas, pancreatitis, bowel perforation, and thoracoabdominal injury associated with rib fracture. However, it is important to note that severe internal injuries can be present with no external signs or symptoms.[37]

Chest injuries include pulmonary contusion, pneumothorax, pleural effusion, rib fractures, and vascular or tracheobronchial injuries. The most common thoracic injuries seen in child abuse cases are fractured ribs and underlying organ injury resulting from the fractures. Penetrating chest injuries may be seen as well and usually present as catastrophic injuries.[44] Implausible or unlikely reasons for chest injuries, such as falling out of bed, sibling stepping on infant, or rolling onto a child sleeping in bed, should raise suspicions of child abuse[40] (**Table 4-12**).

Table 4-12. Suspicious Thoracic and Abdominal Injuries

History	— Unsubstantiated story of how injury occurred — Child fell out of bed — Someone rolled onto sleeping child — Sibling stepped on infant
Signs and Symptoms the Child may Manifest	— Vomiting — Abdominal pain — Abdominal tenderness — Hematuria — Emesis — Absence of bowel sounds
Physical Findings on Examination	— Blunt thoracoabdominal injury — Duodenal hematomas — Pancreatitis — Bowel perforation — Thoracoabdominal injury associated with rib fracture

Evaluation and Treatment

The evaluation and management of acute abdominal injury in children is the same for both accidental and intentional injuries.[40] The stability of the patient should determine the appropriate diagnostic evaluation of the child because CT scans or ultrasounds may be more or less indicated, depending on the child's physiological stability.[45] The initial radiographic assessment of the injured child should include the usual studies of the chest, cervical spine, and abdomen to evaluate for thoracic and abdominal injuries. A CT scan should be performed when internal chest or abdominal injury is suspected and the patient's condition is stable. Ultrasonography is sometimes used to evaluate injuries associated with child abuse, but a CT scan is the preferred diagnostic tool, as it best reveals injuries.[40,46]

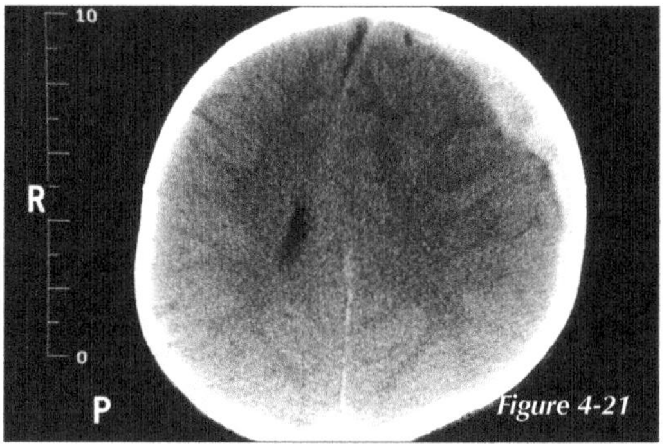

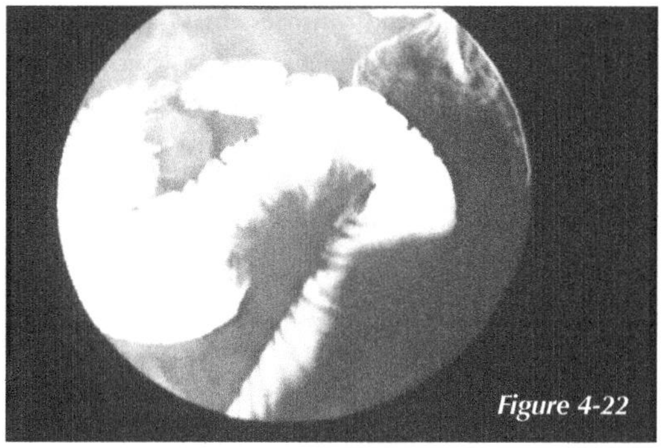

Figure 4-21. Acute subdural with shift. (Contributed by Lawrence R. Ricci, MD; Portland, ME.)

Figure 4-22. Duodenal hematoma. (Contributed by Lawrence R. Ricci, MD; Portland, ME.)

Head Trauma

The most common cause of death in child abuse cases is head injury[47] (**Figures 4-21** and **4-22**). The younger the child, the more predisposed that child is to death from head injury. A study of children aged 2 years and younger admitted for head injury found that 24% of the injuries resulted from inflicted trauma.[48,49] Inflicted head injury accounts for a substantial number of head injuries that require hospitalization in children aged 6½ years and younger.[50]

Inflicted injury to the head results from a variety of mechanisms, including the rotational forces associated with shaking and impact injuries resulting from being slapped, hit, or punched. The head of a small child can be slammed into a hard object, such as a wall, seen with and without shaking, and children can also be dropped from a height onto their heads. Children may suffer penetrating injuries to the head from firearms, knives, or glass. Penetrating injuries have a high potential for serious morbidity and mortality. Fractures of the skull, usually linear, can cause severe concussions and anoxia. Children can suffer asphyxiation as a result of choking, gagging, or both.

Abusive head trauma (AHT) is a category of inflicted head injuries and includes what was formerly referred to as shaken baby syndrome (SBS) or shaken impact syndrome (SIS). AHT accounts for a significant number of cases of head trauma in young children. AHT is associated with shaking and may include impact of the head against a surface. The 3 crucial components typically present when making a diagnosis of AHT are:

— Closed head injury evidenced by altered level of consciousness, convulsions, coma, or death.

— CNS injury evidenced by CNS hemorrhaging, brain contusion, laceration, or concussion.

— Retinal hemorrhages

The occurrence of AHT is unrelated to gender, race, education, or socioeconomic status[51] and can alter a child's normal developmental course by causing neuropsychological deficits.[52] The characteristic presentation of the child with AHT resulting from a shaking or a shaking-impact-type mechanism includes subdural hemorrhage, intraocular hemorrhage, and, often, little evidence of external trauma.[53] AHT can go unidentified because of the absence of external injuries and lack of witnesses other than the perpetrator of the event. Any infant or toddler who presents with an altered level of consciousness should be considered to have head trauma until proven otherwise. Often, the history collected for the child with AHT includes a mechanism of injury that is relatively minor in nature.[49] As with other forms of abuse, the history may be false or misleading, and the uncovered damage is usually disproportionate to the type of injury described by the caregiver. The findings of AHT often involve a changing history; fractures of various ages, particularly rib fractures; subdural hematoma of the brain; and retinal hemorrhages.[54]

Head injuries may also present as seizures, respiratory problems, and disturbed consciousness. Signs and symptoms of AHT may be nonspecific and mimic seizure disorders, infections, or metabolic abnormalities.[55] The physical act of shaking a child may also cause bruises of the upper arms and shoulders depending on the manner in which the child is held. Evaluation of a child with a head injury includes assessment of level of consciousness, because loss of consciousness is a common finding with head injury. A study of 95 children who died from accidental head injury found that 94 had an immediate decrease in the level of consciousness.[49] Nonaccidental head injury is often characterized by subdural hematomas with retinal hemorrhages but little to no external trauma.[56] The presenting signs and symptoms of head trauma are as follows:

— Altered level of consciousness

— Coma

— Vomiting

— Convulsions

— Opisthotonic posturing

— External injuries (may be subtle or not present at all)

— Swelling and bruising of the scalp

— Respiratory compromise

— Apnea

— Hypoventilation

— Cheyne-Stokes breathing

Ophthalmological Findings with Head Trauma

When head injury occurs, an ophthalmological examination is essential because retinal hemorrhage is found in 65% to 95% of children with inflicted head injury.[49] A child's head and its contents are extremely vulnerable to trauma, and the head should not be shaken, slapped, or struck.[57] In the absence of a documented history of major trauma, subdural hematomas (SDHs) and retinal hemorrhages should be considered as highly suspicious for possible child abuse.[58] Shaking a baby or small child can induce intracranial, ocular, and, less often, cervical spine injuries. Shaking trauma can cause SDHs, subarachnoid hemorrhages, and brain contusions. SDH is also a common finding in inflicted CNS injuries which may be caused by the violent shaking of the baby with or without impact to the head, such as when a child is thrown against a stationary object like a mattress, floor, or wall.[23] Nonspecific signs and symptoms of SDHs include irritability, lethargy, or a lack of appetite. Classic signs of increased intracranial pressure (ICP) possibly caused by a SDHs are seizures, vomiting, stupor, and coma.[23,59]

The primary cause of retinal hemorrhage in infants is vaginal delivery while AHT is the next leading cause. Retinal hemorrhages in AHT can be unilateral or bilateral and vary in degree. The severity of retinal hemorrhage often parallels the severity of brain injury.[60] Retinal hemorrhage caused by accidental trauma[49] usually have a significant trauma history witnessed by others, such as a motor vehicle accident (see *Chapter 7, Differential Diagnosis: Conditions That Mimic Child Maltreatment*). Birth-related retinal hemorrhages heal rapidly and are completely resolved within 30 days.[61,62] Retinal hemorrhage in infants aged 1 month or older should raise suspicions that the injury is associated with factors other than birth related trauma.

Retinal hemorrhage is a common fundoscopic finding in AHT,[60,63] but the diagnosis of AHT can be made in the absence of retinal hemorrhage. The presence of extensive bilateral retinal hemorrhages in a child with no known major trauma raises a strong likelihood of AHT. When retinal hemorrhage is present, all other differential diagnoses for hemorrhages should be investigated and eliminated.[54] A tool to evaluate ophthalmic findings in suspected AHT was developed that can be used to improve clinical reporting in head trauma cases.[64] Additionally, **Table 4-13** identifies characteristics of injuries that help to determine their cause as accidental or inflicted.

Table 4-13. Recognizing When a Child's Injury or Illness Is Caused by Abuse

Visible Injury	Characteristic of the Injury
External Eye Injuries	— Common in children; not clear-cut evidence of abuse.
Two Black Eyes	— Seldom occur together accidentally.
Raccoon Eyes	— Associated with accidental and nonaccidental fractures at the base of the skull. — Usually associated with more swelling and skin injury from nonaccidental trauma. — History helps distinguish between accidental and inflicted.
Hyphema	— Traumatic entry of blood into front eye chamber — May result from nonaccidental injury caused by striking eye with a hard object (eg, belt buckle). — Possible complaints of pain in eye; visual problems
Retinal Hemorrhages	— Hallmark of AHT — Only rarely associated with some other mechanism of injury.
Nonaccidental Trauma	— Always considered in child aged younger than 3 years with retinal hemorrhages or any traumatic disruption of globe eye (eg, the lens or retina) or the skin around the eye.

Tin Ear Syndrome

The diagnosis of head injury encompasses injuries to the ears and the eyes. The health care provider should evaluate the child's ear for tin ear syndrome, which results from blunt trauma to one ear. Tin ear syndrome may present with bruising of the injured ear, cerebral edema, and hemorrhagic retinopathy on the same side. There may also be bruising and hemorrhaging in the antitragus and helix; findings are similar to those seen in AHT or whiplash. The mechanism of injury for tin ear syndrome may be inflicted or accidental as in the case of sports injuries. When CT, magnetic resonance imaging (MRI), or plain films of the head are needed in cases of possible head injury, the health care provider should consider adding chest views to look for current rib fractures and evidence of healed fractures.

Physical Examination

Table 4-14 is a guideline for the steps to complete when conducting the physical examination for the child suspected of having head trauma.

Table 4-14. Guidelines for Physical Examination in Head Injury

Skin	— Check torso and neck for fingertip bruising.
Head and Scalp	— Examine and palpate for trauma. — Check for swelling or bruising. — Check ears.
Retinal Examination	— Direct fundoscopic evaluation; assess for retinal hemorrhages. — Indirect ophthalmoscopy (by ophthalmologist) — Check for specific types of hemorrhages. — Check for vitreous bleeding.
Glasgow Coma Scale (GCS)	— Evaluate level of consciousness. — GCS can be difficult to apply in infants and young children.

Adapted from Monteleone J, Brodeur A. Identifying, interpreting, and reporting injuries. In: Monteleone JA, ed. Child Maltreatment: A Clinical Guide and Reference. *2nd ed. St. Louis, MO: GW Medical Publishing; 1998:1-29.*

Radiographic Evaluation of Head Injury

Radiographic findings are important in helping to identify nonaccidental cranial trauma because the clinical presentation of head injury can often be nonspecific or misleading. A CT scan identifies CNS injury and is superior in the acute setting over an MRI for evaluation of acute hemorrhage. While an MRI offers the highest sensitivity and specificity for uncovering subacute and chronic injury, the American Academy of Pediatrics (AAP) recommends delaying the use of an MRI for up to 7 days for children who are acutely ill.[40] An MRI can help determine whether both old and new blood is present within a hemorrhage but may fail to detect acute subdural or subarachnoid hemorrhage.[42] The technique of diffusion-weighted imaging (DWI) reveals nonhemorrhagic posttraumatic infarction much earlier than can be seen with a conventional MRI. A study showed that DWI provided an indicator of severity that was more complete than other imaging modalities. DWI may help to guide management decisions through the identification of children at high risk for poor outcome.[65]

Mouth and Teeth

During the physical examination, the health care provider should pay special attention to the mouth, gums, and mucosal lining of victims of child abuse. Positive findings include palatal petechiae, mucosal tears, lacerations, and abrasions or tears of the frenulum and tongue.[66] The teeth should be examined for chipping, dislocation, cleanliness, and signs of decay. In sexual abuse, the mouth should be examined for signs of trauma and infection secondary to forced oral-genital contact.[66]

There are many ways in which trauma can occur to a child's teeth and mouth structures. A caregiver may become frustrated during feeding and use excessive force to push the bottle nipple into the infant's mouth, thereby causing contusions to the labial frenulum, the tissues of the vestibule, and the alveolar ridge.[24,67] Common oral injuries seen in cases of child abuse include fracture, displaced or avulsed teeth, oral contusions, frenulum tears, lacerations, jaw fractures, and burns.[66]

Poisoning

Accidental poisoning is a common medical emergency in pediatrics. 2010 statistics showed that children aged 3 years and younger accounted for 37.7% of the 2.38 million cases of reported toxin exposures; children younger than 6 years of age accounted for half of the reported cases.[68] Intentional poisoning is a different occurrence than accidental poisoning and is a form of child physical abuse. Intentional poisoning may be used as a type of discipline or punishment with the age of the child most affected under 2 years.[69,70] There are documented incidents of intentional poisonings by adults for the purpose of punishment, amusement, attempted suicide of caregiver and child for reasons decided by the adult, and quieting the child.[71] The common agents that poison children are outlined in **Table 4-15**.

Table 4-15. Common Agents That Poison Children

Common Agents That Poison Children	
Prescription Medications	— Opioids — Sedative-hypnotics — Cardiovascular agents[74]
Nonprescription Medications	— Ipecac — Laxatives
Food Products	— Pepper — Salt — Water — Sugar — Apple juice concentrate — Alcoholic beverages — Vitamin A
Miscellaneous	— Carbon monoxide Household substances — Antifreeze — Lye — Sodium carbonate — Naphtha and other hydrocarbons — Illegal drugs

Adapted from Bays J, Feldman K. Child abuse by poisoning. In: Reece R, Ludwig S, eds. Child Abuse: Medical Diagnosis and Management. *2nd ed. Philadelphia, PA: Lippincott, Williams, and Wilkins; 2001:405-411.*

Intentional poisoning is a less common form of child abuse and may be initially overlooked. The delay in detecting intentional poisoning may be due to a lack of obvious physical cues and historical information.[73] Health care providers often do not consider poisoning in the differential diagnosis and as a result may not obtain appropriate toxicology screens that would determine the presence of poisonous substances.[74]

Intentional poisoning of a child is often more lethal than accidental poisoning and must be considered in any case of abuse.[71] Ideally, the perpetrator's underlying motivation will become clearer through the history taking and physical examination. In such cases, the caregiver often does not mention the possibility of poisoning as the cause of the child's distress and denies the possibility of poisoning as a potential cause when broached by the health care provider.[70]

Physical Examination

The physical examination of the child with suspected poisoning provides direction for treatment and helps to determine whether a decrease in CNS function is drug induced or related to other causes of comas. The main focus of the examination should be on the CNS and autonomic nervous systems (ANS), eye findings, changes in skin or oral and gastrointestinal mucous membranes, and odors. The assessment findings form a collection of signs and symptoms referred to as ***toxidromes.*** Toxidromes include those symptoms produced by exposure to adrenergic, anticholinergic, anticholinesterase, opioid, sedative hypnotic agents, and certain heavy metals. Discovering the child's symptoms and physical responses to the poisoning agent may help to identify a specific toxidrome.[75]

The child who has been a victim of intentional poisoning commonly presents with the following signs: coma, apnea, drowsiness, ataxia, lethargy, vomiting, diarrhea, dehydration, stridor, and red diapers or signs of hemorrhagic diarrhea.[70,71,75] For example, sympathomimetic substances cause increased pulse and pupillary dilation, and cholinergics cause bradycardia and urinary incontinence. **Tables 4-16** and **4-17** include recommendations for what to include in the physical examination of the child suspected of being poisoned (see also **Tables 4-18** to **4-20**).

Table 4-16. Criteria to Include in the Physical Examination of a Suspected Poisoning Victim

Cardiac and Vital Signs	— Pulse — Heart rhythm — Temperature (normal, warm, cool) should be warm — Capillary refill (time in seconds): 2 seconds (normal) — Blood pressure ranges[76] (see **Table 4-17**)
Pulmonary Function	— Assessment of respiration (normal or respiratory distress) — Respiration effort (normal, increased, decreased): normal effort — Breath sounds (equal, asymmetric, wheezing, rales): clear, equal lung sounds bilaterally — Excursion — Visible movement, depth, symmetry — Equal chest excursion — Respiratory pattern — Apnea — Stridor
Neurological Examination	— Pulse — Heart rhythm — Temperature (normal, warm, cool) should be warm — Capillary refill (time in seconds): 2 seconds (normal) — Blood pressure ranges[76] (see **Table 4-17**)
Gastrointestinal and Genitourinary Examination	— Assessment of respiration (normal or respiratory distress) — Respiration effort (normal, increased, decreased): normal effort

(continued)

Table 4-16. Criteria to Include in the Physical Examination of a Suspected Poisoning Victim *(continued)*

Gastro-intestinal and Genitourinary Examination *(continued)*	— Breath sounds (equal, asymmetric, wheezing, rales): clear, equal lung sounds bilaterally — Excursion — Visible movement, depth, symmetry — Equal chest excursion — Respiratory pattern — Apnea — Stridor

Skin Assessment	— Facial and nasal mucosa
	— Mucous membranes
	— Signs of intentional poisoning
	  — Restraint marks
	  — Intravenous (IV) injections sites
	  — Bruises or signs of physical abuse
	  — Burns
	  — Presence of powder on skin

Odors	— Evaluation of odors
	  — Acetone: isopropyl alcohol, phenol, and salicylates
	  — Bitter almond: cyanide
	  — Garlic: heavy metals, organophosphates
	  — Oil of wintergreen: methyl salicylate
	  — Gasoline: hydrocarbons

Adapted from Welliver J. Unusual injuries. In: Ludwig S, Kornberg AE, eds. Child Abuse: A Medical Reference. *2nd ed. New York, NY: Churchill Livingstone, 1992:213-222. Adapted from Bays J, Feldman K. Child abuse by poisoning. In: Reece R, Ludwig S, eds.* Child Abuse: Medical Diagnosis and Management. *2nd ed. Philadelphia, PA: Lippincott Williams & Wilkins; 2001:405-441. Adapted from Coulter K, Scalzo A. Poisoning. In: Monteleone JA, ed.* Child Maltreatment: A Clinical Guide and Reference. *2nd ed. St. Louis, MO: GW Medical Publishing; 1998:315-326.*

Table 4-17. Blood Pressure Ranges

Age	Systolic/Diastolic (mm Hg)
1 month	86/54
1 year	96/65
4 years	99/65
6 years	100/60
8 years	105/60
10 years	110/60
12 years	115/60
14 years	118/60
16 years	120/65

Table 4-18. Identifying Specific Toxicological Syndromes

Poison Syndrome	Symptoms and Signs	Drug
Sympathomimetic	Increased pulse and blood pressure Fever Papillary dilation Sweating Agitation Psychosis	Cocaine Barbiturates Phencyclidine
Sympatholytic	Decreased pulse and blood pressure Hypothermia Small pupils Decreased peristalsis Obtundation Coma	Ethanol Barbiturates Sedative hypnotics Opiates
Cholinergic	Bradycardia Miosis Sweating Hyperperistalsis Salivation Bronchorrhea Urinary incontinence	Organophosphates Carbamates Nicotine
Anticholinergic	Tachycardia Hypertension Fever Papillary dilation Hot dry skin Decreased peristalsis Urinary retention	Tricyclic antidepressants Antihistamines Phenothiazines Atropine Scopolamine

Adapted from Olsen K, Banner W. Emergency management of childhood poisoning. In: Grossman M, Dieckmann R, eds. Pediatric Emergency Medicine: A Clinician's Reference. *Philadelphia, PA: Lippincott Williams & Wilkins; 1991:332-339.*

Table 4-19. Signs Indicating That a Child Has Swallowed a Toxic Substance

—Severe throat pain

—Difficulty breathing

—Behavior changes, such as unusual sleepiness or jumpiness

—Nausea or vomiting

—Stomach cramps

—Lip or mouth burns

—Stains from the poison around lips or mouth

—Clothing stains

—Unusual drooling

—Smell of child's breath

—Unusual eye movements, such as inability to follow an object with the eyes or eyes going around in circles

—Unconsciousness or seizures

—Open or empty container of a toxic substance found near child

Table 4-20. Toxidromes

Toxidrome	Presentation	Vital Sign Changes	Causative Agents
Anticholinergic	Delerium Flushed skin Dilated pupils Urinary retention Decreased bowel sounds Memory loss Seizures "Hot as a hare, dry as a bone, red as a beet, blind as a bat."	Tachycardia Hyperthermia Hypertension	Antihistamines Scopolamine Jimson weed Angel trumpet Benztropine Tricyclic Antidepressants Atropine
Cholinergic	Confusion Weakness Salivation Lacrimation Defecation Emesis Diaphoresis Muscle fasciculations Miosis Seizures	Bradycardia Hypothermia Tachypnea	Organophosphates Carbamates Mushrooms
Hallucinogenic	Disorientation Hallucinations Visual illusions Panic reaction Moist skin Hyperactive bowel sounds Seizures	Tachycardia Tachypnea Hypertension	Amphetamines Cannabinoids Cocaine Phencyclidine (PCP)
Opiate/Narcotic	Altered mental status Unresponsiveness Miosis Shock	Shallow respirations Slow respiratory rate Bradycardia Hypothermia Hypotension	Opiates Propoxyphene Dextromethorphan
Sedative/ Hypnotic	Coma Stupor Confusion Sedation Progressive deterioration of CNS function	Apnea	Barbiturates Benzodiazepines Ethanol Anticonvulsants
Sympathomimetic	Delusions Paranoia, diaphoresis Piloerection Mydriasis Hyperreflexia Seizures Anxiety	Tachycardia Bradycardia (if pure alpha agonist) Hypertension	Cocaine Amphetamines Methamphetamine Phenylpropanolamine Ephedrine Pseudoephedrine Albuterol Ma huang

Reprinted with permission from Florida Poison Information Center Jacksonville. Toxidromes. Florida Poison Information Center Jacksonville Web site. http://www.fpicjax.org/Toxidromes.htm. Accessed June 23, 2013.

Laboratory Data

Many poisons can be detected in the urine or blood; therefore, laboratory data can help to confirm the diagnosis of poisoning. Ordering specific tests for poisoning is based on the history and physical examination. A toxicology screen can detect a number of drugs including alcohol; marijuana; opioids, such as heroin and codeine; aspirin; acetaminophen; amphetamines; benzodiazepines, such as diazepam and chlordiazepoxide; and cocaine.[77] It is possible to get serum blood levels on some drugs, such as acetaminophen, phenytoin (Dilantin), theophylline, digoxin, and lithium. Also, an electrocardiogram (ECG) may reveal toxicity in medications that affect the electrical activity of the heart. Laboratory tests also include serum osmolality, glucose, electrolytes, creatinine, and blood urea nitrogen (BUN) to determine if other organs might be affected by poisoning.[75]

Specific Examination Issues Related to Cases of Suspected Sexual Abuse

The physical examination of the suspected child victim of sexual abuse is a fundamental component of the overall health care evaluation. The focus of the evaluation should be on the child's health status and determining whether or not there are physical findings consistent with the abuse. In most cases of sexual abuse, the examination reveals normal or nonspecific genital or anal findings.[1,78] Additionally, in the majority of cases, there is a low likelihood of forensic evidence due to the dynamics of child sexual abuse and the typical pattern of a time lapse between the actual abuse and the child's disclosure of the situation to others[79-82] (see *Chapter 6, Sexually Transmitted Infection in the Setting of Child Maltreatment; Chapter 11, Sexual Abuse of Adolescents;* and *Chapter 20, Forensic Nursing*).

Time Frame for Forensic Examination

With the exception of stranger rape, most cases of child sexual abuse do not present as an acute assault situation. A sexual assault examination is usually completed if alleged contact occurred within 72 hours from the time of the evaluation. This timeframe has been set based on experience with adult sexual assault victims and the likelihood of finding useful forensic evidence during the examination.[83,84] The child suspected of having been sexually abused should receive a full health care evaluation, to include a complete physical examination to inspect the genitalia for suspicious findings and to determine treatment for any conditions resulting from the sexual contact.[83-85] One of the best predictors of discovering abnormal findings in the female genital examination is the timeframe between the actual assault and the examination.[86,87] The closer the examination is to the actual assault, the better the possibility of finding physical evidence of the assault.[79,81,88] As time passes, the likelihood of finding traces of forensic evidence on the child or clothing is decreased. A physical examination can be delayed pending further investigation in situations where sexual contact occurred more than 72 hours before the health care visit and there are no immediate physical complaints, such as discharge or bleeding. In this situation, the focus of the evaluation shifts from the collection of forensic evidence to the identification of possible physical findings, since forensic evidence has usually disappeared from the child by this time.[79,83,88]

The Examination Conducted within 72 Hours of Alleged Sexual Assault

The examination of a child victim of sexual abuse within 72 hours of alleged contact should focus on determining physical findings that can confirm sexual contact and the collection of forensic specimens that may still be present on or in the child's body, clothing, or other environmental materials, such as linens or upholstery. The examiner should use a forensic evidence collection kit, at times called a rape kit, when there is reason to believe that evidence of trace elements and seminal products may be present[84,89] (**Figure 4-23**). It is essential that all evidence be collected and packaged appropriately because it will be examined in a crime laboratory and possibly used as evidence in legal proceedings; therefore, only practitioners who have experience in the collection and preservation of forensic evidence shouls use a rape kit.

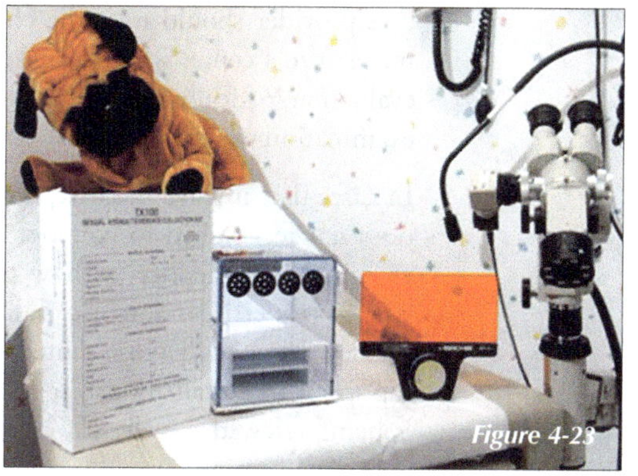

Figure 4-23. *Sexual assault kit and tools. Children's Assessment Center; Houston, Texas. (Contributed by Paul Kuntz, Photographer, Texas Children's Hospital; Houston, TX.)*

The child's body should be inspected for the presence of semen and saliva using an ultraviolet (UV) light, a Wood's lamp, or another alternate light source. Any areas suspected of having such evidence should be swabbed and then the swabs dried to preserve the evidence. Swabs with specimens collected from the mouth, vagina or penis, and rectum are dried, packaged appropriately, and, following the proper chain of evidence, given to police for transport to the police crime laboratory. The clinician should collect any debris on the child's body and send it to the crime laboratory by way of the police as well. The child's clothing should be placed into paper bags for crime laboratory analysis (see *Chapter 5, Laboratory Findings, Diagnostic Testing, and Forensic Specimens in Cases of Child Sexual Abuse*).

Anal and genital injuries are rarely found during the physical examination of the suspected victim of child sexual abuse,[84,90] since most injuries to the genital and anal tissues resulting from sexual abuse are superficial and heal quickly.[78,90] Superficial injuries in children heal in 48 to 72 hours. Injuries resulting from sexual abuse may be fresh if less than 72 hours have passed between the assault and the examination, whereas injuries older than 72 hours will be in various stages of healing. Specific physical or emotional signs of sexual abuse at the time of the child's examination may include:

— Vaginal or penile discharge

— Indications of sexually transmitted infections (STIs) (eg, discharge)

— Acute rectal or vaginal bleeding

— Severe emotional distress in child or caregiver

— Possible pregnancy in the pubertal child

Examiner Expertise

The question often arises as to whether a health care provider who does not usually conduct a child sexual abuse evaluation has the ability to appropriately evaluate a child in cases where sexual abuse is suspected. To evaluate possible abuse findings, the health care provider must be knowledgeable of normal genital anatomy as well as variations in genital and anal tissue that are consistent with abuse. Health care providers who are inexperienced with sexual abuse evaluations have diagnosed normal variations in anatomy as findings of abuse. It is best for all aspects of a sexual abuse evaluation that the clinician be someone who understands how to conduct the evaluation and document assessment findings.[84] A health care provider who is not familiar with abuse evaluation may doubt his or her ability to perform the genital examination and may, therefore, be unclear about the nature of the findings of the physical examination. In this case, the health care provider should refer the child to an expert examiner, such as a certified SANE nurse or to a center where sexual abuse evaluations are routinely conducted, for further evaluation.[82] Ideally, a child should undergo only one physical examination because the examination experience can be emotionally upsetting.

In cases that involve the investigation of a possible crime, a health care provider who does not feel skilled to conduct such an evaluation can consult with an experienced examiner for guidance on how to proceed or defer the full examination to someone who has expertise in forensic evaluation. The recommendation may be that the child be evaluated at a child abuse center where health care providers have expertise in performing specialized evaluations. In either case, the examiner would document that the child is being referred to a health care provider or child abuse center that can provide the appropriate examination.[84]

Knowledge of Normal Genital Anatomy and Findings Indicative of Sexual Abuse

A study of pediatric nurse practitioners (PNPs) found concerning differences in the PNP's familiarity with normal genital anatomy and their knowledge of when to report significant findings as suspected child sexual abuse.[7] Other studies examining the knowledge base of family practitioners and pediatricians regarding the identification of child sexual abuse and normal and abnormal genital findings found that physicians and nurse clinicians also had difficulty identifying specific findings of child sexual abuse.[8-10,91] The findings of these studies suggest that practitioners must reestablish their knowledge base of normal anatomy in the context of a general health screening and child sexual abuse evaluations (**Figure 4-24**). Additionally, the health care provider may make referrals to those more experienced with child sexual abuse evaluations as needed.

Stress Associated with Sexual Abuse Evaluations

Studies show that the genital examination is a stressful experience for prepubertal children and adolescents.[5,92,93] The anticipation of a genital examination is usually stress provoking for the child and adolescent as well. Studies of children have also shown that the fear associated with the examination is greater than that associated with a regular doctor visit but that the evaluation is less traumatic when performed in a controlled setting by experienced providers who support the child psychologically[92,93] (see *Appendix 4-1, Genital Evaluation Protocol Script).*

Steward et al[94] found that children were not generally retraumatized by the colposcope examination of the genital area and that the child's anxiety was lessened after completion of the examination. Few data support the examination as a form of revictimization to the child.[12] The genital examination distress scale (GEDS) objectively measures the emotional distress of a child during the anogenital component of the sexual abuse evaluation.[95] The GEDS tool is used while the child undergoes the examination and may help compare different approaches to the examination. Generally, children respond well to the examination when someone talks with them about the purpose of the process and what to expect in the evaluation[96] (see *Appendix 4-2, Genital Examination Distress Scale*).

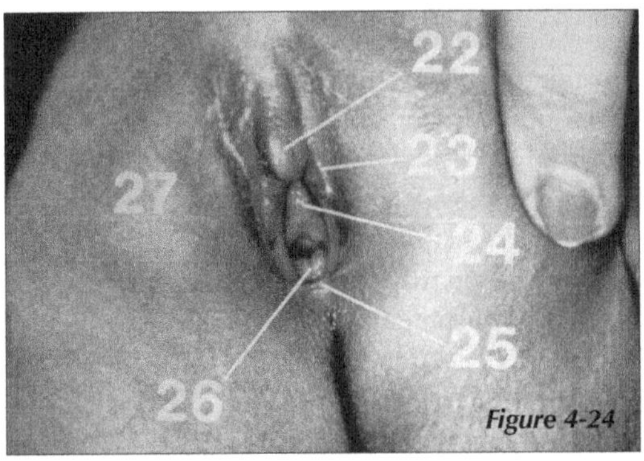

Figure 4-24. *Identifying prepubescent anatomy (answers follow below): 22: clitoris, 23: labia minora, 24: urethral orifice, 25: posterior fourchette, 26: hymen 27: labia majora. Reprinted with permission from Ladson S, Johnson C, Doty R. Do physicians recognize sexual abuse?* Am J Dis Child. *1987;141(4):411-415. © 1987, American Medical Association. All rights reserved.*

Setting

The setting for the medical examination is important. A child who requires immediate medical attention and is brought to a health care institution is typically seen in a hospital emergency room (ER). The examination room should, ideally, be dedicated to child abuse evaluations and have adequate lighting and video colposcopy to facilitate the examination.[3] Other visualization enhancement tools such as lighted magnifying glasses may be used in situations where optimal equipment is unavailable.[3] When the sexual abuse evaluation is not urgent, health care providers can refer the child to a child abuse center. Centers provide for the needs of children and offer a friendly, comfortable environment with clinicians who are experts in evaluating and treating cases of abuse. Child abuse centers have furniture that accommodates children, child friendly lighting, and toys available in the waiting areas (**Figure 4-25**). The employees at child abuse referral centers are experts in dealing with the issues of child sexual abuse and offer the child and caregiver a relaxed environment for the evaluation to take place.

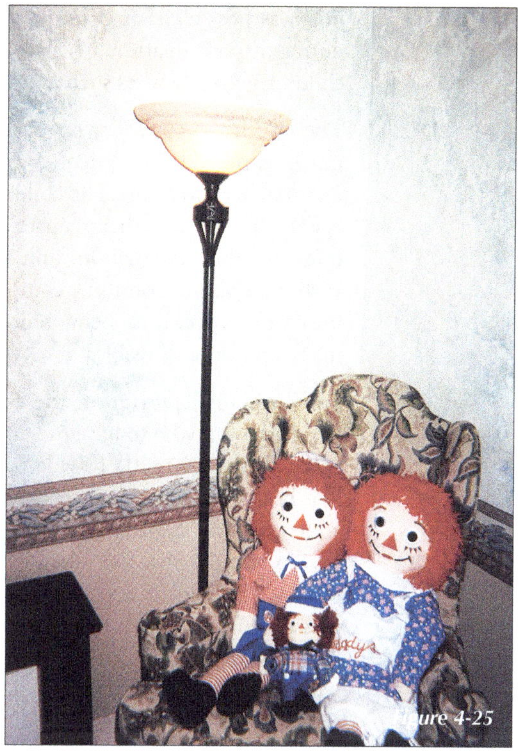

Figure 4-25. *A child abuse center provides a child-friendly setting.*

Preparing the Child for the Interview and Physical Examination

Sexual abuse, at its most basic level, is a violation of trust by an older or more powerful person toward a child.[84] Perpetrators of child sexual abuse are often someone the child knows, such as a family member, neighbor, or an individual met through organized activities or in school.[97] The abuse by a trusted person becomes a form of betrayal to the child; therefore, the child's ability to trust other adults may be marred by the circumstances of the abuse situation.[98]

The interview process is the time for the health care provider to begin to establish a short-term relationship with the child who may have difficulty trusting an adult. Rapport is essential when performing a complete physical examination and collecting forensic evidence. The process of building trust and rapport with the child starts by explaining the importance of the examination.[3,99] Children respond to sincerity, so the examiner should be open, honest, and straightforward and should assure the child that he or she is interested in the child's health and well-being and wants to determine what has happened with the child. In cases of suspected sexual abuse, the practitioner must prepare the child for the examination techniques that may be required to complete the forensic examination.

Children with a history of abuse need to feel like they have some control of the examination process because the health care evaluation involves an adult seeing and touching the child's body. Because the abuser took an element of control from the child's life, it is important to give the child as much control over the examination as possible. Using an approach that builds confidence and trust is essential because physically forcing or coercing a child to undergo an examination against his or her will is never appropriate. Giving the child as much control in the examination as the examiner can potentially reduce anxiety and help gain cooperation during the examination.[100] The need for the physical examination itself is not negotiable, but many aspects of the examination can be negotiated. The child should be allowed to control aspects of the examination as much as possible. For example, the child can decide what gown or clothing to wear during the examination, where to sit, and what parts of the examination to do first. The child may keep clothes such as underwear or socks on as long as possible.

The health care provider should allow the child to participate in the examination as much as possible and encourage the child to become familiar with the examination instruments and room. The child should be allowed to use the stethoscope and listen to his or her heart and then palpate his or her own "belly." The child can choose the time frame for the examination, unless the health of the child is in danger. Some children wish the examination to be completed as quickly as possible, while others wish to take breaks to recover from being touched. The health care provider should give the child as many options as possible.

For the genital portion of the examination, the child can choose what to hold and, within reason, who to have present in the room. It is helpful for the child to see how the colposcope works and, if a video colposcope is used, to view the picture on the screen.[101] The health care provider can show the child how the image is viewed on the colposcope screen by first showing the image of the child's face, hands, or feet. Once the child is comfortable with the instrument and the projection process, then it is appropriate to film the genital area and let the child also view that part of the examination. It is reassuring to the child to see, feel, and hear what the examiner is seeing, hearing, and feeling. The clinician can reassure the child by explaining health considerations, whenever possible, as the examination progresses.

Figure 4-26-a. *Exam Room with colposcope. This system has the ability to visualize anatomy and injury that may not be easily visible to the naked eye.*

Figure 4-26-b. *Colposcope. (Contributed by Nancy D. Kellogg, MD; San Antonio, TX.)*

Use of a Colposcope in the Anogenital Examination

A colposcope is a useful instrument for the detection and recording of genital injury (**Figure 4-26-a** and **b**). It provides a noninvasive method for visualizing the anogenital structures of the male or female child.[3] Colposcopy provides magnification and an excellent light source that is helpful in identifying and capturing injury on film.[102] The health care provider can take still images during the examination by attaching a 35-mm camera to the colposcope. A video camera can be attached to the colposcope to document the examination through still photography or videotape. Video images have advantages over still photography because the variability of the anogenital anatomy is more easily viewed.[103]

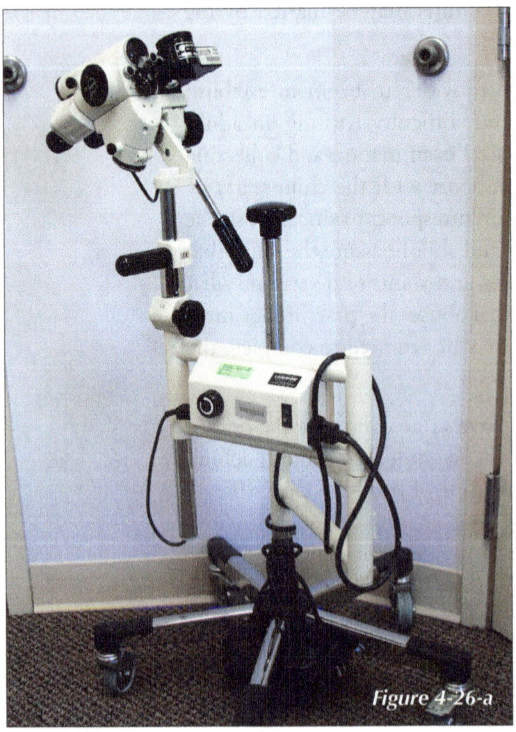

Figure 4-26-a

Allowing the opportunity for a child to observe the genital examination by watching the video colposcope screen causes a demystification of the process for the child and a resultant sense of increased con-

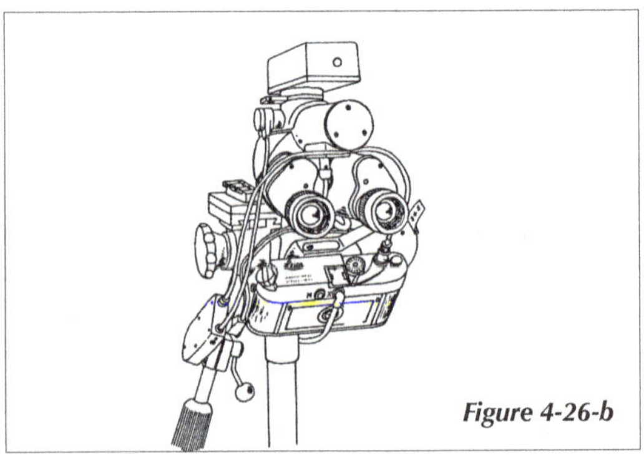

Figure 4-26-b

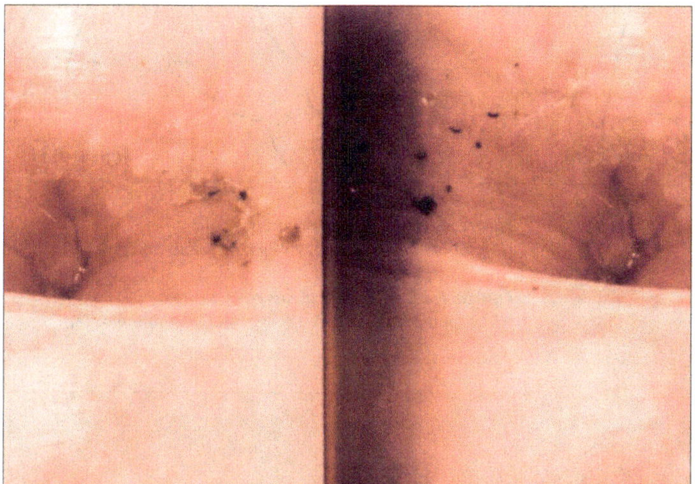

Figure 4-27

Figure 4-27. *Incorrect positioning of patient, photocolposcope, or both for knee-chest position resulting in an inadequate photograph of anus. (Contributed by Nancy D.Kellogg, MD; San Antonio, TX.)*

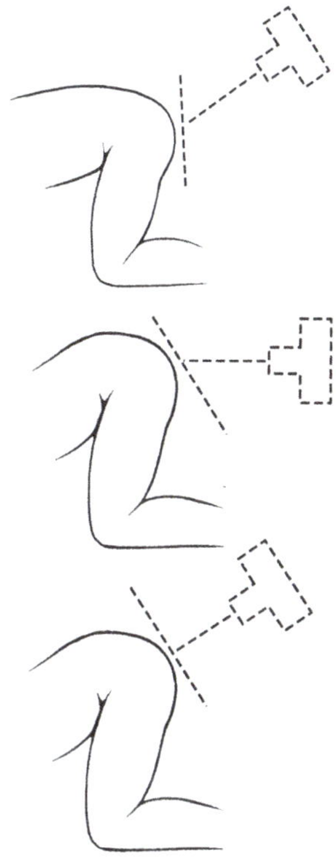

Figure 4-28

Figure 4-28. *Top: incorrect patient position (lower back not lordotic); Middle: incorrect photocolposcope position (colposcope not high enough); Bottom: correct position (lens is at right angle to photograph subject).*

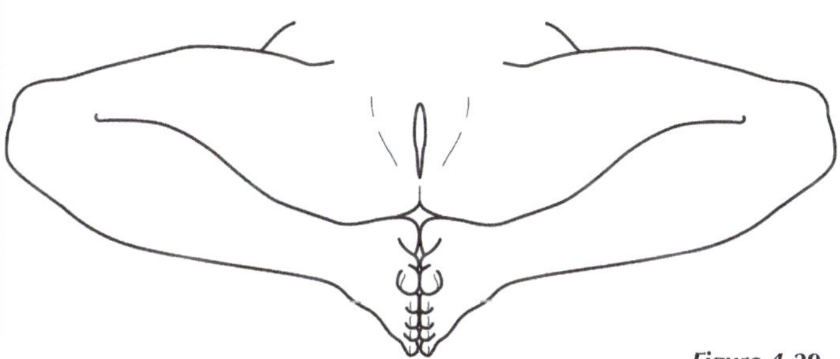

Figure 4-29

Figure 4-29. *Supine frog-leg position. (Contributed by Nancy D. Kellogg, MD; San Antonio, TX.)*

trol over the examination situation.[102] A study of children who underwent video colposcopy found that children generally watched their evaluation and were cooperative and enthusiastic throughout the examination.[80]

Position for Genital Evaluation

For the genital examination, the child should be placed in a comfortable position that also enables the examiner to view the genitalia (**Figures 4-27** and **4-28**). Children can be examined on a caregiver's lap or when sitting or lying on an examination table. Because the examination itself and the position required for viewing the genitalia may mimic the abuse, it is important to avoid any position or situation that reminds the child of the abuse.

In prepubertal and pubertal girls, the most common examination positions include the supine frog-leg, frog-leg while sitting on a person's lap, and prone knee-chest position (**Figures 4-29** and **4-30**). The lithotomy position is acceptable for pubertal girls. For boys, the genital examination may be performed in the sitting, standing, supine, or lateral decubitus position (**Figure 4-31**).[104,105] Visualization of the external genitalia,

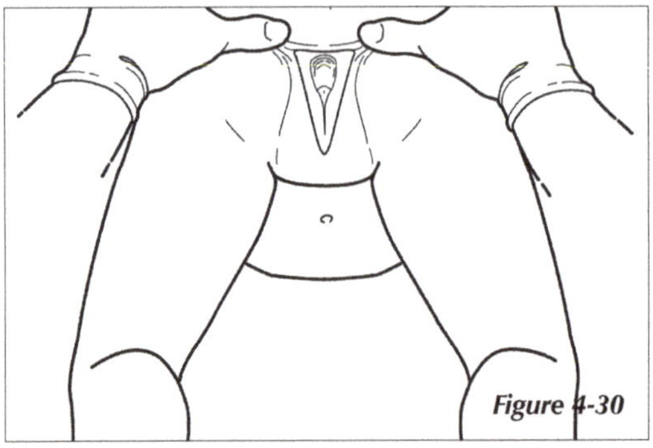

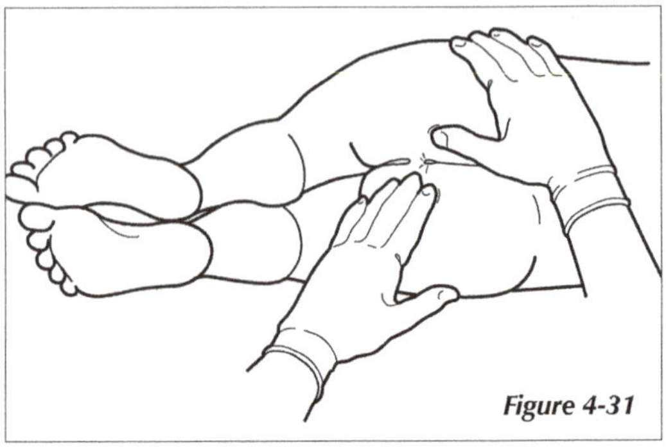

Figure 4-30. *Prone knee-chest position. (Contributed by Nancy D. Kellogg, MD; San Antonio, TX.)*

Figure 4-31. *Lateral decubitus position. (Contributed by Nancy D. Kellogg, MD; San Antonio, TX.)*

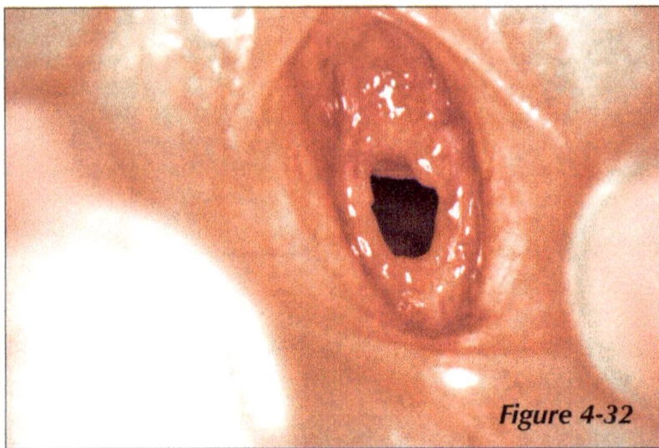

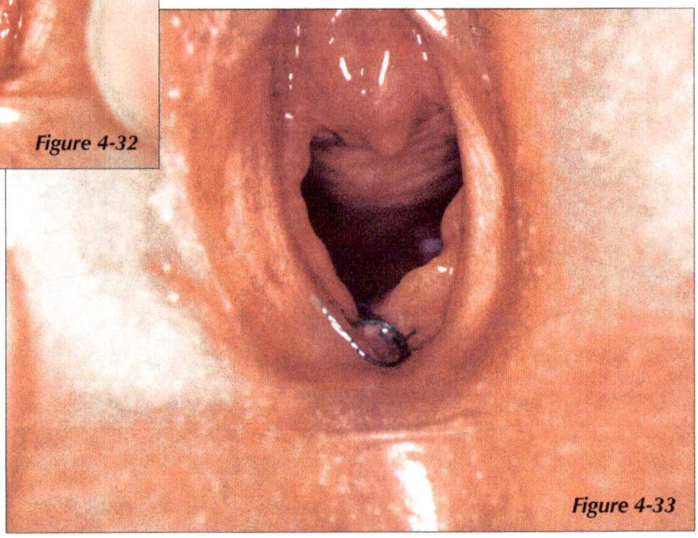

Figure 4-32. *Infant in supine frog-leg position; hymenal orifice is annular with a "bump" at 1 o'clock position and a small "notch" at 10 o'clock position. Hymenal membrane is thin, translucent, and no interruption of scarring present. (Contributed by Carol D. Berkowitz, MD; Torrance, CA.)*

Figure 4-33. *Child examined in supine frog-leg position after genital trauma. Exam reveals suture in place at 6 o'clock position to stop bleeding from injury. Hymenal edge is irregular and asymmetric. (Contributed by Carol D. Berkowitz, MD; Torrance, CA.)*

including the hymen, is all that is required. The position in which the child is examined should be documented in the record.

It is important for the child to be as relaxed as possible to better view the hymen or anus. When relaxed, the health care provider is better able to visualize hymenal edges and the outline of the vaginal opening.[106] Both the supine frog-leg position and knee-chest position with the buttocks raised allow for good visualization of the hymen (**Figures 4-32** and **4-33**). The prone knee-chest position, because of the effects of gravity, is the best to achieve dilatation of the vaginal vault and hymenal orifice but is often the most uncomfortable for the child.[107] Lateral positions can be used if preferred by the child, are commonly used for male examinations, and allow for anal examinations for boys and girls. A good light source is necessary regardless of the positions used.

Anatomy and Terminology Discussed in Child Sexual Abuse

The examination of a child who has been sexually abused requires knowledge of genital and anal anatomy. Such knowledge assists the health care provider in differentiating between normal and abnormal findings and variations between injuries and anatomical variations. Knowledge of proper terminology and clinical findings also assists in documentation.[108] Documentation must be as specific as possible and stated in a language known and used by other health care providers. Basic terms used by health care providers include the following:

— ***Vulva:*** All of the components of the external genitalia to include the mons, labia majora and minora, clitoris, vaginal orifice

— ***Perineum:*** Between the thighs, between the vulva and anus in girls and between the scrotum and anus in boys

— ***Vestibule:*** Between the labia minora, the clitoris, and the posterior fourchette

— ***Posterior fourchette:*** Formed by the posterior joining of the labia minora

— ***Hymenal membrane:*** Recessed in the vestibule; the internal surface of the hymenal membrane marks the beginning of the vagina.

— ***Fossa navicularis:*** Posterior attachment of the hymen and the fourchette

Sexual Abuse Physical Examination

The physical examination in the sexual abuse evaluation always occurs in the context of a complete head-to-toe examination. In cases of suspected sexual abuse, the examiner seeks to determine if there are physical injuries or forensic findings consistent with sexual abuse. A complete examination is necessary despite the expectation that sexual abuse evaluations often reveal minimal to no physical findings. Health care providers must be aware that during the comprehensive examination, a condition unrelated to the suspected sexual abuse may be uncovered. The lack of physical findings in examinations for suspected sexual abuse also reinforces the need for a comprehensive health care evaluation that goes beyond the physical examination and forensic evidence collection. A comprehensive evaluation searches for additional indicators of abuse, such as specific historical information and nonspecific physical and behavioral complaints that are common in children who have been sexually victimized.[109]

Forensic findings may include the perpetrator's body fluids such as semen, saliva, or blood.[66] Conducting a forensic evidence evaluation during the examination is often dependent on the amount of time that has passed between the last occurrence of suspected sexual abuse and the health care evaluation. If sexual abuse occurred less than 72 hours from the time of the examination, the examination focus is on physical findings and collecting forensic specimens that may still be present on or in the child's body, clothing, or other environmental material.

Genital Examination

The findings of the genital examination of children who have been sexually abused are often normal or nonspecific.[86,90,110,111] A lack of physical findings should not be seen as evidence that sexual abuse did not occur. The lack of definitive physical findings in cases of sexual abuse may be related to the nature of the sexual contact that the perpetrator may have engaged the child in during the abuse; the length of time between the abuse and the disclosure and subsequent arrival to a health care setting for evaluation; and the relatively rapid healing observed in the mucous membranes of the child's anogenital tissues.

Examination requires patience, training, and experience because injury is often subtle. Experience is needed to determine the normalcy of genitalia at various developmental stages and ages. The genital examination of males and females begins with visualization of the external genitalia. It is necessary to evaluate Tanner staging for both sexes and then document the child's stage in the record. For the genital evaluation of girls, the Huffman staging system provides a frame-work from which to assess the level of estrogenization of the tissues (**Tables 4-21** and **4-22**) (see *Chapter 11, Sexual Abuse of Adolescents*).

Table 4-21. Huffman Rating

Stage 1	— Birth to about 2 months of life; maternal estrogen effects evident. — Hymen typically appears as follows: — Thick — Pink in color — Moist — Actual secretions may be present. May see small amount of blood as the maternal estrogen effect decreases postnatally.
Stage 2	— Low endogenous estrogen — Occurs from about age 2 months to about 6 or 7 years. Hymen typically appears as follows: — Thin — Translucent or whitish in color — Minimal secretions — Hymen typically appears dry
Stage 3	— Body begins producing more estrogen. Tanner staging gives indications of estrogen effect. — Typically, this stage occurs between the ages of 7 and 13 — Hymen appears as follows: — More pink in color — Thicker — Somewhat lubricated
Stage 4	— This is the premenarcheal stage. — Genitalia more adult-like in appearance — Hymen appears as follows: — Lubricated — Thick — Pink and opaque — Tanner staging consistent with endogenous estrogen production

Adapted from Huffman JW. The Gynecology of Childhood and Adolescence. *Philadelphia, PA: WB Saunders Company; 1969.*

Table 4-22. Adams' Approach to Interpretation of Medical Findings in Suspected Child Sexual Abuse: 2009

This table lists medical and laboratory findings; however, most children who are evaluated for suspected sexual abuse will not have signs of injury or infection. The child's description of what happened to him or her and the child's report of specific symptoms in relationship to the events described is an essential part of the full medical evaluation.

FINDINGS DOCUMENTED IN NEWBORNS OR COMMONLY SEEN IN NON-ABUSED CHILDREN

The presence of these findings generally neither confirms nor discounts a child's clear disclosure of sexual abuse.

Normal variants

1. Periurethral or vestibular bands
2. Intravaginal ridges or columns
3. Hymenal bumps or mounds
4. Hymenal tags or septal remnants
5. Linea vestibularis (midline avascular area)
6. Hymenal notch/cleft in the anterior (superior) half of the hymenal rim (prepubertal girls), on or above the 3 o'clock–9 o'clock line with patient supine
7. Shallow/superficial notch or cleft in inferior rim of hymen below 3 o'clock–9 o'clock line
8. External hymenal ridge
9. Congenital variants in appearance of hymen, including crescentic, annular, redundant, septate cribiform, microperforate, and imperforate
10. Diastasis ani (smooth area)
11. Peri-anal skin tag
12. Hyperpigmentation of the skin of labia minora or peri-anal tissues in children of color, such as Mexican-American and African-American children
13. Dilation of the urethral opening with application of the labial traction
14. "Thickening hymen" (May be due to estrogen effect, folded edge of hymen, swelling from infection, or swelling from trauma. The latter is difficult to assess unless follow-up examination is done.)

Findings commonly caused by other medical conditions

15. Erthema (redness) of the genital tissues (May be due to irritants, infection, or dermatitis.)
16. Increased vascularity ("dilatation of existing blood vessels") of vestibule and hymen (May be due to local irritant or normal pattern in non-estrogenized state.)
17. Labial adhesion (May be due to irritation or rubbing.)
18. Vaginal discharge (There are many infectious and noninfectious causes. Cultures must be taken to confirm if caused by sexually transmitted organisms or other infections.)
19. Friability of the posterior fourchette or commisure (May be due to irritation, infection, or an examiner's traction on the labia majora.)
20. Anal fissures (Usually due to constipation, peri-anal irritation.)
21. Venous congestion or venous pooling in the peri-anal area (Usually due to positioning of child; also seen with constipation.)

Conditions Mistaken for Abuse*

22. ***Urethral prolapse****
23. ***Lichen sclerosus et atrophicus****
24. ***Vulvar ulcers (May be caused by many types of viral infections, including Epstein-Barr virus (EBV) and influenza, or by conditions such as Behcet's disease or Crohn's disease.)****
25. ***Failure of midline fusion, also called perineal groove****
26. ***Rectal prolapse (Often caused by infection, such as Shigella sp.)****
27. ***Complete dilation of the internal and external anal sphincters, less than 2 centimeters in AP diameter, revealing the pectinate line****

(continued)

Table 4-22. Adams' Approach to Interpretation of Medical Findings in Suspected Child Sexual Abuse: 2009 *(continued)*

28. ***Partial dilation of the external anal sphincter, with the internal sphincter closed, causing the appearance of deep folds in the peri-anal skin that can be mistaken for signs of injury****

29. ***Marked erythema, inflammation, and fissuring of the peri-anal or vulvar tissues due to infection with Group A beta hemolytic streptococci****

Conditions Mistaken for Abuse*

22. *Urethral prolapse**

23. *Lichen sclerosus et atrophicus**

24. *Vulvar ulcers (May be caused by many types of viral infections, including Epstein-Barr virus (EBV) and influenza, or by conditions such as Behcet's disease or Crohn's disease.)**

25. *Failure of midline fusion, also called perineal groove**

26. *Rectal prolapse (Often caused by infection, such as Shigella sp.)**

27. *Complete dilation of the internal and external anal sphincters, less than 2 centimeters in AP diameter, revealing the pectinate line**

28. ***Partial dilation of the external anal sphincter, with the internal sphincter closed, causing the appearance of deep folds in the peri-anal skin that can be mistaken for signs of injury****

29. ***Marked erythema, inflammation, and fissuring of the peri-anal or vulvar tissues due to infection with Group A beta hemolytic streptococci****

INDETERMINATE FINDINGS: INSUFFICIENT OR CONFLICTING DATA FROM RESEARCH STUDIES, OR NO EXPERT CONSENSUS

These physical and laboratory findings may support a child's clear disclosure of sexual abuse, if one is given, but should be interpreted with caution if the child gives no disclosure. Report to Child Protective Services may be indicated in some cases.

30. Deep notches or clefts in the posterior/inferior rim of hymen that extend through more than 50% of the width of the hymen

31. Deep notches or complete clefts in the hymen at the 3 o'clock or 9 o'clock location in adolescent girls

32. Marked, immediate anal dilation to an AP diameter of 2 cm or more, in the absence of other predisposing factors such as chronic constipation, sedation, anesthesia, and neuromuscular conditions

33. Genital or anal condyloma accuminata in child, in the absence of other indicators of abuse. ***Lesions appearing for the first time in a child older than 5-8 years may be more suspicious for sexual transmission.****

34. Herpes Type 1 or 2 in the genital or anal area in a child with no other indicators of sexual abuse. ***Isolated genital lesions caused by HSV-2 in a child older than 4-5 years may be more suspicious for sexual transmission.***

FINDINGS DIAGNOSTIC OF TRAUMA AND/OR SEXUAL CONTACT

The following findings support a disclosure of sexual abuse, if one is given, and are highly suggestive of abuse even in the absence of a disclosure, unless a clear, timely, plausible description of accidental injury is provided by the child and/or caretaker. ***Photographs or video recordings of these findings should be reviewed by an expert in a sexual abuse evaluation for a second opinion to assure accurate diagnosis.****

Acute trauma to external genital/anal tissues

35. Acute lacerations or extensive bruising of labia, penis, scrotum, peri-anal tissues, or perineum (May be from unwitnessed accidental trauma or from physical or sexual abuse.)

36. Fresh laceration of the posterior fourchette, not involving the hymen (Must be differentiated from dehisced labial adhesion or failure of midline fusion [see #25]. Posterior fourchette lacerations may also be caused by accidental injury or by consensual sexual intercourse in adolescents.)

(continued)

Table 4-22. Adams' Approach to Interpretation of Medical Findings in Suspected Child Sexual Abuse: 2009 *(continued)*

Residual (healing) injuries
These rare findings are difficult to assess unless an acute injury was previously documented at the same location.

37. Peri-anal scar (May be due to other medical conditions such as Crohn's disease, accidental injuries, or previous medical procedures.)
38. Scar or posterior fourchette or fossa (Pale areas in the midline also be due to linea vestibularis or labial adhesions.)

Injuries indicative of blunt force penetrating trauma (or from abdominal/pelvic compression injury if such history is given)

39. Extensive bruising on the hymen
40. Laceration (tear, partial, or complete) of the hymen (acute)
41. Peri-anal lacerations extending deep to the external anal sphincter (not to be confused with partial failure of midline fusion)
42. Hymenal transection (healed). An area between 4 o'clock and 8 o'clock on the rim of the hymen, where it appears to have been torn through to or nearly to the base, so there appears to be virtually no hymenal tissue remaining at that location. This finding has also been referred to as a "complete cleft" in sexually active adolescents and young adult women.
43. Missing segments of hymenal tissue. Area in the posterior (inferior) half of the hymen, wider than transection, with an absence of hymenal tissue extending to the base of the hymen, which is confirmed using additional position or methods.

Presence of infection confirms mucosal contact with infected and infective bodily secretions; contact most likely to have been sexual in nature

44. Positive confirmed culture for gonorrhea from genital area, anus, or throat in a child outside neonatal period
45. Confirmed diagnosis of syphilis, if perinatal transmission is ruled out
46. Trichomonas vaginalis infection in a child older than 1 year of age, with organisms identified by culture or, in vaginal secretions, by wet mount examination
47. Positive culture from genital or anal tissues for Chlamydia, if child is older than 3 years at time of diagnosis and if specimen was tested using cell culture or comparable method approved by the Centers for Disease Control
48. Positive serology for HIV if perinatal transmission, transmission from blood products, and needle contamination have been ruled out

Diagnostic of sexual contact

49. Pregnancy
50. Sperm identified in specimens taken directly from a child's body

**Changes from the version published in 2007 are in bold italics.*

Adapted from Adams J, Kaplan R, Starling S, et al. Guidelines for medical care of children who may have been sexually abused. J Pediatr Adolesc Gynecol. *2007;20(3):163-172.*

Reprinted from Adams J. Medical evaluation of suspected child sexual abuse: 2009 update. APSAC Advisor. *2010:2-7.*

Reprinted by permission of the American Professional Society on the Abuse of Children, 350 Poplar Avenue, Elmhurst, IL 60126. Email apsac@apsac.org. Web www.apsac.org. Phone 877-402-7722.

The health care provider must carefully observe the genitalia for scarring, tears, abrasions, bruising, decreased amount or absence of hymenal tissue, and contour of the hymenal opening (**Figures 4-34** and **4-35**). It is important to accurately document examination findings of any injury to the area. The location of injuries should be noted in relationship to the face of a clock placed over the child in the anatomical position. The use of a colposcope is paramount to completing a thorough inspection. Keep in

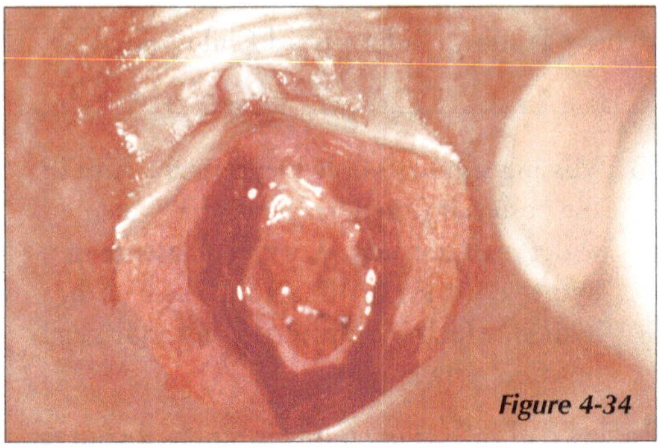

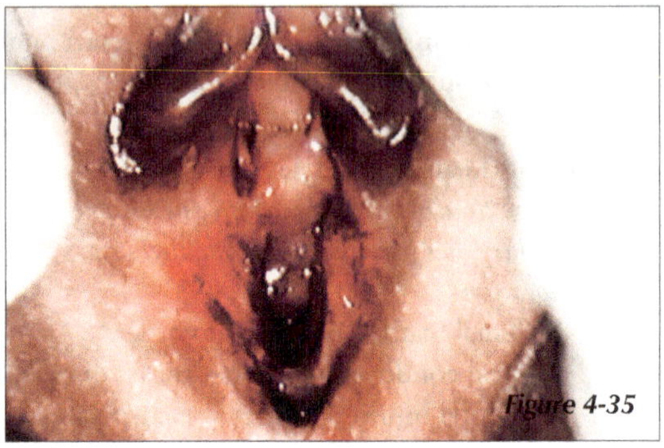

Figure 4-34. *Child whose genital examination reveals bruising on medial aspects of labia minora, hymenal trauma with disruption of hymenal tissue, and fresh blood. (Contributed by Carol D. Berkowitz, MD; Torrance, CA.)*

Figure 4-35. *Infant with significant bruising involving labia minora and labia majora, hymenal trauma with disruption of hymen, and fresh blood. (Contributed by Carol D. Berkowitz, MD; Torrance, CA.)*

mind that the lack of specific physical findings in the examination of suspected sexual abuse does not rule out the diagnosis of child sexual abuse. It is uncommon to find serious physical injury in a child victim of sexual abuse, and any detected injury is usually minor and rarely requires medical intervention. It is a rare case that a child-sexual-abuse-related injury requires suturing.

It is usually difficult for a child to describe sexual activity adequately. Actual penetration of a young child's vagina is unusual, even when a child seems to be describing such an event. What is more common is vulvar coitus, in which the offender rubs an erect penis between the labia for sexual stimulation. To the child, the perception may be penetration. Vulvar coitus can produce abrasions and bruising but does not usually disturb the hymen. If an examination were completed immediately after the abuse, the examination would reveal redness and swelling of the labia. Even short periods of time between the actual abuse and the evaluation will allow for healing of the tissue. Additionally, if the male perpetrator ejaculated during the abuse, a seminal deposit on the genitalia, the abdomen, or lower back of the child might be found if the child has not bathed. If semen or saliva is present on the external genitalia, the area should be swabbed for evidence collection.

In the male examination, the health care provider should document Tanner staging and circumcision status. The health care provider should then inspect the penis, scrotum, testicles, and perineum for signs of trauma, such as bite marks, bruising, abrasions, and suction ecchymosis. When the foreskin is intact, it is advisable to retract the foreskin and inspect the base of the glans.[106]

Evaluation of the Hymen

It is not usually possible to determine whether sexual abuse has occurred by the examination findings.[84] The appearance of the normal hymen in prepubertal and postpubertal children varies. The range of normal variants is wide, and examination techniques and positioning of the child can affect what the examiner sees. Studies have found normal-appearing genital tissues as well as nonspecific findings in children for whom sexual abuse by way of vaginal penetration is known to have occured.[84]

The diameter of the hymen is easy to describe, while thickness and degree of elasticity are more difficult to quantify. The prepubertal hymen has a variety of orifice configurations described as annular, crescentic, fimbriated, cribriform, or septate[84] (**Figures 4-36** to **4-39**). The most common shapes are crescentic and annular. Estrogen affects the hymen as it does all periurethral tissue. Maternal estrogen affects the appearance of the newborn hymen by causing a thick and redundant appearance. The estrogen effect changes after 2 to 3 months and then reappears again as the child approaches puberty. Estrogen creates a thicker and paler appearance of the hymen (**Figures 4-40** and **4-41**).

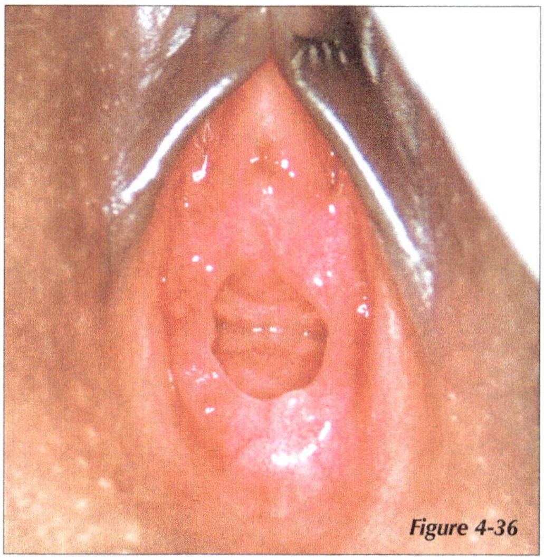

Figure 4-36

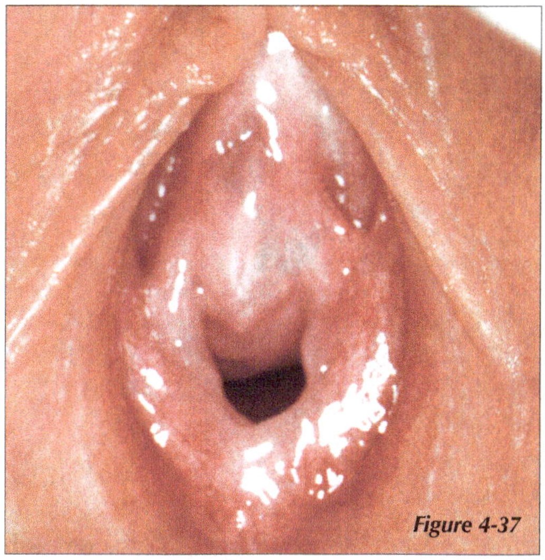

Figure 4-37

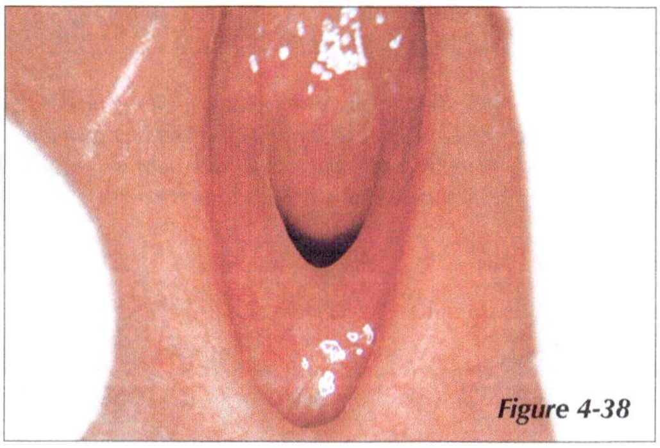

Figure 4-38

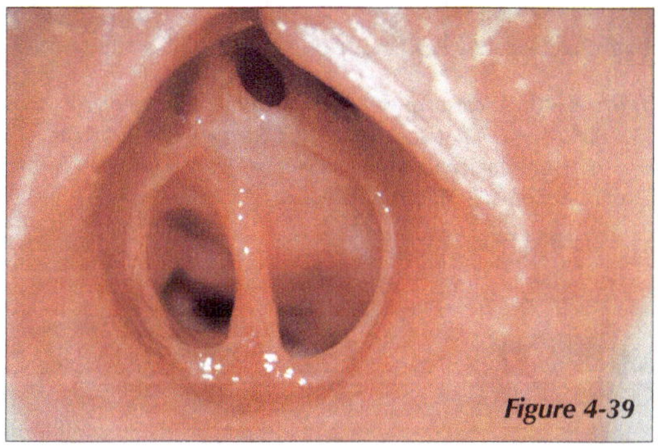

Figure 4-39

Figure 4-36. *Annular hymen, early estrogen. (Contributed by Martin A. Finkel, DO, FACOP, FAAP; Stratford, NJ.)*

Figure 4-37. *Ten-year-old with crescentic hymen. (Contributed by Martin A. Finkel, DO, FACOP, FAAP; Stratford, NJ.)*

Figure 4-38. *Crescentic hymen, translucent edge. (Contributed by Martin A. Finkel, DO, FACOP, FAAP; Stratford, NJ.)*

Figure 4-39. *Septate hymen. (Contributed by Martin A. Finkel, DO, FACOP, FAAP; Stratford, NJ.)*

The prepubertal unestrogenized hymen has an appearance of involuted tissue and tends to appear more vascular and reddened.[84] Normal hymenal appearance varies between thick and elastic and thin and nonelastic.[84]

Visualization of the hymen and the component parts of the vestibule in girls often requires separation and mild labial traction (**Figures 4-42** to **4-44**). The hymen is visualized with positioning and gentle traction only. Traction is applied by grasping the labia majora between the clinician's thumb and forefinger and gently applying traction downward and laterally.[3,106] The clinician applies gentle traction to prevent injury and to make the orifice appear larger. The hymenal membrane of the prepubertal child is innervated and can be sensitive to touch.[84]

An unestrogenized hymenal edge is tender, so touching the hymen with items such as a cotton-tipped applicator or applying too much traction can be uncomfortable for the child. Warm saline solution may be applied by way of a catheter or syringe to "float" the hymen and allow better visualization of the hymenal edges.[3,106] The examiner may also use moistened cotton swabs to move the hymen and enhance visualization. Another technique that may be used to enhance visualization is the gentle insertion of a Foley catheter into the vagina.[84] When using this technique to view the estrogenized hymen, improved visualization occurs by inserting a partially inflated Foley catheter into the vaginal vault behind the hymenal membrane,[107] resulting in mild retraction and stretching of the tissues. A vaginal speculum is never used with children who have not reached puberty. For the prepubertal child who has unexplained bleeding

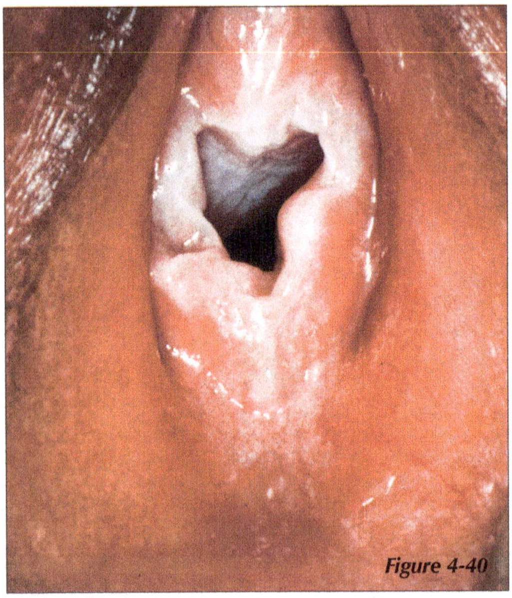

Figure 4-40. *Adolescent genital exam reveals estrogenized hymenal tissue (pink, thick, opaque); orifice appears irregular secondary to significant redundancy of tissue. (Contributed by Carol D. Berkowitz, MD; Torrance, CA.)*

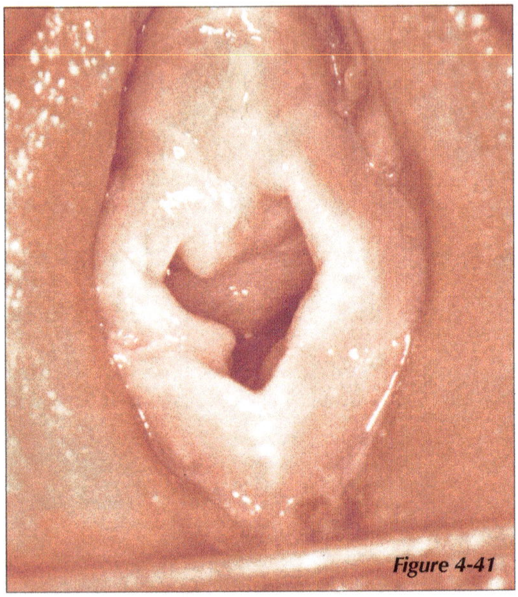

Figure 4-41. *Adolescent genital exam showing estrogenized hymenal tissue (pink, thick, opaque); orifice is irregular owing to areas of redundancy, specifically at 9 o'clock position. (Contributed by Carol D. Berkowitz, MD; Torrance, CA.)*

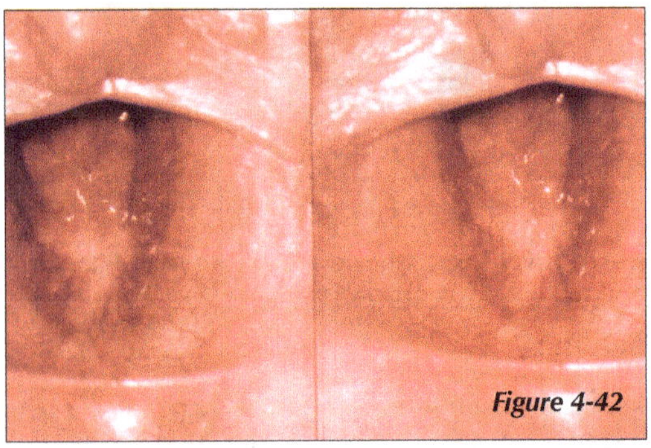

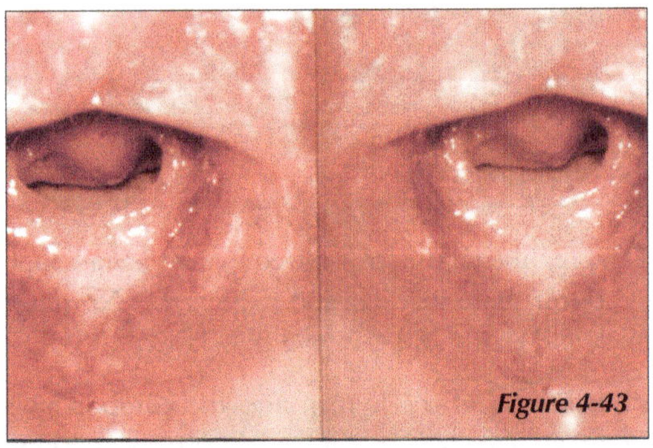

Figure 4-42. *Labial separation. (Contributed by Nancy D. Kellogg, MD; San Antonio, TX.)*

Figure 4-43. *Labial traction (same patient as Figure 4-42). (Contributed by Nancy D. Kellogg, MD; San Antonio, TX.)*

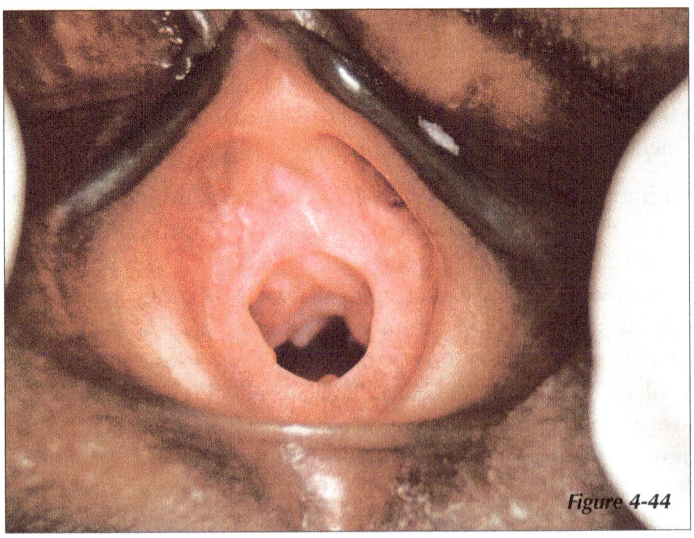

Figure 4-44. *Hymenal appearance with labial traction and separation. (Contributed by Martin A. Finkel, DO, FACOP, FAAP; Stratford, NJ.)*

or other unusual findings, a speculum examination, when indicated, should be done under sedation or anesthesia if there is a true need to evaluate the child's findings more fully.[104]

The penis can cause trauma to the clitoral hood or the fourchette resulting in irritation or discomfort. Periurethral irritation can cause dysuria. Fondling of the female child can create erythema, abrasions, scratches, and edema. Most fondling does not result in serious trauma unless a digit is introduced forcefully into the vagina. Children who are fondled may complain of dysuria after the event. This symptom is related to irritation and inflammation of the urethra.[3]

Anal Examination

It is important that the examiner be knowledgeable of anatomy of the anus and the rectum and the correct technique for completing an anal and rectal examination for suspected sexual abuse. The anatomy of the anus and rectum includes the anal sphincter that is covered with tissue called the anal verge. The hemorrhoidal plexus is located within the loose connective tissue surrounding the external orifice, while the external tissue has symmetrical radiating folds known as the rugae.

The anus and perianal area are evaluated with the child in a frog-leg supine, knee-chest, lithotomy with buttocks separation, or lateral decubitus position.[3] The knee-chest position is more awkward for the child to assume and may be the position in which a child was victimized. The rectum should be carefully inspected for injury using gentle retraction of the gluteal folds during inspection of the tissues.[104] A trained clinician may need to perform an anoscopic examination if acute injury of the rectum is noted. It is typically not necessary to insert a gloved finger into the anus.[106] As the gluteal folds are separated, the perianal muscles typically tighten reflexively; this tightening may also be stimulated by brushing the examiner's hand against the medial aspect of the child's buttock.

Laxity of anal sphincter tone may be noted after chronic abuse, but may also be present in normal situations, such as when stool is present in the distal part of the child's rectum.[3] Abnormal findings that may be indicate abuse include lacerations, bruising, ulcerations, external and internal scarring, bleeding, or fissures. Inflammation is seen as redness, swelling, or tenderness of perianal tissues.[92]

In sexual abuse evaluations, careful inspection for lacerations and abrasions of the anus in various stages of healing is a necessary part of the examination. The anus of a child may or may not be penetrated. Gluteal coitus occurs when the perpetrator rubs the dorsal shaft of the penis over the external anal tissues, causing pressure perceived as penetration. A penile shaft rubbed between the gluteus and over the rectum may cause abrasions, and if ejaculation occurs, seminal products may be present on the tissues and collected.

Differential Diagnosis for Child Sexual Abuse

Several conditions may create findings that mimic findings of sexual abuse. Of course, the given history should support these nonabusive etiologies. Among the more common differential diagnoses are the following:

— Accidental injury (eg, a fall creating bruising or abrasion on the superficial areas in the genital region, such as the mons, labia majora, buttocks, or the penis and scrotum)

— Infection creating vulvovaginitis from organisms such as *Candida albicans* or from pinworms (*Enterobius vermicularis*)

— Diaper dermatitis

— Foreign bodies such as toilet paper placed into the vagina (**Figures 4-45** and **4-46**)

— Labial adhesions secondary to mild inflammation, often related to poor hygiene

— Anal fissures related to constipation

The differential diagnosis for genital findings is presented in more detail in *Chapter 7, Differential Diagnosis: Conditions That Mimic Child Maltreatment.*

Conclusion

The physical examination of a suspected victim of child abuse is an essential part of the complete medical and psychosocial evaluation and treatment plan. The health care provider must consider many aspects of conducting the examination process, such as interview techniques, gathering appropriate assessment findings, and documenting physical examination findings. The data from the physical examination is an important component in the investigation of the allegation of child abuse. Health care providers play an important role in identifying and referring possible victims of child abuse and treating any physical injuries the child may have received during an abusive episode. Therefore, evaluating children suspected of being abused requires expertise over and above that necessary for a usual examination.

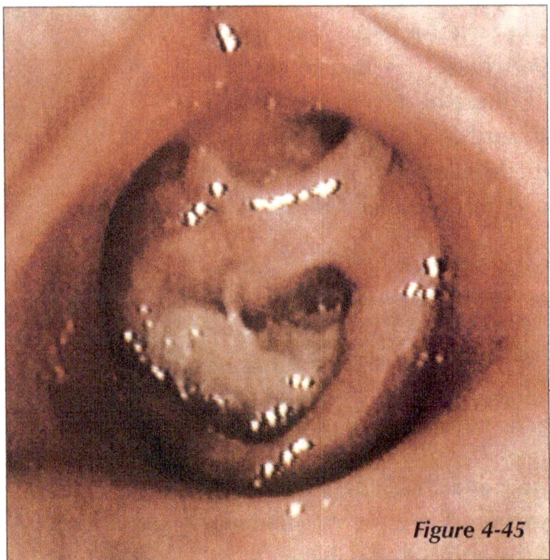

Figure 4-45. *Prepubertal child with foul-smelling, bloody discharge who, on examination, reveals the presence of a foreign body in the vagina just past the hymenal orifice. The foreign body appears to be toilet tissue that had become lodged in the vagina and colonized with bacteria. The presence of the foreign body caused a vulvovaginitis to develop. Foreign body was dislodged with gentle water flushing during exam. (Contributed by Carol D. Berkowitz, MD; Torrance, CA.)*

Figure 4-46. *Another view of foreign body in child from Figure 4-45. (Contributed by Carol D. Berkowitz, MD; Torrance, CA.)*

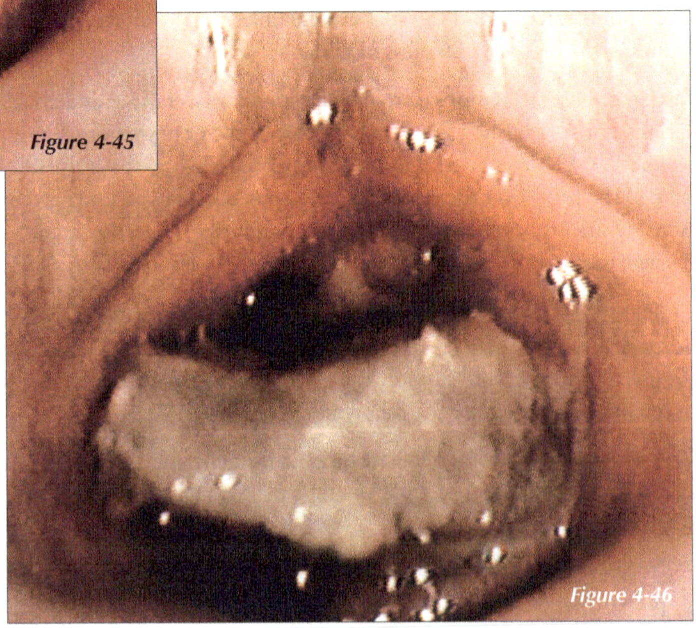

Appendix 4-1: Genital Evaluation Protocol Script

Genital Evaluation Protocol Script

Purpose: *To promote coping with the sensations and emotions felt during genital evaluation*

Outcome: *The child will actively participate in the evaluation*

Procedure Information

Nurse: My name is Ms. Lawson, and I'm going to show you everything Dr. Moore will do when she comes to examine you. Have you ever been to the doctor before?

Child: Yes, Dr. Briggs looks at my ears when they hurt. He gives me medicine that tastes like bubblegum.

Nurse: Has he ever let you look inside his ears?

Child: (Shakes her head no, looks wide-eyed, and leans toward nurse.)

Nurse: Would you like to use this light to look in mine?

Child: (Shakes her head no, pulls away.)

Nurse: Well, how about if mom looks in my ears? (Nurse positions otoscope so mother can see through.)

Child: Here! Let me see!

Nurse: What do you see?

Child: Something shiny and white.

Nurse: What's it doing now? (Nurse insufflates.)

Child: It wiggles! (Child pulls away, exclaims to her mother, and then looks again.)

Nurse: What you saw was my eardrum, and when it wiggled it was because I put a little puff of air on it like this (nurse demonstrates insufflator on child's hand). That's what Dr. Moore will do when she looks in your ears. If your eardrum is shiny like that and it wiggles, it means you're not sick and you don't need medicine. That's the point of this whole thing: to see if what happened made you sick or hurt. If it did, we'll give you what you need to get well.

Child: But I'm not sick. At least, I don't think I am. What do you mean by, "What happened"?

Nurse: Well, remember when you told Ms. Carol about what your granddad did?

Child: She told you?

Nurse: Of course she did. She wants to make sure you're okay. That's why she helped your mom bring you to the doctor. We know that you've done nothing to be ashamed of. What happened is your granddad's mistake—he's the one who did something wrong.

Child: So what happens to him? Oh, I know. The cop said he'd arrest granddad if he hurt me.

Nurse: And what we want to figure out is if he hurt you. Okay?

Child: Okay. (She sits straight, uses matter-of-fact tone of voice.) What's next?

Nurse: Well, next, Dr. Moore will want to look at your eyes.

(continued)

Genital Evaluation Protocol Script *(continued)*

Child: He didn't do anything to my eyes (scornfully).

Nurse: I know, but all your body parts are important—no one part is more important than the other. (Describes and rehearses eye examination, then proceeds through the heart and lung examination, then to the abdominal examination.)

Nurse: Once she's through listening to your lungs, Dr. Moore will check your tummy, so let's practice that part. Will you lie down with your head here?

Child: (Child lies down and looks up expectantly.)

RELAXATION EXERCISE

Nurse: Every 7-year-old girl I ever saw was ticklish. Are you?

Child: (Giggles and says yes.)

Nurse: Would you like to learn a way to not be ticklish when you don't want to be?

Child: Sure!

Nurse: Okay, then bend your knees up (demonstrates). That makes your tummy soft. Now find a spot on the ceiling and take a deep breath—in through your nose—out through your mouth (demonstrates).

Child: (Child tries several times then figures out how to regulate her breathing.)

Nurse: Now that you've figured that out, let's go to the next step. Take another deep breath in—let it out—and let all the muscles in your face get soft. Now take a deep breath in—let it out— and let the muscles in your shoulders get soft.

Child: (Child complies.)

Nurse: (Continues to pace child, gently touching each body part. Mentions each major body part, including her bottom. Pays particular attention to any body part that seems tense. If the child begins to giggle, gives her time to "get the giggles out." When she is completely focused and relaxed, says:) See! I touched you all over—even your tummy—and you didn't even giggle. That's because you can't feel giggly and relaxed at the same time. That will be helpful to you when Dr. Moore goes to the next part of the examination, which is to look at your "privacy" (use child's term). So to get that part done, you have to let this knee go to the wall (tap far knee), and let this muscle get soft (tap inner thigh). Then let this knee come toward me, and let the muscle get soft (positions the child in frog-leg position).

Child: Ooh. Yuk (face tense).

Nurse: Sometimes children tell me that when they separate their knees like this, they feel nervous or embarrassed. (Go through several words describing negative emotional responses. Stop at the one that seems to produce a reaction.)

Child: Yeah, it's like I'm doing something nasty.

Nurse: Lots of kids tell me they feel nasty when they move their legs this way, but you know what to do.

Child: (Looks puzzled.)

Nurse: Oh, you know. Take a deep breath, blow it out, then let the muscles in your legs get soft.

Child: (Child complies.)

(continued)

Genital Evaluation Protocol Script *(continued)*

SENSATION INFORMATION

Nurse: Next, Dr. Moore will look at your privacy. Your privacy is little and hard to see, and it's protected by skin. Dr. Moore will put on these special glasses (show optical visor) to make your privacy look bigger so she can see it. She will move the skin out of the way, like this (pulls a little abdominal skin), so she can see. Then she'll touch your privacy with a Q-tip (allow the child to have one for her own). After that's done, you get to put your knees together and sit up. Dr. Moore will tap on your knees and tickle your feet, and that will be the end of that part. Do you have any questions?

Child: No, I think I'm ready.

Nurse: Okay, then you need to put on a gown. Which one do you want—the white or the blue one?

APPENDIX 4-2: GENITAL EXAMINATION DISTRESS SCALE

Genital Examination Distress Scale

Instructions: Immediately at the end of the medical examination for possible sexual abuse, rate the 7 indices of behavioral distress for the child during the anogenital phase of the procedure. If the behavior was not observed, assign 1 point; score 2 points if the behavior was somewhat displayed; a rating of 3 points should be made if the behavior was definitely displayed.

Not displayed = 1; somewhat displayed = 2; definitely displayed = 3

Rating

____ 1. Nervous behavior (eg, repeated nail biting, lip chewing, leg fidgeting, rocking, fingers in mouth, not listening)

____ 2. Cry (eg, crying sounds, tears or the onset of tears)

____ 3. Restraint (eg, Pressure is used to hold onto the child or physical attempts to keep the child from moving.)

____ 4. Muscular dystrophy (eg, tensing of muscles like clenched fists, facial contortions, or general body tightening)

____ 5. Verbal fear (eg, statement of apprehension or fear, such as "I'm scared," or "I'm worried.")

____ 6. Verbal pain (eg, statement of pain in any tense, such as "That hurt," "Owwwh," "You're pinching me," or "This will hurt")

____ 7. Flail (eg, random movement of arms, legs or body without trying to be aggressive, like pounding fists, throwing arms, or kicking legs)

REFERENCES

1. Adams J. Medical evaluation of suspected child sexual abuse: 2009 update. *APSAC Advisor*. 2010:2-7.
2. Giardino AP, Giardino E. Multidisciplinary teamwork issues related to child sexual abuse. In: Giardino AP, Datner E, Asher J, et al, eds. *Sexual Assault: Victimization Across the Life Span*. St. Louis, MO: GW Medical Publishing; 2003: 173-188.
3. Finkel M. The evaluation. In: Finkel MA, Giardino AP, eds. *Medical Evaluation of Child Sexual Abuse: A Practical Guide*. 2nd ed. Thousand Oaks, CA: Sage Publications; 2002:23-37.
4. Kirschner RH, Stein RJ. The mistaken diagnosis of child abuse: a form of medical abuse? *Am J Dis Child*. 1985;139(9):873-875.
5. Horner G, Scribano P, Curran S, Stevens J. Emotional response to the ano-genital examination of suspected sexual abuse. *J Forensic Nurs*. 2009;5(3):124-130.
6. Horner G. Genitourinary assessment: an integral part of a complete physical examination. *J Pediatr Health Care*. 2007;21(3):162-170.
7. Hornor G, McCleery J. Do pediatric nurse practitioners recognize sexual abuse? *J Pediatr Health Care*. 2000;14(2):45-49.
8. Ladson S, Johnson C, Doty R. Do physicians recognize sexual abuse? *Am J Dis Child*. 1987;141(4):411-415.
9. Lentsch KA, Johnson CF. Do physicians have adequate knowledge of child sexual abuse?: the results of two surveys of practicing physicians, 1986 and 1996. *Child Maltreat*. 2000;5(1):72-78.
10. Dubow SR, Giardino AP, Christian CW, Johnson CF. Do pediatric chief residents recognize details of prepubertal female genital anatomy: a national survey. *Child Abuse Negl*. 2005;29(2):195-205.
11. Mahat G, Scoloveno MA, Cannella B. Comparison of children's fears of medical experiences across two cultures. *J Pediatr Health Care*. 2004;18(6):302-307.
12. Britton H. Emotional impact of the medical examination for child sexual abuse. *Child Abuse Negl*. 1998;22(6):573-579.
13. Gully KJ, Britton H, Hansen K, Goodwill K, Nope JL. A new measure for distress during child sexual abuse examinations: the genital examination distress scale. *Child Abuse Negl*. 1999;23(1):61-70.
14. Lynch L, Faust J. Reduction of distress in children undergoing sexual abuse medical examination. *J Pediatr*. 1998;133(2):296-299.
15. Kellogg NK; The American Academy of Pediatrics Committee on Child Abuse and Neglect. The evaluation of sexual abuse in children. *Pediatrics*. 2005;116(1):506-512.
16. Virginia Department of Social Services. Child abuse and neglect: recognizing, reporting, and responding for educators. Virginia Department of Social Services Web site. http://www.dss.virginia.gov/family/cps/mandated_reporters/cws5691/topic1_1.html. Updated May 24, 2012. Accessed June 23, 2013.
17. Kellogg ND. Evaluation of suspected child physical abuse. *Pediatrics*. 2007; 119(6):1232-1241.

18. Swerdlin A, Berkowitz C, Craft N. Cutaneous signs of child abuse. *J Am Acad Dermatol.* 2007;57(3):371-392.

19. Harris TS. Bruises in children: normal or child abuse? *J Pediatr Health Care.* 2010;24(4):216-221.

20. Kessler DB, Hyden P. Physical, sexual, and emotional abuse of children. *Ciba Found Symp.* 1991;43(1):1-32.

21. Schwartz AJ, Ricci LR. How accurately can bruises be aged in abused children?: literature review and synthesis. *Pediatrics.* 1996;97(2):254-257.

22. Wilson EF. Estimation of the age of cutaneous contusions in child abuse. *Pediatrics.* 1977;60(5):750-752.

23. Farley RH, Reece RM; United States Department of Justice. *Recognizing When a Child's Injury or Illness Is Caused by Abuse.* Washington, DC: United States Department of Justice; 2002.

24. Mouden L. Oral injuries of child abuse. In: Monteleone JA, ed. *Child Maltreatment: A Clinical Guide and Reference.* 2nd ed. St. Louis, MO: GW Medical Publishing; 1998:59-66.

25. Hinchliffe J. Forensic odontology, part 4. human bite marks. *Br Dent J.* 2011;210(8):363-368.

26. Sweet D, Pretty IA. A look at forensic dentistry - part 2: teeth as weapons of violence—identification of bitemark perpetrators. *Br Dent J.* 2001;190(8):415-418.

27. Monteleone J, Brodeur A. Identifying, interpreting, and reporting injuries. In: Monteleone JA, ed. *Child Maltreatment: A Clinical Guide and Reference.* 2nd ed. St. Louis, MO: GW Medical Publishing; 1998:1-29.

28. Robson M, Heggers J. Pathophysiology of the burn wound. In: Carvajal HF, Parks DH, eds. *Burns in Children: Pediatric Burn Management.* St. Louis, MO: Year Book Medical Pub; 1988:27-32.

29. Davis A; United States Department of Health and Human Services, National Institutes of Health, National Institute of General Medical Sciences. Medicines by design. National Institute of General Medical Sciences Web site. http://publications.nigms.nih.gov/medbydesign/chapter2.html. Updated October 27, 2011. Accessed June 23, 2013.

30. Giardino AP, Christian CW, Giardino E. Evaluation of abuse and neglect. In: Giardino AP, Christian CW, Giardino E, eds. *A Practical Guide to the Evaluation of Child Physical Abuse and Neglect.* Thousand Oaks, CA: Sage Publications; 1997:23-59.

31. Giardino AP, Christian CW, Giardino E. Skin: bruises and burns. In: Giardino AP, Christian CW, Giardino E, eds. *A Practical Guide to the Evaluation of Child Physical Abuse and Neglect.* Thousand Oaks, CA: Sage Publications; 1997:61-95.

32. Maguire S, Moynihan S, Mann M, Potokar T, Kemp AM. A systematic review of the features that indicate intentional scalds in children. *Burns.* 2008;34(8):1072-1081.

33. Offiah A, van Rijn R, Perez-Rossello JM, Kleinman PK. Skeletal imaging of child abuse (non-accidental injury). *Pediatr Radiol.* 2009;39(5):461-470.

34. Berkowitz CD. Pediatric abuse: new patterns of injury. *Emerg Med Clin North Am.* 1995;13(2):321-341.

35. Kleinman PK, Marks SC, Richmond JM, Blackbourne BD. Inflicted skeletal injury: a postmortem radiologic-histopathologic study in 31 infants. *Am J Roentgenology.* 1995;165(3):647-650.

36. Kleinman PK, Marks SC. A regional approach to the classic metaphyseal lesion in abused infants: the distal femur. *Am J Roentgenology.* 1998;170(1):43-47.

37. Sirotnak AP, Krugman RD. Physical abuse of children: an update. *Pediatr Rev.* 1994;15(10):394-399.

38. Kocher MS, Kasser JR. Orthopaedic aspects of child abuse. *J Am Acad Orthop Surg.* 2000;8(1):10-20.

39. Landlin LA. Epidemiology of children's fractures. *J Pediatr Orthop B.* 1997;6:79-83.

40. American Academy of Pediatrics. Diagnostic imaging of child abuse. *Pediatrics.* 2009;123(5):1430-1435.

41. American College of Radiology. *ACR-SPR Practice Guideline for Skeletal Surveys in Children.* Reston, VA: American College of Radiology; 2011:3.

42. Belfer R, Klein B, Orr L. Use of the skeletal survey in the evaluation of child maltreatment. *Am J Emerg Med.* 2001;19(2):122-124.

43. Herendeen PM. Evaluation of physical abuse in children: solid suspicion should be your guide. *Adv Nurse Pract.* 2002;10(8):32-36.

44. Cooper A. Thoracoabdominal trauma. In: Ludwig S, Kornberg AE, eds. *Child Abuse: A Medical Reference.* 2nd ed. New York, NY: Churchill Livingstone; 1992:131-150.

45. Ludwig S. Visceral injury manifestations of child abuse. In: Reece RM, Ludwig S, eds. *Child Abuse: Medical Diagnosis and Management.* 2nd ed. Philadelphia, PA: Lippincott Williams & Wilkins; 2001:157-175.

46. Shenoi R. Abdominal and thoracic trauma. In: Giardino AP, Lyn MA, Giardino ER, eds. *A Practical Guide To The Evaluation Of Child Physical Abuse And Neglect.* 2nd ed. New York: Springer; 2010:207-229.

47. Ross AH, Abel SM, Radisch D. Pattern of injury in child fatalities resulting from child abuse. *Forensic Sci Int.* 2009;188(1):99-102.

48. Duhaime AC, Christian CW, Rorke LB, Zimmerman RA. Nonaccidental head injury in infants: the "shaken-baby syndrome." *N Engl J Med.* 1998;338(25):1822-1829.

49. Duhaime AC, Partington MD. Overview and clinical presentation of inflicted head injury in infants. *Neurosurg Clin N Am.* 2002;13(2):149-154.

50. Reece R, Sege R. Childhood head injuries: accidental or inflicted? *Arch Pediatr Adolesc Med.* 2000;154(1):11-15.

51. Lancon JA, Haines DE, Parent AD. Anatomy of the shaken baby syndrome. *Anat Rec.* 1998;253(1):13-18.

52. Goldberg KB, Goldberg RE. Review of shaken baby syndrome. *J Psychosoc Nurs Ment Health Serv.* 2002;40(4):38-41.

53. Fulton DR. Shaken baby syndrome. *Crit Care Nurs Q.* 2000;23(2):43-50.

54. Kivlin JD. Manifestations of the shaken baby syndrome. *Curr Opin Ophthalmol.* 2001;12(3):158-163.

55. Loh JK, Chang DS, Kuo TH, Howng SL. Shaken baby syndrome. *Kaohsiung J Med Sci.* 1998;14(2):112-116.

56. Horner G. Physical abuse: recognition and reporting. *J Pediatr Health.* 2005;19(1):4-11.

57. Johnson, CF. Child maltreatment 2002: recognition, reporting and risk. *Pediatr Int.* 2002;44(5):554-560.

58. Fung EL, Sung RY, Nelson EA, Poon WS. Unexplained subdural hematoma in young children: is it always child abuse? *Pediatr Int.* 2002;44(1):37-42.

59. Yates D, Rifna A, Hill J. Guidelines: assessment, investigation, and early management of head injury: summary of NICE guidance. *BMJ.* 2007;335(7622):719.

60. Levin A V, Christian CW. The eye examination in the evaluation of child abuse. *Pediatrics.* 2010;126(2):376-380.

61. Anteby II, Anteby EY, Chen B, Hamvas A, McAlister W, Tychsen L. Retinal and intraventricular cerebral hemorrhages in the preterm infant born at or before 30 weeks' gestation. *J AAPOS.* 2001;5(2):90-94.

62. Emerson MV, Pieramici DJ, Stoessel KM, Berreen JP, Gariano RF. Incidence and rate of disappearance of retinal hemorrhage in newborns. *Ophthalmology.* 2001;108(1):36-39.

63. Morad Y, Wygnansky-Jaffe T, Levin AV. Retinal haemorrhage in abusive head trauma. *Clin Experiment Ophthalmol.* 2010;38(5):514-520.

64. Ng WS, Watts P, Lawson Z, Kempe A, Maguire S. Development and validation of a standardized tool for reporting retinal findings in abusive head trauma. *Am J Ophthalmol.* 2012;154(2):333-339.

65. Suh DY, Davis PC, Hopkins KL, Fajman NN, Mapstone TB. Nonaccidental pediatric head injury: diffusion-weighted imaging findings. *Neurosurgery.* 2001;49(2):309-318.

66. Kellogg N; The American Academy of Pediatrics Committee on Child Abuse and Neglect. Oral and dental aspects of child abuse and neglect. *Pediatrics.* 2005;116(6):1565-1568.

67. Kempe C. Uncommon manifestations of the battered child syndrome. *Am J Dis Child.* 1975;129:1265.

68. Bronstein AC, Spyker DA, Cantilena LR. 2010 Annual report of the American Association of Poison Control Centers' national poison data system (NPDS): 28th annual report. *Clin Toxicol (Phila).* 2011;49(10):910-941.

69. Pray WS. Reversing the effects of poisoning. *United States Pharmacist.* 1997;22(2):1-5.

70. Welliver J. Unusual injuries. In: Ludwig S, Kornberg AE, eds. *Child Abuse: A Medical Reference.* 2nd ed. New York, NY: Churchill Livingstone; 1992:213-222.

71. Bays J, Feldman K. Child abuse by poisoning. In: Reece R, Ludwig S, eds. *Child Abuse: Medical Diagnosis and Management.* 2nd ed. Philadelphia, PA: Lippincott Williams & Wilkins; 2001:405-441.

72. Bond GR, Woodward RW, Ho M. The growing impact of pediatric pharmaceutical poisoning. *J Pediatr.* 2012;160(2):265-270.

73. Black J, Zenel JA. Child abuse by intentional iron poisoning presenting as shock and persistent acidosis. *Pediatrics.* 2003;111(1):197-199.

74. Litovitz T, Klein-Schwartz W, Rodgers GC Jr, et al. 2001 Annual report of the American Association of Poison Control Centers toxic exposure surveillance system. *Am J Emerg Med.* 2002;20(5):391-452.

75. Coulter K, Scalzo A. Poisoning. In: Monteleone JA, ed. *Child Maltreatment: A Clinical Guide and Reference.* 2nd ed. St. Louis, MO: GW Medical Publishing; 1998:315-326.

76. Hogstel MO, Curry LC. Body organ and system assessment. In: Hogstel MO, Curry LC, eds. *Practical Guide to Health Assessment Through the Life Span.* 3rd ed. Philadelphia, PA: FA Davis Company; 2001:89.

77. Cunha JP. Poisoning. Emedicinehealth Web site. http://www.emedicinehealth.com/poisoning/article_em.htm. Accessed February 17, 2013.

78. Heger A, Ticson L, Velasquez O, Bernier R. Children referred for possible sexual abuse: medical findings in 2384 children. *Child Abuse Negl.* 2002;26(6-7):645-659.

79. Christian CW, Lavelle JM, De Jong AR, et al. Forensic evidence findings in prepubertal victims of sexual assault. *Pediatrics.* 2000;106(1):100-104.

80. Palusci VJ, Cyrus TA. Reaction to videocolposcopy in the assessment of child sexual abuse. *Child Abuse Negl.* 2001;25(11):1535-1546.

81. Girardet R, Bolton K, Lahoti S, et al. Collection of forensic evidence from pediatric victims of sexual assault. *Pediatrics.* 2011;128(2):233-238.

82. Murphy SB, Potter SJ, Stapleton JG, Wieseon-Martin D, Pierce-Weeks J. Findings from sexual assault nurse examiners (SANE): a case study of New Hampshire's pediatric SANA database. *J Forensic Nurs.* 2010;6:163-169.

83. Adams JA. Evolution of a classification scale: medical evaluation of suspected child sexual abuse. *Child Maltreat.* 2001;6(1):31-36.

84. Finkel MA, DeJong AR. Medical findings in child sexual abuse. In: Reece RM, Ludwig S, eds. *Child Abuse: Medical Diagnosis and Management.* 2nd ed. Philadelphia, PA: Lippincott Williams & Wilkins; 2001:286.

85. The American Academy of Pediatrics Committee on Child Abuse and Neglect. Guidelines for the evaluation of sexual abuse of children: subject review. *Pediatrics.* 1999;103(1):186-191.

86. Adams JA, Harper K, Knudson S, Revilla J. Examination findings in legally confirmed child sexual abuse: it's normal to be normal. *Pediatrics.* 1994;94(3):310-317.

87. Muram D. Anal and perianal abnormalities in prepubertal victims of sexual abuse. *Am J Obstet Gynecol.* 1989;161(2):278-281.

88. Thackeray JD, Hornor G, Benzinger EA, Scribano PV. Forensic evidence collection and DNA identification in acute child sexual assault. *Pediatrics.* 2011;128(2):227-232.

89. Palusci VJ, Christian CW. Forensic evidence in child sexual abuse. In: Finkel MA, Giardino AP, eds. *Medical Evaluation of Child Sexual Abuse: A Practical Guide.* Elk Grove Village, IL: American Academy of Pediatrics; 2009.

90. Horner G. A normal ano-genital exam: sexual abuse or not? *J Pediatr Health Care.* 2010;24(3):145-151.

91. Fraser JA, Mathews B, Walsh K, Chen L, Dunne M. Factors influencing child abuse and neglect recognition and reporting by nurses: a multivariate analysis. *Int J Nurs Stud.* 2010;47(2):146-153.

92. Hennigen L, Kollar LM, Rosenthal SL. Methods for managing pelvic examination anxiety: individual differences and relaxation techniques. *J Pediatr Health Care.* 2000;14(1):9-12.

93. Lazebnik R, Zimet GD, Ebert J, et al. How children perceive the medical evaluation for suspected sexual abuse. *Child Abuse Negl.* 1994;18(9):739-745.

94. Steward M, Schmitz M, Steward D, Joye N, Reinhart M. Children's anticipation of and response to colposcopic examination. *Child Abuse Negl.* 1995;19:997-1005.

95. Fischer H. The genital examination distress scale (GEDS) [Letter to the Editor]. *Child Abuse Negl.* 1999;23(12):1205.

96. Lawson L. Preparing sexually abused girls for genital evaluation. *Issues Compr Pediatr Nurs.* 1990;13(2):155-164.

97. Child Welfare Information Gateway. *National Child Abuse and Neglect Data System (NCANDS) Summary of Key Findings for Calendar Year 2000.* Washington, DC: Child Welfare Information Gateway; 2000.

98. Finkelhor D, Browne A. The traumatic impact of child sexual abuse: a conceptualization. *Am J Orthopsychiatry.* 1985;55(4):530-541.

99. De San Lazaro C. Making paediatric assessment in suspected sexual abuse a therapeutic experience. *Arch Dis Child.* 1995;73:174-176.

100. Giardino AP, Finkel MA, Giardino ER, Seidl T, Ludwig S. *A Practical Guide to the Evaluation of Sexual Abuse in the Prepubertal Child.* Newbury Park, CA: Sage Publications Inc; 1992.

101. Mears CJ, Heflin AH, Finkel M, Deblinger E. Adolescents' responses to video colposcopy and educational information provided during a sexual abuse evaluation. *J Adolesc Health.* 1997;20(2):128.

102. Finkel M. Physical examination. In: Finkel MA, Giardino AP, eds. *Medical Evaluation of Child Sexual Abuse: A Practical Guide.* 2nd ed. Thousand Oaks, CA: Sage Publications; 2002:39-98.

103. Ricci LR. Documentation of physical evidence in child sexual abuse. In: Finkel MA, Giardino AP, eds. *Medical Evaluation of Child Sexual Abuse: A Practical Guide.* 2nd ed. Thousand Oaks, CA: Sage Publications; 2002:99-110.

104. Lahoti SL, McClain N, Girardet R, McNeese M, Cheung K. Evaluating the child for sexual abuse. *Am Fam Physician.* 2001;63:883-892.

105. McClain N, Girardet R, Lahoti S, Cheung K, Berger K, McNeese M. Evaluation of sexual abuse in the pediatric patient. *J Pediatr Health Care.* 2000;14:93-101.

106. Botash AS. Examination for sexual abuse in prepubertal children: an update. *Pediatr Ann.* 1997;26(5):312-320.

107. Levitt C. Further technical considerations regarding conducting and documenting the child sexual abuse medical examination. *Child Abuse Negl.* 1998;22(6):567-571.

108. The Terminology Subcommittee of the APSAC Task Force on Medical Evaluation of Suspected Child Abuse. *Practice Guidelines: Descriptive Terminology in Child Sexual Abuse Evaluations.* San Diego, CA: APSAC; 1995.

109. Ludwig S. Child abuse. In: Fleisher GR, Ludwig S, Henretig FM, Ruddy RM, Silverman BK eds. *Textbook of Pediatric Emergency Medicine.* 4th ed. Philadelphia, PA: Lippincott Williams & Wilkins; 2000:1669-1704.

110. Adams JA. Evolution of a classification scale: medical evaluation of suspected child sexual abuse. *Child Maltreat.* 2001:6(1):31-36.

111. Adams JA, Kaplan RA, Starling SP, et al. Guidelines for medical care of children who may have been sexually abused. *J Pediatr Adolesc Gynecol.* 2007;20(3):163-172.

Chapter 5

Laboratory Findings, Diagnostic Testing, and Forensic Specimens in Cases of Child Sexual Abuse

Stacey A. Mitchell, DNP, MBA, RN, SANE-A, SANE-P
Diana K. Faugno, MSN, RN, CPN, SANE-A, SANE-P, FAAFS, DF-IAFN
Tracy Evanson, PhD, PHCNS-BC

Key Points

1. It is imperative that the health care provider checks with the laboratory slated to analyze forensic specimens to be sure that he or she follows the appropriate protocols. While the types of specimens are relatively uniform, the techniques for testing may vary. Each crime laboratory functions differently and may request evidence be packaged in a certain manner.

2. In addition to assessing clothing for traces of bloodstains and seminal fluids, the health care provider should pay close attention to the condition of the clothing. Tears or missing buttons may be evidence of force or indicate a struggle and may help to corroborate the child's history of the event.

3. A nondestructive screening technique, such as an alternate light source (ALS), may be used to identify areas that should be swabbed for evidence.[1] Various types of commercial light sources are available through evidence supply companies. Before purchasing such a light, the health care provider should ensure that the ALS allows for the possible fluorescence of a multitude of substances.

4. Swabs should be specific to the body area assaulted (eg, oral, anal, vaginal), and 2 swabbed specimens should be collected from each area. However, the health care provider should use his or her own discretion when deciding if all or additional locations should be swabbed.

5. Photography is considered 1 of the 3 necessary forms of documentation alongside written or narrative descriptions and diagrams that pinpoint location, size, shape, and quantity of injuries.

6. The chain of custody, or chain of evidence, is the record that details the individuals who gain custody and control of a particular piece of evidence.[2] The chain begins with the health care provider(s) who collects a given piece of physical evidence from the child.[2] It is the health care provider's responsibility to document the proper collection and packaging of each item and ensure that the integrity of the contents is maintained.

Introduction

When evaluating a child for sexual abuse, several findings help the health care provider to make a diagnosis. For example, the presence of certain sexually transmitted infections (STIs) in the prepubertal child beyond the neonatal period substantiates that sexual contact has occurred.[3] The history provided by the child and the caregivers often points to a specific perpetrator. Thorough evidence collection, according to established guidelines, for forensic specimen collection and laboratory testing plays an important role in identifying the perpetrator as well as confirming sexual contact and ensuring appropriate medical treatment of the child. Even though it is uncommon to find visible physical evidence in cases of suspected sexual abuse, such evidence is extremely important when identified.[4] Physical evidence of sexual abuse may include injuries, bodily fluids, hairs, and other specimens, such as torn clothing. It is the Emergency Nurses Association's (ENA) position that it is within the nurse's role to not only provide emotional and physical care to victims of violence, but to also evaluate the child, collect evidence, preserve the chain of custody, and document findings in the medical record.[5] The specialty of forensic nursing focuses on the forensic aspects of health care as related to victims, perpetrators, and families of both who experience violence, crime, and traumatic accidents.[6] The American College of Emergency Physicians (ACEP) supports clinical forensic programs as an excellent option for acute and chronic sexual assault evaluations, in part because of the standardized examination and evidence collection process.[7]

According to other studies, it is unlikely to reveal positive laboratory results for acute sexual assault after 24 hours; however, Thackeray et al[8] recommend that collecting evidence in the prepubertal child should be completed anyway as DNA technology continues to advance. It is important to recognize that failing to conduct evidence collection will result in missed opportunities.[8,9] This chapter focuses on the process used to collect evidence in cases where sexual abuse of a child is suspected and as indicated by the history and physical assessment. This chapter will also review the laboratory testing involved in the evidence collection process and the standard procedures for retrieving samples to be tested for STIs.

Evidence Collection

The evidence collection process is as important as the other components of the medical-forensic examination, including consent, history, physical assessment, treatment, and discharge process. The health care provider must be competent in the procedures used to recover and preserve biological evidence. It is imperative that the health care provider checks with the laboratory slated to analyze the forensic specimens to be sure that he or she follows the appropriate protocols. While the types of specimens are relatively uniform, the techniques for testing may vary. Each crime laboratory functions differently and may request evidence be packaged in a certain manner. Samples gathered may include objects such as clothing and bed linens as well as oral, vaginal, or anal swabs. In some cases, fluids, such as seminal fluid and saliva, may be recovered from the skin. Epithelial cells may also be found on the child. The examiner should consider swabbing areas such as bruises and the external genitalia as well. Many jurisdictions now have specialized kits for drug screens when drug-facilitated assault is suspected.

The medical-forensic examination should be conducted systematically. By beginning at the head and progressing toward the feet, each body part can be assessed and evidence collected. Several tools are available to the clinician to facilitate identification and thorough collection of specimens, including a sexual assault evidence collection kit, an alternate light source, toluidine blue dye, and equipment specific for magnification and image capturing (**Table 5-1**) (see *Chapter 4, The Physical Examination in the Evaluation of Suspected Child Maltreatment: Physical Abuse and Sexual Abuse Examinations*).

Table 5-1. Tools Used for Evidence Collection
— Sexual assault evidence collection kit
— Paper bags
— ALS or other multi-wave light source
— Magnification and image capturing
— Digital camera
— Colposcope
— STI Testing
— Culture
— Nucleic amplification testing (urine or swab)

Evidence Collection Kits

Many jurisdictions use a standardized kit to collect forensic evidence in cases of sexual assault. Examples of kits that may be used include the sexual assault collection kit or the sexual assault forensic kit (SAFE), sometime referred to as the Vitullo kit. These kits are designed to bring continuity to the examination process so that evidence is collected and preserved in a similar manner, regardless of who collected it.[10] Although kits vary from state-to-state and manufacturer-to-manufacturer, they basically contain the same types of containers for evidence recovery (**Table 5-2**). All sexual assault evidence collection kits contain detailed instructions outlining the collection and packaging of each item and envelopes specifically marked as to what should be put in them. Common protocol requires the examiner to seal and initial each item of evidence so that the writing is half on the seal and half on the box, envelope, or bag. Once filled, the health care provider should return the containers to the kit and then seal it. When the evidence is received in the forensic laboratory, each sealed container is assessed for deviations in the lettering. If none is discovered, then evidence tampering has not occurred (**Figures 5-1** to **5-8**).

A sexual assault evidence collection kit should be used for the medical-forensic examination that occurs acutely; that is, if the assault occurred less than 96 hours before the child's presentation to the facility or if the examiner feels that biological evidence may still be present after 96 hours. The standard time-frames for evidence collection involving pediatric patients has been called into question. As technology evolves, the timing of evidence collection continues to change.[8,11,12]

Table 5-2. Common Contents of Sexual Assault Evidence Collection Kits
— Reference sample swabs or blood card
— Envelopes to place known hair samples
— Envelopes to place pubic hair combings
— Envelope to place pubic hair pullings
— Vaginal swabs
— Rectal swabs
— Oral swab
— Paper bags to collect clothing
— Paper bag to collect underwear
— Swabs to collect suspected biological fluids on the skin
— Additional envelopes for evidence collection or a debris collection sheet (included in some, but not all, kits)

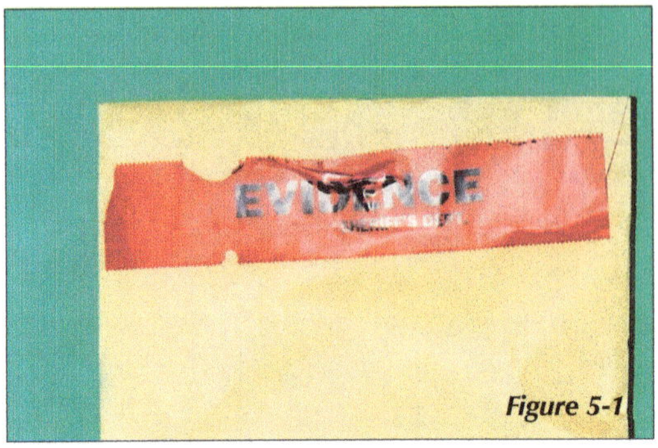

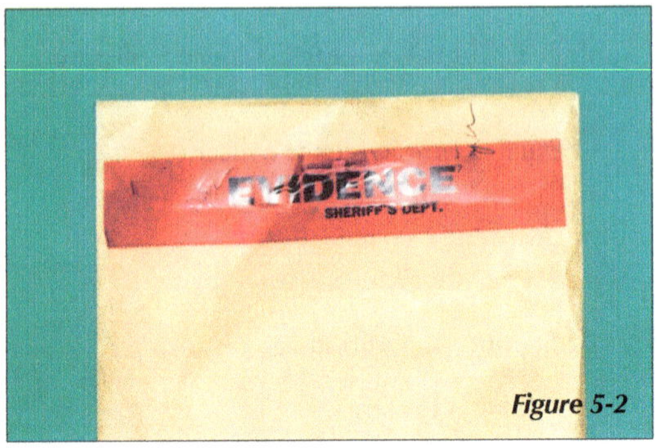

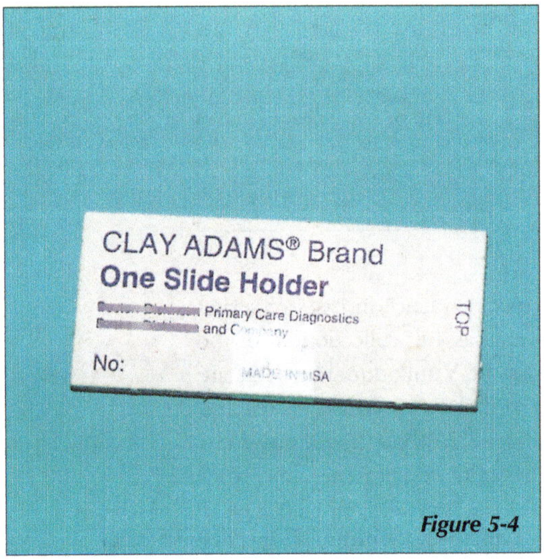

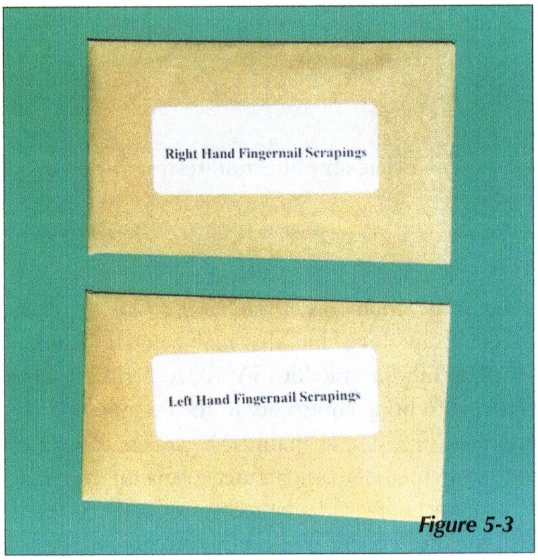

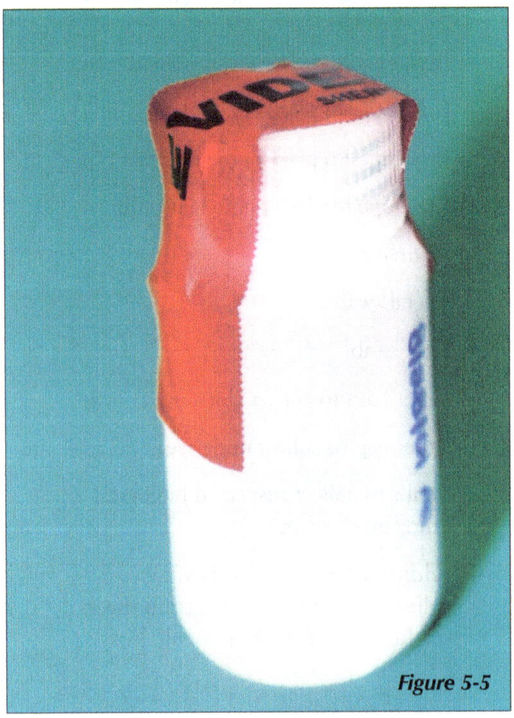

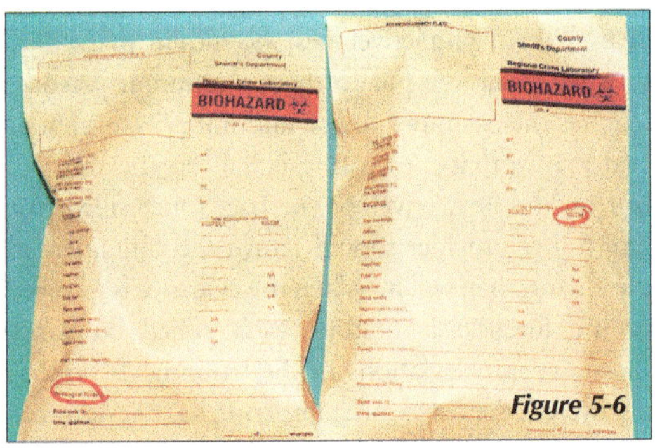

Figure 5-1. *Improperly sealed envelope (no name, date, or time).*

Figure 5-2. *Properly sealed envelope (includes name, date, and times). Evidence tape should go around the corners of the bag for correct sealing.*

Figure 5-3. *Envelopes for fingernail scrapings. Many programs are using swabs instead of scraping.*

Figure 5-4. *Slide holder.*

Figure 5-5. *Improperly sealed urine container (no initials on the seal or bottle).*

Figure 5-6. *Sexual assault kit envelopes.*

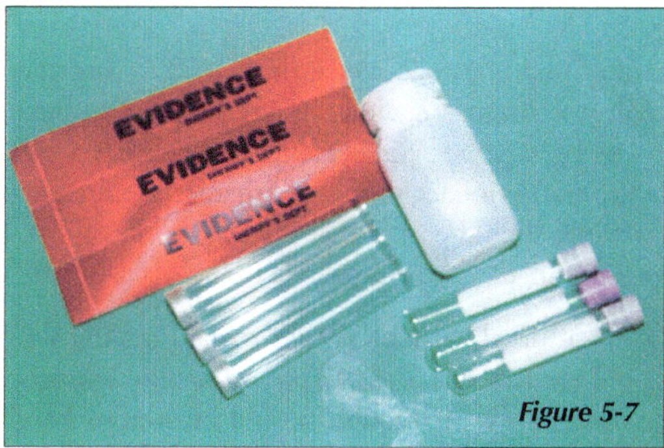

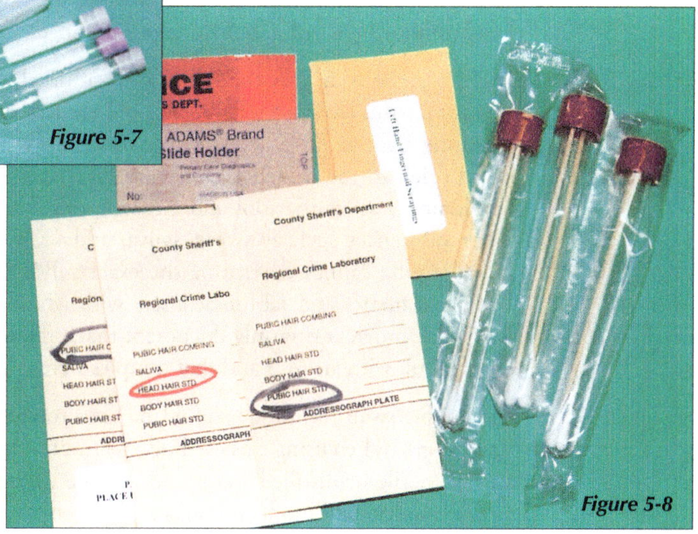

Figure 5-7. *Contents of left envelope in Figure 5-6.*

Figure 5-8. *Contents of right envelope in Figure 5-6.*

The clinician must make his or her decision to collect or not collect evidence based on the history given by the child or caregivers, physical findings, and any other pertinent circumstances that may arise. It is imperative that the examiner employs critical thinking skills during this phase of the medical-forensic evaluation to ensure the best possible outcomes.

Clothing

All clothing worn by a child during a sexual assault, particularly the underwear, may contain evidence and must be collected. In addition to assessing clothing for traces of bloodstains and bodily fluids, the health care provider should pay close attention to the condition of the child's clothing. Tears or missing buttons may be evidence of force or indicate a struggle and may help to corroborate the child's history of the event.

Clothing that has bloodstains or seminal fluid is tested for deoxyribonucleic acid (DNA) to identify a suspect. Whenever possible, linens should also be collected from the crime scene because they may have evidence of semen, blood, hair, or fibers on them. The health care provider should make every effort to secure the child's clothing, even if the child has already changed before the commencement of the medical-forensic examination because important physical evidence may be present on the clothing and the opportunity for preservation of evidence must not be missed. Clothing and bed linens are the most likely sources of forensic evidence of blood or semen.[13]

Clothing should be carefully removed in order to protect foreign materials adhered to them. The child should stand on a clean sheet or the debris-collection sheet provided in the evidence collection kit and should remove each piece of clothing so as to not shake or discard anything onto the floor.[2] Any clothing that is wet or damp should be air-dried before packaging; it may be hung on a clothes hanger or placed on butcher paper to dry while the examination continues. After drying, each piece of clothing should be placed an individual paper bag. The top of the bag should then be folded over, sealed with tape, and labeled with the examiner's initials.[2]

Evidence Present on the Skin

Biological evidence deposited on the skin should be collected so that DNA testing may be performed. A nondestructive screening technique, such as an alternate light source (ALS), may be used to identify areas to be swabbed for evidence.[1] Various types of commercial light sources are available through evidence supply companies. Before purchasing such a light, the health care provider should ensure that the ALS allows for the possible fluorescence of a multitude of substances.

By shining the ALS over the body, areas of dried substances that remain on the skin may absorb the ultraviolet light, become excited, and then fluoresce or glow, thereby indicating areas of possible evidence.[14] Such areas of reaction should be swabbed and placed dried in the evidence collection kit.[10] It is important to note that the ALS is a preliminary screening tool and a reaction does not confirm the presence of semen. Other substances such as sweat, saliva, and urine fluoresce under this light as well; therefore, one cannot determine the exact substance by light alone.[14-16] Other fluids such as cosmetics and fabric cleansers with whiteners also fluoresce.[14] Therefore, the health care provider can only document that a fluorescent reaction occurred during the examination with an ALS and that samples were collected.

The double swab technique should be used to collect samples from areas of reaction (**Table 5-3**). When using this method, the health care provider should immerse a cotton swab in sterile or distilled water and roll the tip over the surface of the skin, using a circular motion and moderate pressure[17] to rehydrate the dried material. A second dry swab should then be rolled over the surface in the same manner as the first to allow the retrieval of any additional material. The double swab technique may be used to collect any type of biological evidence left on the skin (eg, saliva, blood, seminal fluid). The cotton applicators should be allowed to dry and then packaged together in the same envelope. The health care provider should label the envelope with the location of the area swabbed, seal the envelope, and then place it in the evidence collection kit. The process should be repeated for each area of reaction.

Bite Marks

Bite marks may be found in cases of sexual abuse as well as physical abuse. Bite mark evidence has been accepted in courts of law based upon 2 premises: (1) each person's dentition is presumed to be unique and (2) the uniqueness of dentition is accurately

Table 5-3. Double Swab Technique

1. Identify the area to be swabbed.
2. Immerse one sterile cotton swab in either sterile or distilled water.
3. Roll the moistened swab over the skin surface, using a circular motion and moderate pressure.
4. Take a second dry swab, which should remain dry, and roll the swab over the same surface area.
5. Roll the swabs with the collected samples over a slide if required by a specific protocol. If slide is not required by protocol, allow swabs to dry and then package the swabs in an envelope.
6. Seal, label, and place the envelope in the evidence collection kit.

Adapted from Sweet D, Lorente M, Lorente J, et al. An improved method to recover saliva from human skin: the double swab technique. J Forensic Sci. *1997;42(2):320-322.*

preserved in the injured skin or in objects.[18] The child should be examined closely because findings may be subtle and overlooked, especially if the wound is almost healed. Bite marks should be suspected when injuries such as ecchymosis (bruising), abrasions, or lacerations form an oval or elliptical pattern.[19] Traditionally, bite-mark evidence has been used to develop comparative evidence between the identified pattern and a potential suspect. A forensic odontologist should be consulted in the event possible bite marks are identified.

The American Board of Forensic Odontology (ABFO) has developed guidelines for bite-mark evidence.[18] The health care provider should photograph the bite mark at a 90-degree angle to avoid distorting the proportion of the bite,[19] and should place a No. 2 ABFO ruler, an L-shaped ruler specially designed for bite-mark photography, next to the bite mark.[19] The examiner should photograph the injury with and without the ABFO ruler.

In addition to providing a means through which a perpetrator's identity may be confirmed, a bite mark may provide biological evidence.[17,20] After obtaining images of the wound, the nurse should swab the area for saliva using the double swab technique. Chain of custody must be maintained throughout this portion of the medical-forensic examination (see *"Chain of Custody"* later in this chapter for further discussion).

Oral, Vaginal, and Anal Specimens

If the child victim of suspected sexual abuse presents for an acute evaluation, samples should be collected from each body area indicated in the assault. Swabs should be specific to the body area assaulted (eg, oral, anal, vaginal), and 2 to 3 swabbed specimens should be collected from each area. However, the health care provider should use his or her own discretion when deciding if all or additional orifices should be swabbed. The swabs should be tested for sperm, acid phosphatase, prostate specific protein, and prostate specific antigen (P30).[15,21] The health care provider may prepare a saline wet mount of specimens from the designated orifices and immediately examine the specimens for the presence of nonmotile and motile sperm.[10]

Oral Specimens

Oral swabs should be collected in cases of fellatio. The health care provider should use several cotton applicators to swab the buccal pouch and along the bottom edges of the teeth and gums.[10] Some protocols may require that an oral rinse be collected for which the child should be asked to rinse his or her mouth with a small amount of sterile or distilled water and then to spit the contents into a sterile cup. Some kits provide the sterile cup needed for the oral rinse. The provider should consider collecting oral samples in cases where there is limited history.[8] (**Figures 5-9-a** and **b**)

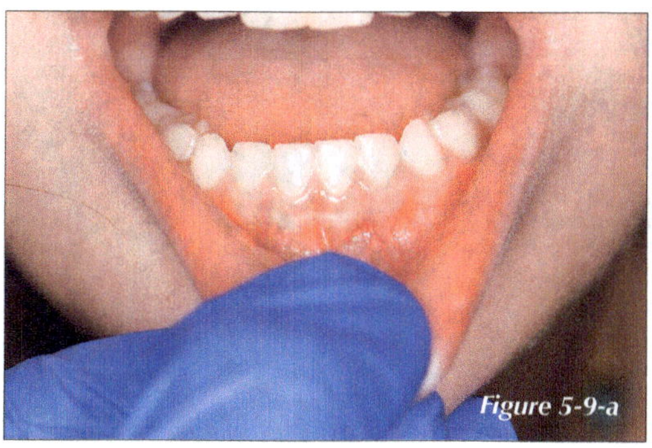

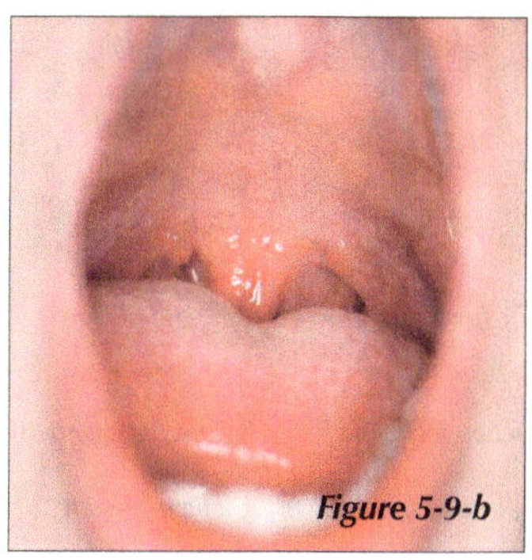

Figures 5-9-a and b. *Observing for any injury or medical findings in the oral cavity of a child.*

Vaginal Specimens

In the event of suspected vaginal penetration or vulvar coitus, the health care provider should collect samples from the external genitalia, as opposed to the vagina or cervical os (**Figures 5-10** to **5-12**). To minimize discomfort for the prepubertal child, the health care provider should use a Mini-tip culturette® swab rather than a large cotton tipped applicator.[21] The lack of estrogenization of the hymenal tissue causes greater sensitization of that area. To decrease fears the child may have, the health care provider may allow the child to see the swabs before using them. This would be done in pubertal girls if a culture must be collected to test for sexually transmitted diseases, and not just as evidence collection. The applicator should be carefully inserted into the vaginal vault. Because of the increased sensitivity, the clinician must take care so as not to touch

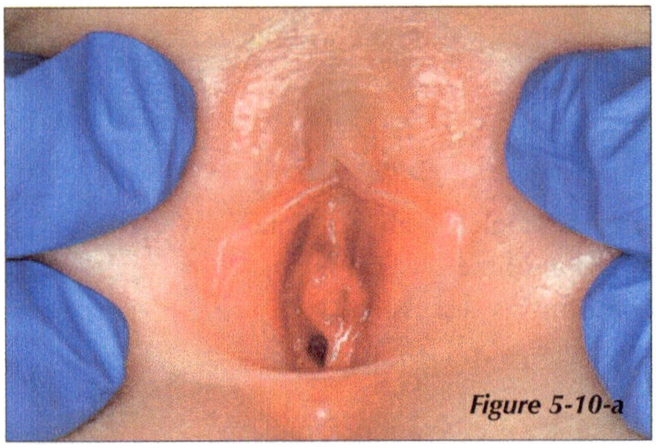

Figure 5-10-a

Figures 5-10-a and b. *Labial separation.*

Figure 5-10-c. *Labial separation with the hymen not opened and the an asymmetrical Labia Minora.*

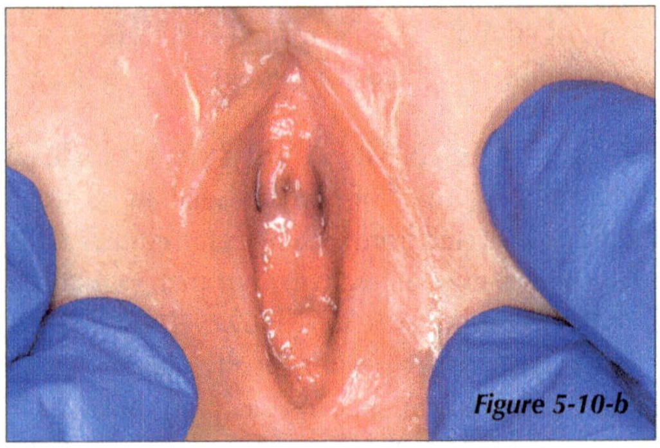

Figure 5-10-b

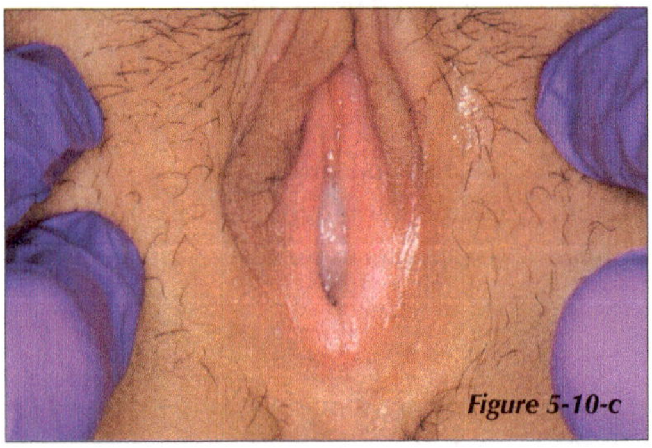

Figure 5-10-c

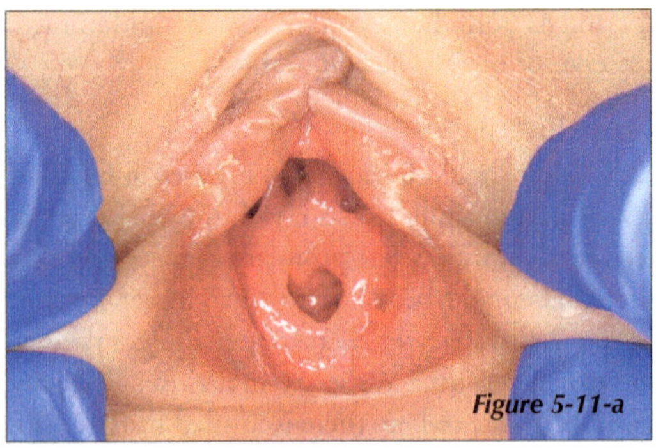

Figure 5-11-a

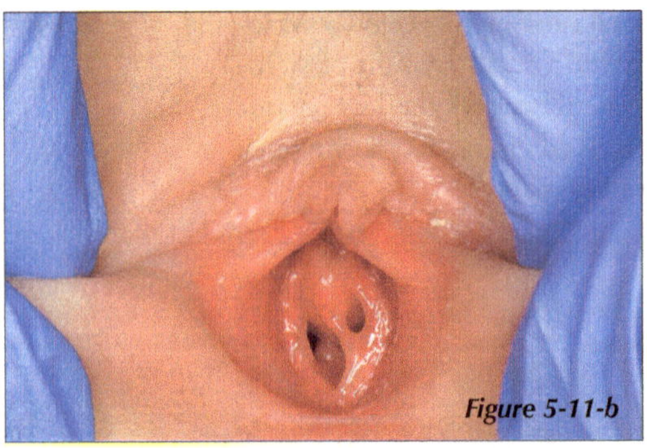

Figure 5-11-b

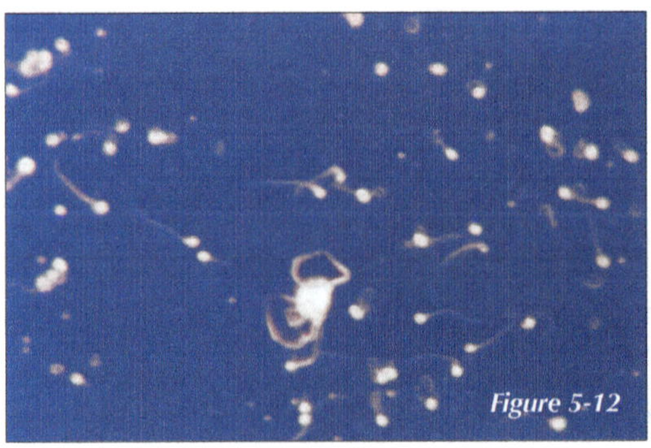

Figure 5-12

Figure 5-11-a. *Labia traction technique exposing the hymen and urethral openings.*

Figure 5-11-b. *Labia traction technique exposing a septate hymen.*

Figure 5-12. *Identifying motile sperm by using a light-staining microscope.*

the applicator while retrieving samples.[13] During the adolescent examination, the nurse should obtain samples from the cervical os and the posterior fornix. The swabs should be dried and then packaged in the envelope provided as part of the evidence collection kit. Care must be taken to ensure that each swab is placed in the correct package. The nurse should seal and label the envelope and then place it in the kit.

Anal Specimens

For suspected anal penetration, the nurse should obtain samples from the anal and rectal area by inserting the swab beyond the external folds of the anus.[10] As a result of the pull of gravity, seminal fluid may drain and pool in or around the anus. The examiner should consider retrieving anal swabs in the event of vaginal penetration, for the same reason. Several cotton applicators are required when collecting evidence from the anal and rectal area. The health care provider should collect external samples from the perianal area after the child has been examined for trauma. Once the external samples are collected, the health care provider should then collect the internal samples. To collect the internal samples, the health care provider should insert the cotton swab into the anus and then rotate the swab several times. The applicators should be dried and then packaged according to chain of evidence.

Blood Specimens

At times, it might be necessary to obtain a sample from the child for DNA comparison. This reference sample is used to distinguish between the child's DNA profile and the perpetrator's DNA profile.[10] Most evidence collection kits are moving away from blood samples and using buccal swabs that can be placed into the kit. If blood is required, it is often in the form of a blood card instead of a tube of blood. The type of reference sample required is based upon individual crime laboratory requirements. To obtain a blood card, the health care provider should prick the child's finger with a lancet. Drops of blood should then be placed on the card, as per the instructions that accompanied the card. The blood card must be air-dried and then placed in the evidence collection kit.

A buccal swab is a non-invasive sample that may be obtained. To obtain a buccal swab, the health care provider should ask the child or adolescent to rinse his or her mouth with tap water. Using a cotton swab with gentle pressure, the clinician should swab the inner cheek area.[10] The swab should be air-dried and placed in the correct envelope. The clinician should seal and label the envelope and then place it in the evidence collection kit.

Hair Samples

There is great controversy regarding whether or not the hair should be obtained. In the child abuse examination, the technique of pulling the child's hair is generally no longer used.

Identification of Motile Sperm

The identification of motile sperm is often left to the crime laboratory analyst. Protocols for viewing sperm are based upon jurisdictions in each community.

Forensic Photography

The use of photodocumentation in the medical-forensic examination enables the court to see the victim through the eyes of the examiner. Photography should be considered 1 of the 3 necessary forms of documentation alongside written or narrative descriptions and diagrams that pinpoint location, size, shape and quantity of injuries. Each form of documentation builds on and supports the other. Photography does not take the place of good documentation.[2] Each image must be a true and accurate representation of the child at the time of the examination (see *Chapter 2, Presentation and Overview of the Evaluation of Child Maltreatment* and *Chapter 9, Documenting the Evaluation of Suspected Child Maltreatment Cases*). **Table 5-4** lists equipment used in forensic photography.

Table 5-4. Forensic Digital Photography Equipment List

— Camera bag or hard case
— Digital camera body
  — Max resolution
  — Zoom features
  — Manual focus
  — USB connectivity
  — Battery source and charger
— Lens
— External flash
  — Ring flash or top-mounted flash
  — Through-the-lens capability
  — 3D balanced fill flash
  — Matrix metering
— Storage media
  — Memory card
  — Memory stick
  — Compact disc
— Flash cord
— Tripod
— Filters
  — UV filters
  — No. 15 yellow filter for fluorescent UV light photography
  — No. 18 red filter for reflective UV light photography
— Scales and labels
  — 6-inch scales of various colors
  — ABFO ruler
  — Micro scales
  — Identification cards
— Extra batteries
— Magic markers
— Camera cleaning cloth

Photographing Nongenital Injuries

Photographs of nongenital injuries should be taken in a series. It is recommended that the health care provider include one overall, head-to-toe photograph of the child to mark the beginning of the series, capture trauma and any evidence in the form of disheveled clothing, and identify the patient. The next photograph in the series is called an orientation photograph. This photograph orients the examiner to the general location of a particular injury or finding (**Figures 5-13** to **5-14**). The final photograph in the series is called a close-up photograph. This photograph is taken of the injury itself and includes the greatest detail. The examiner should obtain 2 close-up photographs, one taken with and one without a rule to indicate the size of the injury.[2] In the case of multiple injuries, the health care provider should take orientation and close-up photographs of each injury.[22]

Photographing Genital Injuries

A system designed to magnify the genitals and allow for image capture is a necessary tool in the medical-forensic examination (see *Chapter 4, The Physical Examination in the Evaluation of Suspected Child Maltreatment: Physical Abuse and Sexual Abuse Examinations*).

Becoming adept at forensic photography requires much practice; however, with practice, the health care provider can perfect his or her ability to obtain optimal photographs. The photographer should be familiar with the type of camera being used and have a good working knowledge of specific settings and functions. Exploring various techniques, taking practice shots using various camera settings, reviewing practice photographs, and attending photography classes are a few ways in which a health care provider can improve his or her skills (**Figures 5-15** to **5-17**). The health care provider must be aware that there is only one opportunity to document acute injuries, and it is important not to miss that chance.

Chain of Custody

The chain of custody, or chain of evidence, is the record that details the individuals who gain custody and control of a particular piece of evidence.[2] The chain begins with the health care provider(s) who collects a given piece of physical evidence from the child.[2] It is the health care provider's responsibility to document the proper collection and packaging of each item and ensure that the integrity of the contents is maintained.

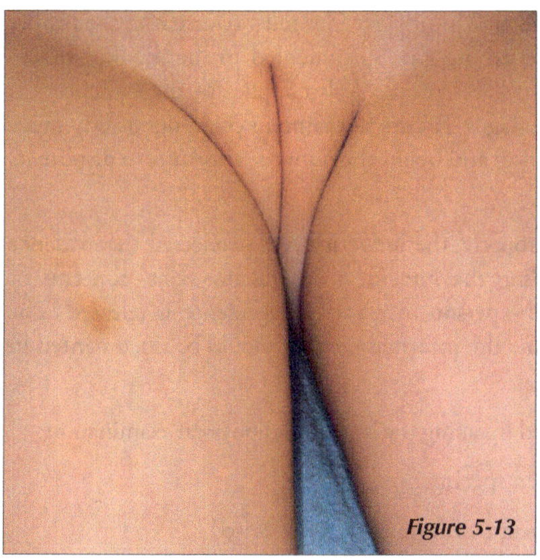

Figure 5-13

Figure 5-13. *4 year-old girl with a bruise on the top of the right thigh.*

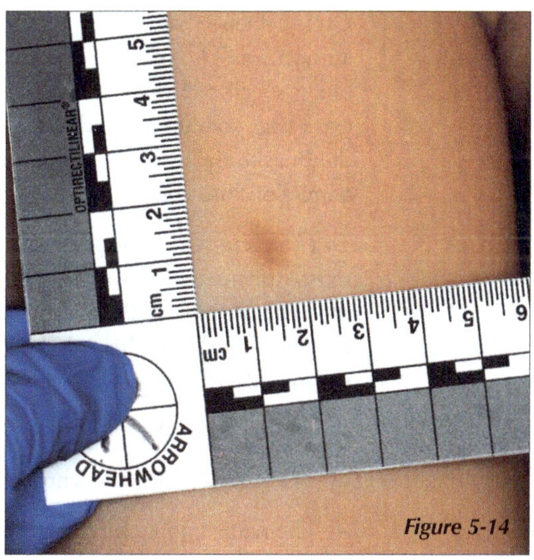

Figure 5-14

Figure 5-14. *Close-up photograph of a bruise on the thigh.*

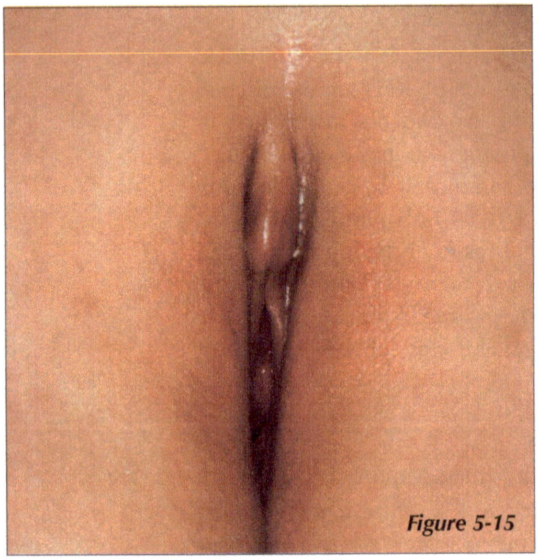

Figure 5-15

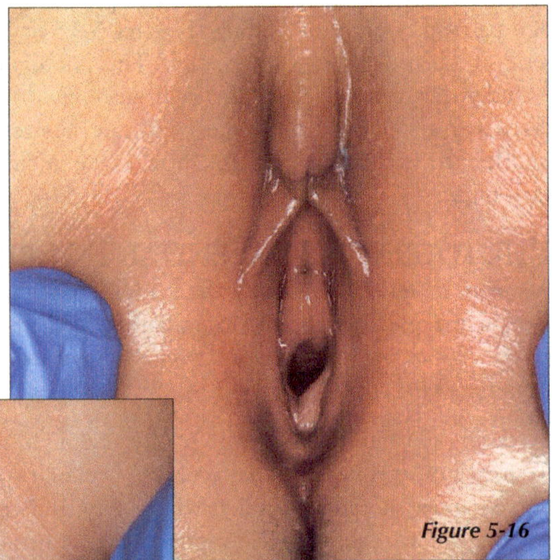

Figure 5-16

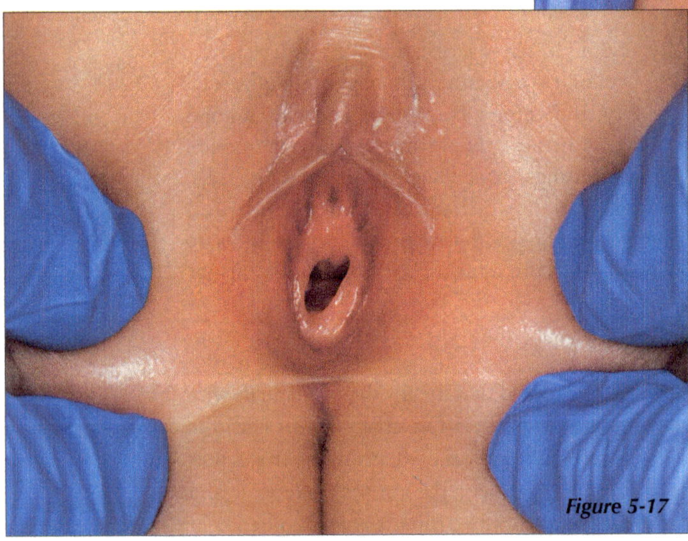

Figure 5-17

Figure 5-15*. A photograph of the genital area before any toughing or separation is preformed.*

Figure 5-16*. A close-up photograph of the labia separation.*

Figure 5-17*. A close-up photograph of the genital traction exposing the annular hymen and the vestibule.*

Once evidence has been collected, the health care provider must release it to the proper authorities. The release of any evidence must be documented in the medical record or on specific chain of custody forms. This protocol also applies to the evidence kit, extra bags containing clothing, and images. Failure to maintain chain of custody raises doubt as to the integrity of the evidence[2] and opens the door for attorneys to dispute its admission into court.[23]

To complete the chain of custody properly, the individual who collected the evidence must document information regarding the intactness of evidence seals, contents of the evidence kit, and the name of the person to whom the evidence is released. The following guidelines help to determine the information that should be documented in the medical record[7]:

— The names of all personnel involved in taking the history and physical examination

— The names of anyone who handled specimens

— The name and identity of the officer to whom the kit is released

—The name of the agency to which the officer belongs

—The date the kit is transferred to the officer

—A comprehensive list of evidence collected

Laboratory Testing of Forensic Evidence

The forensic laboratory scientist has the ultimate authority when it comes to processing evidence. Once evidence is received by the laboratory, it is dispersed to the appropriate department within the laboratory for evaluation. For example, the forensic biology department of the laboratory would receive evidence that is to be examined for the presence of bodily fluids and would conduct subsequent DNA testing on any such findings elicited from the evidence.

Detecting the Presence of Seminal Fluid

The probative evidence, evidence associated most closely with a crime, such as underwear or bed linens, collected in cases of sexual abuse must be examined for the presence of seminal fluid and other body secretions by the forensic biology laboratory department. Preliminary testing or screening is necessary to identify potential body fluids on evidence included in the evidence collection kit or submitted separately. Several methods are used to determine the presence of seminal fluids. If the health care provider made slides using swabs with samples collected from the mouth, anus, vagina, or other locations, the scientist will view the slides under a microscope. When evaluating other pieces of evidence, the scientist conducts a visual inspection of the items, looking for bloodstains and the characteristic stiff, off-white, crusty appearance of seminal fluid stains. The visual inspection of such items can be an arduous task considering the amount of evidence, such as bed linens, underwear, and other articles of clothing, that may be submitted to the laboratory.

The eye alone is unreliable when attempting to identify the presence of fluids in evidence.[24] Depending on the item, the forensic scientist may choose to examine it with an ALS. Just as the health care provider uses the ALS to identify areas of potential evidence on skin, forensic laboratory personnel use an ALS to highlight areas of interest on clothing and other materials.[14] Once a stain is detected, it is tested for acid phosphatase and P30. Acid phosphatase is found in seminal fluid and in very low levels in the vagina. Quantification of acid phosphatase is necessary to verify ejaculation.[15] P30, also verifies the presence of seminal fluid; however, the protein is found only in male urine and in seminal fluid[25]; making its presence in a stain a more significant finding than that of acid phosphatase. Still, the scientist tests for both. Once the presence of seminal fluid is established, the scientist takes a sample from the swab or fabric and makes a slide for microscopy visualization. After sperm are identified, the scientist proceeds with DNA testing of the sample in order to confirm the identity or to identify a potential perpetrator.

Blood and Saliva

Blood typing, secretor status, and, most significantly, DNA testing provide invaluable identifying information in cases of sexual abuse. Blood typing is usually conducted through the testing of blood samples. However, for 80% of the population, blood typing may also be conducted through the testing of saliva and semen samples. Determining whether a saliva or semen sample yields information as to typology establishes one's secretor status. While a determination of blood type and secretor status cannot identify an assailant, it may help exclude a person of interest if the evidence does not demonstrate the same typology (A, B, or O status) as that individual.[26] However, with advances in forensic science, DNA analysis is able to identify a specific perpetrator with a high degree of certainty.[15]

Deoxyribonucleic Acid Profiling

DNA testing is an invaluable tool for identifying and eliminating suspects in cases of suspected sexual abuse. DNA is the genetic code found in the nucleus of cells in all living things. Each person receives half of his or her DNA from his or her biological mother and half from his or her biological father. With the exception of identical twins, each individual is genetically unique.[2] About 99% of human DNA is the same, while the remaining 1% makes each person different. It is that 1% that is significant in terms of forensic testing.

Short tandem repeat (STR) typing is one type of forensic testing being done in crime laboratories across the country. In STR testing, a region of DNA that has a short sequence is copied over and over.[2] Typically, there are 13 markers, or areas, of repeated patterns that are examined to produce a profile that is unique enough to establish an identity.[2]

Blood, hair with tissue at the root, skin cells, muscle cells, and sperm cells contain DNA. The DNA is extracted from the swabs of unknown samples (eg, vaginal and anal swabs) and from known reference samples of the involved individuals. The forensic scientist then prepares the samples for amplification, or copying, by placing the material on a gel and then applies an electric current effectively separating the samples so they may be evaluated with the aid of computer software.[24,27,28] As a result, someone may be included or eliminated as a donor of the sample. In the case of an inclusion, statistics are computed to determine how rarely or commonly the particular DNA profile is found in the population.

Y-STR testing is another type of DNA testing that is used in forensic laboratories. This type of profiling is particularly useful because male DNA and female DNA may now be separated. Therefore, when using Y-STR profiling, the forensic scientist isolates patterns only found on the male Y-chromosome.[2] The resulting Y-chromosome profile is then searched against other Y-chromosome profiles in DNA databases for matches.[2]

The use of DNA typing has major implications with respect to law enforcement investigations. At state forensic laboratories throughout the United States, scientists are creating a databank or a database of DNA profiles. These profiles are those of convicted felons, criteria for inclusion varies in each state, and used for comparison with each subsequent case that is submitted by law enforcement.[28] Investigators may request the scientist to compare DNA profiles from cases in which the identity of the suspect is unknown against the profiles included in the database. If the unknown profile matches one in the database, the scientist has achieved what is referred to as a *cold hit.* DNA databases have allowed for cases once thought unsolvable to be reopened with the possibility of identifying the perpetrator. Law enforcement agencies are finding success and have brought many perpetrators to justice as a result.

Testing for Sexually Transmitted Infection: Collecting Samples

Testing for sexually transmitted infections (STI) is important for several reasons: (1) The presence of an STI may be the only evidence that sexual contact has occurred in some cases of child sexual abuse, (2) Testing is important in addressing the overall health of the child, (3) Identifying and treating these infections will prevent adverse health outcomes.

Many of these infections are asymptomatic; therefore, consideration must be given when developing protocols for testing. STIs are identified through cultures, nucleic amplification testing, and serological testing, and, as a result, specimens must be collected properly in order to identify a particular infection. Samples may be collected up to 2 weeks after an exposure.[29]

Specimen collection may be traumatic for the child and an unnecessary expense when testing is done indiscriminately. The clinician should decide whether or not to collect specimens as well as which sites (eg, oral, anal, vaginal, penile, or conjunctival) to asses on an individual basis in conjunction with the facility's established protocols. Testing is recommended under the following circumstances[30]:

— The child is symptomatic.

— The suspected offender is known to have an STI or to be at a high risk for one.

— The suspect has had multiple partners or a past history of an STI.

— There is a history of forced sexual assault, genital-to-genital contact, or possible ejaculation.

— There is evidence that suggests penetration has occurred.

— Another household member is known to have an STI.

— There is a high prevalence of STIs in the community.

The examiner should consider obtaining specimens to test for diseases such as gonorrhea, chlamydia, syphilis, hepatitis, herpes, and human immunodeficiency virus (HIV). Specimen collection may vary depending on which disease is suspected. Testing should be performed in response to the history given by the child, risk of exposure, and any current symptoms. When conducting the child sexual abuse examination, the examiner should have the appropriate tools readily on hand so samples can be quickly obtained (see *Chapter 6, Sexually Transmitted Infection in the Setting of Maltreatment*).

Conclusion

In the child sexual abuse examination, evidence collection is one piece of the process. Various specimens may be collected from the child based upon the history and physical examination. Proper evidence collection is necessary to facilitate a positive outcome; however, the examination represents one component of the investigation, which is a collaborative effort among agencies. The crime laboratory processes the evidence collected by the examiner. Law enforcement uses the information gained to appropriately investigate the case. This results in better-informed decisions about the protection of and treatment for the child. Protocols must be established with area agencies with whom the examiner interacts so that evidence can be collected properly, preserved, and handled. Evidence must be obtained in a manner that is useful to everyone, especially those who will be processing it in the crime laboratory, and the chain of custody must be documented. Therefore, communication and collaboration are essential to ensure the integrity of the evidence and its admittance into the courtroom.

References

1. Eldredge K, Huggins E, Pugh L. Alternate light sources in sexual assault examinations: an evidence-based practice project. *J Forensic Nurs.* 2012;8(1):39-44.

2. Savino JO, Turvey BE. *Rape Investigation Handbook.* New York, NY: Elsevier; 2005:75:134-136.

3. Shapiro RA, Makoroff KL. Sexually transmitted diseases in sexually abused girls and adolescents. *Curr Opin Obstet Gynecol.* 2006;18(5):492-497.

4. Edinburgh L, Saewyc E, Levitt C. Caring for young adolescent sexual abuse victims in a hospital-based children's advocacy center. *Child Abuse Negl.* 2008;32(12):1119-1126.

5. Emergency Nurses Association. Position statement: forensic evidence collection. Emergency Nurses Association Web site. http://www.ena.org/SiteCollectionDocuments/Position%20Statements/Forensic%20Evidence.pdf. Updated 2010. Accessed September 20, 2009.

6. International Association of Forensic Nurses. What is forensic nursing? International Association of Forensic Nurses Web site. http://www.iafn.org/displaycommon.cfm?an=1&subarticlenbr=137. Accessed September 20, 2009.

7. American College of Emergency Physicians. *Evaluation and Management of the Sexually Assaulted or Sexually Abused Patient.* Dallas, TX: United States Department of Health and Human Services, Health Resources and Services Administration, Maternal and Child Health Bureau; 1999:7-8-121.

8. Thackeray JD, Hornor G, Benzinger EA, Scribano PV. Forensic evidence collection and DNA identification in acute child sexual assault. *Pediatrics.* 2011;128(2):227-232.

9. Mayntz-Press KA, Sims LM, Hall AM, Ballantyne J. Y-STR profiling in extended interval (> or = 3 days) postcoital cervicovaginal samples. *J Forensic Sci.* 2008;53(2): 342-348.

10. United States Department of Justice Office of Violence Against Women. *A National Protocol for Sexual Assault Medical Forensic Examinations: Adults/Adolescents.* NCJ 206554. Washington, DC: United States Department of Justice Office of Violence Against Women; 2004:93-98.

11. Maiquilla SM, Salvador JM, Calacal GC, et al. Y-STR DNA analysis of 154 female child sexual assault cases in the Philippines. *Int J Legal Med.* 2011;125(6):817-824.

12. Girardet R, Bolton K, Lahoti S, et al. Collection of forensic evidence from pediatric victims of sexual assault. *Pediatrics.* 2011;128(2):233-238.

13. Hammer RM, Moynihan B, Pagliaro EM. *Forensic Nursing: A Handbook for Practice.* Sudbury, MA: Jones & Bartlett Publishers; 2006:295,297,564.

14. Wawryk J, Odell M. Fluorescent identification of biological and other stains on skin by the use of alternative light sources. *J Clin Forensic Med.* 2005;12(6):296-301.

15. Sakelliadis El, Spiliopoulou CA, Papadodima SA. Forensic investigation of child victim with sexual abuse. *Indian Pediatr.* 2009;46:144-151.

16. Christian C, Giardino A. Forensic evidence collection. In: Finkel MA, Giardino AP, eds. *Medical Evaluation of Child Sexual Abuse: A Practical Guide.* 2nd ed. Thousand Oaks, CA: Sage Publications Inc; 2002:131-145.

17. Sweet D, Lorente M, Lorente JA, et al. An improved method to recover saliva from human skin: the double swab technique. *J Forensic Sci.* 1997;42(2):320-322.

18. Martin-de las Heras S, Valenzuela A, Valverde AJ, Torres JC, Luna-del-Castillo JD. Effectiveness of comparison overlays generated with DentalPrint software in bite mark analysis. *J Forensic Sci.* 2007;52(1):151-156.

19. Kellogg N; the American Academy of Pediatrics Committee on Child Abuse and Neglect. Oral and dental aspects of child abuse and neglect. *Pediatrics.* 2005;116(6);1565-1568.

20. Sweet D, Lorente M, Lorente J, Valunzuela A, Villanueva E. An improved method to recover saliva from human skin: the double swab technique. *J Forensic Sci.*1997;42:320-322.

21. Finkel M, De Jong A. Medical findings in child sexual abuse. In: Reece RM, Ludwig S, eds. *Child Abuse: Medical Diagnosis and Management.* 2nd ed. Philadelphia, PA: Lippincott Williams & Wilkins; 2001:207-286.

22. Ricci LR, Shapiro RA. Photodocumentation and other technologies. In: Reece RM, Christian CW, eds. *Child Abuse: Medical Diagnosis and Management.* 3rd ed. Elk Grove Village, IL: American Academy of Pediatrics; 2009:755-792.

23. Lynch VA. *Forensic Nursing.* New York, NY: Elsevier Health Sciences; 2005:348.

24. Saferstein R. *Criminalistics: An Introduction to Forensic Science.* 8th ed. Upper Saddle River, NJ: Prentice Hall; 2004:349, 377-380.

25. Young KL, Jones JG, Worthington T, Simpson P, Casey PH. Forensic laboratory evidence in sexually abused children and adolescents. *Arch Pediatr Adolesc Med.* 2006;160:585-588

26. Ferris LE, Sandercock J. The sensitivity of forensic tests for rape. *Med Law.* 1998;17(3):330-350.

27. O'Connor T. DNA Analysis: typing and identification. http://www.aspu.edu/oconnort/3210/3210lect07.htm. Published 2006. Accessed October 1, 2009.

28. DNA Initiative. About forensic DNA. DNA Initiative Web site. http://www.dna.gov/basics/. Accessed October 1, 2009.

29. Centers for Disease Control and Prevention. Sexual assault and STDs: sexually transmitted diseases treatment guidelines, 2010. Centers for Disease Control and Prevention Web site. www.cdc.gov/std/treatment/2010/sexual-assault.htm. Updated January 28, 2011. Accessed June 15, 2013.

30. Centers for Disease Control and Prevention. Sexually transmitted disease treatment guidelines 2006. Centers for Disease Control and Prevention Web site. http://www.cdc.gov/std/treatment/2006/sexual-assault.htm. Accessed September 27, 2009.

Chapter 6

Sexually Transmitted Infection in the Setting of Maltreatment

Erin Endom, MD
Annie Lewis-O'Connor, NP-BC, PhD, MPH
Marisa V. Atendido, MSN, CRNP
Angelo P. Giardino, MD, PhD

Key Points

1. Urine nucleic acid amplification tests (NAATs) can be used as a confirmatory test for sexually transmitted infections (STIs) in girls; samples for confirmatory tests should be obtained from different NAATs. To confirm test results in boys, urethral cultures must be obtained.
2. STI testing should not be uncomfortable. When significant injuries are present, the health care provider should consider an evaluation under anesthesia. For the prepubescent child, speculum examinations are strictly prohibited; if deemed necessary because of injury or the need to rule out a foreign body, the examination should be performed under anesthesia and in consultation with experienced providers. Medical providers that conduct examinations and evaluations for sexual abuse should have relevant advanced training. Skills should include the ability to conduct the examination without any resulting discomfort to the child. When injuries are present or an evaluation is needed for a foreign body, the child should be brought to the operating room and evaluated under anesthesia. Based on the history and review of systems, the medical provider should consider the need for STI testing, recognizing that many tests and testing methodologies are available and that some methodologies have a higher sensitivity and specificity than others.
3. The prepubertal child and adolescent differ with regard to the transmission, presentation, identification, and assessment of STIs.
4. The examination of the prepubertal child includes inspection of the external genitalia for signs of trauma, inflammation, and discharge and should include a visual examination of the vaginal vestibule. Again, for the prepubescent child, a speculum examination is strictly prohibited and a speculum should never be used; the one exception being under anesthesia to rule out a foreign body or exploration of bleeding of unknown etiology.
5. Infection with *Neisseria gonorrhoeae (N. gonorrhoeae)* does not confer immunity. Many cases may manifest without symptoms or with discharge. Infants born to women who have tested positive for *N. gonorrhoeae* rarely have the organism isolated when they are aged 1 to 6 months. Outside of the perinatal period, gonorrhea in a prepubertal child should be treated as highly suspect for sexual abuse and warrant a thorough evaluation.
6. The emotional stigma associated with the diagnosis of an STI is often paramount to the young child's caregiver. Offering emotional support and providing evidence-based education will provide the best opportunity to de-escalate fears and concerns.

Introduction

An important component of the health care evaluation for suspected sexual abuse, assault, or both in the prepubertal child and the adolescent is the identification of STIs, formerly sexually transmitted diseases (STDs), in the child or adolescent being evaluated. The American Academy of Pediatrics (AAP)[1] and the Centers for Disease Control and Prevention (CDC)[2] have issued guidelines to assist the clinician in deciding what circumstances warrant the evaluation of children and adolescents for STIs during the examination. In some cases, the STI may be the presenting indicator of abuse, while in other cases, the presence of an STI may serve to confirm the child's history of inappropriate sexual contact or support the concerns that an inappropriate sexual contact occurred when there is no disclosure. Estimates vary, but 3% to 13% of children evaluated for STIs will test positive.[1,3-7]

The thinking around STI screening in the setting of sexual maltreatment has evolved over the past decades. For example, all prepubertal children suspected of having been the victim of sexual abuse are screened for STIs using urine NAATs or, if discharge is present, a culture. Additionally, it is best to have the child evaluated by a medical provider trained in conducting sexual abuse evaluations, such as those available at a child advocacy center (CAC) or by a medical provider on a child protection team.[1,2]

This chapter provides a critical thinking framework to guide the health care provider through the process of evaluating a child for suspected sexual abuse and takes into consideration which patients should be tested for which diseases within the context of a health care history and physical examination. This chapter also focuses on several STIs that the clinician should consider during the evaluation process, realizing that actions taken during evaluation have legal, ethical, moral, and forensic implications (see *Chapter 5, Laboratory Findings, Diagnostic Testing, and Forensic Specimens in Cases of Child Sexual Abuse*). Listed below, in alphabetic order, are the specific infections addressed in this chapter:

— Bacterial vaginosis (BV)

— Chancroid

— Chlamydia

— Gonorrhea (GC)

— Hepatitis B (HBV)

— Herpes genitalis

— Human immunodeficiency virus (HIV) and acquired immune deficiency syndrome (AIDS)

— Human papillomavirus ([HPV], condylomata acuminata, or genital warts)

— Pediculosis pubis

— Pelvic inflammatory disease (PID)

— Syphilis

— Trichomoniasis

Each infection has its own characteristic clinical presentation, diagnosis, and treatment, and is discussed individually in this chapter. **Table 6-1** details the incidence of each infection in populations of sexually abused children. **Table 6-2** addresses the likelihood of a given infection being an indicator of sexual abuse in prepubertal children and non-sexually active adolescents.

Table 6-1. Incubation Periods, Clinical Manifestations, Transmission, and Diagnosis of STIs

	GONORRHEA *Neisseria gonorrhoeae*	CHLAMYDIAL INFECTIONS *Chlamydia trachomatis*
Incubation Period	3 to 5 days	5 to 7 days
Clinical Manifestations	— Vaginitis, urethritis, pharyngitis, proctitis — Rare: arthritis, conjunctivitis — Most pharyngeal (throat) and rectal infections and as many as 50% of vaginal infections in children may be asymptomatic	— Most prevalent sexually transmitted infection in the United States — In adults and adolescents: urethritis and mucopurulent cervicitis, which can lead to pelvic inflammatory disease; however, most infections in adults and children are asymptomatic
Transmission	— Through sexual contact — Exception: neonatal conjunctivitis is acquired by the infant from his/her mother at delivery — No evidence of transmission by fomites (eg, via toilet seats, dirty towels)	— Sexually, in children 3 years of age or older — Perinatally acquired infection (mother-to-infant) may last in the vagina and rectum for up to 3 years or longer — No evidence of transmission by fomites
Diagnosis	— Culture of *N. gonorrhoeae* using selective media with confirmation by at least 2 different methods using different principles (eg, sugar fermentation, enzyme substances, serological, or DNA hybridization) — Use of DNA probes or other nonculture methods, including Gram's stain smears or vaginal or urethral discharges, is not recommended because other bacteria may be misidentified as *N. gonorrhoeae.*	— Isolation of the organism in tissue culture only with microscopic identification of the characteristic inclusions with fluorescent antibody staining — Nonculture methods, including enzyme immunoassays (EIAs), direct fluorescent antibody (DFA) tests, and DNA probes, are not approved for use in children. Use at these sites has led to many false positive tests.
Prevalence Range in Children Evaluated for Sexual Abuse[3-5,8,9]	1% to 2.8%	0.5% to 1.3%
Prevalence Range for Women Evaluated for Sexual Assaults[10]	0% to 26.3%	3.9% to 17%

(continued)

Table 6-1. Incubation Periods, Clinical Manifestations, Transmission, and Diagnosis of STIs *(continued)*

	SYPHILIS *Treponema pallidum*	TRICHOMONIASIS *Trichomonas vaginalis*
Incubation Period	Primary infection: 10 to 90 days, usually 3 to 4 weeks Secondary: 6 weeks to 6 months after the primary lesion heals	5 to 28 days
Clinical Manifestations	— Primary syphilis: chancre—a painless ulcer at the site of inoculation (eg, penis, vulva, vagina, rectum); the chancre heals spontaneously after 1 to 2 weeks. — Secondary syphilis: diffuse rash, fever, enlarged lymph nodes, mucous patches — Latent syphilis: asymptomatic, although positive serological findings may persist for years	— Vaginitis — In males, infection appears to be asymptomatic, but *T. vaginalis* may cause some cases of nonspecific urethritis.
Transmission	— Through sexual contact; the chancre and mucous patches are very infectious. — Infants may acquire congenital syphilis from their mothers. The presentation is similar to secondary syphilis.	— Through sexual contact — Has not been found in children 1 year of age or older without history of sexual contact. — Infants can acquire infection from mother at delivery; can cause vaginitis. — Perinatally acquired infection may persist for 6 to 9 months after birth. — No evidence of transmission by fomites

(continued)

Table 6-1. Incubation Periods, Clinical Manifestations, Transmission, and Diagnosis of STIs *(continued)*

	SYPHILIS *Treponema pallidum*	TRICHOMONIASIS *Trichomonas vaginalis*
Diagnosis	— Identification of *T. pallidum* in lesions by dark-field microscopy or by staining with fluorescein-conjugated monoclonal antibody — The most common methods used are serological: rapid plasma reagin (RPR) test; Venereal Disease Research Laboratory (VDRL) reaginic antibody test; and fluorescent treponemal antibody absorption (FTA-ABS) test, a test for a specific anti-*T. pallidum antibody.* — Positive results on an RPR or VDRL test in a child who does not have a history of congenital syphilis — RPR and VDRL test results will be negative after effective treatment; FTA-ABS remains elevated for the lifetime of the patient.	— Microscopic identification of the organism in vaginal fluid — Culture methods may be more sensitive, but not widely available. — The finding of trichomonads in urine collected for another purpose is not sufficient for accurate diagnosis because the urine could be contaminated. — *Trichomonas hominis* is a normal inhabitant of the bowel that is not sexually transmitted.
Prevalence Range in Children Evaluated for Sexual Abuse[3-5,8,9]	0.15% to 1.5%	0.5% to 2.5%
Prevalence Range in Women Evaluated for Sexual Abuse[10]	0 to 5.6%	0 to 19%

(continued)

Table 6-1. Incubation Periods, Clinical Manifestations, Transmission, and Diagnosis of STIs *(continued)*

	BACTERIAL VAGINOSIS (BV) *Gardnerella vaginalis, Bacteroides species and other anaerobic bacteria, and Mycoplasma hominis*	HERPES *Herpes simplex virus (HSV), types 1 and 2*
Incubation Period	5 to 28 days	2 to 5 days
Clinical Manifestations	— BV is not really an infection, but a disturbance of the normal vaginal flora, which is replaced by the organisms listed. — Clinically presents as gray, foul-smelling vaginal discharge, but may be asymptomatic.	— Painful vesicular lesions that become ulcers on the vulva, vagina, penis, and perirectal area. — May be associated with inguinal lymphadenopathy (disease of the lymph nodes in the groin) and fever.
Transmission	— Through sexual and nonsexual contact — Probably related to poor hygiene in some young children.	— Through sexual contact — Primarily HSV-2, although 10% of genital herpes in adults can be due to HSV-1. — Young children with herpetic gingivostomatitis (herpetic infection of the gum tissues), a primary, nonsexually acquired infection caused by HSV-1, may autoinoculate (infect themselves) in the genital area. There should be a history of stomatitis (sores in the mouth) in the previous 2 weeks.

(continued)

Table 6-1. Incubation Periods, Clinical Manifestations, Transmission, and Diagnosis of STIs *(continued)*

	Bacterial Vaginosis (BV) *Gardnerella vaginalis, Bacteroides species and other anaerobic bacteria, and Mycoplasma hominis*	Herpes *Herpes simplex virus (HSV), types 1 and 2*
Diagnosis	— Microscopic identification of "clue cells," which are epithelial cells studded with bacteria in vaginal secretions; a positive "whiff" or amine test, which is the release of a characteristic fishy odor when 10% potassium hydroxide (KOH) is added to the vaginal fluid; and a vaginal fluid pH of >4.5 — The latter test should only be done in adolescents, as there are no vaginal pH standards for prepubertal children. — Culture of *G. vaginalisis* not indicated and is not diagnostic for BV. *G. vaginalis* can be normal vaginal flora and has been isolated in 5% to 15% of normal children who have not been abused.	— Isolation of the virus from the lesions — No commercially available antibody tests will reliably differentiate between HSV-1 and HSV-2
Prevalence Range in Children Evaluated for Sexual Abuse[3-5,8,9]	7%[§]	0.1% to 0.5%
Prevalence Range in Women Evaluated for Sexual Abuse[10]	10% to 64%[11,12]	Not available

(continued)

Table 6-1. Incubation Periods, Clinical Manifestations, Transmission, and Diagnosis of STIs *(continued)*		
	HUMAN PAPILLOMAVIRUS (HPV) *Condyloma acuminata, venereal wart*	AIDS *Human immunodeficiency virus (HIV)*
Incubation Period	4 to 12 weeks, but may be clinically inapparent for up to 18 months	Seroconversion: 6 weeks after exposure; more than 90% of individuals will be HIV positive by 6 months. Development of AIDS: 5 to 10 years
Clinical Manifestations	— Flesh- to purple-colored papillomatous growths in the anogenital region	— Children who are HIV positive before developing AIDS are asymptomatic. — Some individuals develop an acute retroviral syndrome, similar to influenza, with lymphadenopathy after infection. — Has not been described in children with acquired HIV infection
Transmission	— Sexually, perinatally, and probably, but rarely, nonsexually — Major confounding variable is the long period after infection before the lesions become visible to the naked eye, which could be as long as 18 months	— Sexually, perinatally, and via blood transfusion, intravenous drug abuse (IVDA), and sharing needles — Approximately 30% of infants born to HIV-positive mothers will develop HIV infection but may not develop clinical AIDS for 5 years or longer. — Acquisition by sexual abuse needs to be differentiated from perinatal infection because risk factors for maternal infection and sexual abuse are similar.

(continued)

Table 6-1. Incubation Periods, Clinical Manifestations, Transmission, and Diagnosis of STIs *(continued)*

	HUMAN PAPILLOMAVIRUS (HPV) *Condyloma acuminata, venereal wart*	AIDS *Human immunodeficiency virus (HIV)*
Diagnosis	— Clinical: HPV DNA-typing of the lesions is not generally available.	— Serological: presence of HIV antibody, detection of p24 antigen. Child being evaluated for HIV after abuse needs to be tested for 6 months. Consider HIV testing if the child is from an area of high HIV prevalence, if the abuser is in a high-risk group (eg, IVDA, crack user), or if another STI is present.
Prevalence Range in Children Evaluated for Sexual Abuse[3-5,8,9]	0.7% to 1.8%	Not available
Prevalence Range in Women Evaluated for Sexual Abuse[11,12]	0.6% to 2.3%	Not available

[§]*Difficult to quantify because the presence of* G. vaginalis *alone is not diagnostic of BV.*
Reprinted from Hammerschlag MR. Sexually Transmitted Diseases and Child Abuse: Portable Guides to Investigating Child Abuse. *Washington, DC: US Department of Justice, Office of Justice Programs and Office of Juvenile Justice and Delinquency Preventions; 1996.*

Table 6-2. Implications of Commonly Encountered Sexually Transmitted Infections for the Diagnosis of Sexual Abuse

	DIAGNOSTIC	HIGHLY SUSPICIOUS	SUSPICIOUS
Confirmed STI organism	Gonorrhea* Syphilis* HIV‡ *C. trachomatis**	*Trichomonas vaginalis*	Condyloma acuminata (anogenital warts) Herpes†‡ (genital location)

**If not perinatally acquired.*
‡*If not perinatally or transfusion acquired.*
†‡*Unless there is a clear history of autoinoculation.*
Adapted from Kellogg N; The American Academy of Pediatrics Committee on Child Abuse and Neglect. The evaluation of sexual abuse in children. Pediatrics. *2005;116(2):506-512.*

Other less common STIs that will not be discussed but may need to be considered in the differential diagnosis of genital findings include chancroid, lymphogranuloma venereum (LGV), and highly contagious skin diseases, such as scabies, streptococcal infections, and *molluscum contagiosum* (**Figures 6-1** to **6-13**). These entities should be considered when the clinical presentation is atypical and the more typical infectious diseases have been eliminated or ruled out.

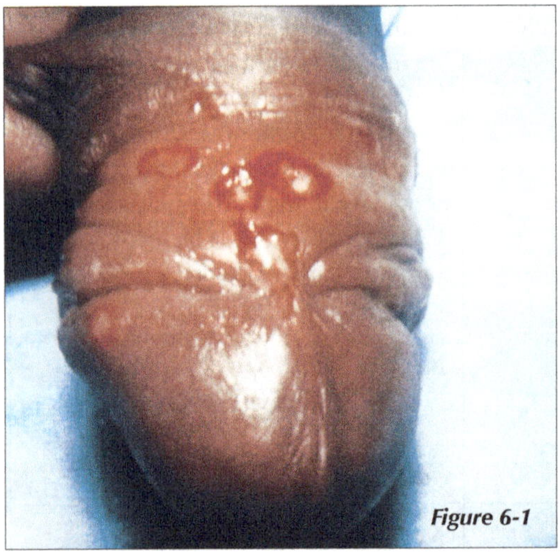

Figure 6-1. *Chancroid ulcers. (Contributed by the Centers for Disease Control and Prevention [CDC]; Atlanta, GA.)*

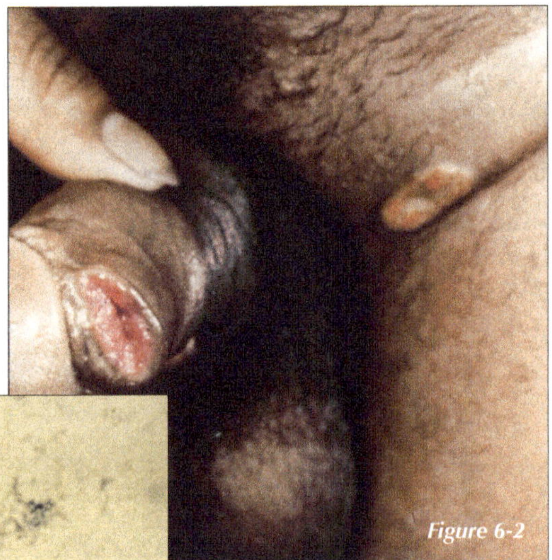

Figure 6-2. *Chancroid, male. Regional adenopathy. (Contributed by CDC; Atlanta, GA.)*

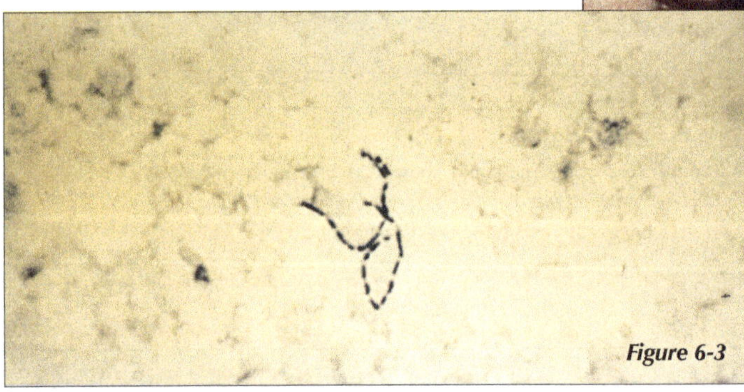

Figure 6-3. *Chancroid. Gram stain of* Haemophilus ducreyi. *(Contributed by CDC; Atlanta, GA.)*

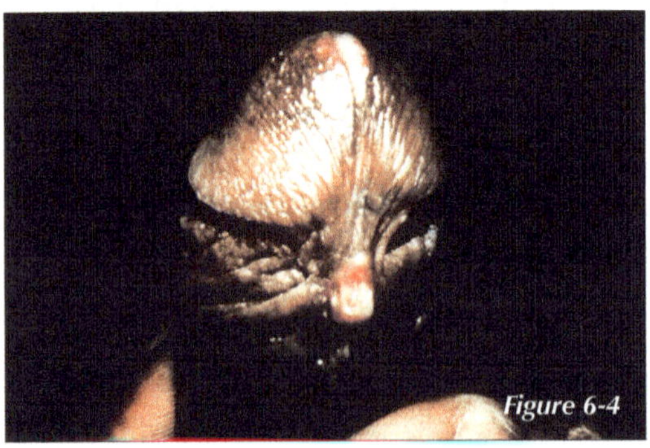

Figure 6-4. *Lymphogranuloma (LGV) primary lesion. (Contributed by CDC; Atlanta, GA.)*

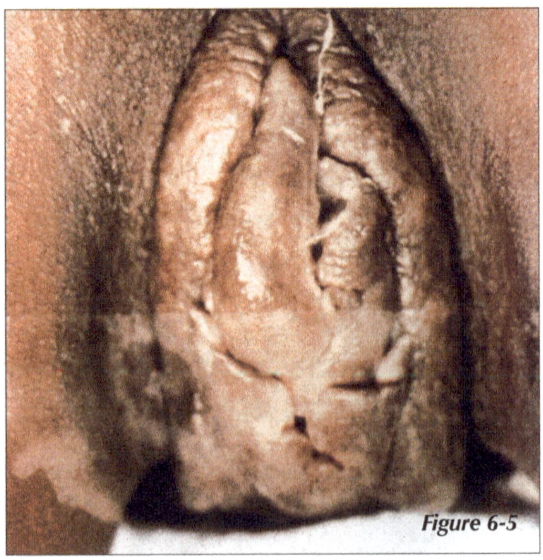

Figure 6-5. *Chronic LGV in female. Genital elephantiasis. (Contributed by CDC; Atlanta, GA.)*

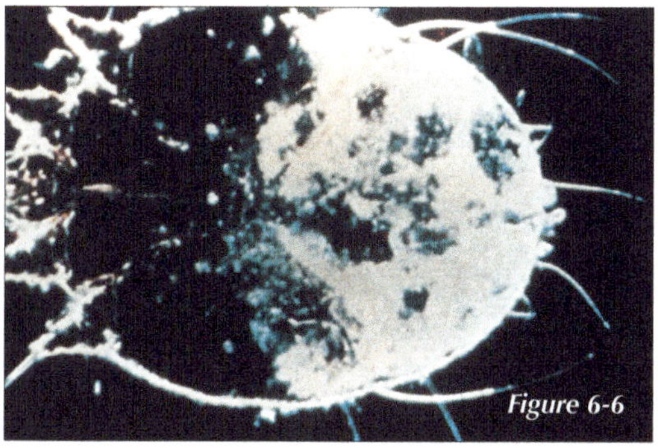

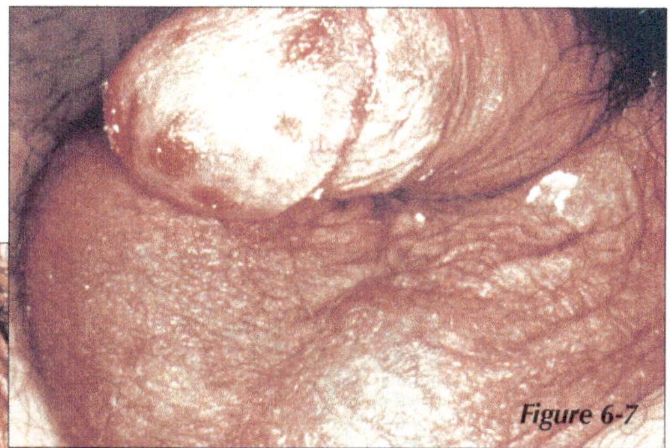

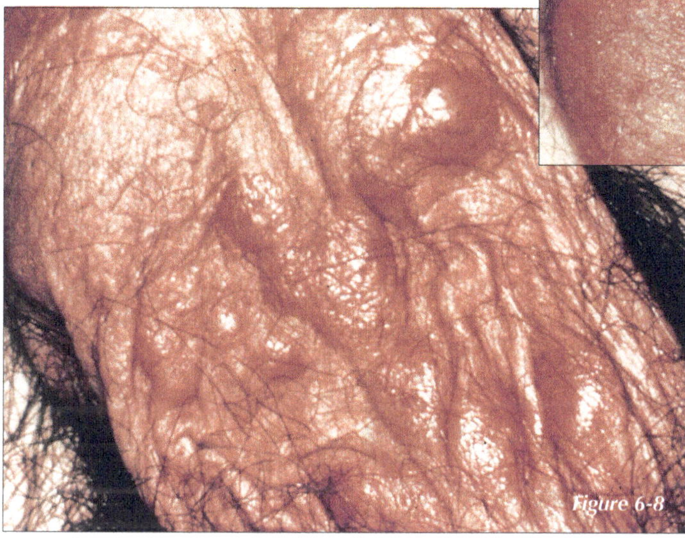

Figure 6-6. *Scabies mite. (Contributed by CDC; Atlanta, GA.)*

Figure 6-7. Scabies. *(Contributed by CDC; Atlanta, GA.)*

Figure 6-8. Scabies. *(Contributed by CDC; Atlanta, GA.)*

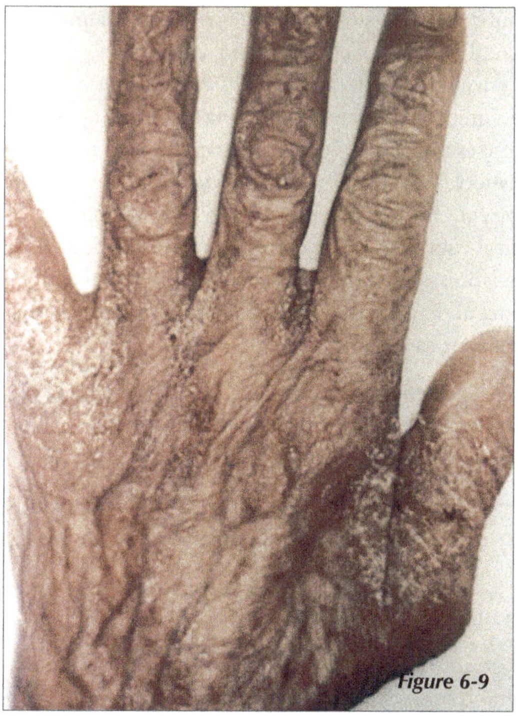

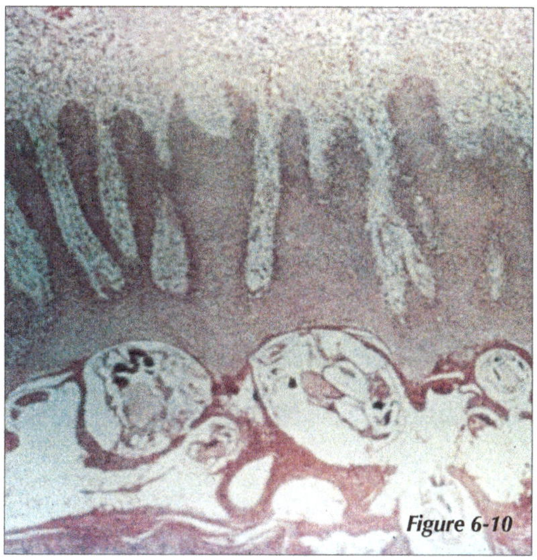

Figure 6-9. Scabies causing eczema-like skin condition. *(Contributed by CDC; Atlanta, GA.)*

Figure 6-10. Histologic section of a scabies mite burrow. *(Contributed by CDC; Atlanta, GA.)*

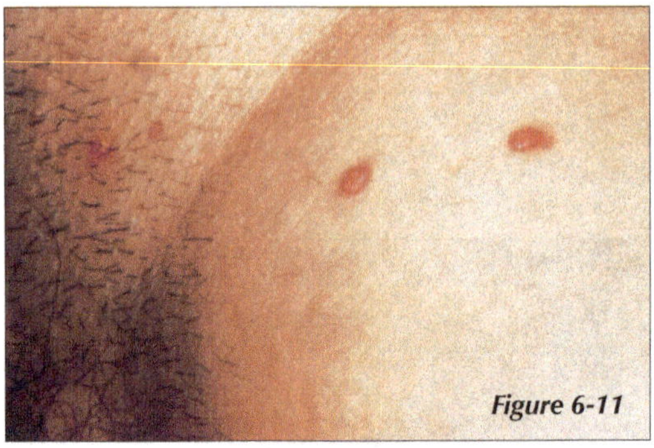

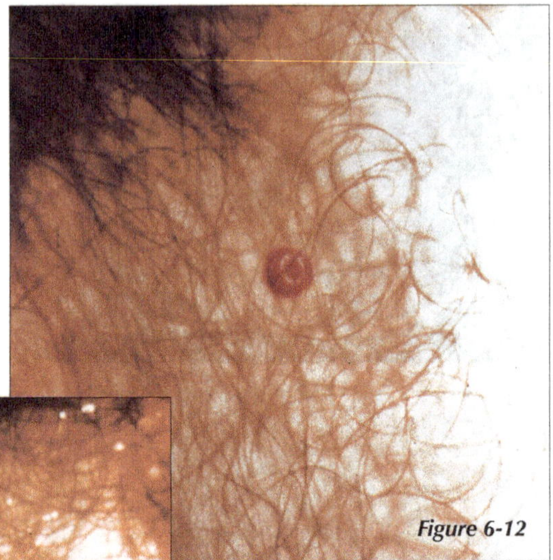

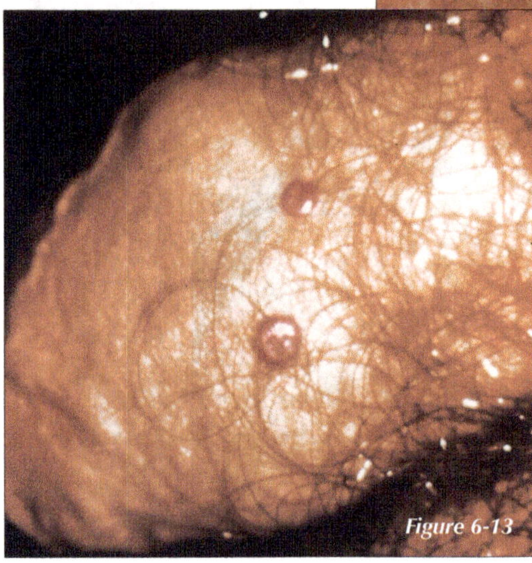

Figure 6-11. Molluscum contagiosum, *vulva and thighs. (Contributed by CDC; Atlanta, GA.)*

Figure 6-12. Molluscum contagiosum. *(Contributed by CDC; Atlanta, GA.)*

Figure 6-13. Molluscum contagiosum, *penis. (Contributed by CDC; Atlanta, GA.)*

Screening for STIs occurs in the context of a focused history, review of systems, and comprehensive physical examination. Prepubertal children and adolescents, as well as their caregivers, may experience anxieties about the impending examination. The clinician should take the time to use a gradual and sensitive trauma-informed approach with the patient before and during the examination, telling the patient what to expect and allowing opportunities for questions or pauses.[13,14] (see *Chapter 4, The Physical Examination in the Evaluation of Suspected Child Maltreatment: Physical Abuse and Sexual Abuse Examinations*). Important clinical issues should be taken into consideration when evaluating a child's or adolescent's risk for having acquired an STI from a sexual assault. Hammerschlag et al[15-17] and Girardet et al[7] have synthesized the clinical material in this complicated area and summarize each issue as follows:

— The possibility of vertical transmission (from mother to child during birth) and the extent to which vertical transmission can be used to explain an STI (eg, prolonged colonization after perinatal acquisition)

— The regional variation of STIs in the adult population (potential perpetrators) and the observation that variation may exist among different populations within the same region

— Timing of examination related to time of suspected contact

— Range of incubation periods and symptom presentation, which can be several days, as with GC or chlamydia, to several months to years, as with HPV

— Controversy concerning symptomatic versus asymptomatic infection, especially in the prepubertal child

— Inability to differentiate preexisting infections from those caused by a sexual assault

— Controversy regarding the extent to which infections in the prepubertal child and non-sexually active adolescent may be related to nonsexual spread.[16]

There are challenging issues regarding adolescents suspected of having been sexually maltreated and the evaluation regarding an associated STI after such contact. These issues are related to characteristics seen in the pubertal and postpubertal populations, which can be defined by determining the following:

— If the adolescent has engaged in consensual sexual behaviors

— The influences of substances (alcohol, drugs, or both) in the sexual encounter

— Whether neglect occurred, specifically if the supervising adults failed to protect the adolescent

— The significance of age difference between the adolescent and the sexual contact (eg, a 14- and 16-year-old versus a 15- and 26-year-old)

— What constitutes mandatory reporting versus what is protected under emancipated minor laws

— What is considered consent

Although these challenges exist, there is a clear need for the identification and treatment of STIs. The CDC[2] recognizes this need as more important for the physical and psychological well-being of the adolescent victim than for actual legal considerations. The CDC and AAP have issued guidelines for clinicians who evaluate adolescent victims of sexual abuse; these include information about the initial examination, follow-up examinations, and need for prophylaxis[18](**Table 6-3**).

Table 6-3. Recommendations for Prophylaxis of the Evaluation of Sexually Transmitted Infection in Adolescents and Adults*

Recommended Regimens
Ceftriaxone 250 mg IM in a single dose
or
Cefixime 400 mg orally in a single dose
plus
Metronidazole 2 g orally in a single dose
plus
Azithromycin 1 g orally in a single does
or
Doxycycline 100 mg orally twice a day for 7 days

**Drug dosage recommendations listed herein are those of the authors and are not endorsed by the United States Public Health Service or the United States Department of Health and Human Services. Adapted from Centers for Disease Control and Prevention. Sexually transmitted diseases treatment guidelines 2010.* MMWR. *2010;59(RR-12):1-110. Centers for Disease Control and Prevention Web site. http://www.cdc.gov/std/treatment/2010/toc.htm. Updated January 28, 2011. Accessed September 29, 2013. Adapted from American Academy of Pediatrics Committee on Infectious Diseases; Pickering LK, Long SS.* Report of the Committee on Infectious Diseases. *28th ed. Oak Grove Village, IL: American Academy of Pediatrics; 2009.*

The first step in clinically assessing a child for STIs is to ask questions of both the child and parent during the history-taking process about specific symptoms. It is essential to have a direct, yet sensitive approach when asking questions because the trauma of sexual abuse and assault can make the child, family, and adolescent uncomfortable.

When to Test for Sexually Transmitted Infections in the Setting of Suspected Maltreatment

The health care provider must take several factors into consideration when deciding whether a suspected child victim of sexual abuse should be tested for STIs. The likelihood of positive cultures for gonorrheal and chlamydial infection is very low in prepubertal children; regardless, the standard of practice today is to screen all children who are suspected of having been a victim of sexual abuse. It is important to note that some children do not disclose all the details of the assault. Any child with anal, vaginal, or oral penetration should be tested for gonorrhea and chlamydia; samples should be collected from all orifices and submitted for testing.[1,2,19-21] STI screening can be achieved by first performing a urine NAAT screening for gonorrhea and chlamydia. In prepubertal children, empiric treatment is deferred. While the standard for legal prosecution in cases of suspected sexual abuse remains culture with typing for gonorrhea and chlamydia, the standard for child protective services (CPS) supports immunoassay testing. A positive culture, specifically typed, does not need to be repeated. Cultures have good specificity but are not as sensitive as immunoassay testing, so a negative culture may represent a false-negative result.

Urine collection is less invasive than immunoassay testing. Collection of urine specimens requires a dirty collection, meaning the specimen should be obtained before any clean-catch urine testing. Different types of NAAT testing may be used to confirm the results of cultures. NAATs include polymerase chain reaction (PCR), thermomechanical analysis (TMS), and strand displacement amplification (SDA), all of which have good sensitivity but a higher rate of false positives, or lower specificity. If a child's NAAT test result is positive, then the health care provider should consider confirming the results by culture or another NAAT test that uses a different target. For example, if a urine PCR result is positive, then the health care provider might consider confirming the results by performing SDA or TMS urine testing. When possible, the health care provider should ask the laboratory to retain a small amount of the original urine sample for confirmatory testing. The confirmatory NAAT test may use an alternate target on the original sample.

Urine NAATs can be used for a confirmatory test in girls but not boys. To confirm test results in boys, urethral cultures must be obtained.[2,22] The following factors should be taken into consideration while deciding when to test prepubertal children for STIs, what STIs to test for, and which anatomic sites to test[2,23]:

— Child with chief complaint or caregiver with reason to believe that a sexual assault occurred

— Appropriateness of oral, anal, and vaginal screening should be considered— oral and rectal screening for evidence should be considered when assault occurred 24 hours or less before examination; however, in the child population, the standard of practice is to swab all orifices if there is a strong suspicion of contact abuse or sexual assault.

— Local incidence of STIs in the adult population

— Abuser with risk factors for an STI (eg, substance abuse, history of sexual assault, homelessness)

— Evidence of symptoms—screening for STIs in children may occur in both symptomatic and asymptomatic children.

— Age of the child

— Amount of time lapsed since last sexual contact

— Family member or sibling with an STI: when one sibling tests positive for an STI, consideration should be given to testing other children in the home.

— Request or concerns of child or family

The CDC[2] advises that the decision to test prepubertal children for STIs in the sexual abuse evaluation should be made on a case-by-case basis and individualized based on risk, history, and concern for the child's safety (**Table 6-4**). Indicators for testing according to CDC guidelines include the following:

— Known STI or a high risk for STIs in suspected offender

— Symptomatic child

— High prevalence of STIs in the community

— Evidence or suspicion of anogenital or oral penetration or ejaculation

— STIs in siblings or other children in the household

Table 6-4. General Guide for the Testing of Sexually Transmitted Infections in Prepubertal Children

Suspected of Having Been Sexually Abused	**The decision to test must be made on an individual basis predicated on suspected risk. Single examination may be sufficient if:** — Abuse occurred over an extended period. — Last suspected episode of abuse occurred well before the medical evaluation.
Initial Visit and 2-Week Follow-Up Examination	**Visual inspection of genital, perianal, and oral area for the following:** — Genital discharge — Odor — Bleeding — Irritation — Warts — Ulcerative lesions
	Cultures for *N. gonorrhoeae:* — Vagina — Urethra, in boys (Meatal specimen is adequate if urethral discharge present.) — Pharynx, in both girls and boys — Anus in both girls and boys

(continued)

Table 6-4. General Guide for the Testing of Sexually Transmitted Infections in Prepubertal Children *(continued)*

Initial Visit and 2-Week Follow-Up Examination	**Cultures for *C. trachomatis:*** — Vagina — Anus, in both girls and boys — If urethral specimen, meatal specimen indicated when urethral discharge is present — Not recommended, pharyngeal specimens in either girls or boys
	Culture and vaginal wet mount for *T. vaginalis:* — Vagina — BV, as suggested by presence of clue cells exclusively or in conjunction with a positive whiff test
	Serum sample for *T. pallidum,* HIV, and hepatitis B surface antigen (HBsAg): — Case-by-case basis — Requires immediate evaluation and preservation for subsequent analysis
Recommendations for Postexposure Assessment of Children within 72 Hours of Sexual Assault*	— Review local epidemiology of HIV and AIDS and assess risk for HIV infection in the assailant. — Evaluate circumstances of assault that may affect risk for HIV transmission. — Consult with a specialist in treating HIV-infected children if postexposure prophylaxis is considered. — If the child appears to be at risk for HIV transmission from the assault, discuss postexposure prophylaxis with the caregiver(s), including its toxicity and its unknown efficacy. — If caregivers choose for the child to receive antiretroviral postexposure prophylaxis, provide enough medication until the return visit at 3 to 7 days after initial assessment to reevaluate child and to assess tolerance of medication; dosages should not exceed those for adults. — Perform HIV antibody test at original assessment, 6 weeks, 3 months, and 6 months. — Review local epidemiology of HIV and AIDS and assess risk for HIV infection in the assailant. — Evaluate circumstances of assault that may affect risk for HIV transmission. — Consult with a specialist in treating HIV-infected children if postexposure prophylaxis is considered.

(continued)

Table 6-4. General Guide for the Testing of Sexually Transmitted Infections in Prepubertal Children *(continued)*

Recommendations for Postexposure Assessment of Children within 72 Hours of Sexual Assault*	— If the child appears to be at risk for HIV transmission from the assault, discuss postexposure prophylaxis with the caregiver(s), including its toxicity and its unknown efficacy. — If caregivers choose for the child to receive antiretroviral postexposure prophylaxis, provide enough medication until the return visit at 3 to 7 days after initial assessment to reevaluate child and to assess tolerance of medication; dosages should not exceed those for adults. — Perform HIV antibody test at original assessment, 6 weeks, 3 months, and 6 months.
12 Weeks After Last Suspected Sexual Exposure	— Observe 12-week period to allow time for antibodies to infectious agents to develop if baseline tests are negative. — Interpret results of HBsAg carefully because hepatitis B (HBV) can be transmitted nonsexually. — Presumptive treatment for STIs is not recommended in prepubertal children unless symptomatic for several reasons. —Low prevalence of most STIs following abuse or assault —Lower risk for ascending infection in girls before puberty —Increased ability to ensure follow-up care with children — Take patient or caregiver concerns into consideration as an indication for treatment.

**May vary according to local laws.*
Adapted from Centers for Disease Control and Prevention. Sexually transmitted diseases treatment guidelines 2002. MMWR. *2002;51(RR06):72-74. Centers for Disease Control and Prevention Web site. http://www.cdc.gov/mmwr/preview/mmwrhtml/rr5106a1.htm. Published May 10, 2002. Accessed September 21, 2013.*

Asymptomatic Versus Symptomatic Infections

The prepubertal child and the adolescent differ anatomically and physiologically with regard to the transmission, presentation, and best means of identification of STIs.[2] **Table 6-5** lists differences between female children and female adults that affect the identification of STIs. Controversy exists regarding how common asymptomatic infections are in prepubertal children versus adolescents. Anatomical and physiological changes associated with puberty cause some of the differences seen in the frequency of asymptomatic infections between the prepubertal child and the adolescent.

With regard to STIs, asymptomatic infections are more common in the adolescent than the prepubertal child. Symptoms of STIs in the prepubertal child vary and manifest in several ways, including vaginal or urethral discharge; genital itching and irritation, such as vulvovaginitis or urethritis; and genital lesions and growths, depending on the specific etiology. Asymptomatic genital infections have been observed to be uncommon in prepubertal children. In the adolescent patient, however, chlamydial infections are often asymptomatic, while GC, HPV, and herpes are usually symptomatic. When symptomatic, the adolescent patient may experience vaginal discharge of varying colors

Table 6-5. Differences Between Female Adults and Female Children Affecting the Diagnosis of Sexually Transmitted Infections

Characteristics	Adults	Children	Effect on Diagnosis or Treatment
Vaginal pH	Less than 4.5 (acidic)	6.6 to 7.5 (alkaline)	Vagina supports a different flora. Example: Alkaline pH is hostile to yeast. Vaginal yeast infections are rare in children.
Vaginal mucosa	Stratified squamous	Columnar epithelium	Pathogens such as *N. gonorrhoeae* and *C. trachomatis* infect columnar epithelium and cause vaginitis in children instead of cervicitis.
Vaginal mucous glands	Present	Absent	Child's vagina is probably a more hostile environment to some pathogens such as *T. vaginalis* because of a lack of vaginal mucus.
Normal vaginal flora	Lactobacilli	Gram-positive cocci and anaerobic gram-negatives are more common; flora resembles that of postmenopausal women.	Gram-positive cocci and gram-negative anaerobes can "cross react" with immunofluorescent stains for *C. trachomatis*. Gram-negative enteric pathogens are more likely to cause vaginitis in prepubertal children.
Vaginal length	11 cm to 12 cm	4 cm to 5 cm	Cuboidal mucosa closer to external genitalia might increase the likelihood of STI microorganisms entering the vagina without actual penile penetration.
Vaginal anatomy	Thick protective labia; elastic distensible vaginal structure	Comparatively thin labia; rigid, nonelastic, thin-walled vagina	Sexual activity is probably more likely to cause bleeding and mucosal disruption in children, possibly increasing the likelihood of infection with HIV after exposure.

Reprinted with permission from Jenny C. Sexually transmitted diseases and child abuse. Pediatr Ann. *1992;21(8):497-503.*

and quantities, irregular bleeding, itching or irritation in the genital area, genital lesions or growths, a nonspecific odor, generalized urinary complaints, and mild to severe pain in the vagina or lower abdomen. Adolescent males are more likely to complain of dysuria, urethral discharge, and genital lesions or growths. In both females and males, genital lesions may be painless or extremely painful, depending on the etiology.

In addition to genital complaints resulting from the presence of STIs, problems with the perianal area and rectum in prepubertal children and adolescents are possible, depending on the type of sexual contact and the infecting organism involved. The presence of symptoms such as anorectal pain, tenesmus, and rectal discharge suggest the existence of proctitis.[2]

Specific Infections

Bacterial Vaginosis

General Overview and Epidemiology

BV is a heterogeneous clinical entity marked by a disorder of vaginal flora that represents a polymicrobial syndrome in which several bacterial species interact to alter the vaginal ecosystem.[17,24] A shift in the ecosystem leads to a decrease in lactobacilli, usually predominant in the vagina, and an increase in anaerobes, such as *Mobiluncus* species, *Gardnerella vaginalis* (*G. vaginalis*), *Bacteroides* species, peptostreptococci, and *Mycoplasma hominis*.[24] BV is the most common cause of vaginitis and vaginal discharge in postpubertal women, accounting for 40% to 50% of cases, compared to vulvovaginal candidiasis, which is seen in 20% to 25% of cases, and trichomoniasis, in 15% to 20% of cases.[24-26] This nonspecific infection is probably the most common cause of vaginal discharge in female children as well.[17] Its prevalence and incidence are difficult to obtain, but BV has been found in 10% to 25% of women in gynecological and obstetric clinics and in up to 64% of women seen in STI clinics. BV is not treated in male partners.[25,26] Although BV is not considered to be an STI and is often found in nonsexually active women, it is thought to be associated with sexual activity because vaginal penetration may be the factor that alters the ecosystem, leading to an overgrowth of bacteria. BV has been shown to increase the risk of acquiring HIV and other STIs.[27] BV may be present after the sexual abuse of children and in adolescents who have been sexually assaulted, but its significance as an indicator of sexual exposure is unclear.[2,17,26] Clinicians caring for victims of sexual assault should assess for BV and treat patients, keeping in mind that in cases of acute sexual assault, the patient may not present with symptoms in the first 48 hours following the assault.

Clinical Finding

BV may be asymptomatic in prepubertal children and adolescents. Symptoms are present in up to 50% of adolescents and adult women with BV.[19] However, a 2007 study of participants in the National Health and Nutrition Examination Survey (NHANES), aged 14 to 49 years, found a 29.2% prevalence of BV; only 15.7% of women with BV reported symptoms.[27] Common symptoms in both prepubertal and postpubertal females include an unpleasant "fishy" odor in the vaginal area or in the urine; a grayish-white, thin, and creamy vaginal discharge; and vulvar irritation, redness, and itching. The physical examination of the adolescent female patient should include a complete pelvic examination. The patient's external genitalia may reveal the homogenous gray-white discharge either at the introitus before inserting a speculum or adherent to the vaginal walls or cervical fornices during the pelvic examination. Other clinical signs such as inflammation and erythema are usually not seen when BV exists on its own.[24,26]

Diagnosis

Diagnosis of BV is confirmed by specific diagnostic findings because clinical signs and symptoms are not reliable on their own to make such a determination. In the prepubertal child, vaginal discharge is examined for the presence of ***clue cells***, which are defined as vaginal squamous epithelial cells covered with bacteria obscuring the normally well-defined edges of an epithelial cell. With adolescent patients, the health care provider should determine vaginal pH, perform microscopy for clue cells, and perform the whiff test to aid in the diagnosis. Health care providers should use these tests together and correlate findings with clinical symptoms to diagnose BV. Diagnosis of BV in adolescents requires 3 of the following 4 clinical criteria: (1) characteristic discharge, (2) positive whiff test, (3) pH greater than 4.5, and (4) presence of clue cells. Other tests, including a deoxyribonucleic acid (DNA) probe-based test for high concentrations of *G. vaginalis* (eg, Affirm™ VP III [Becton Dickinson; Sparks, Maryland]), a proline-aminopeptidase test card (eg, Pip Activity Test Card™ [Quidel; San Diego, California]), and a test for elevated sialidase activity in vaginal fluid (eg, OSOM® BVBLUE® [Sekisui Diagnostics; Lexington, Massachusetts]) have acceptable performance characteristics compared with Gram stain.[2] Because of the polymicrobial nature of the infection, vaginal culture is of little value and Pap smears are unreliable in the diagnosis of BV.[24]

In the prepubertal child, samples for the tests are obtained with a cotton swab from the vaginal discharge itself. In the adolescent, samples may be obtained with a swab from the vaginal sidewalls or cervical fornices, avoiding the cervix itself, or the opening of the vaginal canal. For pH testing, the sample can be applied directly to the pH paper. A result greater than 4.5 is consistent with BV. When using microscopy technique, the sample should be applied to a slide, a drop of saline solution added, a cover slide placed over the sample, and 10 fields visualized under high power (400°). The presence of clue cells (at least 20%) indicates BV.

When using the whiff test, the sample is placed on a slide or in a test tube and a drop of 10% potassium hydroxide solution (KOH) is added to the sample. An odor of fish is referred to as a positive whiff test and diagnostic of BV. A separate sample should be collected for the whiff test because KOH lyses the epithelial cells of a sample.

Treatment and Follow-up

The treatment guidelines for BV are summarized in **Table 6-6**. The CDC supports prophylactic treatment for BV in adolescents after a sexual assault, especially because follow-up of these patients can be difficult. However, it is important to review with the patient the possible gastrointestinal side effects of treatment. If a follow-up plan seems likely, prophylactic treatment may be deferred (**Table 6-7**). Follow-up can take place when patients come back for other reasons related to the sexual assault and involves identifying patient follow-through with prescribed medication regimens and resolution of symptoms. The treatment of male partners is not necessary.[2,28]

Table 6-6. Recommendations for the Treatment of Bacterial Vaginosis*

Prepubertal	Metronidazole 15 mg/kg/day (maximum 1 g/day) in 2 divided doses for 7 days
Adolescent	**Recommended regimens:** Metronidazole 500 mg orally twice daily for 7 days *or* Metronidazole gel 0.75%, one full applicator (5 g) intravaginally once daily for 5 days *or* Clindamycin cream 2%, one full applicator (5 g) intravaginally at bedtime for 7 days
	Alternative Regimens: Clindamycin 300 mg orally twice daily for 7 days *or* Clindamycin ovules 100 g intravaginally once at bedtime for 3 days

**Drug dosage recommendations listed herein are those of the authors and are not endorsed by the United States Public Health Service or the United States Department of Health and Human Services.*
Adapted from American Academy of Pediatrics Committee on Infectious Diseases; Pickering LK, Long SS. Report of the Committee on Infectious Diseases. *28th ed. Oak Grove Village, IL: American Academy of Pediatrics; 2009.*
Adapted from Centers for Disease Control and Prevention. Sexually transmitted diseases treatment guidelines 2006. MMWR. *2006;55(RR11):1-94.*

Table 6-7. Initial Examination*	
Initial Examination	The following procedures should be included: — Cultures for *N. gonorrhoeae* and *C. trachomatis* from specimens collected from any sites of penetration or attempted penetration. — NAATs approved by the United States Food and Drug Administration (FDA) (as a substitute for culture). NAATs offer the advantage of increased sensitivity. If an NAAT test is used, a positive test result should be confirmed by a second test. Confirmation tests should consist of a second FDA-licensed NAAT that targets a different sequence from the initial test. Enzyme immunoassay (EIA), nonamplified probes, and direct fluorescent antibody (DFA) tests are not acceptable alternatives for culture because false-negative test results occur more often with these nonculture tests. False-positive test results may occur as well. — Wet mount (WM) and culture of a vaginal swab specimen for *T. vaginalis* infection. If vaginal discharge, malodor, or itching is evident, the WM also should be examined for evidence of BV and candidiasis. — Collection of a serum sample for immediate evaluation for HIV, HBV, and syphilis (see *Prophylaxis, Risk for Acquiring HIV Infection,* and *Follow-Up Examination for 12 Weeks After Assault*).
Follow-Up Examinations	Although it is often difficult for persons to comply with follow-up examinations weeks after an assault, such examinations are essential for the following reasons: — Detect new infections acquired during or after the assault. — Complete HBV immunization, if indicated. — Complete counseling and treatment for other STIs. Examination for STIs should be repeated within 1 to 2 weeks of the assault. Because infectious agents acquired through assault may not have produced sufficient concentrations of organisms to result in positive test results at the initial examination, a culture (or cultures), a WM, and other tests should be repeated at the follow-up visit unless prophylactic treatment was provided. If treatment was provided, testing should only be done if the survivor reports having symptoms. If treatment was not provided, a follow-up examination should be conducted within a week to ensure that results of positive tests can be discussed promptly with the survivor and that treatment can be provided. Serologic tests for syphilis and HIV infection should be repeated 6, 12, and 24 weeks after the assault if initial test results were negative and these infections are likely to be present in the assailant (see *Risk of Acquiring HIV Infection*).
Prophylaxis	Many specialists recommend routine preventive therapy after a sexual assault because follow-up of survivors of sexual assault can be difficult and because these patients may be reassured if offered treatment or prophylaxis for possible infection. The following prophylactic regimen is suggested as preventive therapy: — Postexposure HBV vaccination, without hepatitis B immune globulin (HBIG), should adequately protect against HBV. HBV vaccine should be administered to sexual assault victims at the time of the initial examination if they have not been previously vaccinated. Follow-up doses of vaccine should be administered 1 to 2 and 4 to 6 months after the first dose. — An empiric antimicrobial regimen for Chlamydia, gonorrhea, trichomoniasis, and BV may be administered. *(continued)*

Table 6-7. Initial Examination* *(continued)*	
Recommended Regimen	Ceftriaxone 125 mg intramuscularly in a single dose ***plus*** Metronidazole 2 g orally in a single dose ***plus*** Azithromycin 1 g orally in a single dose *or* Doxycycline 100 mg orally twice daily for 7 days. **Note:** For patients requiring alternative treatments, see the sections in this chapter that specifically address those agents. The efficacy of these regimens in preventing gonorrhea, trichomoniasis, BV, and C. trachomatis genitourinary infections after sexual assault has not been evaluated. Clinicians should counsel patients regarding the possible benefits, as well as the possible toxicity, associated with these treatment regimens. Gastrointestinal side effects can occur with this combination. Providers may also consider antiemetic medications if prophylaxis is administered, particularly if emergency contraception is also provided.
Other Management Considerations	At the initial examination and, if indicated, at follow-up examinations, patients should be counseled regarding the following: — Symptoms of STIs and the need for immediate examination if symptoms occur — Abstinence from sexual intercourse until STI prophylactic treatment is completed — United States Public Health Service or the United States Department of Health and Human Services

**Drug dosage recommendations listed herein are those of the authors and are not endorsed by the United States Public Health Service or the United States Department of Health and Human Services.*

Adapted from American Academy of Pediatrics Committee on Infectious Diseases; Pickering LK, Long SS. Report of the Committee on Infectious Diseases. *28th ed. Oak Grove Village, IL: American Academy of Pediatrics; 2009.*

Adapted from Centers for Disease Control and Prevention. Sexually transmitted diseases treatment guidelines 2006. MMWR. *2006;55(RR11):1-94.*

Chlamydia

General Overview and Epidemiology

Chlamydia organisms are obligate intracellular bacterial parasites.[29-33] Three species exist: (1) *Chlamydophila psittaci (C. psittaci)*, which causes human infection from infected birds; (2) *Chlamydophila pneumoniae (C. pneumoniae)*, which causes pneumonia, pharyngitis, and bronchitis; and (3) *Chlamydia trachomatis* (*C. trachomatis*), which, in the United States, is most often associated with genital tract infections. Infection with *C. trachomatis* does not confer immunity to subsequent infection.[2] Both acute and chronic inflammatory responses are seen with chlamydial infection. It has been estimated that between 2% and 30% of pregnant women have a cervical chlamydial infection; however, a prevalence of only 0.5% was found in a recent study of an urban pregnant population in Germany.[34] Infants born through an infected birth canal can acquire interstitial pneumonia and inclusion conjunctivitis and may manifest urogenital tract and rectal infection.[35] The organism may persist in the child's nasopharynx and oropharynx for nearly 2½ years and in the vagina and rectum for 1 to 3 years after birth.[33,36,37] The AAP[1] considers nonvertically transmitted chlamydial infection in prepubertal children to be highly suspicious of sexual abuse and recommends reporting such cases to CPS for complete investigation.

Chlamydial infection is the most common STI in the United States with an estimated 4 million new cases occurring each year in the United States[36] and up to 90 million new cases per year worldwide.[34] The highest infection rate (5% to 20%) is found among sexually active adolescents and young women.[2,34,36] Rectal and vaginal infection in prepubertal children suspected of having been sexually abused is relatively infrequent, with less than 5% prevalence.[16,17,38] Positive cultures for the organism have been found in 2% to 3% of sexually abused children,[36] while a 2009 study of female children suspected of being victims of sexual assault reported positive *C. trachomatis* tests (including culture and NAATs) in 3.1% of the study population.[7,39]

Approximately 66% to 75% of postpubertal females and 50% of postpubertal males infected with chlamydia are symptom-free.[2,34,40] This accounts for the high incidence and prevalence of this infection. When chlamydial infection is diagnosed in adolescents, clinicians should be alert to the possibility of transmission through sexual assault, while keeping in mind that the infection could also have been acquired through consensual intercourse.

Symptoms

Prepubertal Children

Symptoms in the prepubertal child differ from those in the adolescent and adult. There is debate concerning symptomatology in older children infected with *C. trachomatis*, specifically around the prevalence of asymptomatic infection. Asymptomatic infection with chlamydia may occur in prepubertal children.[21,38,41,42]

Symptomatic chlamydial infection in female children may be associated with a history of vaginal discharge, a chief complaint of discharge or irritation, or a history of sexual abuse.[21] Symptomatic ascending infections of the prepubertal girl's uterus and fallopian tubes have not been reported,[37] and there does not seem to be evidence that supports PID. When symptomatic, a chlamydial infection in a prepubertal child may present as vulvovaginitis in females, with redness, inflammation, and vaginal discharge, and as urethritis in both males and females.[37,43] These children may also be completely asymptomatic, which supports standardized screening when there is concern for sexual abuse.[43] There is little information concerning chlamydia-positive boys who are suspected of having been abused.

Adolescents

Adolescent patients infected with chlamydia may be asymptomatic or minimally symptomatic, which is consistent with patterns seen in 70% of adult women. Diagnosis often occurs when screening at-risk populations or because a sexual contact develops symptoms.[2,29,33] Of those that do present with symptoms, those symptoms include:

— Abnormal, often mucopurulent, vaginal discharge

— Irregular bleeding, including postcoital

— Dysuria

— Vaginal pain

— Lower abdominal pain

Symptomatic adolescent males usually complain of urethral discharge and dysuria. *C. trachomatis* is the most common organism identified in nongonorrheal urethritis in males.[44]

Chlamydial infections in the adolescent female genital tract may develop into an ascending infection spreading to the uterus (endometritis) and fallopian tubes (salpingitis), at times without clinically apparent cervicitis[34] (see *"Pelvic Inflammatory Disease"*). Severe cases can present with pain, fever, and chills. Long-term complications include tubal scarring, chronic pelvic pain, infertility and extra-uterine pregnancy.[34]

Clinical Findings

Prepubertal Children

The examination of the prepubertal child includes inspection of the external genitalia for signs of inflammation and discharge.[44,45] An internal examination is strictly prohibited, and a speculum should never be used in a prepubescent child with only one exception: under anesthesia to rule out a foreign body or exploration of bleeding of unknown etiology. Vulvitis or vulvovaginitis may be present in which mucous membranes appear inflamed and may be friable. Prepubertal children found to have a chlamydial infection may be asymptomatic upon presentation and may disclose a history of vaginal discharge.[1,20,44] Cultures for both *chlamydia* and gonorrhea should be obtained from the external vaginal orifice, rectal area, and oral pharynx when sexual abuse is suspected.[1]

Adolescents

Examination of the adolescent female includes inspection of the external genitalia for the presence of discharge or inflammation. On initial visualization, the discharge may come from the vagina, the urethra, or the Skene gland. Bartholinitis, inflammation of the Bartholin gland, may also suggest chlamydial infection (**Figures 6-14** and **6-15**).

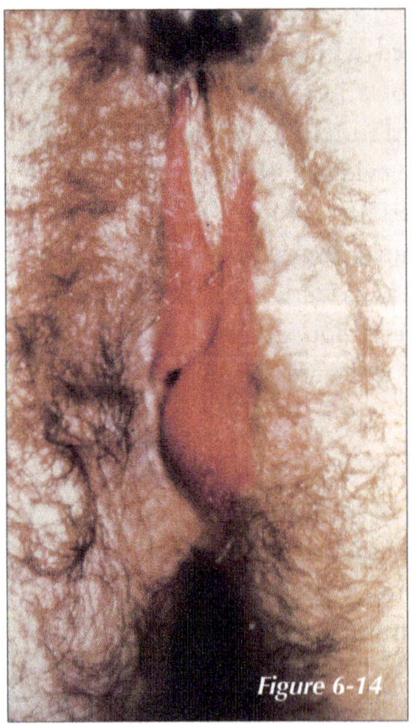

Figure 6-14. *Bartholin abscess. (Contributed by CDC; Atlanta, GA.)*

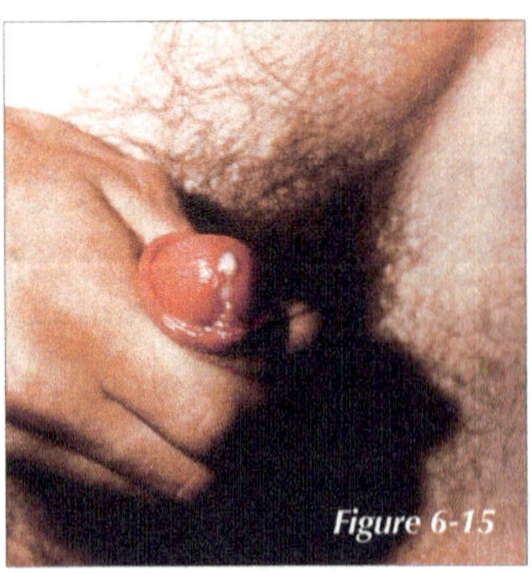

Figure 6-15. *Conococcal urethritis. (Contributed by CDC; Atlanta, GA.)*

Internal examinations are conducted on adolescents that are sexually active; however, urine NAATs are increasingly becoming standard of practice. In cases where PID is being considered, a speculum examination is usually conducted, though the speculum examination is not always necessary. In cases where circumstances necessitate internal examination, symptomatic adolescents may experience pain in specific genital areas, both externally and internally. Clinicians should examine the entire cervix for abnormal discharge, bleeding, and lesions. A cervix that appears edematous and bloody, even when touched lightly with an application swab, is highly suspicious for chlamydial infection or other STIs. Samples for microscopic viewing should come from the posterior or lateral fornices of the cervix or other places where the discharge is free from obscuring blood. In the presence of abnormal discharge, microscopy may also show a few to "too-numerous-to-count" white blood cells (WBCs) per high power field.

Chlamydial infection is always considered in an adolescent male patient who has a urethral discharge, which in isolated chlamydial urethritis is mucopurulent or purulent and may be minimal. Other symptoms include dysuria, urinary frequency, and urethral pruritus or pain.[46,47] 50% to 70% of infected males are asymptomatic.[47]

Diagnosis

A cell culture is the gold standard for testing to confirm the diagnosis of chlamydial infection.[48] This is essential in the context of sexual victimization because of the forensic nature of the examination. Rapid tests are not adequate from a legal standpoint, especially for prepubertal children; however, they carry much weight from a CPS viewpoint. The technique to obtain the culture involves the use of nonwooden, synthetic swabs because cotton swabs with wooden shafts may contain substances that are toxic to chlamydial organisms. The timing of the sexual assault or contact is significant when testing for the presence of chlamydial organisms because it may take up to 2 weeks from time of contact to produce sufficient concentrations of the organism to result in a positive test. Testing may need to be repeated in a subsequent visit if the assault was a recent one and prophylactic treatment was not provided during the initial evaluation.[2] Children are not treated until confirmatory testing is complete because the risk for worsening symptoms or ascending disease is unlikely.

NAATs are a newer form of evaluation for *C. trachomatis* and *N. gonorrhoeae* that may be performed on either vaginal swabs or first-catch urine specimens. NAATs may be more sensitive at detecting vaginal *C. trachomatis* than standard culture techniques, since standard techniques are associated with low sensitivity and difficulties regarding maintaining organism viability during transport.[7,22] A multicenter review conducted by the CDC found that NAAT testing more than doubled the detection of *C. trachomatis* in girls evaluated for STIs, from 1.5 % to 3.1% as compared to culture alone.[2,7] At this time, NAATS are not approved by the United States Food and Drug Administration (FDA) for use in children. The 2006 CDC treatment guidelines recommended NAAT use in the setting of suspected sexual abuse if culture is not available, and if positive results can be confirmed.[38] For cases where a prepubertal child is suspected of having been the victim of sexual abuse, a urine NAAT is completed first; if the NAAT is positive, then confirmatory cultures are completed. In some cases, a second NAAT is completed using a different amplification. The sensitivity of NAAT testing of urine appears to be equal to that of cultures of vaginal swabs and offers a less invasive method of diagnosis that helps to reduce patient anxiety and discomfort.[22] While vaginal culture remains the forensic standard for diagnosis of *C. trachomatis* and *N. gonorrhoeae*, these results suggest that urine NAAT testing may be acceptable as a forensic standard in the future.[22] EIA and DFA, which are nonculture, nonamplified tests, should not be used due to the risk of false-positive results.[2]

Prepubertal Children

The health care provider should use a microswab to collect samples from the prepubertal child because the typical adult-sized swabs are not easily introduced into the smaller prepubertal genital structures. The health care provider should moisten the swab and then rub the swab against the vaginal mucosa to collect a sample, while diligently avoiding the hymen. For young boys, a urine NAAT is performed; a cultural is sent if urethral discharge is present. Urethral swabs are no longer performed.

Adolescents

When collecting a sample from the adolescent, a culture can be obtained from the endocervical canal after excess cervical discharge is removed from the area. The swab should be placed 1 cm to 2 cm into the endocervix, rotated several times, and then removed from the vagina and placed in the appropriate culture medium for immediate transport.

The CDC recommends obtaining specimens from other sites of penetration or attempted penetration to test for chlamydial infection, including anal swabs in both boys and girls. Pharyngeal specimens are not recommended as the yield is low, and some culture systems do not distinguish between *C. trachomatis* and *C. pneumoniae*.[2,38]

Treatment and Follow-Up

The treatment recommendations for chlamydial infection are the same for both female and male patients, as summarized in **Table 6-8**. Table 6-7 details the CDC-recommended regimen for chlamydial prophylaxis after an assault. Follow-up includes assessing patients for symptom resolution or symptom development and compliance

Table 6-8. Treatment of *Chlamydia Trachomatis* Infection*

Uncomplicated Genital Infection in Children Age 8 Years or Older, Adolescents, Adult Men, and Adult Nonpregnant Women*	Azithromycin 1 g orally in a single dose *or* Doxycycline 100 mg orally twice daily for 7 days Alternative Regimens: Erythromycin base 500 mg orally 4 times daily for 7 days *or* Erythromycin ethylsuccinate 800 mg orally 4 times daily for 7 days *or* Ofloxacin‡ 300 mg orally twice daily for 7 days *or* Levofloxacin 500 mg orally for 7 days
Recommended Regimen for Children who Weigh Less than 45 kg	Erythromycin base or ethylsuccinate 50 mg/kg/day orally divided into 4 doses daily for 14 days
Recommended Regimen for Children Who Weigh More Than 45 kg but Are Younger Than Age 8 Years	Azithromycin 1 g orally in a single dose
Uncomplicated Genital Infection in Pregnant Women	Azithromycin 1 g orally in a single dose *or* Amoxicillin 500 mg PO 3 times daily for 7 days
Alternative Regimens	Erythromycin base 500 mg orally 4 times daily for 7 days *or* Erythromycin base 250 mg orally 4 times daily for 14 days *or* Erythromycin ethylsuccinate 800 mg orally 4 times daily for 7 days *or* Erythromycin ethylsuccinate 400 mg orally 5 times daily for 14 days
Infants who Have Conjunctivitis	Erythromycin base or ethylsuccinate 50 mg/kg/day (maximum dose, 500 mg) orally divided into 4 doses daily for 14 days†‡
Infants who Have Pneumonia	Erythromycin base or ethylsuccinate 50 mg/kg/day (maximum dose, 500 mg) orally divided into 4 doses daily for 14 days

**Drug dosage recommendations listed herein are those of the authors and are not endorsed by the United States Public Health Service or the Unites States Department of Health and Human Services.*

‡*Ofloxacin and other quinolone antibiotics are contraindicated for pregnant and lactating women and for children and adolescents younger than age 18 years.*

†‡*An association between oral erythromycin and infantile hypertrophic pyloric stenosis (IHPS) has been reported in infants aged younger than 6 weeks who were treated with this drug. Infants treated with erythromycin should be followed for signs and symptoms of IHPS. Data on use of other macrolides (eg, azithromycin and clarithromycin) for the treatment of neonatal chlamydia infection are limited. The results of one study involving a limited number of patients suggest that a short course of azithromycin, 20 mg/kg/day orally, one dose daily for 3 days may be effective.*

Adapted from American Academy of Pediatrics Committee on Infectious Diseases; Pickering LK, Long SS. Report of the Committee on Infectious Diseases. *28th ed. Oak Grove Village, IL: American Academy of Pediatrics; 2009.*

Adapted from Centers for Disease Control and Prevention. Sexually transmitted diseases treatment guidelines 2002. MMWR. *2002;51(RR06):72-74. Centers for Disease Control and Prevention Web site. http://www.cdc.gov/mmwr/preview/mmwrhtml/rr5106a1.htm. Published May 10, 2002. Accessed September 21, 2013.*

with prescribed medication regimens. Patients with incomplete treatment should be offered the option to be retreated. When treating postpubertal patients, single-dose therapy increases the rate of treatment success over multidose regimens, primarily because of compliance issues for adolescent patients, and makes repeat testing unnecessary. If repeat testing is done for any reason, it should be delayed until 4 to 6 weeks after initial treatment to avoid false-positive results.

Gonorrhea

General Overview and Epidemiology

An estimated 700 000 people are infected with gonorrhea annually.[2] The CDC reports that gonorrhea rates are declining and are at the lowest level on record; however, the rates are declining at a slower rate in minorities.[49] Adolescents and young adults aged 15 to 24 years have the highest incidence of gonorrhea infection.[3] Approximately 50% of adolescent and adult females and a similar percentage of adolescent and adult males are thought to remain asymptomatic for a varied period of time when infected with gonorrhea. *N. gonorrhoeae* infection frequently occurs together with *C. trachomatis* infection.[2]

Gonorrhea is caused by *N. gonorrhoeae*, a gram-negative bacterium that infects mucous membranes with a preference for the columnar epithelium of the genitourinary tract[50,51] (**Figures 6-16** to **6-20**). *N. gonorrhoeae* has antigenic diversity that allows it to survive host defenses and develop resistance to various antibiotics as well. Sexual contact is the most common means of transmission, including the mucous membranes of the genitalia, rectum, and oropharynx.[1] Infants born through an infected birth canal may

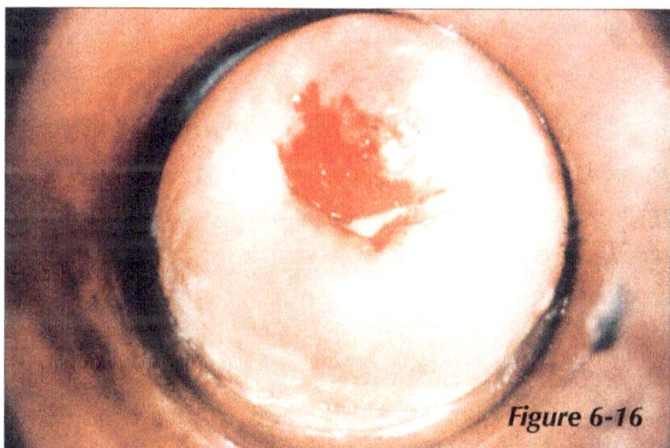

Figure 6-16. Gonococcal cervicitis. *(Contributed by CDC; Atlanta, GA.)*

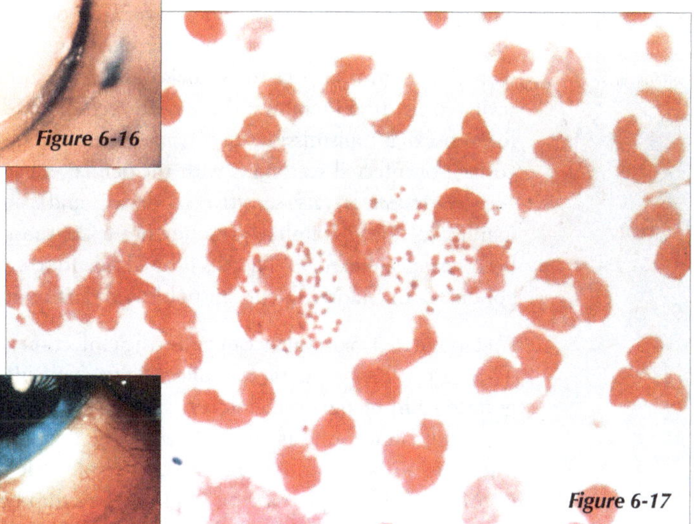

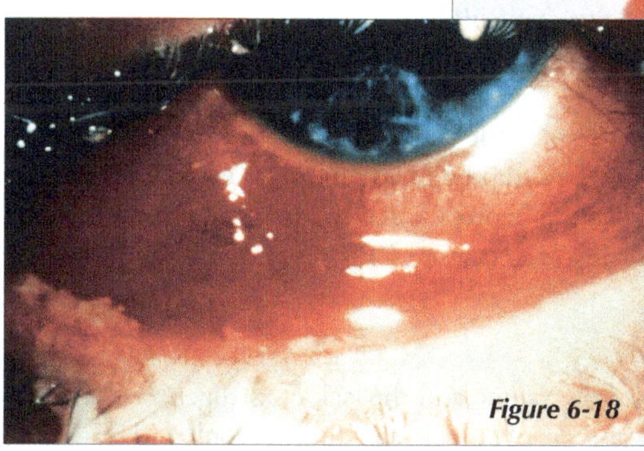

Figure 6-17. N. gonorrhoeae. *Gram's stain of urethral discharge. (Contributed by CDC; Atlanta, GA.)*

Figure 6-18. *Gonococcal ophthalmia. (Contributed by CDC; Atlanta, GA.)*

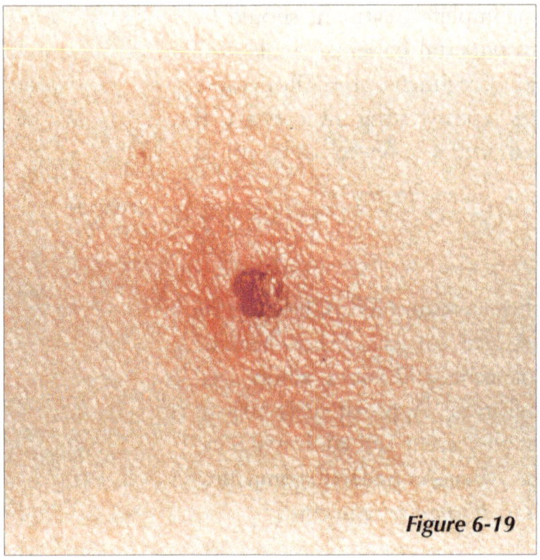

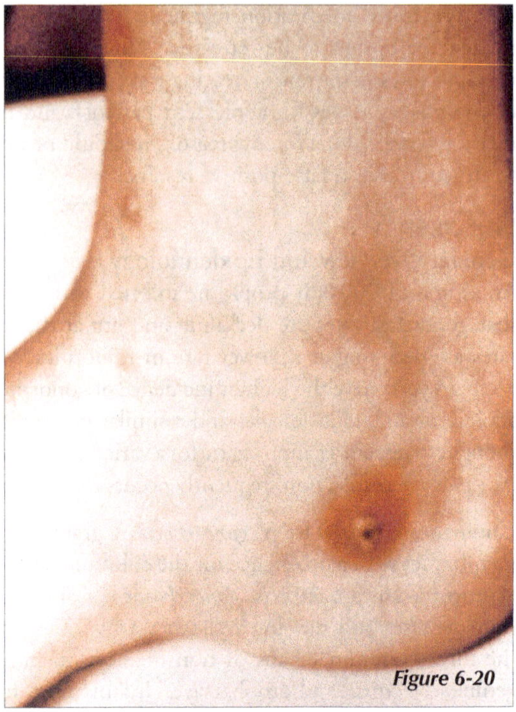

Figure 6-19. *Disseminated gonorrhea; skin lesion. (Contributed by CDC; Atlanta, GA.)*

Figure 6-20. *Disseminated gonorrhea; skin lesion. (Contributed by CDC; Atlanta, GA.)*

contract the infection from their mothers and present with a purulent exudative acute conjunctivitis within 1 week of birth.

Infection with *N. gonorrhoeae* does not confer immunity. Most cases are symptomatic even in the prepubescent child, although asymptomatic infections may occur. Infants born to women who test positive for *N. gonorrhoeae* rarely have the organism isolated when they are aged 1 to 6 months because of the rarity of asymptomatic infection[51]; therefore, outside of the perinatal period, gonorrhea in a prepubertal child should be treated as highly suspect for sexual abuse and warrant a thorough evaluation. In peer-reviewed medical literature, there is no credible evidence outside of the neonatal period for nonsexual transmission of *N. gonorrhoeae* to children. Gonorrhea is spread by direct contact of infected secretions with the genital, anal, or pharyngeal mucous membranes. *N. gonorrhoeae* is very sensitive to drying and cool temperatures, so transmission by inanimate objects is unlikely. Gonorrhea is the most common STI in children who have been sexually abused.[2,50] There is limited scientific evidence for nonsexual transmission of gonorrhea in children[52]; current published data on incidence and prevalence are lagging.

An estimated 3% prevalence of gonorrhea infection is noted among abused children.[17,21,53] There are selective criteria for collecting vaginal cultures because of the low incidence of gonorrhea in prepubertal children who have asymptomatic vaginal infection. Rectal and pharyngeal infections are more likely to be asymptomatic. Definitive advice on genital infections in boys is not available, as a result of few case reports. Asymptomatic gonococcal urethritis in prepubertal boys is believed to be uncommon.[17] The AAP[1] considers nonvertically transmitted gonorrhea infection in prepubertal children to be highly suspect of sexual abuse and recommends reporting such cases to CPS for complete investigation.

Symptoms and Clinical Findings

Prepubertal Children

In prepubertal girls, the alkaline pH of the vagina and the lack of estrogenization allow vaginal infection to occur and appear as a purulent vulvovaginitis. Prepubertal boys may have a purulent urethral discharge and dysuria. The perianal tissues and oropharynx might also be involved and may or may not appear red and inflamed.

Adolescents

Estrogenization of the adolescent protects the vaginal area from *N. gonorrhoeae*,[54] but the organism ascends further to infect the cervix and can cause a purulent cervicitis.[42] Adolescent females may complain of symptoms similar to those associated with chlamydia, including abnormal vaginal discharge, vaginal irritation or itching, irregular bleeding, dysuria, vaginal pain, and lower abdominal pain. Adolescent males may have moderate to large amounts of urethral discharge and dysuria. Pain, tenderness, and testicular swelling characterize the acute epididymitis that may develop. If perianal and rectal tissues are infected and symptomatic, painless mucopurulent anorectal discharge or, rarely, tenesmus may develop. Manifestations of tenesmus, an acute proctitis, include pain on stooling, itching, and bleeding. The pharynx is infrequently infected, but when it is, swollen, exudative tonsils and cervical adenopathy are present.[42]

Adolescent female patients may have visible discharge from the vagina, urethra, or Skene glands. Discharge is typically a purulent yellowish-green color. Bartholinitis may also be present. Cervical discharge is the same color and microscopic evaluation may reveal several to too-numerous-to-count WBCs per high power field. When bleeding is seen, particularly bleeding of the cervical body itself, the clinician should have a high index of suspicion for gonorrhea. As with symptomatic chlamydial infections, gonorrheal infection may also cause pain during the speculum and bimanual examinations. When cervical motion tenderness is present, there is concern for PID, and close monitoring is warranted. In adolescent males, a purulent urethral discharge with a yellowish-green color is suspicious for gonorrhea. Generalized penile and scrotal edema is not common but is more likely in gonorrhea than with chlamydial infection.

Diagnosis

The gold standard diagnostic tool used for the diagnosis of *N. gonorrhoeae* is a culture[1,17,55]; however, NAATs are considered highly sensitive and specific and may be used as well. Some health care providers may request 2 different NAAT amplification tests. In the event that the health care provider determines that a culture is necessary, the provider should know that rapid tests are not adequate for forensic purposes, especially in prepubertal children, but are used for the sexual abuse evaluation of pubertal girls and boys. The examiner should take samples for culture from the vagina in prepubertal females, carefully avoiding the hymen; from the endocervical canal in adolescent females; and from the urethra in adolescent males. Specimens should be collected from the pharynx and anus of both boys and girls as well.[2] Fresh purulent drainage from the vagina may also be sent for culture and, when available, a Gram stain can be performed. This is done in the same way as when testing for chlamydial infection. The media used to test for gonorrhea vary from modified Thayer-Martin, used for urethral samples, to selective Thayer-Martin, used for endocervical samples. Additionally, these media differ from the cell culture media used to test for *C. trachomatis*. Nonselective chocolate agar plates are still used when culturing for gonorrhea. Samples are obtained for microscopy in the same way they are for *C. trachomatis*. It is possible that blood may be seen in the culture area, which should be avoided when sampling.

NAATs are a newer form of evaluation for *C. trachomatis* and *N. gonorrhoeae* which may be performed on either vaginal swabs or first-catch (dirty) urine specimens. NAATs may be more sensitive at detecting vaginal *C. trachomatis* than standard culture techniques, due to low sensitivity and the difficulty of maintaining organism viability during transport.[7,22] While data in prepubertal children is limited,[1] a multicenter review conducted by the CDC found that NAAT testing more than doubled the detection of *C. trachomatis* in girls evaluated for STIs, from 1.5% to 3.1%, as compared to culture alone.[7] The sensitivity of NAAT testing of urine appears to be equal to that of vaginal swabs, offering a less invasive method of diagnosis and reducing patient anxiety and discomfort.[22] While vaginal culture remains the forensic standard for diagnosis of *C. trachomatis* and *N. gonorrhoeae*, these results suggest that urine NAAT testing may be acceptable as a forensic standard in the future.[22]

Treatment and Follow-up

Table 6-9 summarizes treatment guidelines for gonorrhea infection. Table 6-7 presents the prophylaxis regimen for adolescent patients after an assault. There is no need for retesting if symptoms resolve and treatment regimens are completed. Any follow-up

<table>
<tr><th colspan="2">Table 6-9. Treatment of Gonococcal Infection[*‡]</th></tr>
<tr><td>Uncomplicated Genital Infection in Adolescents and Adults</td><td>Cefixime 400 mg orally in a single dose
or
Ceftriaxone 125 mg intramuscularly in a single dose
or
Ciprofloxacin 500 mg orally in a single dose[†‡]
or
Ofloxacin 400 mg orally in a single dose[†‡]
or
Levofloxacin 250 mg orally in a single dose[†‡]
or
Cefpodoxime 400 mg orally in a single dose
or
Spectinomycin 2 g intramuscularly in a single dose
plus
Azithromycin 1 g orally in a single dose
or
Doxycycline 100 mg orally twice a day for 7 days
plus if chlamydial infection is not ruled out
Azithromycin 1 g orally in a single dose
or
Doxycycline 100 mg orally twice daily for 7 days</td></tr>
<tr><td>Disseminated Gonococcal Infection in Adolescents or Adults</td><td>Ceftriaxone 1 g intramuscularly or intravenously every 24 hours
Alternative Regimens:
Cefotaxime 1 g intravenously every 8 hours
or
Ceftizoxime 1 g intravenously every 8 hours
or
Ciprofloxacin 400 mg intravenously every 12 hours[†‡]
or
Ofloxacin 400 mg intravenously every 12 hours[†‡]
or
Levofloxacin 250 mg intravenously daily[†‡]
or
Spectinomycin 2 g intramuscularly every 12 hours</td></tr>
</table>

(continued)

Table 6-9. Treatment of Gonococcal Infection*‡ *(continued)*

Disseminated Gonococcal Infection in Adolescents or Adults	All of the preceding regimens should be continued for 24 to 48 hours after improvement is evidenced, at which time therapy may be switched to one of the following regimens to complete at least 1 week of antimicrobial therapy: Cefixime 400 mg orally twice daily *or* Ciprofloxacin 500 mg orally twice daily†‡ *or* Ofloxacin 400 mg orally twice daily†‡ *or* Levofloxacin 500 mg orally once daily†‡
Disseminated Gonococcal Infection in Adolescents or Adults	Ceftriaxone 1 g intramuscularly or intravenously every 24 hours **Alternative Regimens:** Cefotaxime 1 g intravenously every 8 hours *or* Ceftizoxime 1 g intravenously every 8 hours *or* Ciprofloxacin 400 mg intravenously every 12 hours†‡ *or* Ofloxacin 400 mg intravenously every 12 hours†‡ *or* Levofloxacin 250 mg intravenously daily†‡ *or* Spectinomycin 2 g intramuscularly every 12 hours
	All of the preceding regimens should be continued for 24 to 48 hours after improvement is evidenced, at which time therapy may be switched to one of the following regimens to complete at least 1 week of antimicrobial therapy: Cefixime 400 mg orally twice daily *or* Ciprofloxacin 500 mg orally twice daily†‡ *or* Ofloxacin 400 mg orally twice daily†‡ *or* Levofloxacin 500 mg orally once daily†‡
Meningitis in Adolescents or Adults	Ceftriaxone 1 g to 2 g intravenously every 12 hours for 10 to 14 days ***plus*** Azithromycin 1 g orally in a single dose *or* Doxycycline 100 mg orally twice daily for 7 days
Endocarditis in Adolescents or Adults	Ceftriaxone 1g to 2 g intravenously every 12 hours for a minimum of 28 days ***plus*** Azithromycin 1 g orally in a single dose *or* Doxycycline 100 mg orally twice daily for 7 days

(continued)

Table 6-9. Treatment of Gonococcal Infection*‡ *(continued)*

Uncomplicated Genital Infection in Children	Ceftriaxone 125 mg intramuscularly in single dose *or* Spectinomycin 40 mg/kg (maximum dose, 2 g) intramuscularly in single dose ***plus*** Erythromycin base or ethylsuccinate 50 mg/kg/day (maximum 2 g/day) orally in divided doses for 14 days *or* Cefixime 8 mg/kg (maximum 400 mg) orally in single dose *or* Azithromycin 20 mg/kg (maximum 1 g) orally in single dose
Disseminated Gonococcal Infection in Children without Complications	Ceftriaxone 50 mg/kg/day (maximum 1 g/day) intravenously *or* intramuscularly once daily for 7 days
Meningitis in Children	Ceftriaxone 50 mg/kg/day intravenously or intramuscularly twice daily for 10 to 14 days ***plus*** Erythromycin base or ethylsuccinate 50 mg/kg/day (maximum 2 g) orally in 4 divided doses for 14 days
Endocarditis in Children	Ceftriaxone 50 mg/kg/day intravenously or intramuscularly twice daily for minimum of 28 days ***plus*** Erythromycin base or ethylsuccinate 50 mg/kg/day (maximum 2 g) orally in 4 divided doses for 14 days
Neonatal Gonococcal Ophthalmia Prevention (When Mothers Are Known to Have Gonococcal Infection)	Ceftriaxone 25 to 50 mg/kg (maximum 125 mg) intravenously *or* Intramuscularly in single dose

**Drug dosage recommendations listed herein are those of the authors and are not endorsed by the United States Public Health Service or the United States Department of Health and Human Services.*

‡*Concomitant treatment for* C. trachomatis *should be administered to all patients outside the neonatal period. Children may be treated with erythromycin 40 mg/kg/day orally (maximum 2 g/d) in 4 divided doses for 7 days or azithromycin 10 mg/kg orally (maximum 1 g) in a single dose. Neonates should have tests performed for* C. trachomatis *infection.*

†‡*Quinolones should not be used for infections in men who have sex with men (MSM) or in those with recent foreign travel or partner travel. In addition, use of quinolones is probably inadvisable for treating infections acquired in California, Hawaii, and in other areas with increased prevalence of quinolone resistance.*

Adapted from American Academy of Pediatrics Committee on Infectious Diseases; Pickering LK, Long SS. Report of the Committee on Infectious Diseases. *28th ed. Oak Grove Village, IL: American Academy of Pediatrics; 2009.*

Adapted from Centers for Disease Control and Prevention. Sexually transmitted diseases treatment guidelines 2002. MMWR. *2002;51(RR06):72-74. Centers for Disease Control and Prevention Web site. http://www.cdc.gov/mmwr/preview/mmwrhtml/rr5106a1.htm. Published May 10, 2002. Accessed September 21, 2013.*

testing should also be delayed for 4 to 6 weeks to avoid false-positive results. Clinicians should again consider the timing of the assault as it relates to testing for gonorrhea when deciding on initial and follow-up testing.

Pelvic Inflammatory Disease

General Overview and Epidemiology

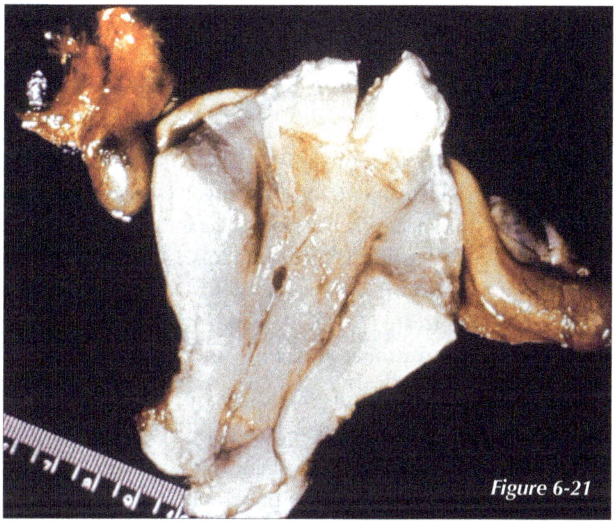

Figure 6-21

Figure 6-21. Pathology specimen from patient with PID. (Contributed by CDC; Atlanta, GA.)

PID (**Figure 6-21**) is a polymicrobial infection that produces an inflammation of the female upper genital tract and can involve the uterus (endometritis, parametritis—an inflammation of the connective tissue adjacent to the uterus termed *parametrium*), fallopian tubes (salpingitis), ovaries (oophoritis), and peritoneum (peritonitis and perihepatitis). PID may lead to the formation of a tubo-ovarian abscess (TOA).[56] Infections are usually caused by organisms such as *N. gonorrhoeae*, *C. trachomatis*, and the organisms causing BV, either alone or together; other vaginal and gastrointestinal (GI) flora may also be involved as well. PID may ascend into the upper genital tract of adolescent females but is not known to occur in prepubertal girls. Adolescents and young adult women seem to be at particularly high risk for this condition. Pubertal females may be at higher risk because of a lack of local immunity and immaturity of the epithelial lining of the cervix.

The incidence of PID appears to have peaked in the 1980s at approximately 1 million cases per year but appears to be decreasing. Its true incidence and prevalence, however, are difficult to evaluate.[57-59] Adolescent females are more susceptible to PID for a number both behavioral (multiple or older sexual partners, inconsistent barrier contraceptive use) and physiologic (cervical ectopy with exposed transformation zone of columnar epithelium, thought to facilitate the attachment of pathogens) reasons.[42,58,60] Adolescent females account for about one quarter of all cases and have a 10-fold higher risk for acquiring PID compared with adult females. From 20% to 40% of pubertal females with chlamydial infection and 10% to 40% of those with gonorrhea develop PID if these infections are not treated effectively.[60] In the context of sexual abuse of pubertal females, PID is a particularly important complication because of the serious long-term consequences that include chronic pelvic pain (18%), infertility (20%), and increased risk of ectopic pregnancy (9%).[2,61]

Clinical Findings

Females with PID may have all of the symptoms seen with chlamydial infection and gonorrhea, along with more extensive symptoms of fever, chills, generalized fatigue, anorexia, abdominal pain, nausea, and vomiting. A distinguishing feature found on bimanual pelvic examination is the presence of cervical motion tenderness. Patients may also have fullness or masses on palpation of the fallopian tubes and ovaries, especially in cases of TOA. Uterine and ovarian tenderness is also possible. Other signs include a guarding-like posture, resulting from attempts to minimize movement of the pelvic region, and an ill-appearing general appearance.

Diagnosis

There is not 1 single factor that confirms PID; therefore, the health care provider should take into consideration the entire clinical picture when making a diagnosis. Minimal diagnostic criteria include lower abdominal tenderness, bilateral or unilateral adnexal tenderness, and cervical motion tenderness.[2] Fever, elevated WBC counts, and erythrocyte sedimentation rates (ESR) are consistent with PID as are positive chlamydia and gonorrhea tests. Clinicians should be aware that mild cases of PID or those seen early in the disease process could be subtle with very minimal signs and symptoms.

Treatment and Follow-Up

Treatment for PID involves combination antibiotic therapy, to include aerobic and anaerobic bacterial coverage. Patients may be treated on an outpatient or inpatient basis depending on the severity, but inpatient management is strongly recommended for cases occurring in pubertal females. Close follow-up is needed for any patient diagnosed and treated for PID, whether managed as an inpatient or outpatient. **Table 6-10** contains treatment guidelines for PID.

Human Papillomavirus

General Overview and Epidemiology

HPV is the most common viral STI in the United States.[2,62] HPV is a double-stranded DNA virus that presents a challenging dilemma to the health care professional evaluating cases of suspected sexual abuse. A large number of people with HPV are asymptomatic and are believed to be shedding the viral pathogen. As the life cycle of HPV takes

Table 6-10. Recommendations for the Parenteral Treatment of Pelvic Inflammatory Disease*

Parenteral Regimen A	Cefotetan 2 g intravenously every 12 hours *or* Cefoxitin 2 g intravenously every 6 hours ***plus*** Doxycycline 100 mg intravenously or orally every 12 hours to complete 14 days
Parenteral Regimen B	Clindamycin 900 mg intravenously every 8 hours ***plus*** Gentamicin loading dose intravenously or intramuscularly (2 mg/kg of body weight) followed by a maintenance dose (1.5 mg/kg) every 8 hours. Single daily dosing may be substituted.
Alternative Parenteral Regimens	Ofloxacin 400 mg intravenously every 12 hours *or* Levofloxacin 500 mg intravenously once daily ***with or without*** Metronidazole 500 mg intravenously every 8 hours *or* Ampicillin/Sulbactam 3 g intravenously every 6 hours ***plus*** Doxycycline 100 mg orally or intravenously every 12 hours

**Drug dosage recommendations listed herein are those of the authors and are not endorsed by the United States Public Health Service or the United States Department of Health and Human Services.*

Adapted from American Academy of Pediatrics Committee on Infectious Diseases; Pickering LK, Long SS. Report of the Committee on Infectious Diseases. *28th ed. Oak Grove Village, IL: American Academy of Pediatrics; 2009.*

Adapted from Centers for Disease Control and Prevention. Sexually transmitted diseases treatment guidelines 2002. MMWR. *2002;51(RR06):72-74. Centers for Disease Control and Prevention Web site. http://www.cdc.gov/mmwr/preview/mmwrhtml/rr5106a1.htm. Published May 10, 2002. Accessed September 21, 2013.*

place in the cells of the squamous epithelium, skin-to-skin contact during sexual contact may cause microabrasions of the epithelium and allow person-to-person transmission even in the absence of visible lesions.[63] Further complicating the clinical picture are the many subtypes of HPV and the growing recognition that several of these subtypes are associated with the onset of cervical cancer in affected women.

Infants born to HPV-infected women through an infected birth canal can acquire the viral infection. In such perinatal cases, HPV may have a prolonged incubation period of up to 3 years, making the possibility of perinatal transmission an important consideration.[2,64,65] Perinatal HPV-exposed infants may have transient mucosal colonization that clears by age 6 weeks.[17,41,42] Other infants may harbor the virus and develop anal or genital warts and, uncommonly, juvenile-onset laryngeal papillomatosis months to years after birth.[66,67] HPV lesions are occasionally seen in the neonate at the time of birth; therefore, operative delivery does not provide complete protection against HPV transmission.[67]

Numerous HPV types have been identified and continue to be closely studied.[68,69] Statistics from epidemiological studies demonstrate HPV is reaching epidemic proportions with over 20 million people infected in the United States and more than 5 million new cases occurring annually.[2,40]

Between 18% and 33% of sexually active female adolescents have tested positive for HPV in various clinical studies of STIs.[70-72] It is difficult to estimate the number of HPV infections in adolescents that occur as a result of sexual assault. The time from initial viral exposure to detection of the infection by the patient or clinician varies widely, making it almost impossible to identify the original source of the infection in adolescents with interim consensual sexual contact. One study found the prevalence of HPV in assault victims to be 0.6% to 2.3%, yet there was no direct evidence that those infections were the result of the assault.[73]

HPV infection, or condyloma acuminata, is present in 1% to 2% of children who have been evaluated for suspected sexual abuse.[17] Children aged younger than 3 years are generally unable to give clear histories of sexual contact which makes the assumption of perinatal transmission problematic.[64,74] The most prudent clinical approach is to always consider the possibility of sexual abuse in children as a differential diagnosis, realizing that younger children may acquire the virus perinatally. The CDC[2] and AAP[1] consider nonvertically transmitted HPV infection as suspicious for sexual abuse and recommends reporting the infection to CPS for full investigation.

Clinical Findings

Prepubertal Children

Genital warts associated with HPV infection, condyloma acuminata, have a predilection for warm, moist areas and appear as flesh- to gray-colored, nonpainful papillomatous growths. Warts can be as small as 1 mm to several square centimeters, if several lesions condense, and may form clusters of multidigitated, papillomatous fibroepitheliomas.[75] The lesions are most commonly found in the perianal area of both boys and girls. In girls they also occur around the urethra; hymen; and posterior fossa, fourchette, or both and may spread onto the labia majora and minora. Boys may have lesions on the corona or shaft of the penis; scrotal lesions are less common.[76] Genital warts have various descriptions. **Figures 6-22** to **6-26** represent the various shapes, sizes, and locations of exophytic warts, including the classic cauliflowerlike growths, fingerlike projections, and smooth papular growths. Flat genital warts are usually subclinical and can be detected by applying acetic acid to the wart, a process that makes the growths more distinct by promoting opacification.[77]

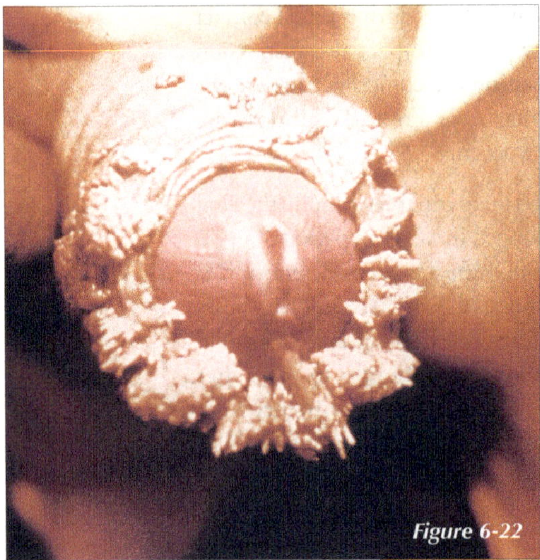

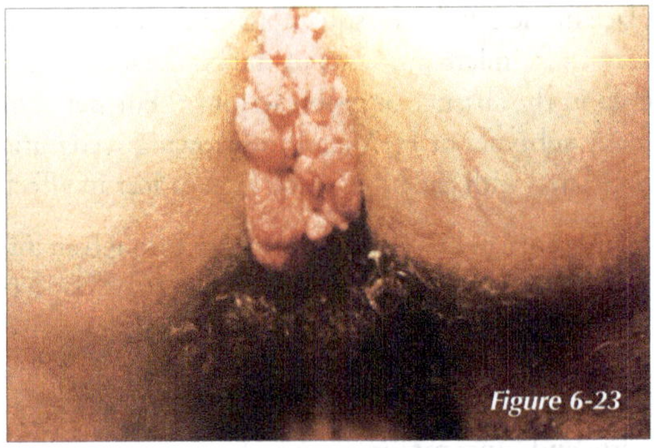

Figure 6-22. Condyloma acuminata, *penile. (Contributed by CDC; Atlanta, GA.)*

Figure 6-23. Condylomata acuminata, *anal. (Contributed by CDC; Atlanta, GA.)*

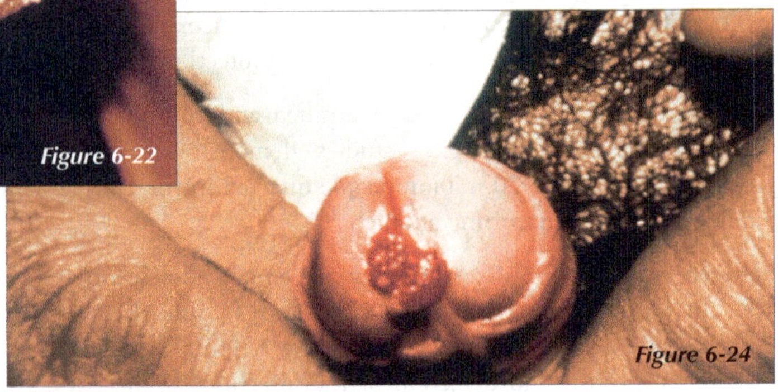

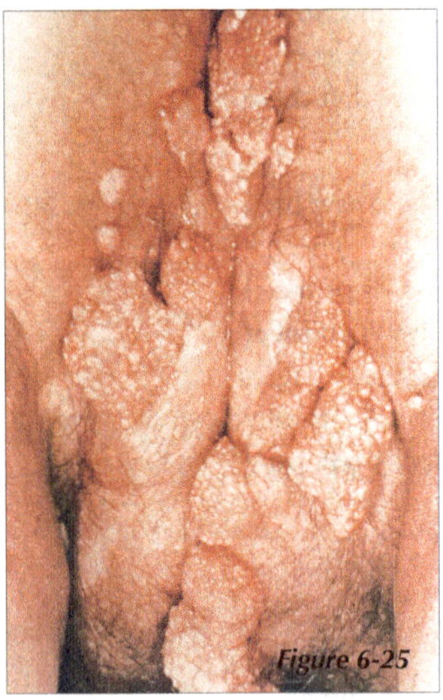

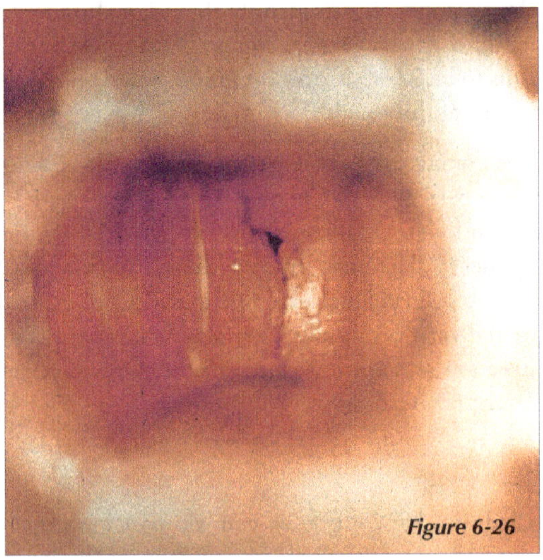

Figure 6-24. Condylomata acuminata, *meatal. (Contributed by CDC; Atlanta, GA.)*

Figure 6-25. Condyloma acuminata, *vulva. (Contributed by CDC; Atlanta, GA.)*

Figure 6-26. Condyloma acuminata, *vaginal. (Contributed by CDC; Atlanta, GA.)*

The appearance of HPV on the vulvar mucous membranes may be subtle and resemble a stippled area on the hymen or medial aspect of the labia minora. In addition to the anogenital area, genital warts may be found on the umbilicus, axilla, mouth, conjunctiva, and webbing between the toes. When HPV infection is subclinical, there may be no obvious warts or signs of infection. For example, a Pap smear may return positive results for HPV while no visible warts are present on examination.

Adolescents

In adolescent females, HPV growths can be located on the vulva, perianal area, vagina, and cervix. Common sites in adolescent males include the prepuce, glans, urethra, penile shaft, scrotum, and perianal area.[77,78] Adolescent females and males may report the presence of growths or bumps anywhere on the external genitalia and perianal region.[77] These growths are usually painless and do not involve bleeding, unless manipulation of those growths has taken place. In the adolescent female, external lesions may coexist in with flat condyloma of the cervix; in the adolescent male, external lesions may coexist on the urethra. Subclinical infection is also possible.

Diagnosis

The diagnosis of HPV is largely based on clinical inspection of the female and male genitalia. Biopsy can be used to confirm the diagnosis in cases that are unclear but is usually unnecessary. In adolescent females, HPV may be initially found on Pap smear and colposcopic examination.[79] Syphilis should be considered in the differential diagnosis because condylomata lata, a clinical manifestation of secondary syphilis infection, can mimic the appearance of condylomata acuminata, in which the etiology is HPV.[80,81] When there is any genital lesion present, screening for syphilis should be included in the workup. Condylomata lata, the wartlike lesions of secondary syphilis, are generally flattened, broad-based lesions with less surface irregularity than the condylomata acuminata. The serological tests for syphilis are positive in cases of condylomata lata. Serological testing for syphilis is recommended in the context of evaluating patients after sexual assault[2] to confirm the status of the patient before the assault. If positive at this time, then it is diagnostic for positive status before the assault.

Treatment and Follow-up

Several options are available for the treatment of genital warts. The goal of therapy is to remove the external warts, keeping in mind that the viral infection with HPV cannot be eradicated. Treatment choice for external warts depends on the location and severity of the growths and ranges from patient- and provider-applied topical agents to cryotherapy and surgical removal.[82] **Table 6-11** contains HPV treatment suggestions. Both prepubertal and pubertal female and male patients may need regular weekly or monthly follow-up depending on the treatment regimen used. It may take several weeks or months to eradicate the warts. There may also be regrowth of external warts, in which case treatment must start over. Adolescent females need close cytological evaluation with Pap smears and possibly colposcopy because cervical cancer is directly linked to HPV infection.[83-88] HPV genotyping tests for oncogenic or high-risk strains are available and have been recommended in some clinical scenarios to guide decisions regarding colposcopy.[89]

Table 6-11. Recommended Treatment of Human Papillomavirus*

External Genital Warts	**Patient-Applied:** Podofilox 0.5% solution should be applied to visible genital warts twice a day for 3 days, followed by 4 days of no therapy. This cycle can be repeated, as necessary, for up to 4 cycles. The total area treated should be less than 10 cm^2, and the total volume of podofilox topical should be less than 0.5 mL per day. *or* Imiquimod 5% cream at bedtime, 3 times per week for up to 16 weeks; the area should be washed with soap and water 6 to 10 hours after application.

(continued)

Table 6-11. Recommended Treatment of Human Papillomavirus* *(continued)*

External Genital Warts	**Provider-Administered:** Cryotherapy with liquid nitrogen or cryoprobe. Repeat applications every 1 to 2 weeks. *or* Podophyllin resin 10% to 25% in a compound tincture of benzoin. A small amount should be applied to each wart and allowed to air dry. The treatment can be repeated weekly, if necessary. To avoid the possibility of complications associated with systemic absorption and toxicity, some specialists recommend that application be limited to less than 0.5 mL of podophyllin or an area of less than 10 cm^2 of warts per session. No open lesions or wound should be present in the treated area. Some specialists suggest that the preparation should be thoroughly washed off 1 to 4 hours after application to reduce local irritation. The safety of podophyllin during pregnancy has not been established. *or* Trichloroacetic acid (TCA) or bichloroacetic acid (BCA) 80% to 90%. A small amount should be applied only to warts and allowed to dry, at which time a white "frosting" develops. If an excess amount of acid is applied, the treated area should be powdered with talc, sodium bicarbonate (ie, baking soda), or liquid soap preparations to remove unreacted acid. This treatment can be repeated weekly, if necessary. *or* Surgical removal either by tangential scissors excision, tangential shave excision, curettage, or electrosurgery.
External Genital Warts: Alternative Treatments	Intralesional interferon *or* Laser surgery
Urethral Meatus Warts	Cryotherapy with liquid nitrogen *or* Podophyllin 10% to 25% in compound tincture of benzoin. The treatment area must be dry before contact with normal mucosa. This treatment can be repeated weekly, if necessary.
Cervical Warts	For women who have exophytic cervical warts, high-grade squamous intraepithelial lesions (SIL) must be excluded before initiating treatment. Management of exophytic cervical warts should include consultation with a specialist.
Vaginal Warts	Cryotherapy with liquid nitrogen. The use of a cryoprobe in the vagina is not recommended because of the risk for vaginal perforation and fistula formation. *or* TCA or BCA 80% to 90% applied to warts. A small amount should be applied only to warts and allowed to dry, at which time a white "frosting" develops. If an excess amount of acid is applied, the treated area should be powdered with talc, sodium bicarbonate (eg, baking soda), or liquid soap preparations to remove unreacted acid. This treatment can be repeated weekly, if necessary.

(continued)

Table 6-11. Recommended Treatment of Human Papillomavirus* *(continued)*

Anal Warts	Cryotherapy with liquid nitrogen *or* TCA or BCA 80% to 90% applied to warts. A small amount should be applied only to warts and allowed to dry, at which time a white "frosting" develops. If an excess amount of acid is applied, the treated area should be powdered with talc, sodium bicarbonate (eg, baking soda), or liquid soap preparations to remove unreacted acid. This treatment can be repeated weekly, if necessary. *or* Surgical removal
Oral Warts	Cryotherapy with liquid nitrogen *or* Surgical removal

**Drug dosage recommendations listed herein are those of the authors and are not endorsed by the United States Public Health Service or the United States Department of Health and Human Services.*
Adapted from American Academy of Pediatrics Committee on Infectious Diseases; Pickering LK, Long SS. Report of the Committee on Infectious Diseases. *28th ed. Oak Grove Village, IL: American Academy of Pediatrics; 2009.*
Adapted from Centers for Disease Control and Prevention. Sexually transmitted diseases treatment guidelines 2002. MMWR. *2002;51(RR06):72-74. Centers for Disease Control and Prevention Web site. http://www.cdc.gov/mmwr/preview/mmwrhtml/rr5106a1.htm. Published May 10, 2002. Accessed September 21, 2013.*

Herpes Simplex Virus

General Overview and Epidemiology

HSV is a large DNA virus with 2 major subtypes. HSV type 1 commonly infects the oral area, causing stomatitis, while HSV type 2 has traditionally more often infected the genitalia. These predilections for infection sites are not absolute, however, and HSV type 1 can infect the genitals, and HSV type 2 can infect the mouth. A recent and significant change in the epidemiology of genital herpes has taken place in recent years; HSV type may now be more prevalent than HSV type 2 in new cases, possibly due to oral-genital contact.[90-92]

In children, an HSV type 1 infection can be spread to the genitals by autoinoculation; however, a genital herpes infection in children should prompt an evaluation for sexual abuse. An HSV-positive mother may transmit the virus to an infant born through the infected birth canal, potentially producing catastrophic, disseminated HSV infection in the neonate; the situation of highest risk is primary infection of the mother near the time of delivery.[93] Mothers known to have HSV are often given suppression medication in the third trimester.[93-96]

Between 16% and 26% of adults in the United States are HSV type 2 seropositive.[90,93,97] HSV type 2 is nearly always sexually transmitted; therefore, seropositivity indicates anogenital infection in nearly all cases.[90] However, according to National Health and Nutritional Examination Survey (NHANES) data from 2005-2008, seroprevalence may be decreasing.[71] Children are known to contract HSV type 2 outside of the perinatal period by sexually abusive contact, which may include manifestations of recurring skin ulcers and vesicles. Infections that may be confused with HSV infections include varicella, herpes zoster, erythema multiforme, impetigo and other streptococcal infections, and syphilis. The AAP[19] considers herpes infections involving the genital areas as suspicious for sexual abuse and recommends that health care providers report these cases to CPS for complete investigation and conduct a thorough family assessment.

Clinical Findings

Prepubertal and postpubertal female and male children with genital herpes complain of painful lesions or sores located anywhere on the external genitalia. They often report pain during urination. Other symptoms include a burning or tingling sensation and lesions that appear as blisters, bumps, or a rash. Anal and genital lesions typically progress from maculopapular lesions to vesicles, ulcers, and finally to lesions that may crust. Lesions tend to heal completely without leaving scars. Approximately 70% of adolescent female patients and 40% of adolescent male patients have systemic complaints in a primary infection. Symptoms may include fever, malaise, and myalgia; meningitis may also occur, with headache, neck pain, and photophobia.[98-101] Genital herpes may be resolved by the time patients come in for a physical examination; therefore, clinicians should assess for a history of symptoms. HSV-infected adults and adolescents may shed the virus intermittently from the cervix or urethra with no evidence of visible lesions. It is currently not known if prepubertal children also shed the virus between recurrences.

Evaluation

The health care provider should perform a complete prenatal and family assessment history when evaluating cases of genital herpes in the prepubertal child. In the adolescent patient, a complete sexual history should be obtained.[99]

For female patients, the evaluation for genital herpes should begin with inspection of the external genitalia. A speculum examination may be performed in the adolescent patient if clinically indicated and tolerated but may need to be deferred secondary to pain and discomfort. Urine NAATs can be used to assess for concomitant infections. The examination of males involves thorough inspection of the external genitalia, taking into consideration that herpes lesions may be found in the perianal region, buttocks and upper thighs.[100,102]

Primary infections are usually severe and painful, with the presence of multiple vesicles or lesions and tender, enlarged inguinal lymph nodes, especially in HSV type 2. HSV type 1 may be less severe, even with a primary infection; therefore, clinicians should attempt to culture all suspicious lesions. Most recurrent infections are less severe in both female and male patients[2,103] (**Figures 6-27** to **6-30**). The course of a genital herpes infection varies among individual patients in terms of the length of time of each stage,

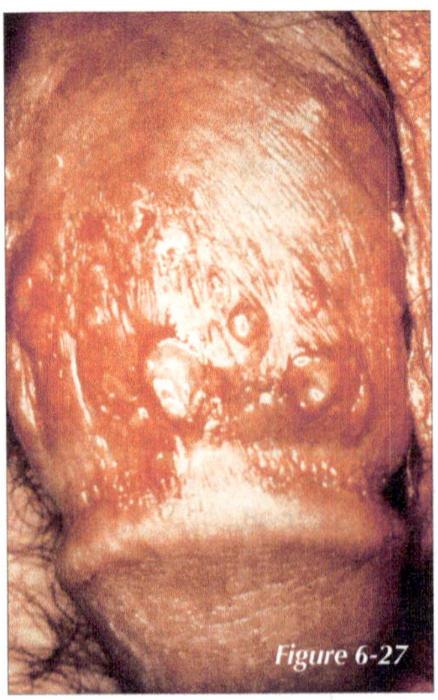

Figure 6-27. *Primary herpes, male. (Contributed by CDC; Atlanta, GA.)*

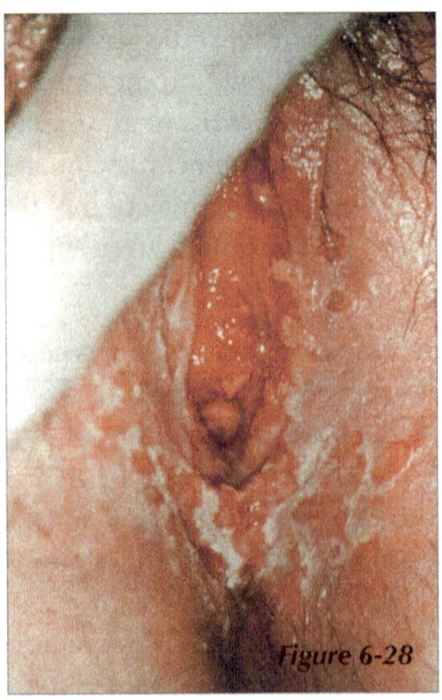

Figure 6-28. *Primary herpes, female. (Contributed by CDC; Atlanta, GA.)*

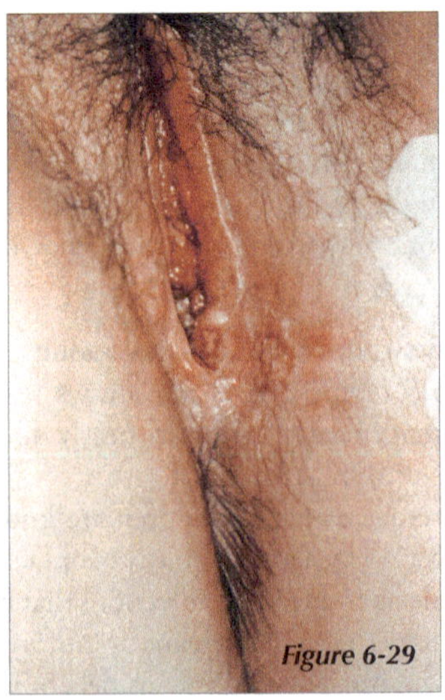

Figure 6-29. *Same patient as Figure 6-28, 4 days later. (Contributed by CDC; Atlanta, GA.)*

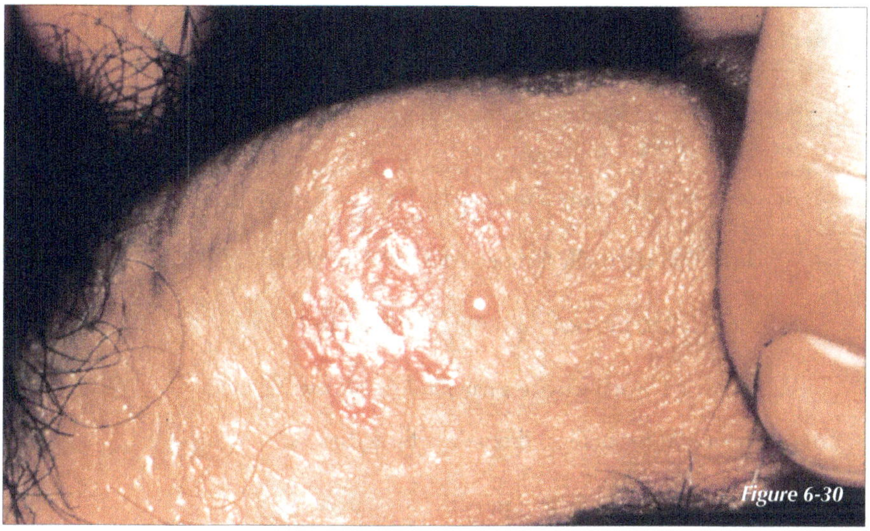

Figure 6-30. *Recurrent herpes, male. (Contributed by CDC; Atlanta, GA.)*

the severity of the infection, and the individual's overall health. In both females and males, systemic symptoms precede the presence of vesicles, followed by lesions that eventually end with crusting and reepithelialization.[98]

Diagnosis

The diagnosis of genital herpes is largely based on patient history and clinical findings. Culture of vesicular material obtained during active viral shedding has been the primary method of confirming HSV infection, with a sensitivity rate of 80% to 90% when primary lesions are cultured, dropping to 25% to 50% with recurrent lesions. In recent years, PCR testing for detection of HSV DNA has been used with sensitivity as high or higher than that of culture,[90,100] and may replace culture as the gold standard for confirmation of diagnosis.[104,105] The ideal culture is obtained directly from an intact vesicle. The health care provider should gently rupture the vesicle using a cotton or dacron swab. When an ulcer is present, samples should be obtained by swabbing the base of the lesion, being sure to remove any crusting before sampling and limit the amount of blood present in the sample. A moderate amount of friction is necessary to obtain an adequate sample for culturing.[98] This is often an uncomfortable procedure for the patient; therefore, the health care provider should assess the need to medicate the patient before the procedure. Samples, which often require the sample to be kept on ice, should be placed in the appropriate medium for transport. PCR testing can be performed on vesicle swabs as well, are less dependent on transport conditions, and potentially faster than viral culture.[100]

Type-specific serologic testing, based on surface glycoprotein-G, can identify HSV infection and differentiate between HSV type 1 and HSV type 2, as well as between recent and preexisting infection.[104,105] This type of testing is recommended to confirm diagnosis in adult patients with healed, recurrent, or atypical symptoms; those with unrecognized infection; and for management of sex partners of individuals with known infection.[100] Data regarding the use of these assays in children is very limited.[105]

Treatment and Follow-Up

The treatment of genital herpes in female and male patients, both prepubertal and pubertal, should emphasize pain management and emotional support as the first priority. This should include the use of topical anesthetics, nonsteroidal antiinflammatory drugs (NSAIDs), and possibly narcotics if severe pain is present (**Table 6-12**). Other palliative

Table 6-12. Treatment of Genital Herpes: First Clinical Episode*

Prepubertal	Acyclovir 80 mg/kg/day (maximum 1.2 g/day) in 3 to 4 divided doses for 7 to 10 days
Adolescents	Acyclovir 400 mg orally 3 times a day for 7 to 10 days *or* Acyclovir 200 mg orally 5 times a day for 7 to 10 days *or* Famciclovir 250 mg orally 3 times a day for 7 to 10 days *or* Valacyclovir 1 g orally twice a day for 7 to 10 days
Episodic Recurrent Infection	Acyclovir 400 mg orally 3 times daily for 5 days *or* Acyclovir 800 mg orally 3 times daily for 2 days *or* Acyclovir 800 mg orally twice daily for 5 days *or* Famciclovir 125 mg orally twice daily for 5 days *or* Famciclovir 1 g PO twice daily for 1 day *or* Valacyclovir 500 mg PO twice daily for 3 days *or* Valacyclovir 1 g PO once daily for 5 days

**Drug dosage recommendations listed herein are those of the authors and are not endorsed by the United States Public Health Service or the United States Department of Health and Human Services.*

Adapted from American Academy of Pediatrics Committee on Infectious Diseases; Pickering LK, Long SS. Report of the Committee on Infectious Diseases. *28th ed. Oak Grove Village, IL: American Academy of Pediatrics; 2009.*

Adapted from Centers for Disease Control and Prevention. Sexually transmitted diseases treatment guidelines 2002. MMWR. *2002;51(RR06):72-74. Centers for Disease Control and Prevention Web site. http://www.cdc.gov/mmwr/preview/mmwrhtml/rr5106a1.htm. Published May 10, 2002. Accessed September 21, 2013.*

measures can also be used, including sitz baths, light application of petroleum jelly, and keeping lesions clean and dry.[98] The goal of antiviral agents is to accelerate the healing process of an acute infection and to decrease the overall number of recurrent infections. Regular follow-up is necessary to ensure that primary herpes infections heal appropriately without complications. Clinicians should evaluate the effectiveness of antiviral treatments and adjust dosages as needed. Patients with a history suspicious for herpes who could not previously be cultured should be advised to return if lesions recur. Sampling recurrent lesions helps to confirm the diagnosis.

The emotional stigma associated with diagnosis is often paramount to the child and his or her caregiver. Offering emotional support and providing evidence-based education will provide the best opportunity to de-escalate fears and concerns. Ongoing counseling and education are essential for all patients who are diagnosed with herpes because it is a lifelong infection requiring ongoing management and social lifestyle modifications. Counseling should be made available to children and their families because it provides needed support and allows clinicians to identify patients who may require referral for further therapy and suppressive treatment.

Trichomoniasis

General Overview and Epidemiology

Trichomonas vaginalis (*T. vaginalis*) is a flagellated protozoon that is a common cause of vaginitis in adult women.[17] Adult and adolescent females and nearly all males infected with *T. vaginalis* may be asymptomatic.[2,106] The extent to which prepubertal children may be asymptomatic is not known. Infants born to *Trichomonas vaginalis*–positive women may become colonized or infected for up to 1 year if not treated.[17,107] After infancy, it is appropriate to assume that a child with *T. vaginalis* has acquired it as the result of sexual abuse.[25] It is important to differentiate *T. vaginalis* from *Trichomonas hominis* (*T. hominis*), a common species that inhabits the human bowel.[108] Distinction may be made by appearance under the microscope based on the length of the undulating membrane. *T. hominis* is often differentiated from *T. vaginalis* by the expert laboratory microscopists looking at a fresh wet mount (WM).[108]

Trichomoniasis affects approximately 7.4 million people annually in the United States.[109] The AAP[1] considers *T. vaginalis* infection outside of infancy to be highly suspicious for sexual abuse and recommends that health care providers report cases to CPS for complete investigation.

Clinical Findings

Prepubertal Children

In the context of the sexual abuse examination, all vaginal discharge should be examined for *T. vaginalis,* which causes vaginitis, by culture.[110] Very little information is available for symptomatology in prepubertal boys.

Adolescents

Approximately 50% or more of adolescent and adult females and more than 75% of adolescent and adult males infected with *T. vaginalis* are asymptomatic.[109] Those adult and adolescent females[106] who have symptoms complain primarily of vaginal irritation or itching and a bubbly cream-colored or green-tinged discharge. Initial presentation may include irregular bleeding, dysuria, vaginal odor, or lower abdominal pain, but these symptoms are not less common. The relatively low numbers of symptomatic males have the same type of discharge and urethral irritation as experienced by females.

The external and internal genitalia of females who have trichomoniasis may reveal slight inflammation and erythema. The presence of a frothy, cream-colored, or green-tinged discharge coming from the vagina or cervix or petechiae of the cervix (strawberry cervix) or friability of the cervix should cause suspicion for trichomoniasis. This same discharge may be seen coming from the urethra in males and should be sampled for microscopic evaluation. A male with this discharge may also have some urethral inflammation and erythema, although this is uncommon.

Diagnosis

The traditional method of diagnosing trichomoniasis is the WM. The discharge should be prepared and examined under the microscope using WM technique. The sample should be combined with a small amount of saline solution, spread gently on a slide, and topped with a cover slide. A diagnosis of trichomoniasis is made when the oval-shaped, motile protozoa are visualized on high-power-field (HPF) microscopy. These protozoa usually have an undulating membrane with visible flagella and are slightly larger than WBCs. There may be a few to multiple protozoa seen microscopically, and WBCs and spermatozoa may be an additional finding.[28] Clinicians should microscopically evaluate samples from any discharge seen in any area from the posterior or lateral fornices in adolescent female patients and from the urethra in adolescent male patients. WM examination has a 60% to 70% sensitivity.[2] False-negative examination may result from low parasite load, delay between specimen collection and microscopic examination (more than 10 to 20 minutes), and clinician skill.[105,109] This method lacks sensitivity in men.[2,109]

T. vaginalis may also be cultured using the Diamond medium; this method is considered the gold standard for diagnosis of trichomoniasis. Culture is more sensitive at detecting *T. vaginalis* than WM, with sensitivity of 95% and specificity of greater than 95%. However, this method has not been as commonly used as WM in clinical settings because it is more expensive and more labor-intensive, requiring incubation and daily microscopic examinations over 3 to 5 days; storage and transport requirements are strict; and results are not immediate as in the WM method.[109] An alternate culture system, the InPouch™ TV culture (IP) (BioMed Diagnostics; White City, OR), has been shown to have 81% sensitivity, compared to 36% sensitivity for WM.[111] Other advantages include lower cost, less stringent storage and transport requirements; potential for more reliable results; and more rapidly available final results compared to the Diamond medium. Additionally, IP does not promote the growth of *T. hominis*, permitting differentiation between the 2 organisms.[112]

Alternative methods of testing have become available in recent years, such as antigen detection and NAATs, with greater sensitivity and specificity than WM. Antigen tests cleared by the FDA include OSOM TV, which uses immunochromatography, and Affirm™ VPIII (Becton Dickinson; Franklin Lakes, NJ), which is a DNA hybridization probe test; both provide results within an hour. APTIMA TV (GenProbe; San Diego, CA) and NuSwab (LabCorp; Burlington, NC) use transcription-mediated amplification (TMA), a form of NAAT.[109] These tests have not been validated or approved for use in children.[105]

Treatment and Management

Trichomoniasis treatment guidelines are discussed in **Table 6-13**. Follow-up includes the assessment for completion of prescribed treatment regimens and resolution of

Table 6-13. Treatment of Trichomoniasis*

Prepubertal	Metronidazole 15 mg/kg/day in divided doses orally every 8 hours for 7 days *or* Tinidazole 50 mg/kg (maximum 2 g) in a single dose
Adolescent	Metronidazole 2 g orally in a single dose *or* Tinidazole 2 g orally in a single dose
Alternative regimen	Metronidazole 500 mg twice daily for 7 days

Adapted from Centers for Disease Control and Prevention. Sexually transmitted disease treatment guidelines 2010. MMWR. *2010;59(RR-12):1-110. Centers for Disease Control and Prevention Web site. http://www.cdc.gov/std/treatment/2010/toc.htm. Updated January 28, 2011. Accessed September 29, 2013.*
Adapted from American Academy of Pediatrics Committee on Infectious Diseases; Pickering LK, Long SS. Report of the Committee on Infectious Diseases. *28th ed. Oak Grove Village, IL: American Academy of Pediatrics; 2009.*
Adapted from Centers for Disease Control and Prevention. Sexually transmitted diseases treatment guidelines 2002. MMWR. *2002;51(RR06):72-74. Centers for Disease Control and Prevention Web site. http://www.cdc.gov/mmwr/preview/mmwrhtml/rr5106a1.htm. Published May 10, 2002. Accessed September 21, 2013.*
**Drug dosage recommendations listed herein are those of the authors and are not endorsed by the United States Public Health Service or the United States Department of Health and Human Services.*

symptoms. Patients should be educated on the side effects of the medication, avoidance of alcohol until medication course is completed, and avoidance of sexual activity. Some patients will need to follow-up with their provider if side effects occur. Repeating treatment is appropriate if clinicians suspect the initially prescribed regimens have failed. Repeat microscopic testing is only needed if symptoms persist or recur after several months.

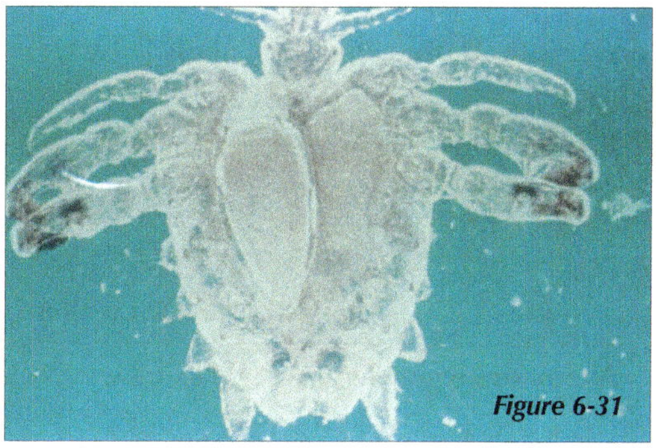

***Figure 6-31**. Female crab louse. (Contributed by CDC; Atlanta, GA.)*

Pediculosis Pubis

General Overview and Epidemiology

Pediculosis pubis may be sexually transmitted through close contact. It is caused by the pubic crab louse, *Pthirus pubis* (*P. pubis*), which is an oval-shaped insect approximately 1 mm to 4 mm in length. The parasite lives on the skin, usually where hair is present, and feeds on host blood. The female pubic louse (**Figure 6-31**) lays about 3 eggs per day, which attach to the shaft of the hair as nits and hatch within 8 to 10 days.[113]

Clinical Findings

Pediculosis pubis is an infection primarily seen in adolescent and adult males and females and is not typically seen in prepubertal children because of the absence of pubic hair. Symptoms usually occur in both females and males, approximately 1 to 2 weeks after initial contact. Patients primarily complain of severe itching throughout all areas of the external genitalia, particularly in areas where there is hair growth. Additionally, the child or a family member may report having actually seen a crab louse in the genital area. Although rare, infestation on eyelashes and eyebrows can occur in both prepubertal children and adolescents.

Diagnosis

During inspection of the external genitalia of female and male patients, clinicians may first notice small yellow-white nits attached to the base of the pubic hair shafts. If such an observation is made, the health care provider should collect the nit as evidence and send the evidence to the laboratory. They may also be viewed more closely by microscope. In the case of prepubertal children, it may be possible to type the DNA from the louse and, if the alleged perpetrator is also infected, attempt to match the louse DNA from the child or adolescent with the comparable louse DNA from the perpetrator. The eyelashes and eyebrows are also inspected, looking for nits and the crab louse. The diagnosis of *P. pubis* infestation is made by considering both the clinical history and clinical findings.

Treatment and Follow-Up

Treatment guidelines for Pediculosis pubis are summarized in **Table 6-14**. Follow-up is required to determine if the infestation was adequately treated. Retreatment may be indicated in 7 to 10 days if nits are still visible, and often a retreatment in 7 to 10 days is prescribed to assure infestation is adequately treated. Pediculosis of eyelashes is treated differently, with ophthalmic ointment to the eyelid margins twice daily for 10 days.[114] Clinicians should advise patients to remove all residual nits with a fine-toothed comb. Articles of clothing and linen should be either dry-cleaned or machine-washed and dried using the heat cycle, or removed from body contact for at least 72 hours.[2] In the context of sexual abuse, all clothing and linen that has come in close contact with the patient and alleged perpetrator should be turned over to the police for forensic evaluation.

Table 6-14. Treatment of Pediculosis Pubis*

Recommended regimens	Permethrin 1% cream rinse applied to affected areas and washed off after 10 minutes *or* Pyrethrins with piperonyl butoxide applied to the affected area and washed off after 10 minutes
Alternative regimens	Malathion 0.5% lotion applied for 8 to 12 hours and washed off *or* Ivermectin 250 mg/kg orally, repeated in 2 weeks

Adapted from Centers for Disease Control and Prevention. Sexually transmitted diseases treatment guidelines 2010. MMWR. *2010;59(RR-12):1-110. Centers for Disease Control and Prevention Web site. http://www.cdc.gov/std/treatment/2010/toc.htm. Updated January 28, 2011. Accessed September 29, 2013.*
Adapted from American Academy of Pediatrics Committee on Infectious Diseases; Pickering LK, Long SS. Report of the Committee on Infectious Diseases. *28th ed. Oak Grove Village, IL: American Academy of Pediatrics; 2009.*
Adapted from Centers for Disease Control and Prevention. Sexually transmitted diseases treatment guidelines 2002. MMWR. *2002;51(RR06):72-74. Centers for Disease Control and Prevention Web site. http://www.cdc.gov/mmwr/preview/mmwrhtml/rr5106a1.htm. Published May 10, 2002. Accessed September 21, 2013.*
**Drug dosage recommendations listed herein are those of the authors and are not endorsed by the United States Public Health Service or the United States Department of Health and Human Services.*

Syphilis

General Overview and Epidemiology

Syphilis is caused by *Treponema pallidum* (*T. pallidum*), a unicellular spirochete that cannot be cultivated in vitro.[115] Congenital infection may be acquired in utero or at the time of delivery. Congenital syphilis infection may cause miscarriage or stillbirth in up to one-fifth of cases.

Following a dramatic decrease in syphilis rates in the United States during the 1990s, the rate increased again during the 2000s. While most pronounced in the population of men who have sex with men, involvement of both men and women of all age groups, including congenital syphilis have been demonstrated.[116,117] The infecting agent, *T. pallidum* enters the body through small skin abrasions and during exposure to mucocutaneous lesions (**Figures 6-32** and **6-33**).[116] Syphilis is then spread through the blood vessels and lymphatics (**Figure 6-34**).[118] Estimates vary based on study, but 0% to 1.8% of children evaluated for suspected sexual abuse are found to have positive serological tests for syphilis.[17,105] The AAP[1] considers syphilis that is not vertically transmitted to be diagnostic of sexual abuse and recommends reporting all cases to CPS for complete investigation.

Infants with congenital syphilis are categorized into 2 groups: (1) early (symptoms before and up to 2 years of age) and (2) late (asymptomatic period followed by symptoms after age 2 years, often presenting at puberty).[119] Early congenital signs and symptoms include mucocutaneous abnormalities, bone findings, and involvement of various organ systems, such as the hematological, hepatic, and renal systems. Late congenital syphilis presents with serious central nervous system, musculoskeletal, and sensory involvement (**Figures 6-35** to **6-39**).

Clinical Findings

Females and males with primary syphilis are usually asymptomatic.[120] Patients may primarily complain of a sore (chancre) anywhere on the external genitalia, yet this ulcer can often go unnoticed (**Figures 6-40** to **6-43**). Chancres may heal over a 4 to 6 week period and are often accompanied by regional lymphadenopathy. Nodes are usually firm and nontender.[120]

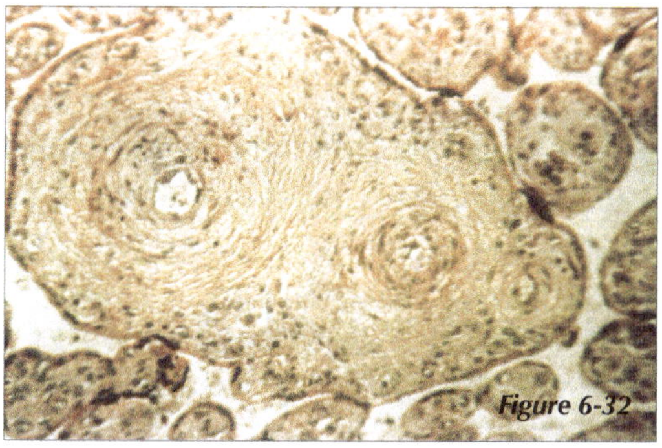

Figure 6-32. *Congenital syphilis; increased size of villi secondary to vasculitis and increased connective tissue. (Contributed by CDC; Atlanta, GA.)*

Figure 6-33. *Congenital syphilis; mucous patches. (Contributed by CDC; Atlanta, GA.)*

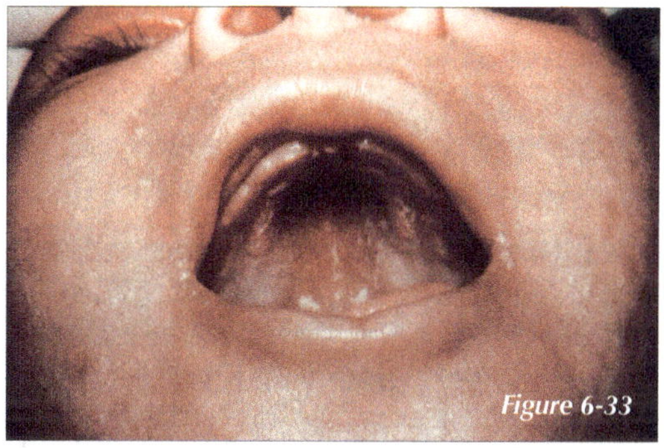

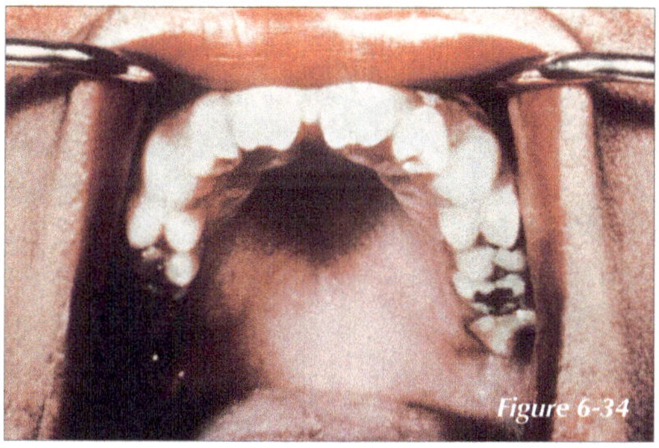

Figure 6-34. *Congenital syphilis; Hutchinson's teeth. (Contributed by CDC; Atlanta, GA.)*

Figure 6-35. *Congenital syphilis; perforation of palate. (Contributed by CDC; Atlanta, GA.)*

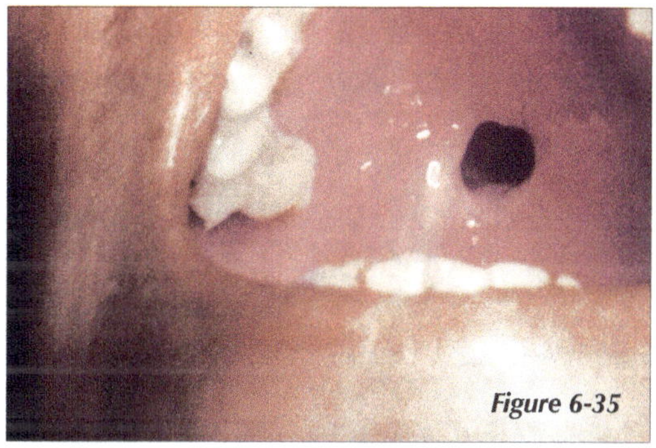

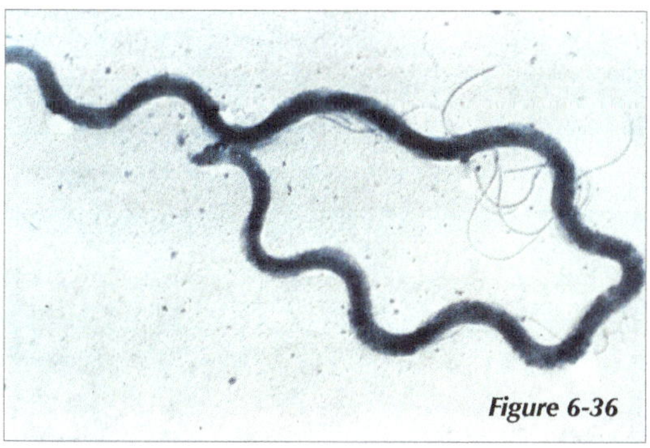

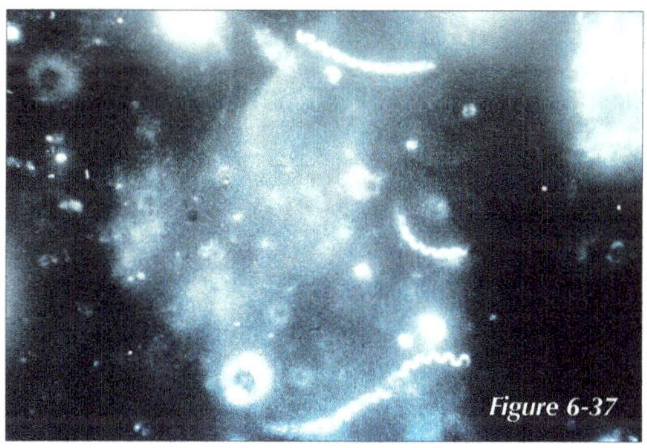

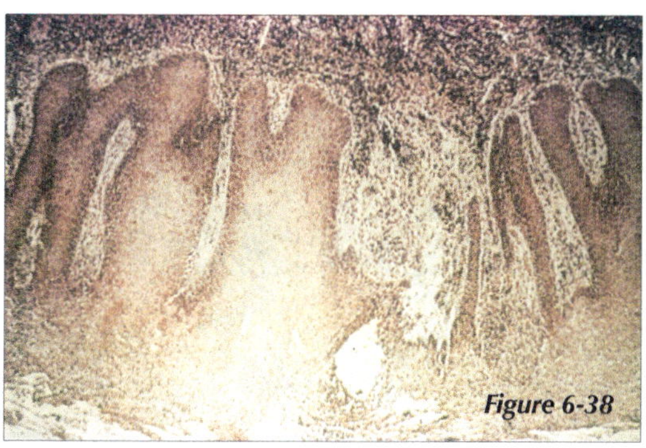

Figure 6-36. *Syphilis;* Treponema pallidum. *(Contributed by CDC; Atlanta, GA.)*

Figure 6-37. *Syphilis;* T. pallidum *on dark field. (Contributed by CDC; Atlanta, GA.)*

Figure 6-38. *Syphilis; migration of polymorphonuclear leukocytes through epidermis, acanthosis (prickle cell layer), elongation of rete ridges, and edema of rete cells. (Contributed by CDC; Atlanta, GA.)*

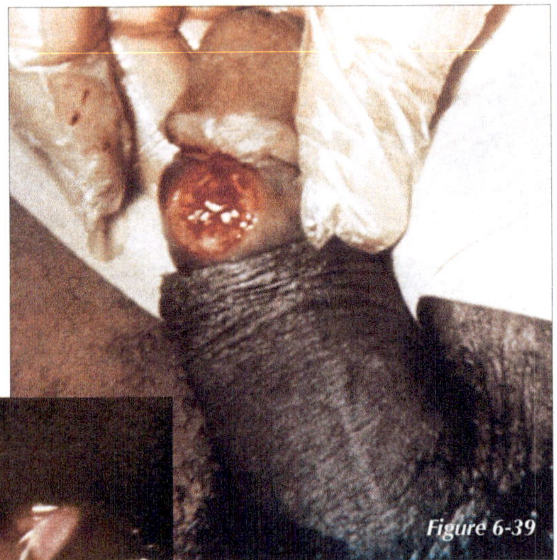

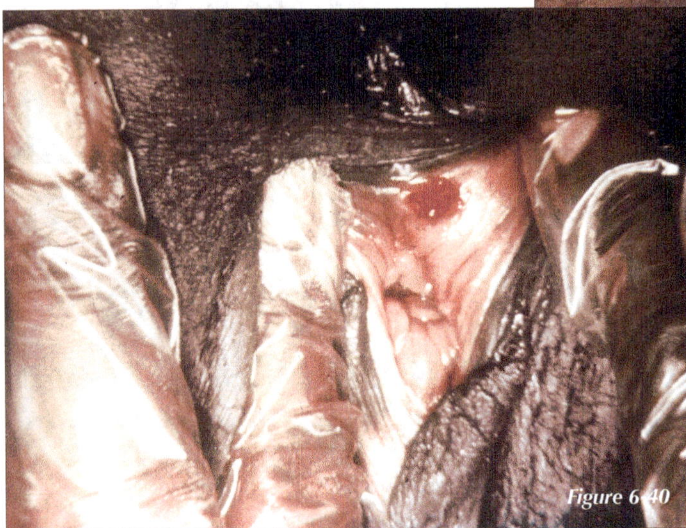

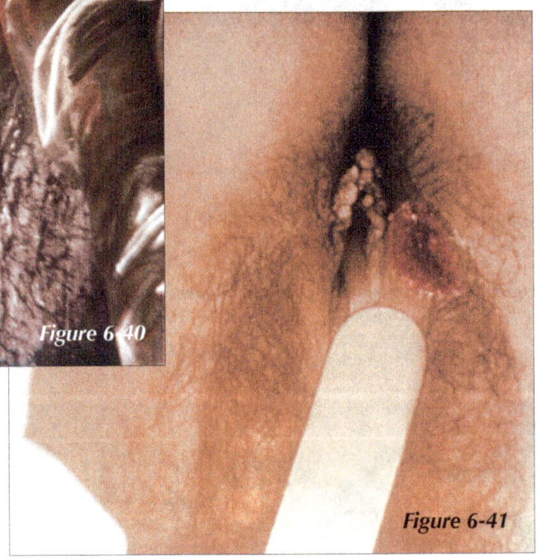

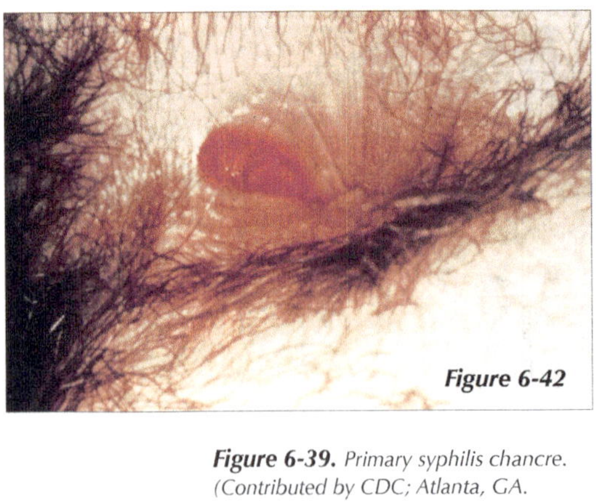

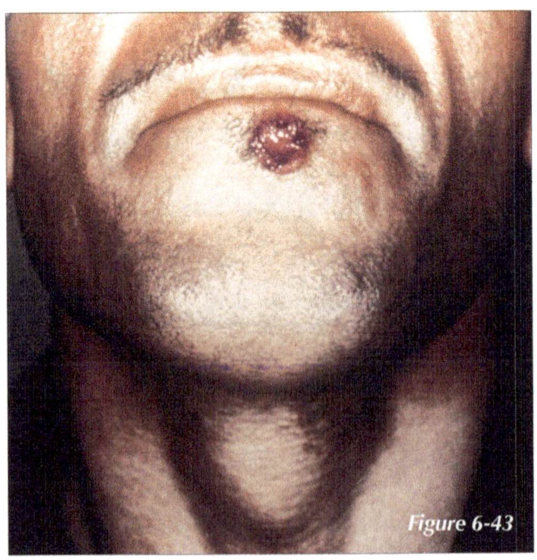

Figure 6-39. Primary syphilis chancre. (Contributed by CDC; Atlanta, GA.

Figure 6-40. Primary syphilis chancre. (Contributed by CDC; Atlanta, GA.)

Figure 6-41. Primary syphilis chancre. (Contributed by CDC; Atlanta, GA.)

Figure 6-42. Primary syphilis chancre of anus. (Contributed by CDC; Atlanta, GA.)

Figure 6-43. Primary syphilis chancre. (Contributed by CDC; Atlanta, GA.)

Between 6 and 8 weeks after initial exposure to syphilis, female and male patients may have the clinical symptoms of secondary syphilis (**Figures 6-44** to **6-50**). Patients primarily complain of a rash on the skin, particularly on the palms of the hands and soles of the feet, and in the mucous membranes. Condylomata lata (**Figure 6-51**), which are hypertrophic granulomatous lesions that may be confused with the condylomata acuminata of HPV, may also occur near the site of the original chancre. Both females and males may complain of genital growths. Although there are classic rashes seen with syphilis, clinicians should be aware that the complaint of any rash could be indicative of secondary syphilis, especially in the context of a history of sexual contact or maltreatment. Children may also present with flu-like symptoms and regional or general lymphadenopathy on physical examination.[118]

Patients with early latent syphilis, occurring within the first year of the infection, and those with late latent syphilis, occurring after the first year, are usually asymptomatic. Female and male patients who develop neurosyphilis (**Figures 6-51** and **6-52**), which can occur at any time during a syphilis infection, may remain asymptomatic or have neurological symptoms, while those with tertiary or late syphilis may have the symptoms of cardiac involvement, neurological disease, or gummata, which are granulomatous lesions of the skin, soft tissue, and bone (**Figures 6-53** and **6-54**). Tertiary syphilis is uncommon today, but can occur 3 to 10 years after initial exposure.[119]

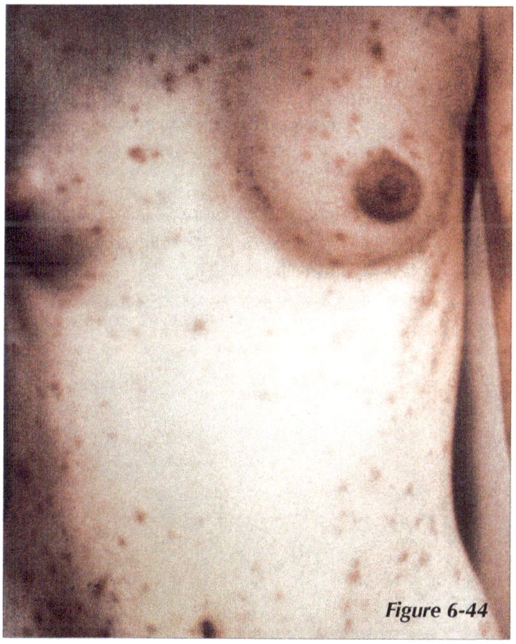

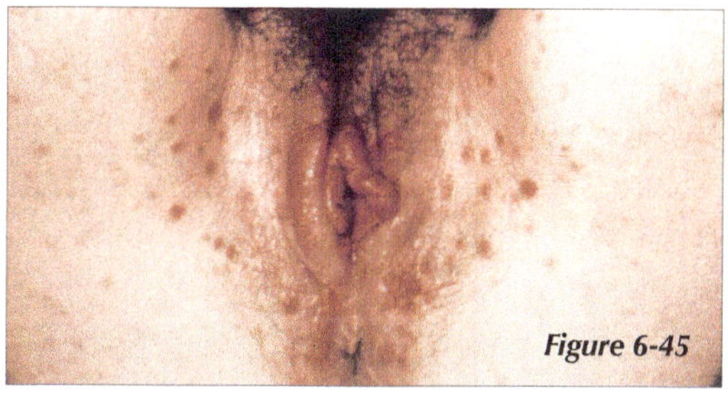

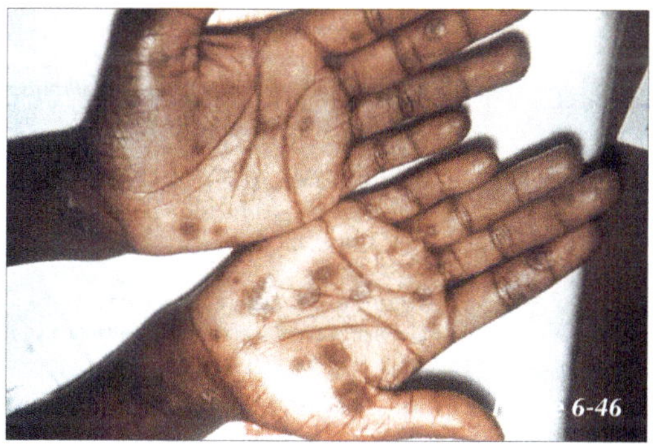

Figure 6-44. *Secondary syphilis; papulosquamous rash. (Contributed by CDC; Atlanta, GA.)*

Figure 6-45. *Secondary syphilis; papulopustular rash. (Contributed by CDC; Atlanta, GA.)*

Figure 6-46. *Secondary syphilis. (Contributed by CDC; Atlanta, GA.)*

Figure 6-47. *Secondary syphilis. (Contributed by CDC; Atlanta, GA.)*

Figure 6-48. *Secondary syphilis. (Contributed by CDC; Atlanta, GA.)*

Figure 6-49. *Secondary syphilis; alopecia. (Contributed by CDC; Atlanta, GA.)*

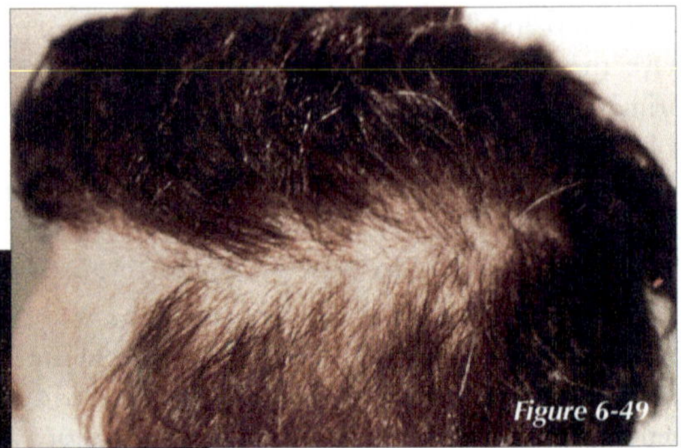

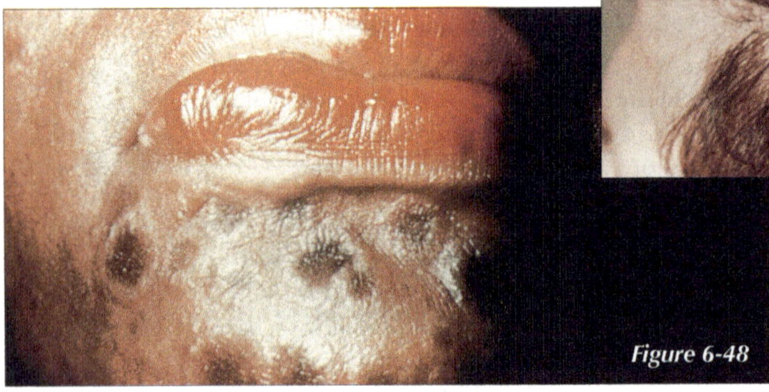

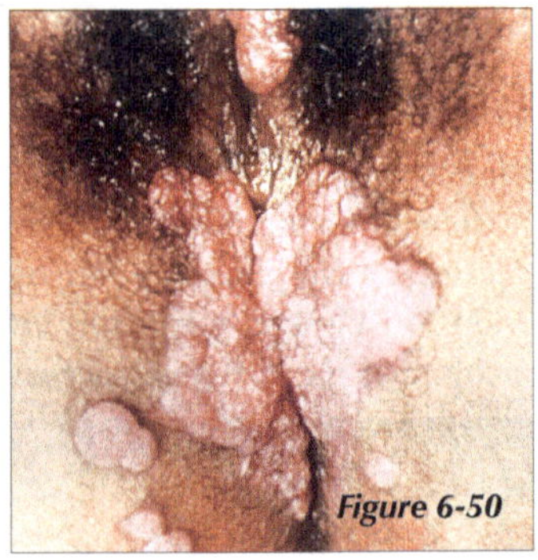

Figure 6-50. *Secondary syphilis; condylomata lata. (Contributed by CDC; Atlanta, GA.)*

Figure 6-51. *Neurosyphilis; spirochetes in neural tissue. (Contributed by CDC; Atlanta, GA.)*

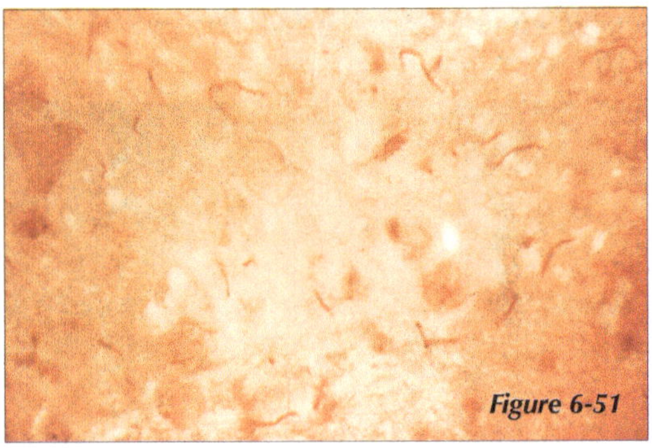

Figure 6-52. *Neurosyphilis; tabes dorsalis, demyelinization of posterior columns and degeneration of dorsal roots. (Contributed by CDC; Atlanta, GA.)*

Figure 6-53. *Late syphilis; serpiginous gummata of forearm. (Contributed by CDC; Atlanta, GA.)*

Figure 6-54. *Late syphilis; ulcerating gumma. (Contributed by CDC; Atlanta, GA.)*

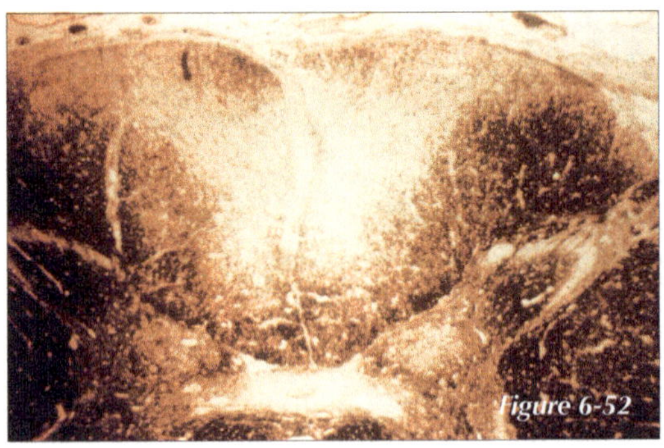

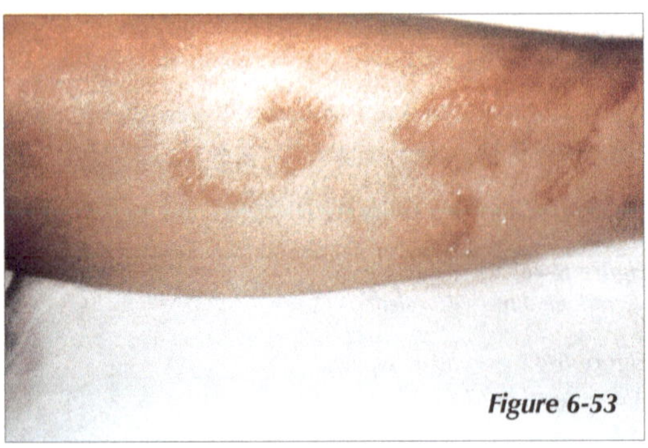

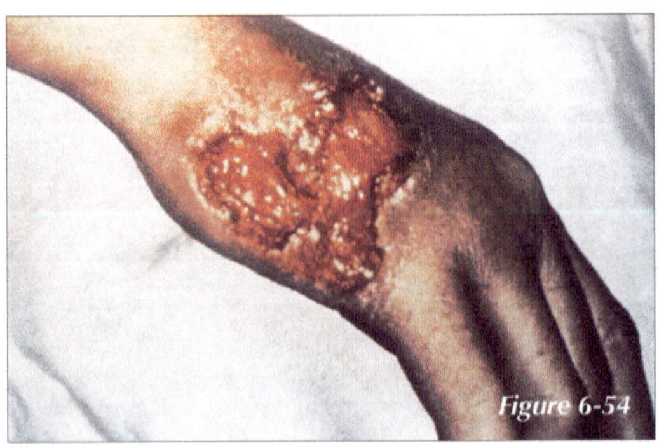

Diagnosis

The diagnosis of syphilis includes an index of suspicion, careful history taking, physical examination, and serological testing. Diagnosis may be established by visualization of spirochetes on dark-field microscopic examination or direct fluorescent antibody staining of fluid from the base of active primary or secondary lesions, if present.[2,105,119] Nontreponemal antibody tests such as the rapid plasma reagin (RPR) and venereal disease research laboratory (VDRL) tests are used for screening purposes of patients at risk for syphilis. If screening tests are positive, a quantitative VDRL test should be done to obtain titers. This test is used to follow the course of syphilis and to ensure adequate treatment. After a positive screening test, a specific treponemal antibody test such as microhemagglutination treponema pallidum (MHA-TP) or fluorescent treponemal antibody absorption (FTA-ABS) should also be done to confirm the diagnosis. Clinicians should be aware that false-positive screening tests may occur and specific tests can be used to clear up any confusion.

Treatment and Follow-Up

A record review should be completed for infants to distinguish acquired from congenital syphilis because evaluation and treatment of congenital disease differs from that of acquired disease.[119] Infants and children with acquired syphilis are treated with benzathine penicillin G, 50 000 units/kg of body weight (up to the adult dose of 2.4 million units), given intramuscularly (IM) as a single dose for primary, secondary, and early latent syphilis.[2,119] Individuals with a history of penicillin allergy should undergo skin testing, desensitization, and treatment with penicillin if at all possible because the efficacy of alternative regimens is poorly defined.[119] The Jarisch-Herxheimer reaction, consisting of fever, malaise, and headache beginning 2 to 12 hours after the initiation of antibiotic therapy, is most common in early disease and is thought to be an effect of endotoxin release from lysing organisms; it usually resolves within 24 hours and does not affect recovery.[119]

Multiple treatment regimens are used when the infection has been present for a year or more, when neurosyphilis is present, or when treatment has failed. All infected individuals should be examined and repeat serological testing (VDRL) completed at 6 and 12 months.[119] Patients with confirmed syphilis should be considered for HIV virus testing as well as screened for other STIs.[2,119]

Children with a history of sexual maltreatment and who are clinically judged to be at risk for syphilis infection should have an initial screening test for syphilis, with follow-up testing at 3 and 6 months. Minimum criteria have been suggested for the selective testing for syphilis in children suspected of having been sexually abused and include the following[121,122]:

— Evidence of an STI

— Lesions with an unclear etiology

— Adolescent age range

— Children from endemic areas or nations

— Parent, family member, or alleged perpetrator with syphilis

— High incidence of syphilis in child's community

If screening for syphilis is initiated and returned results are negative, then follow-up serological testing for syphilis should be repeated 6, 12, and 24 weeks after a sexual assault.[2] Repeat testing should be done at any time after the initial 6 months if clinicians are suspicious of syphilis. **Table 6-15** outlines guidelines for syphilis treatment.

Table 6-15. Guidelines for the Treatment of Syphilis*	
Congenital Syphilis in Infants Aged Younger Than Age 4 Weeks	Crystalline penicillin G 50 000 units/kg per dose intravenously twice daily for 7 days, then 3 times daily to complete a 10 day course *or* Penicillin G procaine 50 000 units/kg/day intramuscularly, once daily for 10 days
Congenital Syphilis in Infants Aged Older Than Age 4 Weeks	**With no neurological involvement and no clinical manifestations of disease:** Benzathine penicillin G* 50 000 units/kg intramuscularly once weekly for 3 weeks *or* Crystalline penicillin G 50 000 units/kg intravenously every 4 to 6 hours for 10 days
	With neurological involvement or clinical manifestations of disease: Crystalline penicillin G* 50 000 units/kg per dose intravenously every 4 to 6 hours for 10 to 14 days Followed by benzathine penicillin G* 50 000 units/kg intramuscularly as a single dose
Primary, Secondary, or Latent Syphilis With Less Than 1-Year Duration	Benzathine penicillin G‡ †‡ 50 000 units/kg intramuscularly as a single dose
Latent Syphilis Greater Than 1 Year or Tertiary Syphilis, Excluding Neurosyphilis	Benzathine penicillin G‡ 50 000 units/kg intramuscularly once weekly for 3 weeks
Neurosyphilis or Syphilitic Eye Disease	Crystalline penicillin G 200 000 to 300 000 units/kg/day (maximum 24 million units/day) in 4 to 6 divided doses or as a continuous infusion for 10 to 14 days *or* Penicillin G procaine 2.4 million units intramuscularly once daily ***plus*** Probenecid 500 mg orally 4 times daily, both for 10 to 14 days
For Penicillin-Allergic Patients	**Uncomplicated Early Syphilis:** Doxycycline 100 mg orally twice daily for 14 days (for children aged older than age 8 years) *or* Erythromycin 10 mg/kg per dose 4 times daily for 14 days *or* Ceftriaxone 1 g intramuscularly or intravenously once daily for 8 to 10 days (optimal dose and duration not well established)

(continued)

Table 6-15. Guidelines for the Treatment of Syphilis* *(continued)*

For Penicillin-Allergic Patients	**Uncomplicated Late Syphilis:** Doxycycline 100 mg orally twice daily for 28 days (for children older than age 8 years) *or* Tetracycline 500 mg orally 4 times daily for 28 days
If Penicillin-Allergic	Undergo testing and desensitization followed by penicillin treatment If treated with nonpenicillin regimens, infants should be evaluated for possible congenital syphilis and treated with penicillin.

**Drug dosage recommendations listed herein are those of the authors and are not endorsed by the United States Public Health Service or the United States Department of Health and Human Services.*
‡Maximum doses: Benzathine penicillin G, 2.4 million units per dose; crystalline penicillin G, 3.4 million units per dose.
†‡If patient is pregnant, some recommend 2 doses of benzathine penicillin 2.4 million units 1 week apart.
Adapted from American Academy of Pediatrics Committee on Infectious Diseases; Pickering LK, Long SS. Report of the Committee on Infectious Diseases. *28th ed. Oak Grove Village, IL: American Academy of Pediatrics; 2009.*
Adapted from Centers for Disease Control and Prevention. Sexually transmitted diseases treatment guidelines 2002. MMWR. *2002;51(RR06):72-74. Centers for Disease Control and Prevention Web site. http://www.cdc.gov/mmwr/preview/mmwrhtml/rr5106a1.htm. Published May 10, 2002. Accessed September 21, 2013.*

Human Immunodeficiency Virus and Acquired Immunodeficiency Syndrome

General Overview and Epidemiology

HIV is a retroviral infection that provides a challenging dilemma to health professionals working with children and adolescents suspected of sexual abuse.[123] Although one can acquire an HIV infection as a result of sexual abuse and sexual assault, the risk is low.[2] However, the seriousness of acquiring HIV makes the risk of this STI a particular concern in the context of the health care evaluation for sexual maltreatment. Issues that arise for the health care provider include whether or not to perform screening tests for the infection and whether or not to initiate postexposure prophylaxis (PEP).[124] The majority of information about what to do in the clinical context of sexual abuse and sexual assault does not come from research in this specific area but instead from extrapolations on data from occupational exposures, which is a less than ideal situation.[2,125] What is known at this point is that the majority of cases of HIV infection in children have been acquired perinatally. Several reports in the pediatric literature indicate a very small number of cases of HIV infection acquired with the sole risk factor of sexual abuse[18,123,124,126] (**Table 6-16**). The risk for an adolescent or adult woman acquiring HIV from a sexual assault is low and dependent on related factors, such as type of assault (ie, oral, vaginal, or anal); presence of oral, vaginal, or anal trauma; ejaculate exposure site; viral load in ejaculate; and the presence of other STIs (eg, syphilis).[2] Although the risk is difficult to determine precisely, a given clinical situation may warrant the need to make a decision about testing and the initiation of antiretroviral agents relatively urgently. Therefore, the CDC[2] recommends a case-by-case approach regarding HIV prophylaxis in instances of sexual abuse and sexual assault. The following selective screening criteria for HIV are suggested because the risk to the prepubertal child of acquiring HIV from sexual abuse is low[17]:

— Presence of STI

— Perpetrator is a member of a high-risk group (ie, homosexual, intravenous [IV] drug abuser, known to be infected with HIV)

Table 6-16. New York State Department of Health Acquired Immune Deficiency Syndrome Institute Estimated Risk of Human Immunodeficiency Virus Transmission Following Different Types of Exposures*

Type of Exposure	Estimated Risk
Percutaneous exposure to infected blood (in HCWs)[25]	0.3% (1 in 333)
Mucous membrane exposure to infected blood (in HCWs)[25]	0.09% (1 in 1100)
Needle-sharing exposure to an infected source[127]	0.67% (1 in 150)
Anal intercourse with an infected source (receptive or insertive)[128,129]	0.5%-3.0% (1-6 in 200)/0.065% (1 in 2000)
Vaginal intercourse with an infected source (receptive/insertive)[129,130]	0.1% (1 in 1000)/0.05% (1 in 2000)
Oral sex with ejaculation with an infected source[131,132]	Conflicting data; however, risk is considered low‡

**These risk estimates depend on many factors, including source viral load, presence of STIs, and the presence of ejaculate.*
‡It is prudent to recommend PEP for receptive oral sex with ejaculation, although discussion about the conflicting data should occur.
Adapted from New York State Department of Health AIDS Institute. Clinical guidelines development program. HIV post-exposure prophylaxis for children beyond the perinatal period. HIV Clinical Resource Web site. www.hivguidelines.org Updated June 2010. Accessed September 24, 2013.

— Perpetrator is known or suspected to have multiple partners or symptoms suggesting immunodeficiency

— Parents have requested HIV screening

— Bloody assault

— Multiple perpetrators

The CDC[2] suggests that for adolescents and adults who have been evaluated for sexual assault, clinicians should consider the following:

— Likelihood of exposure to HIV

— Potential benefits and risks of antiretroviral therapy

— Interval between exposure and initiation of treatment

— HIV status of assailant and, if not known, local epidemiology of HIV and AIDS

If antiviral PEP medications are offered or initiated, the CDC[2] recommends that the health care provider should discuss the following with the patient:

— Efficacy and toxicity of antiretrovirals

— Need for frequent dosing of medications

— Need for close follow-up

— Importance of strict compliance

— Need for immediate initiation for maximal effectiveness

The number of children and adolescents who acquire HIV infection as a result of sexual abuse is very low, and while the number who become HIV positive as a result of sexual assault is not known, it is also believed to be low.[17] At the present time, no universally accepted standard protocols exist related to testing or initiation of postexposure antiretroviral therapy.[133] **Table 6-17** contains the HIV protocol recommended by the CDC. Adherence to HIV PEP in victims of sexual assault is poor at about the 40% range, so ongoing support offered to patients is essential to support adherence to the protocol.[134] The information related to HIV will increase as more study is done, so clinicians should pay close attention and consult with regional experts on this important issue. For the prepubertal child, the AAP[19] considers the presence of HIV infection that is nonvertically transmitted to be indicative of sexual abuse and recommends health care providers report such cases to CPS.

Clinical Findings

The incubation period for HIV infections vary, and may be quite long before symptoms appear. Both males and females infected with the HIV virus can have a wide range of signs and symptoms. Many are asymptomatic, whereas others may initially have mild and vague complaints. Clinicians are referred to major pediatric and adolescent textbooks for a complete discussion of the presentation of HIV and AIDS.

Table 6-17. Recommendations for Postexposure Assessment Related to Human Immunodeficiency Virus

Recommendations for HIV-Related Postexposure Assessment of Children Within 72 Hours of Sexual Assault
— Review HIV/AIDS local epidemiology and assess risk for HIV infection in the assailant.
— Evaluate circumstances of assault that might affect risk for HIV transmission.
— Consult with a specialist in treating HIV-infected children if PEP is considered.
— If the child appears to be at risk for HIV transmission from the assault, discuss PEP with the caregiver(s), including its toxicity and unknown efficacy.
— If caregivers choose for the child to receive antiretroviral PEP (78, 142, 489) provide enough medication to last until the return visit 3 to 7 days after the initials assessment, at which time the child should be reevaluated and tolerance of medication assessed; dosages should not exceed those for adults.
— Perform HIV antibody test at original assessment, 6 weeks, 3 months, and 6 months
Recommendations for Postexposure Assessment of Adolescent and Adult Survivors Within 72 Hours of Sexual Assault*
— Assess risk for HIV infection in the assailant.
— Evaluate characteristics of the assault event that might increase risk for HIV transmission.
— Consult with a specialist in HIV treatment, if PEP is being considered.
— If the survivor appears to be at risk for HIV transmission for the assault, discuss antiretroviral prophylaxis, including toxicity and lack of proven benefit.

**Assistance with PEP-related decisions can be obtained by calling the National Clinician's Post-Exposure Prophylaxis Hotline (PEP Line) (telephone: 888-448-4911).*

Adapted from Centers for Disease Control and Prevention. Sexually transmitted diseases treatment guidelines 2010. MMWR. *2010;59(RR-12):1-110. Centers for Disease Control and Prevention Web site. http://www.cdc.gov/std/treatment/2010/toc.htm. Updated January 28, 2011. Accessed September 29, 2013.*

Diagnosis

HIV infection is diagnosed by serological testing after obtaining informed consent. Initial screening, if it is to be done, should take place after the identification of child sexual maltreatment. Repeat testing is important because negative antibody tests cannot exclude infection that occurred less than 6 months before the test.[135] The CDC[2] recommends repeat HIV testing at 6, 12, and 24 weeks after initial testing in sexual assault cases, along with syphilis testing. A positive antibody test is followed by a more specific test, such as the Western blot or the immunofluorescence assay to confirm HIV infection.

Treatment and Follow-Up

Many medications are used to slow the progression of HIV infection. Patients who are HIV positive require comprehensive medical care to manage the infection, as well as extensive psychosocial support. At the present time, a case-by-case approach is to be followed; routine prophylaxis is not recommended for child victims of sexual maltreatment but may be necessary in individual cases based on the clinical situation of the abuse.[136] A similar case-by-case approach is to be followed for adolescents and adult women who have been sexually assaulted. In the pediatric setting, the patient and family's input is highly valued and serves as a factor in the clinical decision-making process. Because of the rapidly changing recommendations for HIV care, consultation with an infectious disease specialist is recommended to have access to the most current recommendations for therapy.

Hepatitis B Virus

General Overview and Epidemiology

HBV is a DNA virus considered to be both a blood-borne pathogen and an STI. The incidence of HBV has decreased steadily in recent years due to widespread vaccination in infancy; 4033 acute cases were reported in 2008, but it is estimated that the incidence of actual cases is up to 10 times the reported rate.[2] According to the CDC,[137] approximately 60% to 65% of these cases are acquired through sexual transmission. Some acute infections progress to chronic infections with approximately 90% of infants, 25% to 50% of children 1 to 5 years of age, and 5% of older children and adults developing chronic disease.[138] Approximately 2000 to 4000 deaths each year are attributable to HBV infection.[139] The HBV vaccination is highly effective, with protective levels of antibody present in approximately 30% to 55% of recipients after the first dose, 75% after 2 doses, and greater than 90% after 3 doses.[137] Passive immunization with HBIG prevents up to 75% of infections after sexual contact with individuals who have acute HBV infections, and HBV vaccine without HBIG is effective in preventing infections after sexual contact with individuals with chronic infection.[2]

In pediatrics, the majority of infections in prepubertal children occur by way of perinatal infection and person-to-person contact with a chronically infected household member over the first 5 years of life.[2] In adolescents, sexual transmission is most common. Because of the potential long-term consequences of HBV, clinicians should consider its possibility in the context of sexual maltreatment.

Symptoms and Clinical Findings

Those infected with the HBV have a wide range of signs and symptoms, with approximately 30% of individuals remaining asymptomatic. Acutely symptomatic children and adolescents may complain of fatigue, anorexia, nausea, fever, right upper quadrant pain, myalgia, and arthralgias.[140] Clinical findings include liver or spleen tenderness, jaundice, icteric sclera, arthritis, and skin rash.[137,141]

Diagnosis

Several serological tests are available to assess for HBV. A hepatitis B surface antigen (HBsAg) becomes positive during the incubation period and, in most cases, becomes negative during the clinical disease phase. A positive result suggests acute hepatitis B infection, except in cases in which the person is a chronic carrier of the disease, in which case the test will remain positive for life.[141] The antihepatitis B core antigen (anti-HBc) becomes positive after the incubation period when the HBsAg is decreasing. This test can be divided into immunoglobulin M (IgM) and immunoglobulin G (IgG), which is helpful when trying to identify an acute versus older infection. The IgM and IgG are both present when an acute infection is present, while the presence of IgG alone indicates an infection that is at least 6 months old.[141] The health care provider should use the HBsAg and the anti-HBc tests as the baseline tests when initially evaluating a patient for hepatitis B.

Clinicians caring for victims of sexual maltreatment should keep in mind that patients may have been immunized against hepatitis B. A history of having completed the vaccination series may eliminate the need for testing and should provide reassurance. When a patient has been successfully immunized, the HBsAg test will return positive results; this is the only HBV antibody marker present after vaccination.[2] While HBsAg levels decline to low or undetectable levels 10 to 15 years after immunization, immunity persists in nearly all individuals.[141]

Treatment and Follow-Up

Patients who are diagnosed with HBV require long-term care with a gastrointestinal specialist. Much of the care for an acute infection is supportive and palliative, while follow-up is necessary. There is currently no curative treatment for HBV, but medical regimens using antiviral agents, such as lamivudine, adefovir, entecavir, telbivudine and tenofovir, show promise.[142] Unless the perpetrator is known to be acutely infected with HBV, the initiation of the HBV vaccination series in the unimmunized child or adolescent should provide adequate protection. In the unlikely scenario of a perpetrator with a known acute HBV infection, hepatitis B immune globulin (HBIG) along with the initiation of the active vaccination series would be indicated.[2]

Conclusion

The health care evaluation of a child or adolescent in the context of possible sexual abuse or sexual assault requires careful attention to risk for exposure to STIs. In prepubertal children and nonsexually active adolescents, outside of perinatal transmission, the presence of an STI warrants investigation for sexual maltreatment. The CDC guidelines offer a reasonable approach to testing for possible STIs and treatment. Prepubertal children and adolescents differ anatomically and physiologically; therefore, presentation of STIs may differ. Prepubertal children are most often symptomatic with the majority of STIs; asymptomatic infections in adolescents are not uncommon, especially in males. Health care providers should be aware of the forensic-medical issues associated with the evaluation of STIs in the context of sexual abuse evaluations.

References

1. Kellogg N; The American Academy of Pediatrics Committee on Child Abuse and Neglect. The evaluation of sexual abuse in children. *Pediatrics.* 2005;116(2):506-512.

2. Centers for Disease Control and Prevention. Sexually transmitted diseases treatment guidelines 2010. *MMWR.* 2010;59(RR-12):1-110. Centers for Disease Control and Prevention Web site. http://www.cdc.gov/std/treatment/2010/toc.htm. Updated January 28, 2011. Accessed September 29, 2013.

3. Gardner JJ. Comparison of the vaginal flora in sexually abused and nonabused girls. *J Pediatr.* 1992;120(6):872-877.

4. Ingram DL, Everett DV, Lyna PR, White ST, Rockwell LA. Epidemiology of adult sexually transmitted disease agents in children being evaluated for sexual abuse. *Pediatr Infect Dis J.* 1992;11(11):945-950.

5. Robinson AJ, Watkeys JEM, Ridgway GL. Sexually transmitted organisms in sexually abused children. *Arch Dis Child.* 1998;79(4):356-358.

6. White ST, Loda FA, Ingram DL, Pearson A. Sexually transmitted diseases in sexually abused children. *Pediatrics.* 1983;72(1):16-21.

7. Girardet RG, Lahoti S, Howard LA, et al. Epidemiology of sexually transmitted infections in suspected child victims of sexual assault. *Pediatrics.* 2009;124(1):79-86.

8. Schwarcz SK, Whittington WL. Sexual assault and sexually transmitted disease: detection and management in adults and children. *Rev Infect Dis.* 1990;12:S682-S690.

9. White ST, Loda FA, Ingram DL, Pearson A. Sexually transmitted disease in sexually abused children. *Pediatrics.* 1983;72:16-21.

10. Reynolds MW, Peipert JF, Collins B. Epidemiologic issues of sexually transmitted diseases in sexual assault victims. *Obstet Gynecol Surv.* 2000;55:51-57.

11. Committee on Technical Bulletins of the American College of Obstetricians and Gynecologists. ACOG technical bulletin: vaginitis. *Int J Gynaecol Obstet.* 1996;54(226):293-302.

12. Girardin BW, Faugno DK, Seneski PC, Slaughter L, Whelan M. *Color Atlas of Sexual Assault.* St. Louis, MO: Mosby; 1997.

13. Adams JA, Kaplan RA, Starling SP, et al. Guidelines for medical care of children who may have been sexually abused. *J Pediatr Adolesc Gynecol.* 2007;20(3):163-172.

14. Hodas GR. Responding to childhood trauma: the promise and practice of trauma informed care. Child Rescue Web site. http://www.childrescuebill.org/VictimsOfAbuse/RespondingHodas.pdf. Published February 2006. Accessed September 20, 2013.

15. Hammerschlag MR. *Sexually Transmitted Diseases and Child Abuse: Portable Guides to Investigating Child Abuse.* Washington, DC: US Department of Justice, Office of Justice Programs and Office of Juvenile Justice and Delinquency Preventions; 1996.

16. Hammerschlag MR. Chlamydia trachomatis and chlamydia pneumoniae infections in children and adolescents. *Pediatr Rev.* 2004;25(2):43-51.

17. Hammerschlag MR. Sexually transmitted diseases in sexually abused children: medical and legal implications. *Sex Transm Infect.* 1998;74(3):167-174.

18. Centers for Disease Control and Prevention. HIV/AIDS statistics: semi-annual hiv/aids surveillance report. Centers for Disease Control and Prevention Web site. http://www.cdc.gov/hiv/topics/surveillance/resources/reports/pdf/hasr1202.pdf. Accessed January 7, 2014.

19. American Academy of Pediatrics Committee on Child Abuse and Neglect. Guidelines for the evaluation of sexual abuse of children: subject review. *Pediatrics.* 1999;103(1):186-191.

20. Shapiro RA, Schubert CJ, Myers PA. Vaginal discharge as an indicator of gonorrhea and chlamydia infection in girls under 12 years old. *Pediatr Emerg Care.* 1993;9(6):341-345.

21. Siegel RM, Schubert CJ, Myers PA, Shapiro RA. The prevalence of sexually transmitted diseases in children and adolescents evaluated for sexual abuse in Cincinnati: rationale for limited STD testing in prepubertal girls. *Pediatrics.* 1995;96(6):1090-1094.

22. Black CM, Driebe EM, Howard LA, et al. Multicenter study of nucleic acid amplification tests for detection of chlamydia trachomatis and neisseria gonorrhoeae in children being evaluated for sexual abuse. *Pediatr Infect Dis J.* 2009;28(7):608-613.

23. Centers for Disease Control and Prevention. Sexually transmitted diseases treatment guidelines 2002. *MMWR.* 2002;51(RR06):72-74. Centers for Disease Control and Prevention Web site. http://www.cdc.gov/mmwr/preview/mmwrhtml/rr5106a1.htm. Published May 10, 2002. Accessed September 21, 2013.

24. Benrubi G. Bacterial vaginosis: diagnosing and treating the most common vaginal infection. *Female Patient.* August 1999;(suppl):S4-S8.

25. Centers for Disease Control and Prevention. Sexually transmitted diseases treatment guidelines 2006. *MMWR.* 2006;55(RR11):1-94.

26. Hillier S, Holmes K. Bacterial vaginosis. In: Holmes K, Sparling PF, Mardh P, et al, eds. *Sexually Transmitted Diseases.* 3rd ed. New York, NY: McGraw-Hill; 1999:563-586.

27. Koumans EH, Sternberg M, Bruce C, et al. The prevalence of bacterial vaginosis in the United States, 2001-2004: associations with symptoms, sexual behaviors, and reproductive health. *Sex Transm Dis.* 2007;34(11):864-869.

28. American College of Obstetricians and Gynecologists. Vaginitis. *Int J Gynaecol Obstet.* 1996;54(3):293-302.

29. Darville T. Chlamydia. *Pediatr Rev.* 1998;19(3):85-91.

30. Wyrick PB. Intracellular survival by chlamydia. *Cell Microbiol.* 2000;2(4):275-282.

31. Stamm WE. Chlamydia trachomatis. In: Holmes K, Sparling PF, Mardh P, et al, eds. *Sexually Transmitted Diseases.* 4th ed. New York, NY: McGraw-Hill; 2000:575-593.

32. American Academy of Pediatrics. Chlamydial trachomatis. In: Pickering LK, Long SS. *Report of the Committee on Infectious Diseases.* 28th ed. Oak Grove Village, IL: American Academy of Pediatrics; 2009:252.

33. Darville T. Chlamydia infections. In: Remington JS, Klein JO, Wilson CB, Nizet V, Maldonado Y, eds. *Infectious Diseases of the Fetus and Newborn Infant.* 7th ed. Philadelphia, PA: Elsevier Saunders; 2011:600-606.

34. Mylonas I. Female genital Chlamydia trachomatis infection: where are we heading? *Arch Gynecol Obstet.* 2012;285(5):1271-1285.

35. Rours IG, Hammerschlag MR, Ott A, et al. Chlamydia trachomatis as a cause of neonatal conjunctivitis in Dutch infants. *Pediatrics.* 2008;121(2):e321-326.

36. Hammerschlag MR. Chlamydia infection. In: Feigin RD, Cherry JD, Demmler-Harrison GJ, Kaplan SL, eds. *Textbook of Pediatric Infectious Diseases.* 6th ed. Philadelphia, PA: Elsevier; 2009:2655-2667.

37. Jenny C. Sexually transmitted diseases and child abuse. *Pediatr Ann.* 1992;21(8):497-503.

38. Hammerschlag MR. Sexual assault and abuse of children. *Clin Infect Dis.* 2011;53(suppl 3):S103-S109.

39. Hammerschlag MR. Use of NAATs to detect chlamydia in children being evaluated for suspected sexual abuse. National Chlamydia Coalition Web site. http://ncc.prevent.org/products/committee-products/file/RTC-Brief-6.pdf. Published November 2012. Accessed September 25, 2013.

40. Cates W; The American Social Health Association Panel. Estimates of the incidence and prevalence of sexually transmitted diseases in the United States. *Sex Transm Dis.* 1999;26(4):S2-S7.

41. Adams J, Zuckerman AL. Genital complaints in prepubertal girls. Medscape Reference Web site. http://emedicine.medscape.com/article/954024-overview. Accessed 2012.

42. Emans S. Office evaluation of the child and adolescent. In: Emans SJ, Laufer MR, Goldstein DP. *Pediatric and Adolescent Gynecology*. 5th ed. Philadelphia, PA: Lippincott Williams & Wilkins; 2005:1-18.

43. Adams JA. Guidelines for medical care of children evaluated for suspected sexual abuse: an update for 2008. *Curr Opin Obstet Gynecol.* 2008;20(5):435-441.

44. Martin DH. Nongonococcal urethritis: new views through the prism of modern molecular microbiology. *Curr Infect Dis Rep*. 2008;10(2):128-132.

45. American College of Obstetricians and Gynecologists. Pediatric gynecologic disorders. *ACOG Tech Bull 201*. Washington, DC: American College of Obstetricians and Gynecologists; 1995.

46. Lee YS, Lee KS. Chlamydia and male urinary tract diseases. *Korean J Urol.* 2013;54(2):73-77.

47. Wagenlehner FME, Weidner W, Naber KG. Chlamydial infections in urology. *World J Urol.* 2006;24(1):4-12.

48. Hammerschlag MR, Ajl S, Laraque D. Inappropriate use of nonculture tests for the detection of chlamydia trachomatis in suspected victims of child sexual abuse: a continuing problem. *Pediatrics*. 1999;104(5):1137-1139.

49. Centers for Disease Control and Prevention. Trends in sexually transmitted diseases in the United States: 2009 national data for gonorrhea, chlamydia and syphilis. snapshot: sexually transmitted disease. Centers for Disease Control and Prevention Web site. http://www.cdc.gov/std/stats09/figures/trends-figure.htm. Accessed 2012.

50. Darville T. Gonorrhea. *Pediatr Rev.* 1999;20(4):125-128.

51. Sung L, MacDonald NE. Gonorrhea: a pediatric perspective. *Pediatr Rev.* 1998;19(1):13-16.

52. Goodyear-Smith F. What is the evidence for non-sexual transmission of gonorrhoea in children after the neonatal period? a systematic review. *J Forensic Leg Med.* 2007;14(8):489-502.

53. Beck-Sagué CM, Solomon F. Sexually transmitted diseases in abused children and adolescent and adult victims of rape: review of selected literature. *Clin Infect Dis.* 1999;28(suppl 1):S74-S83.

54. Wald ER. Gynecologic infections in the pediatric age group. *Pediatr Infect Dis.* 1984;May/June(suppl 3):S10-S13.

55. American Academy of Pediatrics Committee on Child Abuse and Neglect. Gonorrhea in prepubertal children: subject review (RE9803). *Pediatrics.* 1998;101:1324-1135.

56. Pletcher JR, Slap GB. Pelvic inflammatory disease. *Pediatr Rev.* 1998;19(11):363-367.

57. Centers for Disease Control and Prevention. Other sexually transmitted diseases. Centers for Disease Control and Prevention Web site. http://www.cdc.gov/std/stats11/other.htm. Updated December 13, 2012. Accessed August 4, 2013.

58. Lareau SM, Beigi RH. Pelvic inflammatory disease and tubo-ovarian abscess. *Infect Dis Clin North Am.* 2008;22(4):693-708.

59. Bohm MK, Newman L, Satterwhite CL, Tao G, Weinstock HS. Pelvic inflammatory disease among privately insured women, United States, 2001-2005. *Sex Transm Dis.* 2010;30(3):131-136.

60. Tarr ME, Gilliam ML. Sexually transmitted infections in adolescent women. *Clin Obstet Gynecol.* 2008;51(2):306-318.

61. Benaim J, Pulaski M, Coupey S. Adolescent girls and pelvic inflammatory disease: experience and practices of emergency department pediatricians. *Arch Pediatr Adolesc Med.* 1998;152(5):449-454.

62. American College of Obstetricians and Gynecologists. Genital human papillomavirus infections. *ACOG Tech Bull 193.* Washington, DC: American College of Obstetricians and Gynecologists; 1994.

63. Carter JR, Ding Z, Rose BR. HPV infection and cervical disease: a review. *Aust N Z Obstet Gynaecol.* 2011;51(2):103-108.

64. Cohen BA, Honig P, Androphy E. Anogenital warts in children: clinical and virologic evaluation for sexual abuse. *Arch Dermatol.* 1990;126(12):1575-1580.

65. De Jong AR, Weiss JC, Brent RL. Condyloma acuminata in children. *Am J Dis Child.* 1982;136(8):704-706.

66. Puranen M, Yliskoski M, Saarikoski S, Syrijanen K, Syrjanen S. Vertical transmission of human papillomavirus from infected mothers to their newborn babies and persistence of the virus in childhood. *Am J Obstet Gynecol.* 1996;174(2):694-699.

67. Syrjänen S. Current concepts on human papillomavirus infections in children. *APMIS.* 2010;118(6-7):494-509.

68. Koutsky L. Epidemiology of genital human papillomavirus infection. *Am J Med.* 1997;102(5, suppl 1):3-8.

69. Schiffman M, Castle PE, Jeronimo J, Rodriguez AC, Wacholder S. Human papillomavirus and cervical cancer. *Lancet.* 2007;370(9590):890-907.

70. American College of Obstetricians and Gynecologists. The adolescent obstetric-gynecologic patient. *ACOG Tech Bull 145.* Washington, DC: American College of Obstetricians and Gynecologists; 1990.

71. Centers for Disease Control and Prevention. National health and nutrition examination survey, 2003-2004. Centers for Disease Control and Prevention Web site. http://www.cdc.gov/nchs/about/major/nhanes/nhanes2003-2004/nhanes03_04.htm. Updated August 29, 2012. Accessed September 23, 2013.

72. Dunne EF, Unger ER, Sternberg M, et al. Prevalence of HPV infection among females in the United States. *JAMA.* 2007;297(8):813-819.

73. Reynolds MW, Peipert JF, Collins B. Epidemiological issues of sexually transmitted disease in sexual assault victims. *Obstet Gynecol Surv.* 2000;55(1):51-57.

74. Watts DH, Koutsky LA, Holmes KK, Goldman D, et al. Low risk of perinatal transmission of human papillomavirus: results from a prospective cohort study. *Am J Obstet Gynaecol.* 1998;178(2):365-373.

75. Darville T. Genital warts. *Pediatr Rev.* 1999;20(8):271-272.

76. Frasier LD. Human papillomavirus infections in children. *Pediatr Ann.* 1994;24(7):354-360.

77. Handsfield H. Clinical presentation and natural course of anogenital warts. *Am J Med.* 1997;102(5, suppl 1):16-20.

78. Shew ML, Fortenberry JD. HPV infection in adolescents: natural history, complications, and indicators for viral typing. *Semin Pediatr Infect Dis.* 2005;16(3):168-174.

79. Trofatter KF. Diagnosis of human papillomavirus genital tract infection. *Am J Med.* 1997;102(5, suppl 1):21-27.

80. Deshpande DJ, Nayak CS, Mishra SN, Dhurat RS. Verrucous condyloma lata mimicking condyloma acuminata: an unusual presentation. *Indian J Sex Transm Dis.* 2009;30(3):100-102.

81. Kim JS, Kang MS, Sagong C, Ko JY, Yu HJ. An unusual extensive secondary syphilis: condyloma lata on the umbilicus and perineum and mucous patches on the lips. *Clin Exp Dermatol.* 2009;34(7):e299-301.

82. Beutner K, Ferenczy A. Therapeutic approaches to genital warts. *Am J Med.* 1997;102(5A):28-37.

83. Wright TC, Richart RM. Role of human papillomavirus in the pathogenesis of genital tract warts and cancer. *Gynecol Oncol.* 1990;37(2):151-164.

84. Crum CP, Barber S, Roche JK. Pathobiology of papillomavirus-related cervical diseases: prospects for immunodiagnosis. *Clin Microbiol Rev.* 1991;4(3):270-285.

85. Schiffman MH, Brinton LA. The epidemiology of cervical carcinogenesis. *Cancer.* 1995;15(10 suppl):1888-1901.

86. Turek LP, Smith EM. The genetic program of genital human papillomaviruses in infection and cancer. *Obstet Gynecol Clin North Am.* 1996;23(4):735-758.

87. Ledwaba T, Dlamini Z, Naicker S, Bhoola K. Molecular genetics of human cervical cancer: role of papillomavirus and the apoptotic cascade. *Biol Chem.* 2004;385(8):671-682.

88. Ciesielska C, Nowińska K, Podhorska-Okolów M, Dzięgiel P. The role of human papillomavirus in the malignant transformation of cervic epithelial cells and the importance of vaccination against this virus. *Adv Clin Exp Med.* 2012;21(2):235-244.

89. Massad LS, Einstein MH, Huh WK, et al. 2012 updated consensus guidelines for the management of abnormal cervical cancer screening tests and cancer precursors. *Obstet Gynecol.* 2013;121(4):829-246.

90. Mell HK. Management of oral and genital herpes in the emergency department. *Emerg Med Clin North Am.* 2008;26(2):457-473.

91. Roberts CM, Pfister JR, Spear SJ. Increasing proportion of herpes simplex virus type 1 as a cause of genital herpes infection in college students. *Sex Transm Dis.* 2008;30(10):797-800.

92. Bernstein DI, Bellamy AR, Hook EW 3rd, et al. Epidemiology, clinical presentation, and antibody response to primary infection with herpes simplex virus type 1 and type 2 in young women. *Clin Infect Dis.* 2013;56(3):344-351.

93. Jaiyeoba O, Amaya MI, Soper DE, Kilby JM. Preventing neonatal transmission of herpes simplex virus. *Clin Obstet Gynecol.* 2012;55(2):510-520.

94. Corey L, Wald A. Maternal and neonatal HSV infections. *N Engl J Med.* 2009;361(14):1376-1385.

95. Baker DA. Consequences of herpes simplex virus in pregnancy and their prevention. *Curr Opin Infect Dis.* 2007;20(1):73-76.

96. Watts DH, Brown ZA, Money D, et al. A double-blind, randomized, placebo-controlled trial of acyclovir in late pregnancy for the reduction of herpes simplex virus shedding and cesarean delivery. *Am J Obstet Gynecol.* 2003;188(3):836-843.

97. Fleming DT, McQuillian GM, Johnson RE, et al. Herpes simplex virus type 2 in the United States, 1976 to 1994. *New Engl J Med.* 1997;337(16):1105-1111.

98. Schack L, Neinstein L. Herpes Genitalis. In: Neinstein LS, ed. *Adolescent Health Care: A Practical Guide.* Baltimore, MD: Lippincott Williams & Wilkins; 1996:942-953.

99. Auslander BA, Biro FM, Rosenthal SL. Genital herpes in adolescents. *Semin Pediatr Infect Dis.* 2005;16(1):24-30.

100. Gupta R, Warren T, Wald A. Genital herpes. *Lancet.* 2007;370(9605):2127-2137.

101. Gutierrez K, Arvin AM. Herpes simplex viruses 1 and 2. In: Feigin RD, Cherry JD, Demmler-Harrison GJ, Kaplan SL, eds. *Textbook of Pediatric Infectious Diseases.* 6th ed. Philadelphia, PA: Elsevier; 2009:1993-2022.

102. Centers for Disease Control and Prevention. Genital herpes. Centers for Disease Control and Prevention Web site. http://www.cdc.gov/std/herpes/default.htm. Accessed January 14, 1999.

103. Champion J, Collins J. Reducing STIs screening, treatment, and counseling. *Nurse Pract.* 2012;37(4):40-46.

104. Strick LB, Wald A. Diagnostics for herpes simplex virus: is PCR the new gold standard? *Mol Diagn Ther.* 2006;10(1):17-28.

105. Hammerschlag MR, Guillén CD. Medical and legal implications of testing for sexually transmitted infections in children. *Clin Microbiol Rev.* 2010;23(3):493-506.

106. Centers for Disease Control and Prevention. Trichomoniasis—CDC fact sheet. Centers for Disease Control and Prevention Web site. http://www.cdc.gov/std/trichomonas/stdfact-trichomoniasis.htm. Updated August 3, 2012. Accessed September 24, 2013.

107. Trintis J, Epie N, Boss R, Riedel S. Neonatal Trichomonas vaginalis infection: a case report and review of the literature. *Int J STD Aids.* 2010;21(8):606-607.

108. Garcia LS. Protozoa from other body sites. In: Garcia LS, ed. *Diagnostic Medical Parasitology.* 4th ed. Washington, DC: ASM Press; 2001:106-131.

109. Coleman JS, Gaydos CA, Witter F. Trichomonas vaginalis vaginitis in obstetrics and gynecology practice: new concepts and controversies. *Obstet Gynecol Surv.* 2013;68(1):43-50.

110. Jones JG, Yamauchi T, Lambert B. Trichomonas vaginalis infestation in sexually abused girls. *Am J Dis Child.* 1985;139(8):846-847.

111. Ohlemeyer CL, Hornberger LL, Lynch DA, Swierkosz EM. Diagnosis of trichomonas vaginalis in adolescent females: InPouch TV culture versus wet-mount microscopy. *J Adolesc Health.* 1998;22(3):205-208.

112. Gallion HR, Dupree LJ, Scott TA, Arnold DH. Diagnosis of Trichomonas vaginalis in female children and adolescents evaluated for possible sexual abuse: a comparison of the InPouch TV culture method and wet mount microscopy. *J Pediatr Adolesc Gynecol.* 2009;22(5):300-305.

113. Centers for Disease Control and Prevention. Parasites—lice—body lice. Centers for Disease Control and Prevention Web site. http://www.cdc.gov/parasites/lice/body/biology.html. Accessed September 24, 2013.

114. Nelson A, Neinstein L. Pediculosis pubis and scabies. In: Neinstein L, ed. *Adolescent Health Care: A Practical Guide.* 3rd ed. Baltimore, MD: Lippincott Williams & Wilkins; 1996:969-973.

115. Sung L, MacDonald NE. Syphilis: a pediatric perspective. *Pediatr Rev.* 1998;19(1):17-22.

116. Centers for Disease Control and Prevention. Syphilis. Centers for Disease Control and Prevention Web site. http://www.cdc.gov/std/stats11/syphilis.htm. Updated December 12, 2012. Accessed August 19, 2013.

117. Mattei PL, Beachkofsky TM, Gilson RT, Wisco OJ. Syphilis: a reemerging infection. *Am Fam Physician.* 2012;86(5):433-440.

118. Neinstein L, Himebaugh K. Syphilis. In: Neinstein L, ed. *Adolescent Health Care: A Practical Guide.* 3rd ed. Baltimore, MD: Lippincott Williams & Wilkins; 1996:924-941.

119. Dobson SR, Sánchez PJ. Syphilis. In: Feigin RD, Cherry JD, Demmler-Harrison GJ, Kaplan SL, eds. *Textbook of Pediatric Infectious Diseases.* 6th ed. Philadelphia, PA: Elsevier; 2009:1826-1846.

120. Centers for Disease Control and Prevention. Syphilis. Centers for Disease Control and Prevention Web site. http://www.cdc.gov/std/syphilis/default.htm. Updated August 20, 2013. Accessed September 24, 2013.

121. Bays J, Chadwick D. The serologic test for syphilis in severely abused children and adolescents. *Adolesc Pediatr Gynecol.* 1991;4:148-151.

122. Bays J, Chadwick D. Medical diagnosis of the sexually abused child. *Child Abuse Negl.* 1993;17(1):91-121.

123. Gutman LT, St Claire KK, Weedy C, et al. Human immunodeficiency virus transmission by child sexual abuse. *Am J Dis Child.* 1991;145(2):137-141.

124. Lindegren ML, Hanson IC, Hammett TA, et al. Sexual abuse of children: intersection with the HIV epidemic. *Pediatrics.* 1998;102(4):e46.

125. Moe K, Grau A. HIV prophylaxis within a treatment protocol for sexual assault victims: rationale for the decision. *J Emerg Nurs.* 2001;27(5):511-515.

126. Siegel R, Christie C, Myers M, Duma E, Green L. Incest and Pneumocystis carinii pneumonia in a twelve-year-old girl: a case for early human immunodeficiency virus testing in sexually abused children. *Pediatr Infect Dis J.* 1992;11(8):681-682.

127. Kaplan EH, Heimer R. A model-based estimate of HIV infectivity via needle sharing. *J Acquir Immune Defic Syndr.* 1992;5(11):1116-1118.

128. DeGruttola V, Seage GR 3rd, Mayer KH, et al. Infectiousness of HIV between male homosexual partners. *J Clin Epidemiol.* 1989;42(9):849-856.

129. Varghese B, Maher JR, Peterman TA, et al. Reducing the risk of sexual HIV transmission: quantifying the per-act risk for HIV on the basis of choice of partner, sex act and condom use. *Sex Trans Dis.* 2002;29(1):38-43.

130. European Study Group on Heterosexual Transmission of HIV. Comparison of female to male and male to female transmission of HIV in 563 stable couples. *BMJ.* 1992;304(6830):809-813.

131. Royce RA, Seña A, Cates W Jr, et al. Sexual transmission of HIV [published correction appears in *N Engl J Med.* 1997;337:799]. *N Engl J Med.* 1997;336:1072-1078.

132. Page-Shafer K, Shiboski CH, Dennis H, et al. Risk of HIV infection attributable to oral sex among men who have sex with men and in the population of men who have sex with men. *AIDS.* 2002;16(17):2350-2352.

133. Smith DK, Grohskopf LA, Black RJ, et al. Antiretroviral postexposure prophylaxis after sexual, injection-drug use, or other nonoccupational exposure to HIV in the United States: recommendations from the US department of health and human services. *MMWR.* 2005;54(RR02):1-20. Centers for Disease Control and Prevention Web site. http://www.cdc.gov/mmwr/preview/mmwrhtml/rr5402a1.htm. Accessed October 22, 2013.

134. Chacko L, Ford N, Sbaiti M, Siddiqui R. Adherence to HIV post-exposure prophylaxis in victims of sexual assault: a systematic review and meta-analysis. *Sex Transm Infect.* 2012;88(5):335-341.

135. Belzer M, Neinstein LS. HIV infections and aids. In: Neinstein LS, Gordon C, Katzman D, Rosen D, Woods E, eds. *Adolescent Health Care: A Practical Guide.* 5th ed. Baltimore, MD: Lippincott Williams & Wilkins; 1996:513-544.

136. Vermillion ST, Holmes MM, Soper DE. Adolescents and sexually transmissible diseases. *Obstet Gynecol Clin North Am.* 2000;27(1):163-179.

137. Centers for Disease Control and Prevention, the Advisory Committee on Immunization Practices. A comprehensive immunization strategy to eliminate transmission of hepatitis B virus infection in the United States: recommendations of the Advisory Committee on Immunization Practices (ACIP) part II: immunization of adults. *MMWR.* 2006;55(RR16):1-33.

138. Centers for Disease Control and Prevention. Hepatitis B FAQs for health care professionals. Centers for Disease Control and Prevention Web site. http://www.cdc.gov/hepatitis/HBV/HBVFaq.htm. Accessed November 22, 2010.

139. Wilt TJ, Shamliyan T, Shaukat A, et al. Management of chronic hepatitis B. *Evid Rep Technol Assess.* 2008;(174):1-671.

140. Centers for Disease Control and Prevention. Viral hepatitis. Centers for Disease Control and Prevention Web site. http://www.cdc.gov/ncidod/diseases/hepatitis/b/fact.htm. Accessed January 15, 2002.

141. Mason W, Neinstein LS. Hepatitis. In: Neinstein LS, Gordon C, Katzman D, Rosen D, Woods E, eds. *Adolescent Health Care: A Practical Guide.* 5th ed. Baltimore, MD: Lippincott Williams & Wilkins; 1996:493-512.

142. Papatheodoridis GV, Cholongitas E, Archimiandritis AJ, Burroughs AK. Current management of hepatitis B virus infection before and after liver transplantation. *Liver Int.* 2009;29(9):1294-1305.

Chapter 7

Differential Diagnosis: Conditions That Mimic Child Maltreatment

Frances M. Nadel, MD, MSCE
Angelo P. Giardino, MD, PhD

Key Points

1. The clinician must pay careful attention to the history given, the child's developmental ability, the plausibility of the mechanism of injury described by the caregivers, the pattern of injury observed on examination, and the result of any laboratory and diagnostic testing.
2. Health care providers need to be aware of established cultural practices that are not considered to be abusive. However, he or she should also be aware that some of these practices, such as mollera caida, may cause significant harm; public health education at the community level may be helpful in preventing future injuries.
3. Normally, children quickly withdraw from a heat source that is hot enough to cause burns; therefore, burns that are symmetric, etensive, deep, uniform in severity; have well-demarcated borders; or show a distinctive pattern should raise suspicions for abuse.
4. Broken bones may raise suspicions for child abuse if they are found in a very young, perambulatory child; if there are multiple fractures at different stages of healing; or if the fracture is not consistent with the reported mechanism of injury or the child's developmental abilities.
5. 4 out of 5 deaths in the group of unrecognized abusive head trauma (AHT) might have been prevented had maltreatment been recognized during an earlier health care visit.[1]
6. The fundamental nutritional issues that lie at the root of all failure to thrive (FTT) cases are: (1) too few calories going into the child, (2) too many calories going out of the child, or (3) too many calories being used up by the child.[2]
7. Health care providers should be aware of and learn to distinguish certain dermatological disorders from abuse. For example, over half of African-American children have Mongolian spots,[3] most commonly located on the back and buttocks, that could be confused for child physical abuse.

Introduction

The differential diagnostic process is a form of clinical reasoning and decision making that requires the clinician to obtain a thorough history, complete physical examination, and appropriate laboratory and diagnostic studies. With this information in hand, the clinician considers the various diagnostic possibilities in order to determine which findings support the diagnostic possibility and which do not. Further information may be required to rule a diagnosis in or out. Once all needed information is obtained, a diagnostic impression may be formed with the most likely diagnosis or diagnoses given as the probable cause for the child's signs and symptoms.

Discussing the various diagnostic possibilities that mimic findings in cases of child maltreatment is in no way meant to diminish the need to consider child maltreatment as a possibility. Instead, considering all possibilities highlights the clinical imperative to consider anything relevant to a given clinical situation before arriving at the final diagnosis. Misdiagnosis can have catastrophic consequences for a child who is left with caregivers who have failed to protect the child from injury; however, misdiagnosing child maltreatment in a child and family where it is not present can also have a devastating impact.[4] Differentiating conditions that appear similar to those found in cases of child abuse requires practice and experience; therefore, clinicians may find that consultation with the multidisciplinary team (MDT) at a local or regional center may help during the health care evaluation, especially in complicated or unusual cases.[5]

For the purpose of this discussion, this chapter will focus on the following differential diagnosis considerations:

— Physical abuse in children with injury patterns including bruising, burns, fractures, head trauma, and eye injuries

— Neglect in children with a growth pattern that fails to meet expectations for given age (eg, FTT)

— Sexual abuse in children with sign and symptoms of vulvitis, vulvovaginitis, and vaginitis

Physical Abuse

Many diagnostic possibilities, including physical maltreatment, must be considered when looking for causes of bruises, burns, fractures, head trauma, and eye injuries in children. The clinician must pay careful attention to the history given; the child's developmental ability, the plausibility of the mechanism of injury described by the caregivers, the pattern of injury observed on examination, and the result of any laboratory and diagnostic testing.

The evaluation of cases of suspected child abuse and neglect is often complex and not straightforward. At times, the clinical presentation of children who are physically abused is so clear-cut that other diagnostic possibilities are limited; however, in many cases, the clinical presentation of physical abuse may be less than obvious, include a confusing history, and be without pathognomonic signs of child maltreatment. A more extensive evaluation in these cases is necessary, and an extensive differential diagnosis may be warranted.

Bruising

Bruises that are extensive, multiple, patterned, in unusual locations, or not consistent with the caregiver's reported history or the child's developmental age should raise suspicions for abuse.[6] However, accidental trauma, cultural practices as well as hematological, vasculitic, and inherited disorders may result in findings similar to those seen in cases of child maltreatment.[7,8] Additionally, birthmarks, dermatological conditions, and exposure to skin irritants or even fabric dyes that tattoo the skin may be confused with bruising and child maltreatment. **Table 7-1** lists commonly mistaken etiologies and helpful distinguishing characteristics.

Table 7-1. Factors That May Be Helpful in Distinguishing Conditions That Mimic Child Maltreatment

Mimic Condition	History	Physical Examination Findings	Laboratory Abnormalities
Accidental Bruising	Child is ambulatory	Bruising over bony prominences	None
Coining	Family is Asian, practices alternative medicine	Linear ecchymosis, usually in a Christmas-tree pattern on the back	May have myoglobinuria if extensive bruising
Idiopathic Thrombocytopenic Purpura (ITP)	Often preceded by viral illness	Petechiae with minimal trauma (eg, blood pressure cuff inflation)	Low platelet count with the rest of the complete blood count results normal
Hemophilia	Family history of hemophilia Excessive bleeding at circumcision or cord separation	Bruises in unusual locations Hemarthrosis after minimal trauma	Prolonged partial thromboplastin time (PTT), abnormal factor assay
Ehlers-Danlos (ED)	Family history of ED	Fragile skin with poor wound healing Joint hyperextensibility Elastic skin	Not applicable
Leukemia	May have weight loss, prolonged fever, night sweats, fatigue	Pallor Hepatosplenomegaly Adenopathy Cachexia	Abnormal cells on smear Many other laboratory abnormalities, which may include prolonged prothrombin time (PT), PTT, or both

(continued)

Table 7-1. Factors That May Be Helpful in Distinguishing Conditions that Mimic Child Maltreatment *(continued)*

Mimic Condition	History	Physical Examination Findings	Laboratory Abnormalities
Henoch-Schönlein Purpura (HSP)	Acute onset of a rash that initially may have been urticarial Patient may complain of abdominal and joint pain.	Purpura, often predominately on the buttocks and exterior surfaces of the extremities Swollen joints Scrotal edema or bruising Tender abdomen	Possible eosinophilia, leukocytosis, hematuria
Tattooing	Recent new clothes, especially jeans, pens, markers, removable tattoos	Marks wash off	Not applicable
Mongolian Spots	Present since birth	Not tender Uniform gray-blue color No swelling Takes months to resolve	Not applicable

Adapted from Tunnessen WW Jr. Signs and Symptoms in Pediatrics. *2nd ed. Philadelphia, PA: JB Lippincott; 1988.*

Actual Bruising

Accidental Bruising

Ambulatory children and those learning to walk often have multiple bruises of different ages on their body. The location of bruises and the developmental stage and age of the child help distinguish inflicted from accidental bruising. Two classic studies described bruising in young children who arrived at a health care facility for a well-child care visit and were not suspected to be victims of child abuse. In both studies, bruising increased in children who were older and more ambulatory.[9,10] In fact, bruising was extremely rare in children aged younger than 6 months (0.6%) and in preambulatory infants (2.2%).[10] Bruises in ambulatory children were found on the front of the body and over bony prominences, especially the pretibial region, upper leg, and forehead.

Clinicians are often asked to date the age of a bruise in order to determine if the reported history is consistent with the appearance of the injury. However, a review of the literature demonstrates that clinicians are unable to accurately date a bruise and the color changes seen in bruises over time is highly variable.[11] Location and depth of the bruise as well as the amount of force that caused the bruise all likely contribute to the variability of bruise maturation. Spectrophotometric evaluation of bruises is a promising technique that may help better define the colors of a bruise over time.[12] In this technique, a specialized light source and detector are used to objectively measure the color of the bruise based on its absorption and emission of light.

Folk Remedies

Some folk remedies intended to treat medical ailments may lead to a distinctive pattern of bruising or burns that may be misdiagnosed as maltreatment. For example, cao gio (coining) is an Asian practice often used to treat fever or pain in which a hot coin or spoon is rubbed on a child's back and results in linear bruising (**Figure 7-1**). Cupping is another practice that may be used in many different cultures to treat various ailments.[13] With cupping, a heated cup is placed firmly on the skin, creating a suction-cup effect as it cools. After the cup is removed, a circular ecchymosis or superficial burn may appear. Other folk remedies include, biting the child, shaking infants who have a fallen fontanel (mollera caida), or placing burning incense and yarn on sites of pain (moxibustion). These are established practices of a culture; therefore, they are not considered to be abusive. However, some of these practices, such as mollera caida, may cause significant harm; public health education at the community level may be helpful in preventing future injuries.

Disorders of the Hemopoietic System

Extensive bruises in unusual places or without a consistent mechanism may occur in children as a result of coagulation abnormalities. For example, hemophiliacs may have joint and soft tissue bleeding after minimal trauma. This X-linked disorder is caused by a deficiency in one of the factors responsible for normal clotting (**Figure 7-2**). A history of prolonged bleeding with circumcision or cord separation may be elicited in children with unsuspected hemophilia.[14] Thrombocytopenia, which is a relative decrease in the number of platelets in the blood, or platelet dysfunction may cause generalized petechiae and purpura without a corresponding history of trauma. The most common platelet abnormality in children is idiopathic thrombocytopenic purpura (ITP) (**Figures 7-3** and **7-4**). ITP is caused by an immune-mediated destruction of

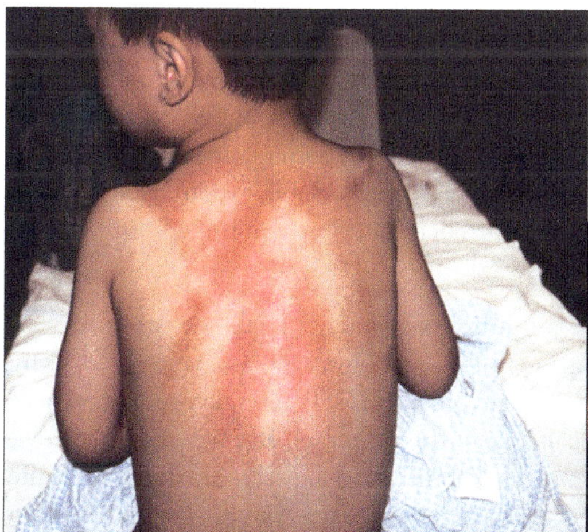

Figure 7-1

Figure 7-1. *Coining. To treat his fever, this child's family practices cao gio. A coin is rubbed up and down the child's back, often in the pattern of a Christmas tree.*

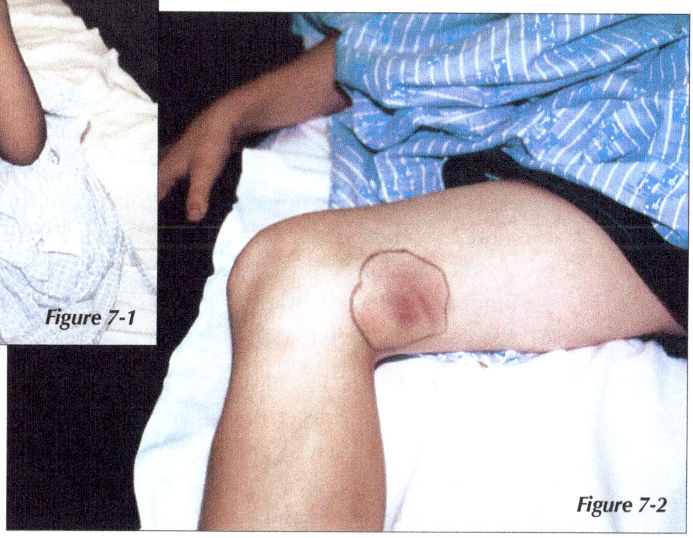

Figure 7-2

Figure 7-2. *Bruising in a child with factor VIII deficiency. This child did not recall any specific trauma to his leg.*

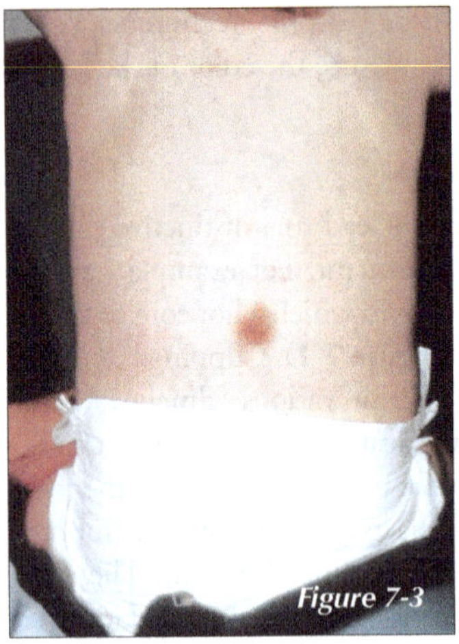

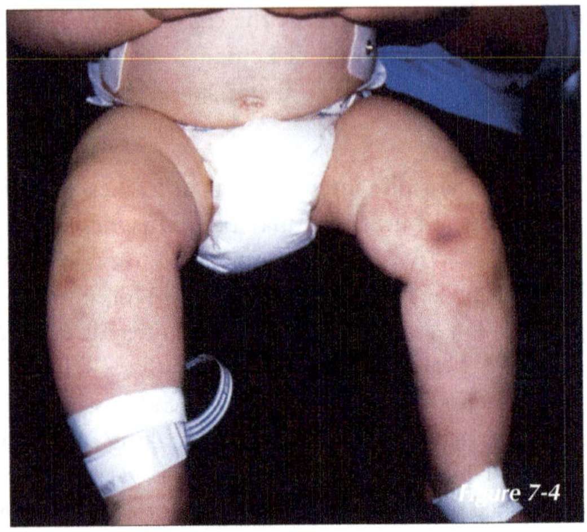

Figure 7-3. *Bruising in a child with new diagnosis of ITP with a platelet count of 13 000.*

Figure 7-4. *Same child in Figure 7-3 with ITP; front view of his legs.*

platelets and is usually self-limited. von Willebrand factor is necessary for normal platelet adherence and function. Platelet dysfunction with prolonged bleeding and easy bruising may result if this factor is abnormal in number or function. Children with leukemia or bone marrow failure from any etiology may also have easy bruising and bleeding because they lack many of the components needed for normal coagulation. A complete blood count (CBC), prothrombin time (PT), and partial thromboplastin time (PTT) laboratory test as well as a consultation with a pediatric hematologist should be considered in children with unexplained bruising.

Deficiencies or dysfunction of vitamin K can cause easy bruising because of abnormal clotting. Newborn babies who did not receive the usual intramuscular injection of vitamin K are at risk for the classic form of hemorrhagic disease of the newborn.[15] These babies are often breastfed, which is a poor source of vitamin K; may have been born at home; and usually present at age 2 to 7 days with nasal, gastrointestinal, and even central nervous system (CNS) bleeding. Additionally, children with gut malabsorption secondary to cystic fibrosis or short bowel syndrome may be deficient in vitamin K. Vitamin K activity may also be inhibited in curious toddlers who ingest rat poison that contains anticoagulant substances. However, the current formulation of rodenticides and the small amounts children accidentally ingest rarely cause symptoms or changes in their coagulation profile.[16] Treatment for this deficiency is vitamin K administration.

Vasculitis

Vasculitic processes causing extensive purpuric lesions may initially be confused with bruising resulting from abuse. A complete history and physical examination are usually sufficient in distinguishing Henoch-Schönlein purpura (HSP), meningococcemia, rickettsial infection, and other causes of palpable purpura from an abusive etiology. Often, more systemic findings such as fever and general malaise will predominate. In HSP, the typical petechial and purpuric rash occurs on bilateral extensor surfaces and is often limited to below the waist (**Figure 7-5**). Arthralgia, arthritis, and abdominal pain are also common findings in HSP.

Inherited defects in collagen synthesis such as Ehlers-Danlos (ED) syndrome or osteogenesis imperfecta (OI) may result in easy bruising and poor wound healing (**Figure 7-6**).[17] There are many types of ED, but the common features in all patients are joint hyperextensibility, skin fragility, and skin elasticity. A complete family history and thorough physical examination are usually sufficient to make these diagnoses.

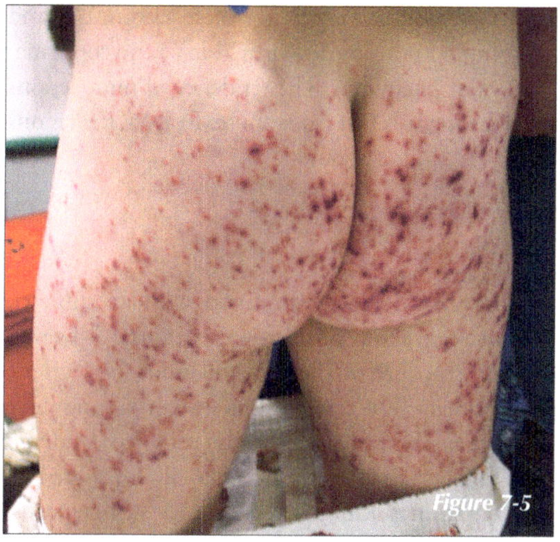

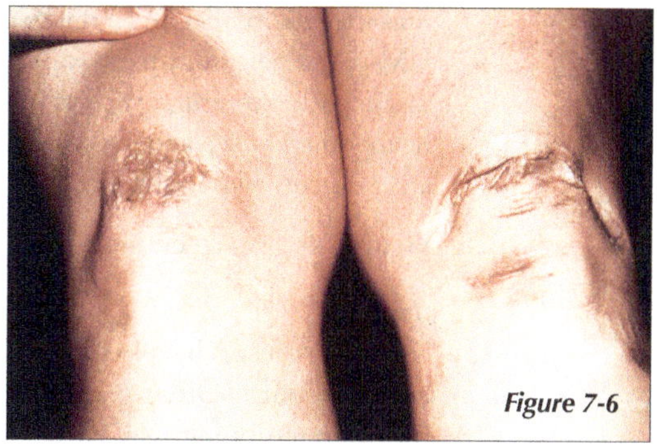

Figure 7-5. Typical rash seen in HSP purpura.

Figure 7-6. Scars from ED. (Contributed by Paul J. Honig, MD; Philadelphia, PA.)

Pseudo-Bruising

Birthmarks

Mongolian spots, birthmarks typically located over the sacrum, back and, less commonly, the face of the legs, may be mistaken for abuse-related bruising. However, unlike bruises, Mongolian spots are not tender; are usually grey and more uniform in color; and, most importantly, have been present since birth. Mongolian spots fade slowly over months to years, unlike bruises, which usually resolve in days to weeks. **Figures 7-7-a** and **b** demonstrate additional examples of pseudo-bruising.

Dermatological Conditions

The sudden appearance of the typical target lesions found in erythema multiforme (EM) or urticaria multiforme (UM) may be confused with bruising (**Figure 7-8**).[18] An erythema-

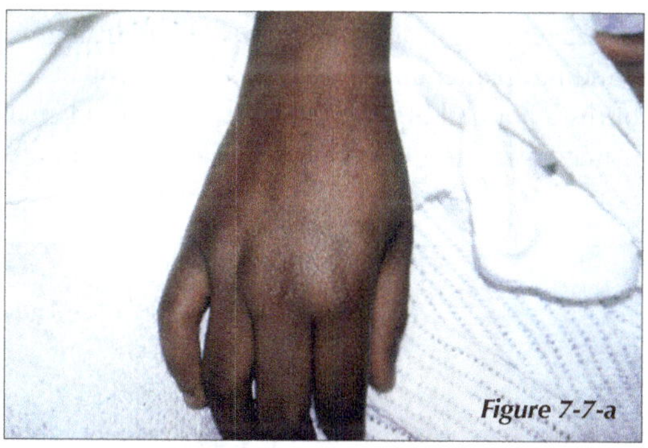

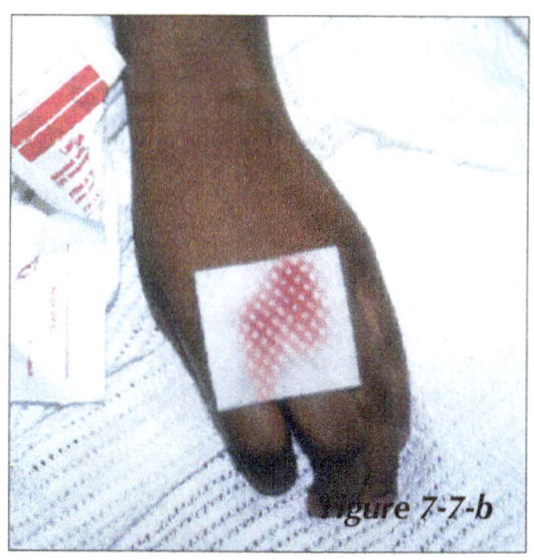

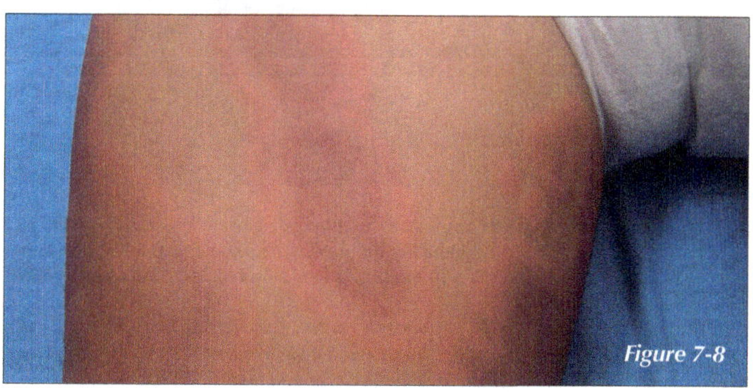

Figure 7-7-a and **b.** Pseudo-bruise. The girl had recently dyed her hair and the "bruise" came off easily with an alcohol swab.

Figure 7-8. Annular wheals with ecchymotic centers seen in UM. (Contributed by Joel Fein, MD; Philadelphia, PA.)

tous irregular border and a dusky or ecchymotic center characterize these lesions. EM and UM may result from many causes, including herpes simplex virus (HSV), mycoplasma, and exposure to drugs, such as sulfonamides or phenytoin. The tendency of more lesions to appear and for plaques to coalesce helps distinguish EM from abuse. In UM, the lesions are transient, with individual lesions lasting less than 24 hours.

Figure 7-9 gives an example of another dermatological disorder.

Toxins

The rash caused by phytophotodermatitis may be easily confused with an inflicted bruise or burn. Often, parents cannot offer an explanation for this injury; however, further questioning may elicit a history of exposure to the juice of limes, figs, celery, or parsnips, all of which contain plant psoralens. When the psoralens-containing juice comes in contact with the child's skin and is exposed to sunlight, the psoralens undergo a photoreaction. A rash results that is initially erythematous, but may then progress to vesicles or even bullae (**Figure 7-10**).[19] Dye from clothing, such as a pair of new jeans, or ink pens may tattoo the skin and be confused with a bruise. Wiping the suspected bruise with an alcohol swab usually serves to differentiate a bruise from dye.

Burns

It is often difficult to distinguish accidental from inflicted burns; however, children normally quickly withdraw from a heat source hot enough to cause burns. Therefore burns that are symmetric, extensive, or deep; uniform in severity; have well-demarcated borders; or show a distinctive pattern should raise suspicions for abuse.[20]

Accidental Burns

Scalds

It is not an uncommon occurrence that a curious preschooler pulls a cup of hot liquid from a table onto him or herself. The resulting burn from the hot liquid is usually located on the face and chest and is triangular in shape with a narrower distal apex. The burn is less severe at the distal aspect resulting from the liquid cooling during its descent. Irregular borders and a surrounding splatter appearance of smaller droplets of burns are seen with accidental scald burns.[18] For children who have repeated accidental burns or injuries, a home evaluation may assist in identifying and modifying unsafe environments or parenting practices.

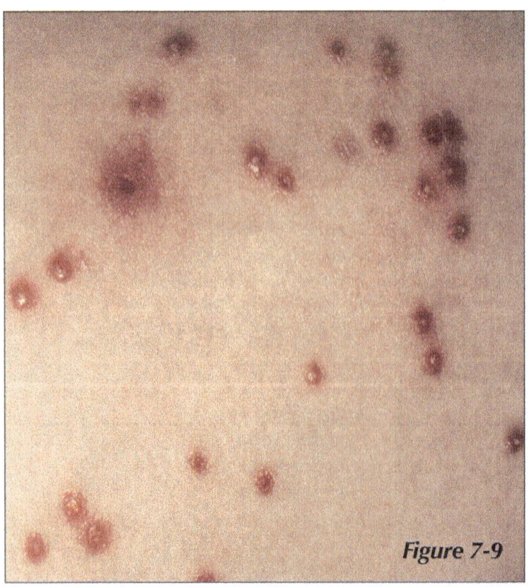

Figure 7-9

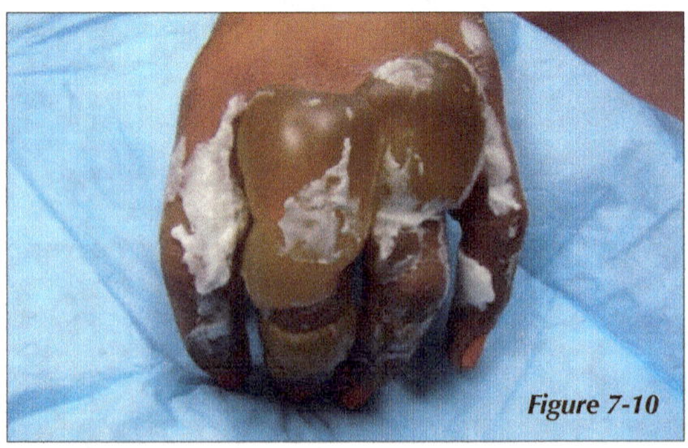

Figure 7-10

Figure 7-9. *Crop of* Molluscum contagiosum *lesions with several demonstrating inflammation surrounding the base of the classic core filled pearly lesions. (Contributed by Paul J. Honig, MD; Philadelphia, PA.)*

Figure 7-10. *Phytodermatitis. This teenager had been making a lime-based drink at the beach, resulting in a bullous rash on her hands the next day. (Contributed by Jennifer Molnar, CRNP; Philadelphia, PA.)*

Patterned Burns

When hot objects come in contact with the skin, a patterned burn may result resembling the actual object. Such patterned burns may be accidental or inflicted. For example, a curious toddler may try to touch, pick up, or run into a hot iron, leaving the distinctive burn of the iron grid. However, one should be concerned about the level of supervision of the child and certainly be more suspicious of abuse if the burn is deep, multiple, or not consistent with the child's developmental abilities when compared with the history offered.

Pseudo-Burns

Infections

The circular lesions of impetigo and ecythema caused by staphylococcal and streptococcal infections may be confused with a cigarette burn (**Figure 7-11**). Impetigo is often more superficial, appears less uniform in shape, and heals more quickly and with less scarring than an inflicted cigarette burn. In addition, the bacteria-caused lesions often occur in crops in various stages of formation from blister to ulcers. Ecythema is similar to impetigo but the infection extends deeper into the dermis.

The craterlike erosions seen in eczema herpeticum may also be confused with inflicted cigarette burns. Children with this condition often appear ill, with multiple vesiculated lesions in areas of eczematous involvement because of a disseminated HSV infection. A scraping of a fresh lesion can be sent for diagnosis. Additionally, bullous impetigo, a localized form of staphylococcal skin infection in infants and young children, may be confused with abuse. The bullae commonly appear in the diaper area and rupture easily, causing an area of moist denuded skin. Extensive areas of infection may be confused with an immersion burn.[21]

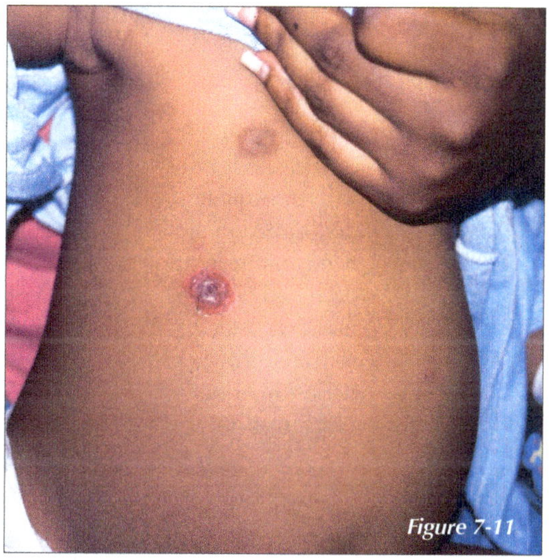

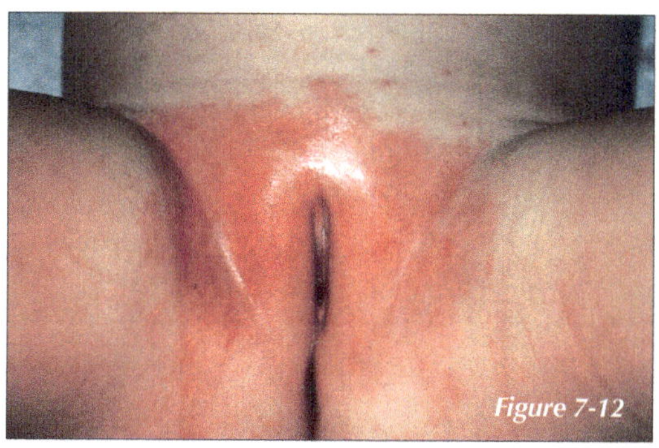

Figure 7-11. *Ecthyma. This patient had several pruritic bug bites that became secondarily infected. Notice the smaller red papule on her left lower quadrant, which may evolve into a similar lesion. The lesion diameter is bigger than would be expected from an inflicted cigarette burn. (Contributed by Martha Stevens, MD, MSCE; Milwaukee, WI.)*

Figure 7-12. *Dermatitis in perineal area secondary to use of super absorbent diapers. (Contributed by Paul J. Honig, MD; Philadelphia, PA.)*

Chemical Irritants

A local contact dermatitis may be confused with an inflicted immersion burn. Diaper dermatitis (**Figure 7-12**) may result from a new diaper cream that is allergenic, ingestion of an irritant,[22] or prolonged exposure to urine from an unchanged diaper. A child with epidermolysis bullosa may raise concern for inflicted burns as well, because of associated extensive unexplained blistering. Epidermolysis bullosa is an inherited disorder characterized by blistering with minimal trauma. Disease severity and age of presentation vary greatly among the disorder's different forms, but the blisters usually appear in areas of friction.

Fractures

Actual Fractures

It is often difficult to distinguish inflicted fractures from accidental fractures. However, broken bones may raise suspicions for child abuse if they are found in a very young, preambulatory child; if there are multiple fractures at different stages of healing; or if the fracture is not consistent with the reported mechanism or the child's developmental abilities.[23] Certain fracture types, such as metaphyseal, or "bucket handle," fractures and rib fractures, may also raise concern for abuse more than others because they are highly associated with the abusive mechanism of shaking.[24] When evaluating skeletal fractures in children, it is important to consider both accidental and abusive etiologies because both may be possible. In addition, birth-related fractures and inherited, metabolic, and infectious disorders may cause some of the same findings found with inflicted trauma. **Table 7-2** describes some mimics of abusive fractures and their distinguishing characteristics.

Table 7-2. Disorders That Mimic Fractures Occurring From Abuse

Disorder	History	Physical Examination Findings	Laboratory Abnormalities	X-ray Findings
Congenital Syphilis[22]	Two-thirds of patients may be asymptomatic at birth. Symptoms may include profuse rhinitis, erythematous rash with subsequent desquamation of hands and feet, or decreased use of limbs, secondary to pain from periosteal or bone inflammation.	Infants may have snuffles, a saddle-nose deformity. Extramedullary hematopoiesis Hepatosplenomegaly FTT	CBC: Anemia Thrombocytopenia Urinalysis (UA): Hematuria proteinuria Elevated liver function tests Cerebrospinal fluid (CSF): Pleocytosis Serological testing: Diagnostic	Diffuse periostitis of long bones Osteochondritis of joints
Fractures from Birth Trauma	Prolonged or difficult delivery, use of forceps, and macrosomia have been associated with fracture from birth.[23,24]	Swelling or extremity disuse may not be found on the newborn screening examination. Callus formation over a healing clavicle fracture may be palpable.		Evidence of fracture healing within 11 to 14 days from birth. The rest of the skeletal survey is without fractures. The clavicle is most commonly fractured, followed by humerus, femur, and skull fractures. Rib fractures are rarely a result of birth trauma.[23-25]

(continued)

Table 7-2. Disorders That Mimic Fractures Occurring From Abuse *(continued)*

Disorder	History	Physical Examination Findings	Laboratory Abnormalities	X-ray Findings
Osteogenesis Imperfecta (OI)	Inherited in autosomal dominant fashion History of early deafness, frequent fractures, easy bruising	Patient may have evidence of poor wound healing, blue sclera, abnormal dentition, joint hypermobility, and hearing impairment	Collagen biochemical studies of skin biopsy confirms diagnosis and type of OI	Multiple fractures at different stages of healing Fracture severity will vary with the different types of OI Osteopenia is a late finding secondary to lack of weight bearing
Rickets	Patients at risk include: premature infants, breast-fed babies not receiving vitamin supplements, and children with liver or kidney disease. Patients may present with seizures or with complaints related to the etiology of rickets.[15]	Prominent costochondral junctions Findings primarily related to the underlying etiology	Normocalcemia Hypocalcemia Hypophosphatemia Elevated alkaline phosphatase	Fraying of metaphyseal and costochondral junctions Epiphyseal widening Periosteal elevation Osteopenia

Accidental Injury

Ambulatory children may have signs and symptoms of a broken bone, and the history provided by the caregiver may point to everyday activities of play and exploration.[25] If the child is older and involved in sport activities, he or she may even have multiple fractures over time. Although there is no magical number of fractures that should be considered to be too many, each child who is brought to a health care provider for evaluation of a fracture should have a complete assessment that considers abuse as a possible etiology. In addition, the clinician must always make sure the history fits the injury and the child's developmental level.

Birth-Related Fractures

In a large study of over 30 000 births, the incidence of fractures attributed to labor and delivery was 0.1%.[26] Macrosomia, shoulder dystocia, difficult or prolonged delivery, and prematurity have been implicated as risk factors for antenatal fractures,[27] with the clavicle being the most commonly fractured bone by far, followed by the humerus, femur, and skull.[26] Rib fractures are extremely rare birth injuries.[28] Birth fractures usually show signs of healing by age 2 weeks, a characteristic that is important to take into consideration when making a determination as to whether the injury is related to abuse.[25]

Inherited and Metabolic Disorders

Osteogenesis imperfecta (OI) is a rare inherited disorder caused by a defect in collagen synthesis. Children with OI may suffer multiple fractures with minimal trauma because of brittle bones. The 4 major types of OI vary in clinical expression. A thorough history and physical examination are usually sufficient in differentiating OI from abuse. Additional findings that suggest OI, include blue sclera, abnormal dentition, short stature, Wormian bones of the skull, joint laxity, easy bruising, perinatal fractures, or a positive family history of OI (**Figure 7-13**).[29] Type IV, a rare form of OI, may not have any of these distinguishing features, which has led to misdiagnosis of abuse. A helpful clue to OI Type IV is continued fractures despite the child having been in the care of different caregivers.[29] However, it is important to remember that children with OI might also be abused. In addition, it is important to consider that OI is much more rare than child abuse; therefore, abuse is much more likely in a young child with a history of multiple unexplained fractures and no other suggestion of OI.[30]

Rare deficiencies in copper and vitamins A and C may cause skeletal changes that mimic abusive injuries. In Menkes syndrome, copper malabsorption leads to characteristic hematological, neurological, and dermatological derangements, as well as metaphyseal bone spurs and diffuse periostitis (**Figure 7-14**). These skeletal anomalies may be confused with a metaphyseal fracture or evidence of an old healing fracture.

Nutritional rickets is the most common form of vitamin D deficiency. Breastfed babies with little sun exposure are particularly susceptible. The periosteal bone formation and metaphyseal changes that occur during the healing phase, referred to as rickets, have been confused with fractures from abuse as have been the fraying that occurs at the costochondral junctions, the so-called rachitic rosary.[31] Regarding laboratory values, calcium levels will be low to normal, phosphate levels low, and alkaline phosphatase (ALP) level high. Vitamin C deficiency, or scurvy, may result in metaphyseal fractures that could be confused with abuse. A complete dietary history and additional typical radiographic changes seen in scurvy help discriminate between the 2 diagnoses.[32]

For many reasons, such as prematurity or prolonged immobilization, osteopenia will make bones more susceptible to fractures with minor trauma. For example, an increase in range-of-motion (ROM) exercises during physical therapy can result in a long bone fracture in a nonambulatory child with spina bifida. Plain radiographs should demonstrate generalized osteopenia.

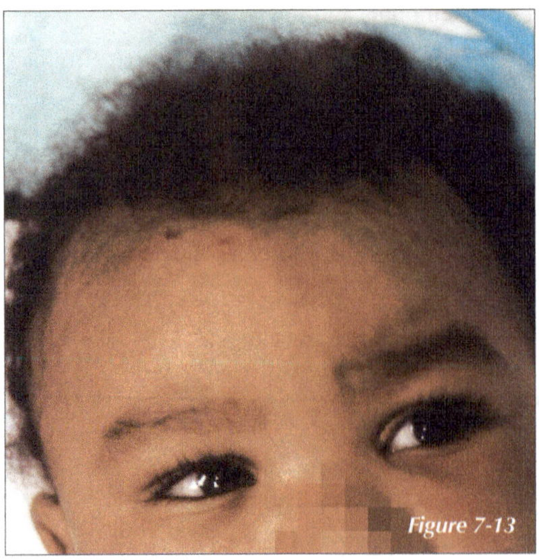

Figure 7-13. *This patient has OI with blue sclera.*

Figure 7-14. *Menkes kinky hair syndrome. (Contributed by Paul J. Honig, MD; Philadelphia, PA.)*

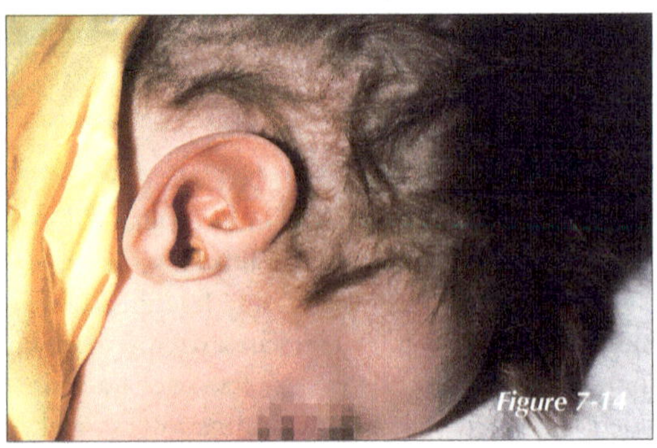

Blount disease is a rare disorder that causes bilateral metaphyseal abnormalities of the proximal tibia as a result of asymmetric growth of the medial aspect. Untreated, this disease can lead to length discrepancy or bowing of the lower extremities.[33] Hereditary sensory neuropathy is a rare inherited disorder in which the child does not feel pain or extremes of temperature. Because these children do not sense painful stimuli, they may not seek treatment until a deformity of a healed fracture is apparent. They may also have extensive bruises, old abrasions, and burns because of their insensitivity to pain.[34]

Pseudo-Fractures

An infant or child may arrive for medical care with pain and an inability to move his or her arm after unwitnessed trauma, a fall, rolling over, or someone pulled on his or her arm. The affected arm is usually held down and in a prone position with some apparent wrist swelling and diffuse tenderness. Though the caregiver is often convinced of a fracture, the child may also have a radial head subluxation, more commonly called a nursemaid's elbow. In children aged under 4 years, the annular ligament surrounding the proximal radius and ulna is lax and a simple pull or rolling may cause the radial head to dislocate. Treatment is a simple maneuver of forearm traction with either supination and flexion or hyperpronation. A palpable click is often felt at the elbow, after which the child will resume use of the arm in about 5 to 10 minutes.

Infections

Congenital syphilis may lead to radiographic findings that raise the suspicion for inflicted injury. Metaphysitis, diffuse periostitis, and pathological fractures associated with congenital syphilis may be confused with abuse.[32] Most children with congenital syphilis are seen within the first 6 months of life and will have serological results that indicate infection with Treponema pallidum (**Figure 7-15**).

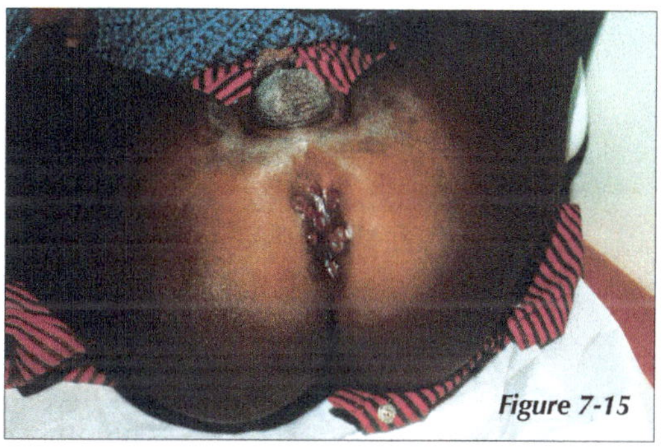

Figure 7-15. *Photograph of prepubertal child's perineum with a perinatally acquired, syphilis-demonstrating skin finding, condyloma lata, surrounding perianal area. (Contributed by Paul J. Honig, MD; Philadelphia, PA.)*

Head Trauma: Accidental or Inflicted

Whether accidentally sustained or intentionally inflicted, head injuries are among the most serious injuries in infants and young children and account for the most traumatic deaths in infants aged younger than one year.[35] A great deal of attention has been focused on the injury mechanisms for both accidental and inflicted head trauma and particular attention has been paid to the unique features of the infant and young child's brain and skull that make them at high risk for morbidity and mortality from head injuries.[36] Head trauma may result in intracranial hemorrhage, including: (1) epidural hemorrhage, which is bleeding in the space between the inner skull bone surface and the dura, frequently due to a direct injury to the middle meningeal artery; (2) subdural hemorrhage, which is bleeding into the space between the inner surface of the dura and arachnoid membranes, typically caused by sheering of the bridging vessels that go from the brain surface to the dura; and (3) subarachnoid hemorrhage, which is bleeding into the space between the inner surface of the arachnoid and the brain surface. Other head injuries may include contusions, such as direct injury to the brain tissue, and intraparenchymal bleeding, such as bleeding directly into substance of the brain.

A growing body of evidence is emerging that highlights the devastating consequences of missed cases of AHT in which the initial evaluation failed to diagnose the nature of the injury only to have the infant or child return later for care with additional injuries. These subsequent injuries could have been prevented if only the child been accurately diagnosed as having been abused during the initial examination.[1,37] Jenny et al[1] retrospectively reviewed medical records of children who were brought to a health care facility with head trauma from a 5-year period of time; of 173 abused children, 54 (31.2%) had been seen by a physician after experiencing AHT injury, yet a diagnosis was not recognized[1] Fifteen of the children (27.8%) sustained additional injury after the diagnosis was missed, and 22 (40.7%) experienced medical complications related to the failure to diagnose the abuse. The article concludes with the tragic assertion that 4 out of 5 deaths in the group of unrecognized AHT might have been prevented had the maltreatment been recognized upon earlier presentation.[1]

Terminology

Discussing head injury and physical abuse inevitably leads to a discussion of shaken baby syndrome (SBS) or shaken infant syndrome (SIS), which is now referred to as AHT.[38] AHT, originally referred to as whiplash syndrome, describes a clinical constellation of findings classically described as subdural hematoma; retinal hemorrhage (found in 65 to 95% of cases); and skeletal fractures, such as metaphyseal fractures and posterior rib fractures (found in 30 to 70% of cases) sustained while a child is shaken violently back and forth. AHT represents a significant injury pattern in the realm of child maltreatment. Although it is associated with the findings listed above, the core injury is to the brain cells themselves, resulting from the application of forces to the child's delicate and developing brain tissue.

AHT has been extended to include cases where the child's head is impacted against a surface, either soft or hard. Diffuse, serious brain injuries result from forces that result in the rotation of the brain about its center of gravity. Such forces exceed those generated in normal childcare activities and are different from the low velocity translational forces, or straight-line movement, that commonly occur in household falls. Immense angular deceleration forces may be generated with sudden striking of the child's head against a surface; these forces act on the brain tissue and cerebral vessels and generate the deleterious effect, which is not specifically from the contact forces applied to the skull.

Concerning Histories for Potential Abusive Head Trauma

There are a number of historical clues that raise suspicion of abuse, particularly in cases of serious head trauma.[39] None of these histories would, by themselves, necessarily mean that abuse has occurred, but the skilled health care professional must consider the clinical situation in light of the history provided by the caregiver when evaluating an infant or child with a head injury. The following factors should raise the suspicion for abuse on the differential diagnosis:

— History of head trauma that is inconsistent or not plausible with the severity of injury on physical and imaging examinations

— History of no trauma with evidence of significant head injury (magical injuries)

— History of self-inflicted trauma incompatible with child's development

— Changing history of the head injury as documented over time by different health professionals during the evaluation

— Caregiver ascribes blame for serious head injuries to a young sibling, playmate, or family pet.

— Delay in seeking treatment

Common Household Injuries and Serious Head Trauma

Clearly, a history of minor trauma that results in serious, life-threatening head injury to an infant or child should be viewed as highly suspicious for AHT, and an evaluation that includes a differential diagnosis of abuse should be performed.

Warrington et al[40] used a large regional data base from the United Kingdom to study the characteristics of injuries to nonambulatory infants over their first 6 months of life, and based on 11 466 parental responses to a mailed questionnaire, characterized the typical minor nature of common household injuries. Household falls appeared common, with 22% of infants (2554 children) experiencing a fall, with 53% falling from a bed, and 12% from a caregiver's arms. Injuries were infrequent and "generally trivial,"[38] with only 14% reporting a visible injury, almost always to the head; 56% suffered a bruise and less than 1% suffered a serious injury described as a concussion or fracture.[40] In a large study of short falls, Chadwick et al[41] reviewed injury databases, peer-reviewed articles, previous literature reviews, and other published materials to calculate the risk of death resulting from falls of less than 1.5 meters among children aged up to 5 years. Chadwick et al[41] arrived at an overall incidence of less than 0.48 deaths per 1 million children and discovered no reliable reports of short-fall deaths among children in childcare centers. A systematic review, conducted by Khambalia of risk factors for unintentional injuries due to falls in children aged birth to 6 years concluded that it is uncommon for children to suffer serious injury from falls of less than 5 feet.[42] Tarantino et al[43] studied the medical records for 167 infants and found significant injuries in 25 (15%), which included skull fractures, other skeletal fractures, and 2 children with intracranial bleeds. The children with intracranial bleeds were later determined to have been abused. After excluding these 2 children, the only risk factor found to be independently associated with injury was being dropped by the caregiver, as opposed to rolling off of a bed or other object.[43] In separate studies, Helfer et al[44,45] and Nimityongskul and Anderson[46] reviewed injuries sustained by children who fell out of bed while in the hospital. Of the approximately 450 children who fell out of beds or cribs from a height of less than 4.5 feet, none was seriously injured; most sustained no identifiable injuries; and all injuries were minor, such as contusions, small lacerations, or an occasional skull or clavicular fracture. A number of studies examined the relationship between the height of free falls and injury and death in children. These studies showed that the predominant injury in falls from heights occurs to the head and skeleton. Musemeche et al[47] reviewed the outcomes of children who fell more than 10 ft, or at least 1 story. Of the 70 records reviewed, the majority of children fell from a height of 1 to 3 stories. Head (54%) and skeletal (33%) trauma were common, but no deaths occurred. Chadwick et al[48] reviewed the outcome of 317 children with a reported fall who were seen at a pediatric trauma center. Interestingly, 7 out of the 100 children who reportedly fell less than 4 ft died of their injuries, whereas no deaths occurred in the 65 children who fell between 5 and 9 ft and only 1 child died who fell between 10 ft and 45 ft. Further analysis of the data showed that the 7 children who died from short falls were victims of abuse whose caregivers falsified their history.

Imaging Work Up

Computed tomography (CT) scans consist of a series of radiologic images that provide sliced views through the area of the body scanned and are often an essential part of the child abuse evaluation. CT scans of the head can identify manifestations of AHT, such as subarachnoid hemorrhage, most subdural hemorrhages, and cerebral edema and infarcts. A CT scan of the head is indicated in any infant or child that may have sustained significant head trauma.[49,50] Unlike x-rays of the skull, CT scans provide images of the brain. Still, x-rays are sensitive indicators of skull fractures; relatively easy and quick to obtain; and, as a result, remain the test of choice for evaluating potential skull fractures.[24,51] Finally, magnetic resonance imaging (MRI) is more sensitive than CT for detecting many injuries but takes longer and may not be available emergently. MRIs can provide images in multiple planes and is generally used as an adjunct to CT in the acute setting in regard to the AHT work up.

Eye Injuries

Retinal Hemorrhages

Although many of the infants and young children who present with retinal hemorrhages are victims of abuse, this injury is not pathognomonic for abuse. Retinal hemorrhages may result from birth, major trauma, infections, blood dyscrasias, metabolic disorders, and intracranial lesions.[52] The shearing and sudden deceleration forces that cause many of the findings in AHT play an important role in the development of retinal hemorrhages (**Figures 7-16** to **7-22**). A baby's relatively large head size, weak neck musculature, and immature myelination put younger children at higher risk for such an injury.[53]

Birth

Approximately 30% of newborns are found to have retinal hemorrhages after delivery.[52] The exact mechanism is not completely understood, and hemorrhages have been found in children after a cesarean section. Retinal hemorrhages from birth resolve relatively quickly, within 7 to 10 days, with no visual deficits. However, some may take longer to heal, occasionally taking as long as 6 weeks postpartum.[54,55]

Trauma

Rarely, retinal hemorrhages have been described after major polytrauma, such as a motor vehicle collision.[52] Although retinal hemorrhages in infants have been described

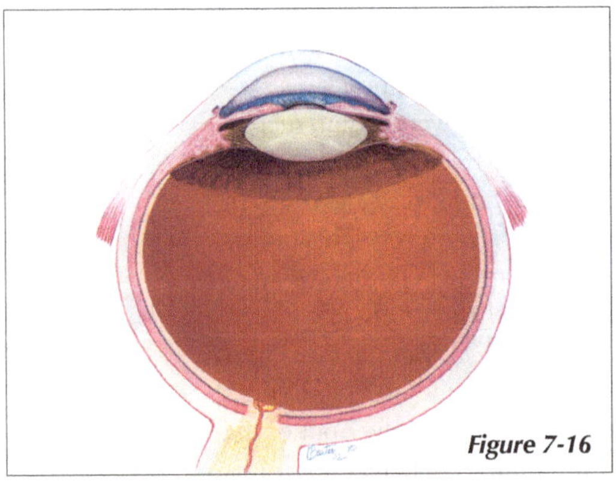

Figure 7-16

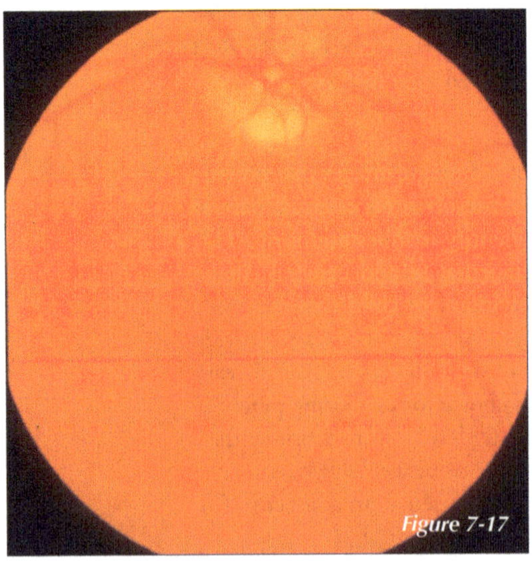

Figure 7-17

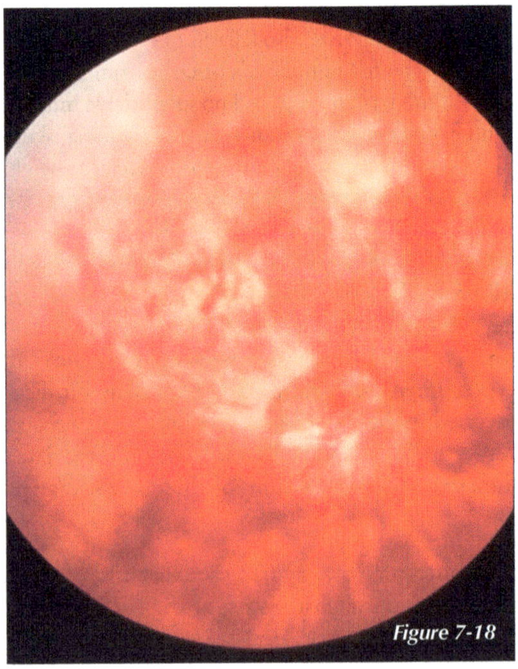

Figure 7-18

Figure 7-16. *Schematic showing the cross section of the human eye. (Contributed by the National Eye Institute, National Institutes of Health; Bethesda, MD.)*

Figure 7-17. *Photograph of an example of a fundoscopic examination showing normal retina and optic nerve in a pediatric patient. (Contributed by Brian J. Forbes, MD, PhD; Philadelphia, PA.)*

Figure 7-18. *Color fundoscopic photo examination demonstrating marked retinal hemorrhages in all layers of the retina in a case of AHT. (Contributed by Brian J. Forbes, MD, PhD; Philadelphia, PA.)*

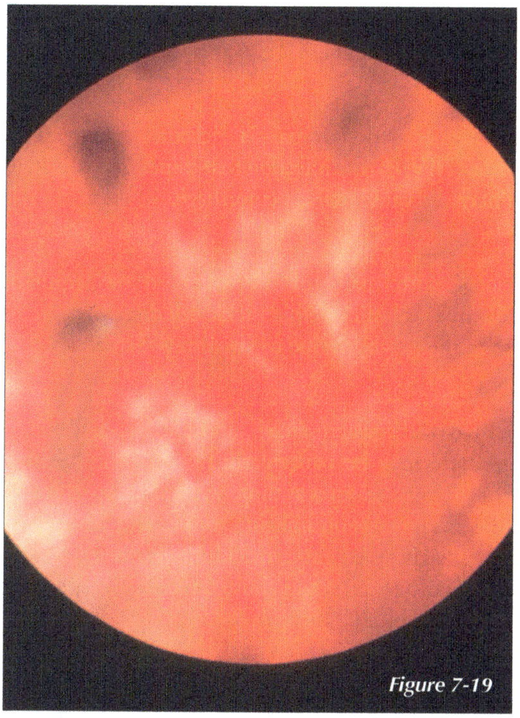

Figure 7-19. *Marked retinal hemorrhages in all layers of retina and optic nerve in a case of AHT. (Contributed by Brian J. Forbes, MD, PhD; Philadelphia, PA.)*

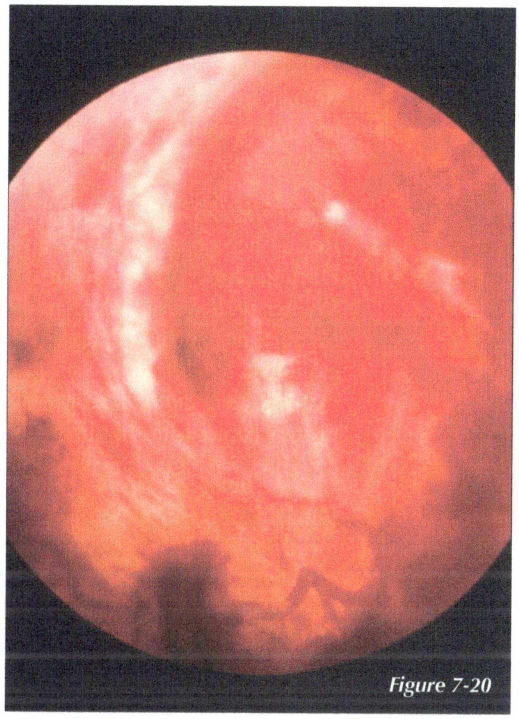

Figure 7-20. *Multiple retinal hemorrhages with a retinal fold in a case of AHT. (Contributed by Brian J. Forbes, MD, PhD; Philadelphia, PA.)*

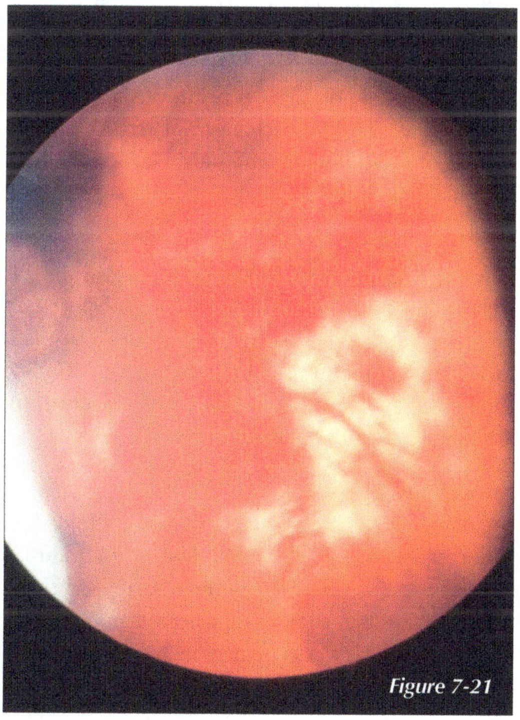

Figure 7-21. *Preretinal hemorrhages in a case of AHT. (Contributed by Brian J. Forbes, MD, PhD; Philadelphia, PA.)*

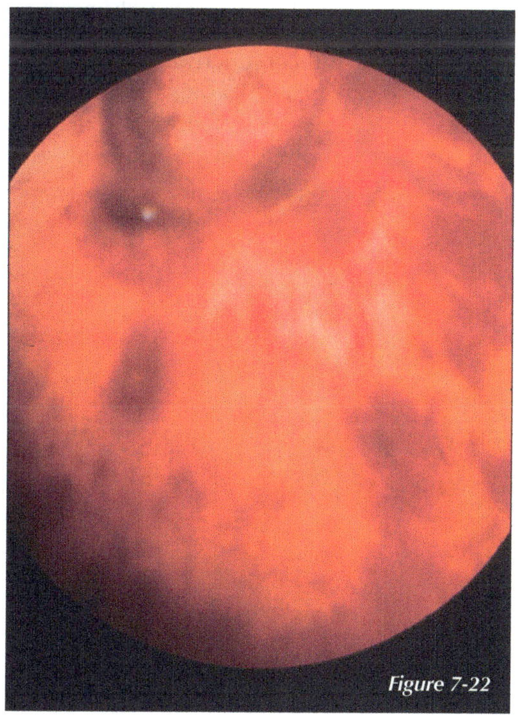

Figure 7-22. *Extensive retinal hemorrhages in all layers in a case of AHT. (Contributed by Brian J. Forbes, MD, PhD; Philadelphia, PA.)*

after household trauma, the mechanisms were not trivial. In such cases, the health care provider should fully explore the possibility of child abuse.[51]

Infections

Retinal hemorrhages have been reportedly associated with malaria, rickettsia, cytomegalovirus, and human immunodeficiency virus (HIV).[56] Any infection that causes disseminated vascular coagulopathy or septic emboli may also cause retinal hemorrhage.

Hematological Disorders

Retinal hemorrhages may be associated with many of the inherited or acquired hematological disorders, including leukemia, aplastic anemia, sickle cell disease, protein C deficiency, and hemorrhagic disease of the newborn due to vitamin K deficiency.[56]

Metabolic Disorders

Retinal hemorrhages have been associated with galactosemia[57] and glutaric aciduria.[58] Distinguishing glutaric aciduria from abuse may be particularly troublesome because children with this disorder have many of the same features as those with AHT, specifically subdural hematomas, irritability, and FTT. Findings on imaging studies and laboratory evaluation are helpful in establishing the diagnosis of glutaric aciduria; however, health care providers should be cognizant that glutaric aciduria and abuse can coexist, especially because babies with this disorder are often irritable and difficult to feed.[58]

Other Etiologies

Retinal hemorrhages are also associated with subdural hematomas, arteriovenous malformations, and subarachnoid hemorrhages.[56] Retinal hemorrhages have been seen in association with severe hypertension, Henoch-Schönlein purpura, postoperative ocular and cardiac surgery, and extracorporeal membrane oxygenation.[55] The role cardiopulmonary resuscitation (CPR) plays in causing retinal hemorrhages is controversial. Autopsy and animal model data do not support CPR as the sole mechanism of retinal hemorrhages.[59] In addition, one prospective study of 43 children found only 1 child who had small punctate retinal hemorrhages after receiving CPR.[60]

Subconjunctival Hemorrhages

Although bruising anywhere in a newborn should raise concerns for abuse, up to one-third of newborns may have subconjunctival hemorrhages after delivery that resolve quickly.[61] Subconjunctival hemorrhages may also occur if the patient has had particularly forceful coughing episodes, as may occur in pertussis. In addition, any coagulation disorder may lead to subconjunctival hemorrhages.

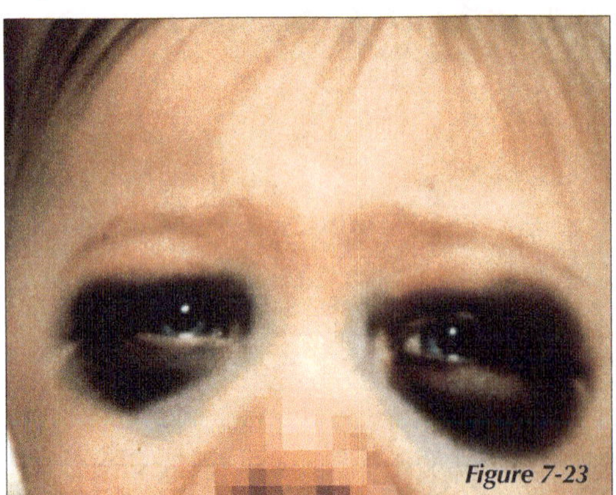

Figure 7-23. *Magical bruising. Orbital neuroblastoma can invade the orbits leading to large periorbital bruising with no or minimal trauma reported. (Contributed by Marc Gorelick, MD; Milwaukee, WI.)*

Periorbital Bruising

Parents may seek care because their child has periorbital bruising without a history of trauma. However, on further questioning, many of these children have had some minor head trauma in the preceding 1 to 2 weeks or may be found to have a bruise on his or her forehead. Characteristic raccoon eyes can result from the pooling of blood in the more dependent infraorbital region. Although an unusual case, neuroblastoma that has metastasized to the orbits may result in periorbital bruising and may also be misdiagnosed as abuse (**Figure 7-23**). Such bruising may be attributed to venous congestion.[62]

Failure to Thrive and Growth Failure

Many situations uncovered in clinical practice may indicate neglect as a possible etiology, including a child who fails to grow as expected; one who lacks routine primary care, a situation in which the caregiver or child seeks medical attention later than would be normally expected, and a child who has poor hygiene. The health care provider should carefully consider the child's basic needs and determine whether or not these are being met.[63]

Children who do not grow according to expected parameters raise concerns about several possible medical conditions and are often said to be experiencing growth failure or manifesting FTT.[64] In general, FTT is a nonspecific term that may be synonymous with growth failure, undernutrition, and growth retardation, depending on a given set of clinical circumstances.[65] Alexander[2] conceptualizes the fundamental nutritional issues that lie at the root of all FTT cases as: (1) too few calories going into the child, (2) too many calories going out of the child, or (3) too many calories being used up by the child. Children are said to suffer from FTT when their growth pattern becomes problematic and their growth parameters demonstrate the following:

- Weight exclusively or weight in addition to weight-for-height measurements follow a curve less than 3%, essentially more than 2 standard deviations from the mean for their age.
- Weight measurements or, less commonly, height and head circumference drop across at least 2 formal growth curves (eg, 95th, 90th, 75th, 50th, 25th, 10th, 5th).
- Fluctuating growth pattern of near-normal periods of growth followed by abnormal delayed periods, producing what has been described as a sawtooth pattern.

Early thinking about FTT categorized the etiologies for this syndrome into organic (medical) and nonorganic (psychosocial) causes.[66,67] Organic etiologies represented bona fide medical conditions as the cause for the growth failure, whereas nonorganic causes were psychosocially related and revolved around neglectful parenting styles and significant environmental stressors in the child's life. Over time, the overlap between these categories was understood, and mixed cases were identified that represented combinations of organic and nonorganic causes in which a medical problem, nutrition issue, or feeding style expressed itself in an environment that was unable to meet the challenges of the child's needs[68] (see *Chapter 8, Clinical Aspects of Child Neglect* for further discussion regarding FTT).

Many medical conditions can lead to FTT, and extensive workups may be needed to rule out various suspected medical conditions.[69] As with any differential diagnostic process, the workup must be tailored to the clinical circumstances of the case. Knowing that many FTT cases are in fact mixed in their cause and understanding that the adequacy of the caregiving environment, with regard to nutritional issues must be assessed, adds to the information the clinician should collect and factor into the differential diagnostic process.

Central to the work-up for FTT are a history, physical examination, and laboratory assessment. The history should focus on signs and symptoms of the various medical conditions and explore the child's nutritional intake.[70] The physical examination should focus on growth parameters, patterns of growth, and findings consistent with various congenital or acquired medical conditions. The physical examination should also evaluate for other findings that may suggest a neglectful environment, such as poor grooming and hygiene, excessive diaper rash, or improper dress for the climate. The laboratory workup should focus on diagnostic possibilities suggested by the history and physical examination and should not be composed of an automatic extensive set of laboratory tests that are not indicated by the history or physical examination because such fishing expeditions rarely yield new or useful information.[68,69] However, once the clinician completes the basic history and physical examination and considers reasonable diagnoses, he or she should then consider possible screening laboratory tests. Reasonable, first-step laboratory evaluations that may be indicated in the preliminary assessment of FTT include the following:

— Complete blood count (CBC), to include hemoglobin (Hbg), hematocrit (Hct), platelet count, white blood count (WBC), and standard red cell indices

— Basic metabolic panel, to include sodium (NA), potassium (K+), chloride (Cl), bicarbonate (HCO3), blood urea nitrogen (BUN), and creatinine

— Erythrocyte sedimentation rate (ESR)

— Urinalysis (UA)

— Bone age radiographs

Other tests and diagnostic studies should be considered based on the clinical situation and diagnostic considerations at hand. Medical conditions to be considered include growth variations, congenital anatomical anomalies, congenital and chromosomal disorders, and organ system disorders.

Growth Variations

Constitutional short stature may be seen in a well-nourished child whose height and weight are at a similar percentile and weight-for-height curve is normal. Normal leanness is seen in an adequately nourished healthy child whose family members demonstrate a propensity for a slender body habitus. Shifting linear growth may be seen in some children as they establish their appropriate formal growth curves, but the FTT workup should be pursued in situations before crossing the 5th percentile.[71] Prematurity affects a child's birth measurements, and adequate assessment requires correction for the child's gestational age for approximately 2 years for weight and 3 years for length or height.[72] Finally, intrauterine growth restriction (IUGR) also affects a child's growth. Symmetric IUGR, in which head circumference, weight, and length are all affected, may occur for various reasons, including prenatal drug and alcohol exposure, congenital infections, and several chromosomal syndromes. Asymmetric or head-sparing IUGR is seen when the weight measurement is decreased out of proportion to the head circumference and often results from insufficient nutrition reaching the growing fetus. Asymmetric IUGR has the best prognosis for postnatal growth if adequate nutrition is provided.

Congenital Anatomical Anomalies

Congenital anomalies may be associated with growth problems for various reasons depending on the impact of the anomaly on the child's growth potential and ability to feed. Cleft lip and cleft palate are among the clearest examples of how a congenital anomaly can affect growth and the child's ability to thrive. Cleft lip and cleft palate are midline craniofacial defects that make proper nutritional intake difficult because the baby cannot create an adequate seal for sucking. Feeding techniques for children with cleft lip and cleft palate have been developed but are challenging. These children also experience frequent otitis media infections that adversely affect growth.

Congenital and Chromosomal Disorders

A large number of identified congenital syndromes include growth failure as a component. Some syndromes have a clearly defined genetic basis. One of the better-understood syndromes is Turner syndrome, or Ulrich-Turner syndrome, which is caused by the complete or partial absence of the X-chromosome in females.[73] With this syndrome, affected children fail to grow as expected, manifest short stature, and fail to undergo pubertal development. Growth failure, however, is rarely the only finding indicating a genetic syndrome. In Turner syndrome the growth failure is also associated with other findings, such as neck webbing; various skeletal anomalies, such as hand or shield chest; and retarded bone age. For the well-recognized syndromes, chromosomal analysis is diagnostic.

Organ System Disorders

Cardiovascular System

With congenital heart disease (CHD), poor cardiovascular function does not provide for the body's tissues to receive adequate oxygen and other nutrients, nor are metabolic waste products adequately removed. Over time, this leads to a clinical situation marked by acidosis, polycythemia, and increased caloric requirements. Growth is impaired secondary to the inability to provide adequate nutrition. Children who develop congestive heart failure (CHF) as part of their clinical picture experience poor cardiac pumping function that also impairs oxygen delivery capacity and other normal metabolic functions, such as removal of waste products. In the setting of impaired cardiac function, the exertion of feeding leads to increased caloric consumption, which only further worsens the growth failure.

Endocrine System

Some endocrinological disorders may affect growth, especially those affecting growth hormone and thyroid hormone. Growth hormone deficiency leads to impaired growth and short stature. Thyroid disorders are among the most common endocrinological disorders that may cause a child to not grow according to expectations. Hyperthyroidism may present as congenital hyperthyroidism in the neonate or, more commonly, can present as an autoimmune thyroid disease or Graves' disease, with tachycardia, nervousness, and weight loss in the face of increased appetite. Hypothyroidism, if present at birth, is usually diagnosed by newborn screening and includes decreased tone, lethargy, poor feeding, and diminished growth. After the neonatal period, hypothyroidism in the child presents primarily as a slowing of linear growth with delayed bone age and often delayed puberty. Serum thyroid function tests are abnormal.

Gastrointestinal System

Children may be born at a normal weight but may experience feeding problems during the first few weeks to months of life. Such problems may be related to incorrect formula preparation, breastfeeding problems, difficulties with mother-infant attachment, and anatomical problems of the airway or esophagus. Gastroesophageal reflux, present to some degree in almost all neonates, may become problematic. The movement of stomach contents into the esophagus may occur with or without vomiting and can interfere with adequate caloric intake. Inflammatory bowel disease (IBD) may manifest itself as a pattern of remitting and relapsing signs and symptoms, including cramping, abdominal pain, diarrhea, blood in the stool, fever, anorexia, weight loss, and growth failure. Severe growth restriction may precede the onset of gastrointestinal symptoms.

Malabsorption of nutrients may lead to growth failure and conditions such as celiac disease with intolerance to gluten; carbohydrate malabsorption with intolerance to sugars such as lactose; cow's milk allergy; soybean allergy; and pancreatic enzyme deficiency, known as Shwachman-Diamond syndrome. The presentation for malabsorption syndromes includes diarrhea, flatulence, bloating, unintended weight loss, and poor growth pattern over time.

Hematological and Oncological Disorders

Malignancies in children can result in abnormal growth patterns based on a number of possible etiologies. These include the direct effects of the neoplasm; a poor metabolic state; loss of appetite secondary to the disease or the treatment of recurrent infections resulting from immunosuppression; chronic diarrhea secondary to the effects of chemotherapy or radiation; and CNS disorders secondary to the disease or the treatment that have an impact on the hypothalamic-pituitary axis, such as irradiation.

Immunological System

Immunodeficiency may be a component of many congenital syndromes. Congenital growth failure may result from recurrent infections that develop and lead to increased work of breathing associated with chronic pneumonia, painful swallowing with chronic candidiasis, and chronic diarrhea with related malabsorption. Children with HIV or acquired immune deficiency syndrome (AIDS) may manifest growth failure for various reasons, including esophagitis, diarrhea from parasitic, viral, or bacterial infections, and malabsorption. Constitutional symptoms, such as malaise, lead to decreased appetite, and a variety of recurrent infections may lead to weight loss.

Autoimmune-type disorders such as juvenile rheumatoid arthritis (JRA), systemic lupus erythematosus (SLE), and dermatomyositis may be associated with growth failure secondary to the presence of malaise, decreased appetite, chronic inflammation, weight loss, gastrointestinal involvement, and chronic steroid use.

Metabolic Disorders

Metabolic disorders typically present with recurring episodes of lethargy, poor feeding, vomiting, and seizures. The laboratory evaluation necessary depends on the clinical situation and the suspected defect. Galactosemia is a well-studied defect that manifests itself in the neonatal period after the initiation of routine feedings that contain the sugar galactose. The child's signs and symptoms include vomiting; diarrhea; jaundice, as demonstrated by an elevated conjugated bilirubin level; poor feeding; abdominal distention with ascites and hepatosplenomegaly; poor weight gain; hypoglycemia; and aminoaciduria.

Renal System

There are several types of renal tubular acidosis (RTA) with various causes, all of which may result in a metabolic acidosis associated with poor growth. With RTA, excess base is present in the urine and the serum bicarbonate level is low. Bacterial urinary tract infection (UTI), if chronic, may lead to kidney damage that significantly affects growth. Renal failure leads to metabolic abnormalities and nutritional restrictions that affect growth. The treatments for these problems may also affect growth.

Respiratory System

Cystic fibrosis (CF) is a multisystem exocrine dysfunction that leads to serious respiratory and gastrointestinal manifestations associated with growth failure. Respiratory involvement includes wheezing, recurrent pneumonia, and sinusitis, while gastrointestinal involvement is seen with pancreatic insufficiency and associated malabsorption. Growth failure results from the combined effects of the increased caloric needs from the respiratory effort and infections as well as decreased nutrition secondary to poor absorption. Chronic lung disease is associated with growth failure because of chronic hypoxia, recurrent pneumonia, and the increased caloric requirement from the work of breathing.

Sexual Abuse

Genital and Anal Findings

The differential diagnosis for anogenital signs and symptoms, such as erythema, excoriation, pruritus, bruising, bleeding, genital discharge, and unusual anogenital appearance, includes both physical and sexual abuse.[74-76] Several conditions affecting the anogenital area may have physical findings similar to those seen in sexual maltreatment and, consequently, could be confused with this type of abuse. As with most differential diagnoses, the diagnostic process should begin with careful attention to the history provided by the child and caregivers. This is especially true with regard to suspected sexual abuse because the presenting complaint often includes various nonspecific behavioral changes. Once the history is obtained, the health care provider should proceed with the diagnostic process by collecting information from the physical examination. The physical examination in potential sexual maltreatment cases frequently does not uncover definitive findings for abuse, and findings that are present are often nonspecific.[77,78] The laboratory evaluation in sexual abuse cases is often not diagnostic unless seminal products or a noncongenitally acquired sexually transmitted infection (STI) is found.[79] Because cases for which sexual abuse is suspected are rarely straightforward, the health care provider may need to consult with an MDT at a regional center to sort out the evaluation findings and to work through the differential diagnoses of the child with anogenital complaints.[80]

Vaginitis, vulvitis, and vulvovaginitis cause a wide range of signs and symptoms referable to the anogenital area.[74,81,82] Vulvitis occurs when the vulvar structures (labia majora, labia minora, clitoris, and components of the vestibule) become inflamed and friable. Vaginitis occurs when the vaginal mucosa becomes inflamed and friable and produces a discharge; bleeding may also occur. Vulvovaginitis is a combination of both entities, with one frequently leading to the other.[83] Males may also have genital inflammation, but this is seen less frequently than in girls. In boys, comparable inflammatory conditions affecting the most distal portion of the penis include phimosis and paraphimosis in the uncircumcised male and urethritis in both circumcised and uncircumcised males. Both male and female children have perianal signs and symptoms that result from inflammation.

The subsequent sections address the differential diagnosis for the following anogenital signs and symptoms in the prepubertal child:

— Anogenital erythema, excoriation, and pruritus

— Bruising in the anogenital area

— Anogenital bleeding or bloody vaginal discharge

— Nonbloody vaginal discharge

— Unusual anogenital appearance, both congenital and acquired

Anogenital Erythema, Excoriation, and Pruritus

Redness in the anogenital tissues and structures may arise from several causes related to inflammation (**Figure 7-24**). A vicious cycle may ensue in which inflammation, irritation, and pruritus lead to repeated scratching of the affected area, which in turn leads to a worsening in the inflammatory process, continuing the cycle.[75,76,84] The health care provider should consider various local conditions, systemic disease, inappropriate genital manipulation, and STIs. Depending on the history and clinical index of suspicion, other diagnostic possibilities could include local irritation, dermatological disorders, infections, and, uncommonly, systemic conditions such as Crohn's disease, Kawasaki syndrome, and Stevens-Johnson syndrome.

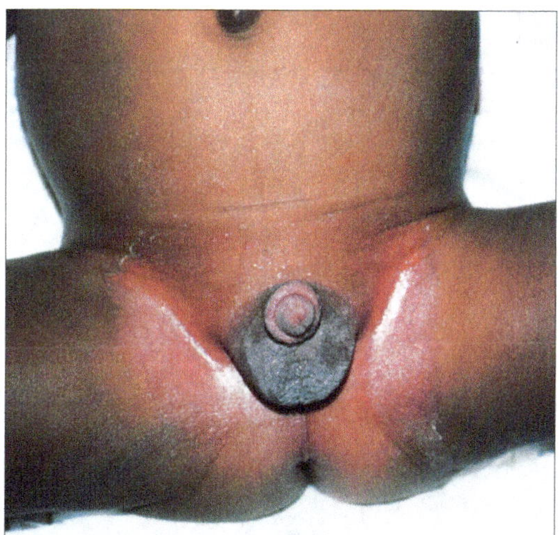

Figure 7-24. *Male infant with perineal erythema and fever, raising concern about bacterial superinfection. (Contributed by Paul J. Honig, MD; Philadelphia, PA.)*

Local Irritation

Poor hygienic practices such as wiping the anogenital area from back to front, instead of front to back, can lead to fecal contamination of the vagina, which can then lead to the development of vaginitis and its accompanying irritation and pruritus.[83] Retained urine in the skin folds of obese children, urinary reflux, and poor drainage of urine into the vagina may lead to inflammation and irritation.[85] Any type of restrictive or poorly ventilated clothing, whether underwear, pants, or tights, may lead to friction and increased heat that can result in inflammation, irritation, pruritus, and erythema.[86] Chemical irritants, including soaps, fragrances, colored toilet tissue, and bubble baths, commonly lead to inflammation in the anogenital area as well. Sandbox vulvitis deserves special mention because it is caused by the entrapment of particles of dirt or sand in the child's vulvar area.[85] In the prepubertal child, the labia majora do not fully surround the vulvar structures, and the child may come into contact with contaminating material while sitting on the ground during outdoor play.

Dermatological Disorders

Contact dermatitis is a skin irritation that results after contact with substances to which the skin is sensitive, typically on an allergic basis.[76] Seborrhea in the genital area is common in infancy, although it may occur at any age, and involves the folds of the diaper area between the labia minora and labia majora. Seborrheic rashes may be pruritic and frequently become secondarily infected from scratching as a result of breaks in the skin's protective barriers. Seborrheic lesions in the genital area appear elevated and erythematous. The yellow, greasy scales of seborrhea are also commonly observed in extragenital areas.[87,88] Psoriasis is a dermatological condition that affects children at any age. The diagnostic lesions vary in size and location and are sharply demarcated, pruritic, erythematous plaques with silvery scales on a flat surface.[86,89]

Lichen sclerosis is an uncommon dermatological condition of unknown etiology that is often seen in the anogenital area. In females, it presents as irregular ivory macules or papules that coalesce to form atrophic hypopigmented plaques in an hourglass or figure-eight pattern.[90-92] In males, lichen sclerosis, known as balanitis xerotica obliterans, presents as a chronic, progressive, atrophic, sclerosing process of the glans and foreskin.[93,94] In both males and females, the skin becomes thin and fissured, may appear reddened and edematous, and is easily traumatized by minimal pressure (**Figure 7-25**).

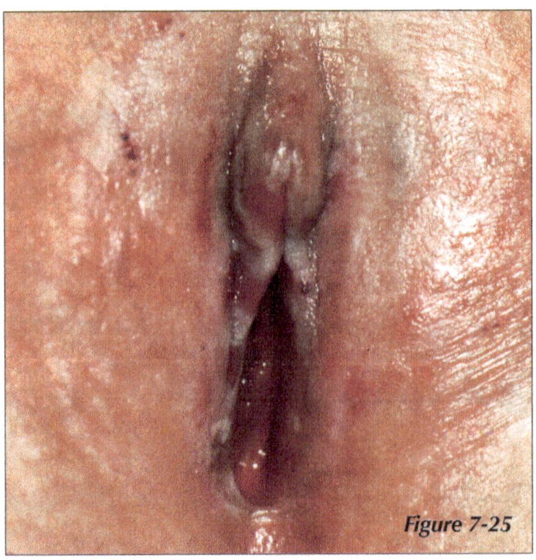

Figure 7-25. *Prepubertal female child's external genitalia demonstrating the friable skin findings seen in lichen sclerosis. (Contributed by Paul J. Honig, MD; Philadelphia, PA.)*

Infections

Infection caused by STIs may lead to local irritation and redness (see *Chapter 6, Sexually Transmitted Infection in the Setting of Maltreatment* for further discussion). Therefore, such findings need to be assessed for possible STIs. Nonspecific vaginitis is a mixed bacterial infection caused by a combination of coliforms, streptococci, Haemophilus vaginalis, and other bacteria.[95] Vaginitis frequently leads to a secondary vulvitis with local irritation, inflammation, erythema, and pruritus.[75] Infestation with pinworms, Enterobius vermicularis, may cause vulvovaginitis as well. The female pinworm resides in the child's intestinal tract and migrates to the perianal area to deposit eggs. This causes pruritus, scratching, and irritation. Pinworms may move from the rectum to the vagina and can introduce fecal flora into the vagina, resulting in a bacterial vulvovaginitis.[86]

Scabies, caused by the parasitic mite Sarcoptes scabiei, results in the development of pruritic erythematous papules with wavy burrows. Additionally, candidal overgrowth in the anogenital area may occur in the following situations: (1) after a course of antibiotics, (2) with diabetes mellitus, (3) when the child is in diapers, and (4) as a result of other risk factors, such as immunodeficiency.[74] Exposure to antibiotics may change the makeup of the vaginal flora that keep the yeast in check.

Finally, perianal streptococcal cellulitis is recognized as an etiology leading to a perianal rash that has an intense confluent erythematous area surrounding the anus.[96] The rash is irregular but well demarcated. The condition may cause painful defecation, blood-streaked stools, and perianal inflammation and irritation (**Figure 7-26**).

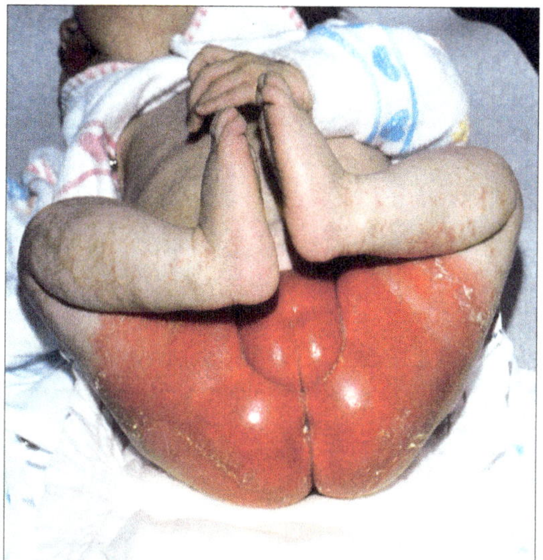
Figure 7-26

Figure 7-26. *An infant's perineum revealing diffuse erythema and swelling consistent with perianal streptococcal cellulitis. (Contributed by Paul J. Honig, MD; Philadelphia, PA.)*

Systemic Conditions

Crohn's disease, an inflammatory bowel disease, may have vulvar or perianal involvement and may be confused with sexual abuse.[89,97] The skin findings associated with Kawasaki syndrome may involve the anogenital area and present with a perineal rash that is painful, erythematous and macular, and that eventually desquamates.[98] Stevens-Johnson syndrome, with its characteristic mucositis, may lead to findings consistent with vulvovaginitis.[99] These serious systemic disorders have other associated findings, so a careful history and physical examination are required to either rule them in or out.

Anogenital Bruising

Anogenital trauma may cause genital or anal bruising. The differential diagnoses for anogenital bruises include both sexual abuse and nonsexually sustained blunt or impaling injuries. Accidental injury should present with a plausible history that details an appropriate mechanism of injury. Additionally, bruising in the genital area may also be seen in a variety of hematological, connective tissue, and dermatological conditions.[100]

Local Injury

A straddle injury occurs as the result of a child falling on a hard object, crushing the soft tissues of the genitalia between the object and the pubic bone. Straddle injuries tend to be anterior (**Figure 7-27**). The hymen, an internal structure, would not be expected to affected by this mechanism of injury because of its relatively recessed position. Impaling or penetrating injuries (**Figures 7-28** and **7-29**), however, such as a fall onto an exposed stick or broom handle, may conceivably injure the hymen. Boys may injure their genitalia if an object, such as a toilet seat, falls on the penis. In addition, zipper injuries to the penis may be seen.

Dermatological Disorders

Mongolian spots are slate blue, well-demarcated areas of hyperpigmentation that are most commonly located on the back and buttocks and may be confused with bruising in infants and toddlers. Over half of African-American children have Mongolian spots.[3]

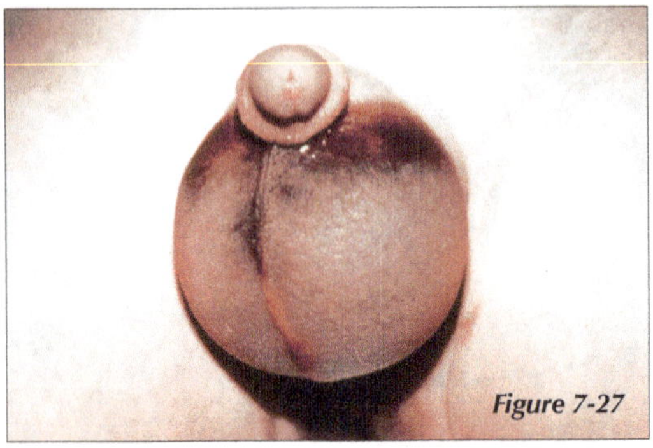

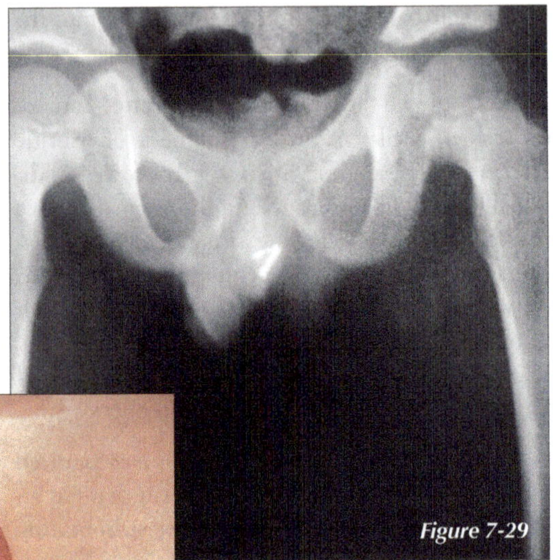

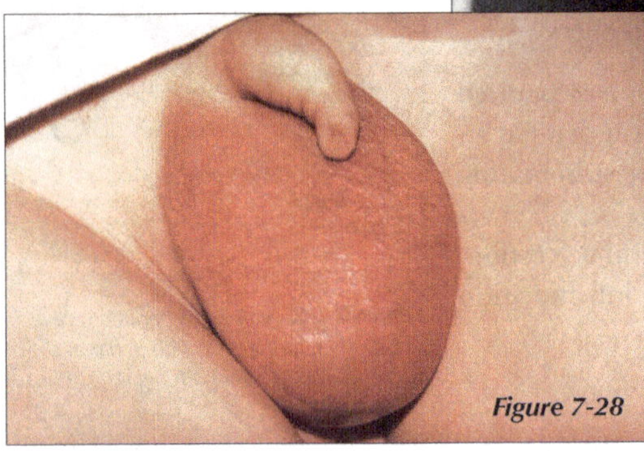

Figure 7-27. *Scrotal hematoma from a straddle bicycle injury. (Contributed by Douglas A. Canning, MD; Philadelphia, PA.)*

Figure 7-28. *Swollen scrotum, tenpenny nail injury. (Contributed by Douglas A. Canning, MD; Philadelphia, PA.)*

Figure 7-29. *Straight pin in bladder caused bladder trauma and urethral injuries. Pin was removed endoscopically from urethra. (Contributed by Douglas A. Canning, MD; Philadelphia, PA.)*

Lichen sclerosis, a dermatological condition, is easily traumatized from minimal pressure and may become blue and discolored as a result. Vascular nevi may give the appearance of bruising secondary to the visible accentuation of the capillary bed. Phytophotodermatitis mimics bruising and burns on the child's skin and has been confused with child physical abuse.[101,102] This photosensitivity reaction occurs when the child's skin comes in contact with plant psoralens and is then exposed to sunlight, leaving a discoloration (see "Toxins") If this is offered as a reason for anogenital bruising, the history must account for contact with the psoralen and exposure of the anogenital skin to sunlight.

Systemic Conditions

Some hematological conditions, including bleeding disorders such as hemophilia, Von Willebrand disease, and idiopathic thrombocytopenic purpura (ITP), may cause anogenital bruising. Bruising in extragenital sites would also be expected and is typical. Appropriate laboratory studies should rule these bleeding disorder causes in or out. In addition, disorders with a vasculitis component may also cause bruising in the anogenital area and would be expected to have other characteristic findings associated with the specific vasculitis, such as generalized lower-extremity petechia with HSP.

Anogenital Bleeding and Bloody Vaginal Discharge

Bleeding in the anogenital area may represent a medical emergency and requires identification and management of the source of the bleeding.[86] Bloody or blood-tinged urethral discharge is a separate clinical entity that may initially be difficult to differentiate from anogenital bleeding. A bloody vaginal discharge, including frank bleeding, requires prompt diagnosis and treatment.

Local Irritation

Bleeding in the anogenital region may result from inappropriate anogenital manipulation from sexually abusive contact. Although sexual abuse should be considered to be the cause of nonaccidental trauma, the differential diagnosis of localized injury and bleeding includes accidental trauma (**Figures 7-30** to **7-33**), superficial abrasions, and friability of the mucosa from a vulvovaginitis. A foul-smelling vaginal discharge raises the possibility of a foreign body, especially if the discharge is bloody.[83] Toilet tissue is the most frequently described foreign body found in a young girl's vagina, the presence of which causes a foul-smelling bloody discharge.

Dermatological Disorders

Bleeding may arise from the effects of pruritic dermatological conditions, such as atopic, contact, and seborrheic dermatitis; psoriasis; and lichen sclerosis.[75,82,89] The related inflammation leads to pruritus and irritation and ultimately to local trauma and bleeding.

Infection

Infections may lead to friable vulvar and vaginal tissues that bleed. A vulvovaginitis-like picture may be seen with STIs contracted during sexual abuse and may present with a characteristic discharge. Less common genital infections may lead to vulvovaginitis as well, including group A b-hemolytic streptococcus, which may cause vaginitis, especially following pharyngitis. Additionally, Shigella and Yersinia cause similar findings and should be considered if diarrhea is present.[74,86,103,104]

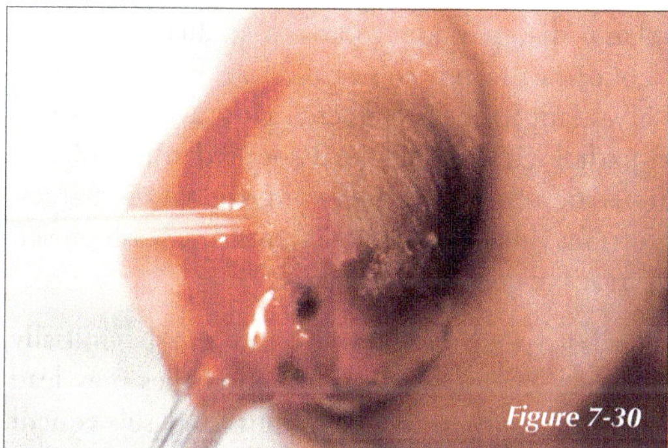

Figure 7-30. Laceration of glans penis. (Contributed by Douglas A. Canning, MD; Philadelphia, PA.)

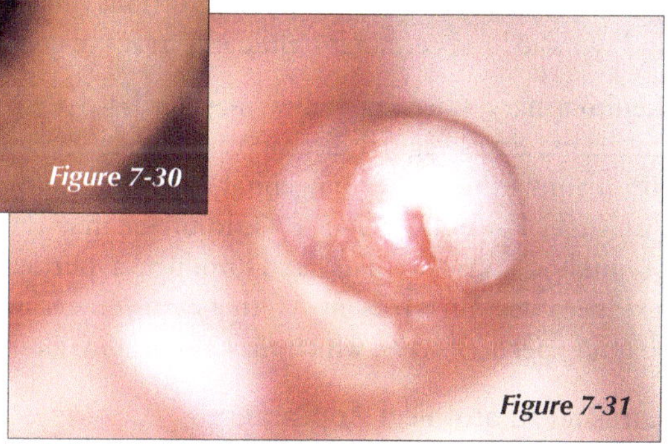

Figure 7-31. Postoperative appearance of laceration of glans penis. (Contributed by Douglas A. Canning, MD; Philadelphia, PA.)

Figure 7-32. Circumcision injury. Child had part of glans removed with the Mogen® clamp. (Contributed by Douglas A. Canning, MD; Philadelphia, PA.)

Figure 7-33. Circumcision injury. Shows postcircumcision cicatrix. (Contributed by Douglas A. Canning, MD; Philadelphia, PA.)

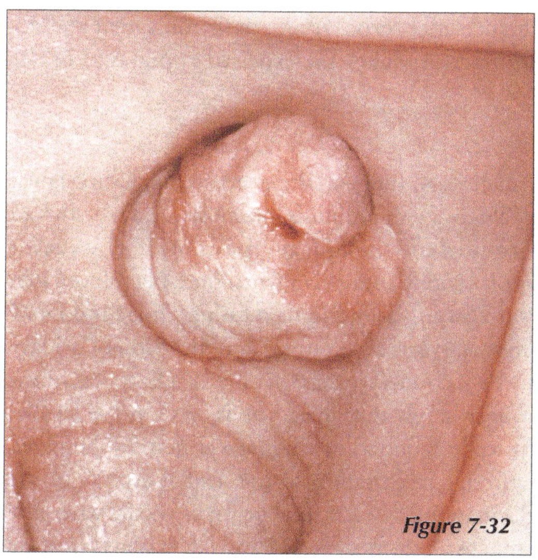

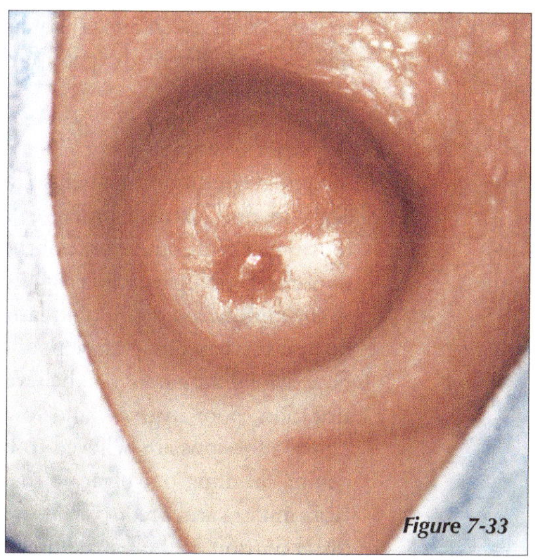

Endocrinological Disorders

What appears to be bleeding from the vagina may actually be menstrual flow from precocious pubertal development in a child. If this is suspected, hormone-producing tumors should be excluded and an endocrinological evaluation completed.[105] Endocrinological reasons for bleeding would be expected to have no signs of genital trauma. In female neonates, there is a well-described bloody discharge that may be transiently observed during the first weeks of life as a result of maternal estrogen withdrawal.

Structural and Neoplastic Disorders

Anatomical structures, such as vaginal polyps and benign growths, may erode and bleed. Vulvar hemangiomas are prone to ulceration and bleeding.[106] Neoplastic conditions such as sarcoma botryoides may present as vaginal bleeding. Sarcoma botryoides is a grapelike malignant tumor that typically arises from the anterior vaginal wall near the cervix and may involve the vagina, uterus, bladder, and urethra.[74,107] Peak incidence is in the first 2 years of life, with most cases presenting before age 5 years. Prognosis is poor unless found early, so all suspicious lesions should be fully evaluated.

Nonbloody Vaginal Discharge

Vaginal discharge is a genital complaint that requires thorough evaluation in the prepubertal child. Nonpathological leukorrhea, a physiological, clear, white, mucoid discharge, may be considered a normal variant in the prepubertal girls, and the skilled examiner should not confuse it with pathological discharges associated with vulvitis, vaginitis, and vulvovaginitis.[74] Infections are often associated with vaginal discharges. Sexually and nonsexually acquired infections, including varicella, measles, scarlet fever, and typhoid, and certain systemic infections may lead to discharge.[76]

Genitourinary tract anomalies may lead to persistent wetness and can be initially misdiagnosed as vaginal discharge. Additionally, such anatomical anomalies may lead to inflammation in the anogenital area, also causing a vulvovaginitis and subsequent discharge. For example, an ectopic ureter may drain into the vagina, cervix, uterus, or urethra; cause wetness; and produce a purulent perineal discharge, especially if a kidney infection is present.[74] Other examples include rectovaginal fistula or an acquired draining pelvic abscess, which may also lead to similar findings.

Unusual Anatomical Appearance

At times, various genital structures may appear abnormal and may simulate the chronic changes observed in anogenital appearance after sexual abuse. Both congenital and acquired anomalies of the genitourinary tract may alter the expected appearance of the genital structures.[76]

Acquired Conditions

Acquired conditions may cause abnormalities in anogenital appearance, including labial agglutination, urethral prolapse, labial abscess, paraphimosis, phimosis, and hair-thread tourniquet syndrome. Some of these acquired conditions may arise from either sexual or nonsexual etiologies. Labial agglutination or adhesions occur when the labia minora join in the midline as a result of inflamed surfaces adhering and then fusing. This fusion may be near total and may cause poor drainage of vaginal secretions and diversion of urinary flow. Labial adhesions are believed to be secondary to the combined effects of vulvar irritation, poor hygiene, and low estrogen levels that make the mucosa more friable. Labial adhesions are believed to be typically acquired in a nonsexual fashion; however, genital fondling or vulvar coitus may result in irritation of the medial aspects of the labia minora and predispose it to agglutination.[108,109] Urethral prolapse occurs when the distal portion of the female urethral mucosa becomes everted and edematous, creating the appearance of a doughnut-shaped structure surrounding the urethral meatus.[110,111] This occurrence is found most commonly in prepubescent black girls, it may be related to an antecedent episode of increased intraabdominal pressure.

Phimosis and paraphimosis are conditions affecting the foreskin of uncircumcised males. Phimosis is a congenital or acquired inflammatory condition of the foreskin resulting in pathological nonretractability that is not consistent with the developmentally normal state of nonretractability seen in most young boys aged under 3 years.[94] If left untreated, phimosis results in inadequate hygiene, severe inflammation, and ulceration of the glans and undersurface of the prepuce.[112] Alternatively, paraphimosis is an acquired inflammatory condition that results when a retracted foreskin is left retracted, which causes venous and lymphatic obstruction. The distal penis becomes swollen and inflamed.

Finally, the uncommon hair-thread tourniquet syndrome affects various appendages and may involve the genitalia. In this situation, fibers of hair or thread become tightly wrapped around external genitalia structures such as the penis, labia minora, and clitoris.[17,113-115] The tourniquet effect leads to various degrees of lymphatic, venous, and arterial obstruction, with subsequent swelling, discoloration, ischemia, and eventually necrosis. Both accidental and intentional cases have been described.[113]

Congenital Conditions

Normal anatomical landmarks may be altered by congenital abnormalities, including imperforate hymen, vaginal septum, distal vaginal agenesis, phimosis, and ambiguous genitalia. Imperforate hymen is a congenital condition in which no hymenal orifice is present. If the imperforate hymen is left untreated, mucocolpos, the retention of vaginal secretions, may develop. Eventually, with the onset of menses, hematocolpos, the retention of menstrual flow, will develop at puberty (**Figure 7-34**).[74,75]

Other congenital anomalies that may alter the appearance of the genitalia include paraurethral cysts, urethral diverticulum, ectopic ureterocele, hymenal or vaginal cysts, vulvar hemangioma, congenital pit, and congenital failure of midline genital fusion.[74,100,106,116]

CONCLUSION

There are very few findings pathognomonic for abuse or neglect. When evaluating children for concerns of physical or sexual abuse, the clinician must also consider the many other conditions that may mimic abusive injuries or neglect. A thorough history should include details about the onset and progression of symptoms, reported mechanism of injury, the presence of absence of systemic symptoms like fever, as well as a thorough past medical and social history to help narrow the diagnostic possibilities. The physical exam should be as thorough, a head-to-toe examination. Laboratory, radiological, and other testing may be helpful in further delineating the most likely diagnosis. The health care provider must then combine these components together to assess the likelihood of abuse or an alternative diagnosis and act accordingly.

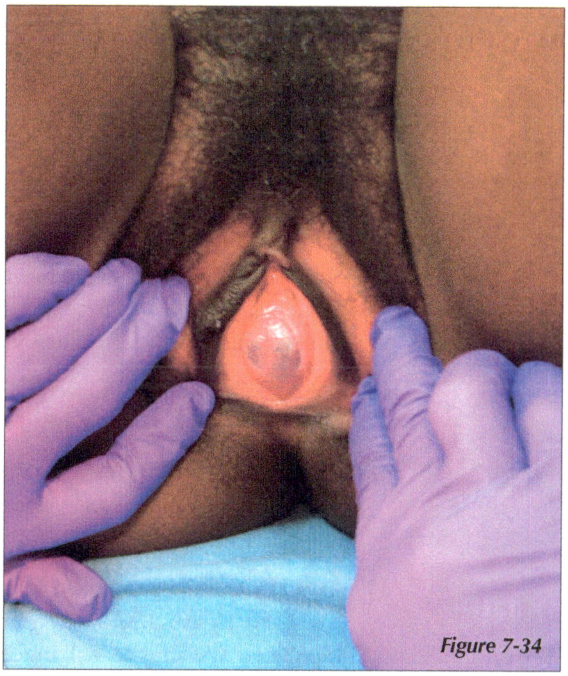

Figure 7-34

Figure 7-34. *Hematocolpos. This girl was born with an imperforate hymen, leading to entrapped menstrual blood with the onset of puberty.*

References

1. Jenny C, Hymel KP, Ritzen A, Reinert ST, Hay TC. Analysis of missed cases of abusive head trauma. *JAMA*. 1999;281(7):621-626.
2. Alexander RC. Failure to thrive. *APSAC Advisor*. 1992;5:1–11-12.
3. Behrman RE, Kliegman RM. The fetus and the neonatal infant: Physical examination of the newborn infant. In: Behrman RE, Vaughan VC, eds. *Nelson Textbook of Pediatrics*. 12th ed. Philadelphia, PA: WB Saunders Co; 1983:322-416.
4. Kirschner RH, Stein RJ. The mistaken diagnosis of child abuse: a form of medical abuse? *Am J Dis Child*. 1985;139(9):873-875.
5. Hibbard RA. Triage and referrals for child sexual abuse medical examinations from the sociolegal system. *Child Abuse Negl*. 1998;22(6):503-513.
6. Altemeier WA III. A pediatrician's view: interpreting bruises in children. *Pediatr Ann*. 2001;30(9):517-518,520.
7. Jenny C, Reece RM. Cutaneous manifestations of child abuse. In: Reece RM, Christian CW, eds. *Child Abuse: Medical Diagnosis and Management*. 3rd ed. Chicago: American Academy of Pediatrics; 2009:19-51.
8. Laposata ME, Laposata M. Children with signs of abuse: when is it not child abuse? *Am J Clin Pathol*. 2005;123(suppl 1):S119-S124.
9. Carpenter RF. The prevalence and distribution of bruising in babies. *Arch Dis Child*. 1999;80(4):363-366.
10. Sugar NF, Taylor JA, Feldman KW; The Puget Sound Pediatric Research Network. Bruises in infants and toddlers: those who don't cruise rarely bruise. *Arch Pediatr Adolesc Med*. 1999;153(4):399-403.
11. Maguire S, Mann MK, Sibert J, Kemp A. Can you age bruises accurately in children?: a systematic review. *Arch Dis Child*. 2005;90(2):187-189.
12. Mimasaka S, Ohtani M, Kuroda N, Tsunenari S. Spectrophotometric evaluation of the age of bruises in children: measuring changes in bruise color as an indicator of child physical abuse. *Tohoku J Exp Med*. 2010;220(2):171-175.
13. Ravanfar P, Dinulos JG. Cultural practices affecting the skin of children. *Curr Opin Pediatr*. 2010; 22(4):423-431.
14. Scott JP, Montgomery RR. Hereditary clotting factor deficiencies. In: Stanton, B, St Geme, J, Schor N, Behrman RE, eds. *Nelson Textbook of Pediatrics*. 19th ed. Philadelphia, PA: WB Saunders Co; 2011:1699.
15. Wetzel RC, Slater AJ, Dover GJ. Fatal intramuscular bleeding misdiagnosed as suspected nonaccidental injury. *Pediatrics*. 1995;95(5):771-773.
16. Caravati EM, Erdman AR, Scharman EJ, et al. Long-acting anticoagulant rodenticide poisoning: an evidence-based consensus guideline for out-of-hospital management. *Clin Toxicol (Phila)*. 2007;45(1):1-22.
17. Bays J. Conditions mistaken for child physical abuse. In: Reece RM, Ludwig S, eds. *Child Abuse: Medical Diagnosis and Management*. 2nd ed. Philadelphia, PA: Lippincott Williams & Wilkins; 2001:177-206.

18. Giardino AP, Christian CW, Giardino EW. Skin: bruises and burns. In: Giardino AP, Christian CW, Giardino EW, eds. *A Practical Guide to the Evaluation of Child Abuse and Neglect.* Thousand Oaks, CA: Sage Publications, Inc; 1997:61-95.

19. Mehta AJ, Statham BN. Phytophotodermatitis mimicking non-accidental injury or self-harm. *Eur J Pediatr.* 2007;166(7):751-752.

20. Maguire S, Moynihan S, Mann M, Potokar T, Kemp AM. A systematic review of the features that indicate intentional scalds in children. *Burns.* 2008;34(8):1072-1081.

21. Porzionato A, Aprile A. Staphylococcal scalded skin syndrome mimicking child abuse by burning. *Forensic Sci Int.* 2007;168(1):e1-4.

22. Leventhal JM, Griffin D, Duncan KO, et al. Laxative-induced dermatitis of the buttocks incorrectly suspected to be abusive burns. *Pediatrics.* 2001;107(1):178-179.

23. Kemp AM, Dunstan F, Harrison S, et al. Patterns of skeletal fractures in child abuse: systematic review. *BMJ.* 2008;337(21):a1518.

24. Kleinman PK. *Diagnostic Imaging of Child Abuse.* 2nd ed. St. Louis, MO: Mosby; 1998.

25. Rivara FP, Parrish RA, Mueller BA. Extremity injuries in children: predictive value of clinical findings. *Pediatrics.* 1986;78(5):803-807.

26. Bhat BV, Kumar A, Oumachigvi A. Bone injuries during delivery. *Indian J Pediatr.* 1994;61(4):401-405.

27. Groenendaal F, Hukkelhoven C. Fractures in full-term neonates. *Ned Tijdschr Geneeskd.* 2007:151(7):424.

28. van Rijn RR, Bilo RA, Robben SG. Birth-related mid-posterior rib fractures in neonates: a report of three cases (and a possible fourth case) and a review of the literature. *Pediatr Radiol.* 2009;39(1):30-34.

29. Giardino AP, Christian CW, Giardino EW. Evaluation of fractures and skeletal injuries. In: Giardino AP, Christian CW, Giardino EW, eds. *A Practical Guide to the Evaluation of Child Abuse and Neglect.* Thousand Oaks, CA. Sage Publications Inc; 1997:61-95.

30. Jenny C; the American Academy of Pediatrics Committee on Child Abuse and Neglect. Evaluating infants and young children with multiple fractures. *Pediatrics.* 2006;118(3):1299-1303.

31. Bloom E, Klein EJ, Shushan D. Feldman KW. Variable presentations of rickets in children in the emergency department. *Pediatr Emerg Care.* 2004;20(2):126-130.

32. Stewart GM, Rosenberg NM. Conditions mistaken for child abuse: part I. *Pediatr Emerg Care.* 1996;12(2):116-121.

33. Thompson GH, Scoles PV. Torsional and angular deformities. In: Behrman RE, Kliegman RM, Jenson HB, eds. *Nelson Textbook of Pediatrics.* 16th ed. Philadelphia, PA. WB Saunders Co; 2000:2069-2070.

34. Scott KR, Kothari MJ. Hereditary neuropathies. *Semin Neurol.* 2005;25(2):174-184.

35. Faul M, Xu L, Wald MM, Coronado VG. Traumatic Brain Injury in the United States: Emergency Department Visits, Hospitalizations and Deaths 2002-2006. Atlanta, GA: Centers for Disease Control and Prevention, National Center for Injury Prevention and Control; 2010.

36. Reece RM, Nicholson CE. *Inflicted Childhood Neurotrauma*. Elk Grove, IL: American Academy of Pediatrics; 2003.

37. Skellern CY, Wood DO, Murphy A, Crawford M. Non-accidental fractures in infants: risk of further abuse. *J Paediatr Child Health*. 200;36(6)L590-592.

38. Lazoritz S, Palusci VJ, eds. *The Shaken Baby Syndrome: A Multidisciplinary Approach*. New York City, NY: The Hayworth Maltreatment & Trauma Press; 2001.

39. Kellogg ND; The American Academy of Pediatrics Committee on Child Abuse and Neglect. Evaluation of suspected child physical abuse. *Pediatrics*. 2007;119(6):1232-1241.

40. Warrington SA, Wright CM; The Avon Longitudinal Study of Parents and Children Study Team. Accidents and resulting injuries in premobile infants: data from the ALSPAC study. *Arch Dis Child*. 2001;85(2):104-107.

41. Chadwick DL, Bertocci G, Castillo E, et al. Annual risk of death resulting from short falls among young children: less than 1 in 1 million. *Pediatrics*. 2008;121(6):1213-1224.

42. Khambalia A, Joshi P, Brussoni M, et al. Risk factors for unintentional injuries due to falls in children aged 0-6 years: a systematic review. *Inj Prev*. 2006;12(6):378-385.

43. Tarantino CA, Dowd MD, Murdock TC. Short vertical falls in infants. *Pediatr Emerg Care*. 1999;15(1):5-8.

44. Helfer RE, Slovis TL, Black M. Injuries resulting when small children fall out of bed. *Pediatrics*. 1977;60(4):533-535.

45. Lyons TJ, Oates K. Falling out of bed: a relatively benign occurrence. *Pediatrics*. 1993;92(1):125-127.

46. Nimityongskul P, Anderson LD. The likelihood of injuries when children fall out of bed. *J Pediatr Orthop*. 1987;7(2):184-186.

47. Musemeche CA, Barthel M, Cosentino C, Reynolds M. Pediatric falls from heights. *J Trauma*. 1991;31(10):1347-1349.

48. Chadwick DL, Chin S, Salerno C, Landsverk S, Kitchen L. Deaths from falls in children: how far is fatal? *J Trauma*. 1991;31(10):1353-1355.

49. Le TH, Gean AD. Imaging of head trauma. *Seminars in Roentgenology*. 2006;41(3): 177-189.

50. Rubin DM, Christian CW, Bilaniuk LT, Zazyczny KA, Durbin DR. Occult head injury in high-risk abused children. *Pediatrics*. 2003;111(6):1382-1386.

51. Cattaneo C, Marinelli E, Di Giancamillo A, et al. Sensitivity of autopsy and radiological examination in detecting bone fractures in an animal model: implications for the assessment of fatal child physical abuse. *Forensic Sci Int*. 2006;164(2-3):131-137.

52. Togioka BM, Arnold MA, Bathurst MA, et al. Retinal hemorrhages and shaken baby syndrome: an evidence-based review. *J Emerg Med*. 2009;37(1):98-106.

53. Duhaime AC, Alario AJ, Lewander WJ, et al. Head injury in very young children: mechanisms, injury types, and ophthalmologic findings in 100 hospitalized patients younger than 2 years of age. *Pediatrics*. 1992;90(2, pt 1):179-185.

54. Levin AV. Ocular manifestations of child abuse. In: Reece RM, Ludwig S, eds. *Child Abuse: Medical Diagnosis and Management*. 2nd ed. Philadelphia, PA: Lippincott Williams & Wilkins; 2001:97-107.

55. The Ophthalmology Child Abuse Working Party. Child abuse and the eye. *Eye.* 1999;13:3-10.

56. Aryan HE, Ghosheh FR, Jandial R, Levy ML. Retinal hemorrhage and pediatric brain injury: etiology and review of the literature. *J Clin Neurosci.* 2005;12(6):624-631.

57. Levy HL, Brown AE, Williams SE, de Juan E Jr. Vitreous hemorrhage as an ophthalmic complication of galactosemia. *J Pediatr.* 1996;129(6):922-925.

58. Morris AA, Hoffmann GF, Naughten ER, Monavari AA, Collins JE. Glutaric aciduria and suspected child abuse. *Arch Dis Child.* 1999;80(5):404-405.

59. Gayle MO, Kissoon N, Hered RW, Harwood-Nuss A. Retinal hemorrhage in the young child: a review of etiology, predisposed conditions, and clinical implications. *J Emerg Med.* 1995;13(2):233-239.

60. Odom A, Christ E, Kerr N, et al. Prevalence of retinal hemorrhages in pediatric patients after in-hospital cardiopulmonary resuscitation: a prospective study. *Pediatrics.* 1997;99(6):e3.

61. Katzman GH. Pathophysiology of neonatal subconjunctival hemorrhage. *Clin Pediatr (Phila).* 1992;31(3):149-152.

62. Caron H, Pearson A. Neuroblastoma. In: Voute PA, Barrett A, Stevens MCG. eds. *Cancer in Children.* 5th ed. Oxford, United Kingdom: Oxford University Press; 2005:337-352.

63. Dubowitz H, Giardino AP, Gustavson E. Child neglect: guidance for pediatricians. *Pediatr Rev.* 2000;21(4):111-116.

64. Zenel JA. Failure to thrive: a general pediatrician's perspective. *Pediatr Rev.* 1997;18(11):371-378.

65. Wilcox WD, Nieburg P, Miller DS. Failure to thrive: a continuing problem of definition. *Clin Pediatr (Phila).* 1989;28(9):391-394.

66. Cantwell HB. The neglect of child neglect. In: Helfer ME, Kempe RS, Krugman RD, eds. *The Battered Child.* 5th ed. Chicago, IL: University of Chicago Press; 1997:347-373.

67. Helfer RE. The neglect of our children. *Pediatr Clin North Am.* 1990;37(4):923-942.

68. Homer C, Ludwig S. Categorization of etiology of failure to thrive. *Am J Dis Child.* 1981;135(9):848-851.

69. Berwick DM, Levy JC, Kleinerman R. Failure to thrive: diagnostic yield of hospitalisation. *Arch Dis Child.* 1982;57:347-351.

70. Gahagan S, Holmes R. A stepwise approach to evaluation of undernutrition and failure to thrive. *Pediatr Clin North Am.* 1998;45(1):169-187.

71. Bithoney WG, Dubowitz H, Egan H. Failure to thrive/growth deficiency. *Pediatr Rev.* 1992;13(12):453-459.

72. Brandt L. Growth dynamics of low birth weight infants with emphasis on the perinatal period. In: Falkner F, Tanner JM, eds. *Human Growth: Neurobiology and Nutrition, Vol I.* New York, NY: Plenum; 1979.

73. Weidemann HR, Kunze J, Grosse HR. *Clinical Syndromes.* 3rd ed. London: Mosby; 1997.

74. Emans SJH, Goldstein DP. *Pediatrics and Adolescent Gynecology.* 3rd ed. Boston, MA: Little Brown & Co; 1990.

75. Wilson MD. Vaginal discharge and vaginal bleeding in childhood. In: Carpenter SE, Rock JA. *Pediatric and Adolescent Gynecology.* Philadelphia, PA: Lippincott-Raven; 1992:139-151.

76. Woodruff JD. Vulvar disease in the prepubertal child. In: Carpenter SE, Rock JA. *Pediatric and Adolescent Gynecology.* Philadelphia, PA: Lippincott-Raven; 1992:123-137.

77. Adams JA. Evolution of a classification scale: medical evaluation of suspected child sexual abuse. *Child Maltreat.* 2001;6(1):31-36.

78. Kellogg ND, Parra JM, Menard S. Children with anogenital symptoms and signs referred for sexual abuse evaluations. *Arch Pediatr Adolesc Med.* 1998;152:634-641.

79. American Academy of Pediatrics Committee on Child Abuse and Neglect. Guidelines for the evaluation of sexual abuse of children: subject review (RE9819). *Pediatrics.* 1999;103(1):186-191.

80. Kini N, Lazoritz S. Evaluation for possible physical or sexual abuse. *Pediatr Clin North Am.* 1998;45(1):205-219.

81. Jaquiery A, Stylianopoulos A, Hogg G, Grover S. Vulvovaginitis: clinical features, aetiology, and microbiology of the genital tract. *Arch Dis Child.* 1999;81(1):64-67.

82. Koumantakis EE, Hassan EA, Deligeoroglou EK, Creatsas GK. Vulvovaginitis during childhood and adolescence. *J Pediatr Adolesc Gynecol.* 1997;10(1):39-43.

83. Paradise JE, Campos JM, Friedman HM, Frishmuth G. Vulvovaginitis in premenarcheal girls: clinical features and diagnostic evaluation. *Pediatrics.* 1982;70:193-198.

84. O'Brien TJ. Paediatric vulvovaginitis. *Australas J Dermatol.* 1995;36(4):216-218.

85. Tunnessen WW. *Signs and Symptoms in Pediatrics.* 2nd ed. Philadelphia, PA: Lippincott; 1988.

86. Altchek A. Recognizing and controlling vulvovaginitis in children. *Contemp Pediatr.* 1985;2:59-70.

87. Gordon IB. Pediatric gynecology and adolescent issues: infections and skin disorders of the genitalia. In: Behrman RE, Vaughan VC, eds. *Nelson Textbook of Pediatrics.* 12th ed. Philadelphia, PA: WB Saunders Co; 1983:1515-1530.

88. Williams TS, Callen JP, Owen LG. Vulvar disorder in the prepubertal females. *Pediatr Ann.* 1986;15:588-605.

89. Quint EH, Smith YR. Vulvar disorders in adolescent patients. *Pediatr Clin North Am.* 1999;46(3):593-606.

90. Albers SE, Taylor G, Huyer D, Oliver G, Krafchik BR. Vulvitis circumscripta plasmacellularis mimicking child abuse. *J Am Acad Dermatol.* 2000;42(6):1078-1080.

91. Berth-Jones J, Graham-Brown RAC, Burns DA. Lichen sclerosus. *Arch Dis Child.* 1989;64:1204-1206.

92. Loening-Baucke V. Lichen sclerosus et atrophicus in children. *Am J Dis Child.* 1991;145(9):1058-1061.

93. Laymon CW, Freeman D. Relationship of balanitis xerotica obliterans to lichen sclerosis et atrophicus. *Arch Derm Syphilol.* 1944;49(1):57-59.

94. Rickwood AMK, Hemalatha V, Batcup G, Spitz L. Phimosis in boys. *Br J Urol.* 1980;52:147-150.

95. Preminger MK, Pokorny SF. Vaginal discharge: a common pediatric complaint. *Contemp Pediatr.* 1998;15:115-122.

96. Mogielnicki NP, Schwartzman JD, Elliott JA. Perineal group a streptococcal disease in pediatric practice. *Pediatrics.* 2000;106(2):276-281.

97. Clayden G. Anal appearance and child sexual abuse. *Lancet.* 1987:620-621.

98. Fink CW. A perianal rash in Kawasaki disease. *Pediatr Infect Dis.* 1983;2(2):140-141.

99. Emans SJ. Vulvovaginitis in the child and adolescent. *Pediatr Rev.* 1986;8(1):12-19.

100. Bays J, Jenny C. Genital and anal conditions confused with child sexual abuse trauma. *Am J Dis Child.* 1990;144(12):1319-1322.

101. Coffman KB, Boyce WT, Hansen RC. Phytophotodermatitis simulating child abuse. *Am J Dis Child.* 1985;139(3):239-240.

102. Dannaker CJ, Glover RA, Goltz RW. Phytophotodermatitis: a mystery case report. *Clin Pediatr (Phila).* 1988;27(6):289-290.

103. Murphy TV, Nelson JD. Shigella vaginitis: report of 38 patients and review of the literature. *Pediatrics.* 1979;63(4):511-516.

104. Watkins S, Quan L. Vulvovaginitis caused by *Yersinia enterocolitica. Pediatr Infect Dis.* 1984;3(5):444-445.

105. Breen JL, Maxson WS. Ovarian tumors in children and adolescents. *Clin Obstetr Gynecol.* 1977;20(3):607-623.

106. Levin AV, Selbst SM. Vulvar hemangioma simulating child abuse. *Clin Pediatr.* 1988; 27(4):213-215.

107. Imai A, Horibe S, Tamaya T. Genital bleeding in premenarcheal children. *Int J Gynaecol Obstet.* 1995;49:41-45.

108. Berkowitz CD, Elvik SL, Logan MK. Labial fusion in prepubescent girls: a marker for sexual abuse? *Am J Obstet Gynecol.* 1987;156(1):16-20.

109. McCann J, Voris J, Simon MA. Labial adhesions and posterior fourchette injuries in childhood sexual abuse. *Am J Dis Child.* 1988;142(6):659-663.

110. Johnson CF. Prolapse of urethra: confusion of clinical and anatomic characteristics with sexual abuse. *Pediatrics.* 1991;87(5):722-725.

111. Lowe FC, Hill GS, Jeffs RD, Brendler CB. Urethral prolapse in children: insights into etiology and management. *J Urol.* 1986;135(1):100-103.

112. Dodson AI. *Urological Surgery.* St. Louis, MO: CV Mosby; 1970.

113. Barton DJ, Sloan GM, Nichter LS, Reinisch JF. Hair-thread tourniquet syndrome. *Pediatrics.* 1988;82:925-928.

114. Press S, Schachner L, Paul P. Clitoris tourniquet syndrome. *Pediatrics.* 1980;66(5):781.

115. Singh B, Kim H, Wax SH. Strangulation of glans penis by hair. *Urology.* 1978;11(12):170-172.

116. Adams JA, Horton M. Is it sexual abuse? confusion caused by a congenital anomaly of the genitalia. *Clin Pediatr.* 1989;28(3):146-148.

Chapter 8

Clinical Aspects of Child Neglect

Tanya S. Hinds, MD, FAAP
Angelo P. Giardino, MD, PhD
Ann L. O'Sullivan, PhD, CPNP, FAAN

Key Points

1. Despite year-to-year variation in child maltreatment rates, occurrences of neglect consistently exceed physical and sexual abuse.[1]

2. Epidemiologically, predictors for substantiated child maltreatment and neglect include a male caregiver, poverty, and a high child care burden.[2] Socioeconomic status is inversely correlated with neglect.[1] Protective factors, which lower the risk of substantiated child maltreatment, include higher levels of support from family and friends; married status; higher income; and a high school diploma, at least.[2]

3. The notion of neglectful families being essentially isolated has given rise to the conceptualization of social impoverishment as a risk factor for child neglect. An impoverished environment often lacks the consistent supportive relationships that provide a source of nurturance and feedback to the family and provide a protective barrier against neglectful behavior.[3,4]

4. Failure to thrive (FTT) is an inadequate intake of calories relative to a child's need to maintain normal growth. FTT was classically described as either organic or nonorganic based on the underlying cause of the condition. Categorizing FTT based on the classification of organic or nonorganic was eventually seen to be less than complete. Taking a more holistic approach, Homer and Ludwig[5] described many cases of FTT as mixed FTT.

5. Acute consequences of neglect may range from exposure to environmental hazards to hunger, unidentified or untreated medical problems, and death. Over the short-term period, Hildyard et al[6] note that preschool- and school-aged survivors of physical and emotional neglect have more severe cognitive, language, and academic deficits and experience more attachment disorders, social isolation, and internalizing behavior compared to their physically abused peers. School-aged children who experience abuse or neglect are also at increased risk for behavioral problems as adults.

Introduction

A particular focus of this chapter is on the evaluation and management of forms of neglect likely to be identified in the health care setting. Typically, the role of health care provider includes a definition of the profession, which helps to guide clinical practice. In 1958, Virginia Henderson was asked by the Nursing Service Committee of the International Council of Nurses (ICN) to prepare a pamphlet on nursing. The definition included in her pamphlet continues to guide nursing clinical practice and is particularly relevant to nurses' work with children and families with regard to neglect. The definition states, "The unique function of the nurse is to assist the individual, sick or well, in the performance of those activities contributing to health or its recovery (or to a peaceful death) that he/she [*sic*] would perform unaided if he/she [*sic*] had the necessary strength, will, or knowledge."[7]

This chapter focuses on the health care evaluation and management of the following forms of neglect:

— ***Physical neglect:*** Inadequate food, clothing, shelter; avoidance of obvious environmental dangers

— ***FTT:*** Inadequate growth when compared to peers

— ***Medical neglect:*** Failure to access or provide reasonable health and medical care

Defining Neglect

Neglect is the most common form of child maltreatment. As a clinical entity, neglect spans a wide continuum of suboptimal caregiving from slightly-less-than-adequate parenting when measured against a generally accepted community standard to severely dangerous omissions in care that are likely to cause death.[8] Zuravin[9] identified at least 12 types of neglect including:

1. Refusal or delay in providing physical health care
2. Refusal or delay in providing mental health care
3. Supervisional neglect
4. Custody refusal
5. Custody-related neglect
6. Abandonment or desertion
7. Failure to provide a stable home
8. Neglect of personal hygiene
9. Housing hazards
10. Inadequate housing sanitation
11. Nutritional neglect
12. Educational neglect

Table 8-1 lists the various forms of child neglect generally recognized by child welfare experts.[10]

The unifying principle underlying each category is that a child's basic needs are not being met as a result of caregiver inattention or omission,[11] resulting in actual or potential harm to a child.

Each state defines neglect in various ways, ranging from statutes containing detailed listings of what constitutes neglect to broad inclusive language describing neglectful caregiving (**Table 8-2**).

Table 8-1. Types of Neglect	
PHYSICAL NEGLECT	
Safety	Conspicuous inattention to avoidable hazards in the home; inadequate nutrition, clothing, or hygiene; and other forms of reckless disregard of the child's safety and welfare, such as driving with the child while intoxicated and leaving a young child unattended in a motor vehicle
MEDICAL NEGLECT	
Refusal of health care	Failure to provide or allow needed care in accordance with recommendations of a competent health care professional for a physical injury, illness, medical condition, or impairment
Delay in health care	Failure to seek timely and appropriate medical care for a serious health problem that any reasonable layman would have recognized as needing professional medical attention
CUSTODY-RELATED NEGLECT	
Abandonment	Desertion of a child without arranging for reasonable care and supervision; this category includes cases in which children were not claimed within 2 days and when children were left by parents, substitutes, or both who gave no or false information about their whereabouts
Expulsion	Other blatant refusals of custody, such as permanent or indefinite expulsion of a child from the home without adequate arrangements for care by others, or refusal to accept custody of a returned runaway
Inadequate supervision	Child left unsupervised or inadequately supervised for extended periods or allowed to remain away from home overnight without the parent, substitute, or both knowing or attempting to determine, the child's whereabouts
Other custody issues	Custody-related forms of inattention to the child's needs other than those covered by abandonment or expulsion; for example, repeated shuttling of a child from one household to another because of apparent unwillingness to maintain custody or chronically and repeatedly leaving a child with others for days or weeks at a time
EMOTIONAL NEGLECT	
Inadequate nurturance or affection	Marked inattention to the child's needs for affection, emotional support, attention, or competence
Chronic or extreme abuse or IPV	Chronic or extreme spousal abuse or other IPV in the child's presence
Permitted abuse of drugs, alcohol, or both	Encouraging or permitting drug or alcohol use by the child; cases of the child's use of drugs, alcohol, or both are included if it appears that the parent or guardian had been informed of the problem and had not attempted to intervene.

(continued)

Table 8-1. Types of Neglect *(continued)*

EMOTIONAL NEGLECT	
Permitted other maladaptive behavior	Encouragement or permittance of other maladaptive behavior (eg, severe assaultiveness, chronic delinquency) in circumstances in which the parent or guardian has reason to be aware of the existence and seriousness of the problem, but does attempt to intervene
Refusal of psychological care	Refusal to allow needed and available treatment for a child's emotional or behavioral impairment or problem in accordance with competent professional recommendation
Delay in psychological care	Failure to seek or provide needed treatment for a child's emotional or behavioral impairment or problem that any reasonable layman would have recognized as needing professional psychological attention (eg, severe depression, suicide attempt)
Other emotional neglect	Other inattention to the child's developmental needs, emotional needs, or both not classified under any of the above forms of emotional neglect, such as markedly overprotective restrictions that foster immaturity or emotional overdependence or chronically applying expectations clearly inappropriate in relation to the child's age or level of development
EDUCATIONAL NEGLECT	
Permitted chronic truancy	Habitual truancy averaging at least 5 days per month is classifiable under this form of maltreatment if the parent or guardian has been informed of the problem and has not attempted to intervene.
Failure to enroll or other truancy	Failure to register or enroll a child of mandatory school age, causing the school-aged child to remain at home for nonlegitimate reasons (eg, to work, to care for siblings) an average of at least 3 days per month.
Inattention to special education need	Refusal to allow or failure to obtain recommended remedial education services or neglect in obtaining or following through with treatment for a child's diagnosed learning disorder or other special education need without reasonable cause

Reprinted from Gaudin JM Jr. Child Neglect: A Guide for Intervention. *Washington, DC: United States Department of Health and Human Services, Administration for Children and Families, Westover Consultants (Contract No HHS-105-89-1730); 1993.*

However, most state statutes and research literature agree on 9 components of neglect that revolve around a conceptualization of what comprises a child's basic needs. Neglect exists when these basic needs are not met and may be seen in cases that demonstrate the following[12]:

— Inadequate food

— Inadequate clothing

— Inadequate shelter

— Inadequate supervision

— Inadequate medical care

— Inadequate emotional care

— Inadequate education

— Exploitation

— Exposure to unwholesome circumstances

Table 8-2. Variations in State Definitions of Neglect

State	Definition
Detailed	
Arkansas	**Citation: Ann Code § 12-18-103** "Neglect" means failure or refusal to: — Prevent abuse of the child when the person knows or has reasonable cause to know the child is or has been abused — Provide necessary food, clothing, shelter, and education required by law, or medical treatment necessary for the child's well-being — Take reasonable action to protect the child from abandonment, abuse, sexual abuse, sexual exploitation, neglect, or parental unfitness when the existence of the condition was known or should have been known — Provide for essential and necessary physical, mental, or emotional needs of the child, including the failure to provide a shelter that does not pose a risk to the health or safety of the child — Provide for the child's care and maintenance; proper or necessary support; or medical, surgical, or other necessary care — Assume responsibility for the care and custody of the child or to participate in a plan to assume such responsibility — Appropriately supervise the child that results in the child being left alone at an inappropriate age or in inappropriate circumstances creating a dangerous situation or a situation that puts the child at risk of harm "Neglect" shall also include: — Causing a child to be born with an illegal substance in the child's bodily fluids or bodily substances as a result of the pregnant mother knowingly using an illegal substance before the birth of the child — At the time of the birth of a child, the presence of an illegal substance in the mother's bodily fluids or bodily substances as a result of the pregnant mother knowingly using an illegal substance before the birth of the child — An "illegal substance" is a drug that is prohibited to be used or possessed without a prescription. — A test of the child's or the mother's bodily fluids or bodily substances may be used as evidence to establish neglect.

(continued)

Table 8-2. Variations in State Definitions of Neglect *(continued)*

State	Definition
Detailed	
California	**Citation: Welf and Inst Code § 300** A child may be considered dependent when: —The child has suffered, or there is a substantial risk that the child will suffer, serious physical harm or illness as a result of: —The failure or inability of the parent or guardian to adequately supervise or protect the child —The willful or negligent failure of the parent or guardian to adequately supervise or protect the child from the conduct of the custodian with whom the child has been left —The willful or negligent failure of the parent or guardian to provide the child with adequate food, clothing, shelter, or medical treatment —The inability of the parent or guardian to provide regular care for the child due to the parent's or guardian's mental illness, developmental disability, or substance abuse —The child's sibling has been abused or neglected, and there is a substantial risk that the child will be abused or neglected. The court shall consider the circumstances surrounding the abuse or neglect of the sibling, the age and gender of each child, the nature of the abuse or neglect of the sibling, the mental condition of the parent or guardian, and any other factors the court considers probative in determining whether there is a substantial risk to the child.
Colorado	**Citation: Rev Stat §§ 19-1-103; 19-3-102** The term "child abuse or neglect" includes any case in which a child is in need of services because the child's parent has failed to provide adequate food, clothing, shelter, medical care, or supervision that a prudent parent would take. A child is "neglected" or "dependent" if: —The parent, guardian, or legal custodian has subjected the child to mistreatment or abuse or has allowed another to mistreat or abuse the child without taking lawful means to stop such mistreatment or abuse and prevent it from recurring —The child lacks proper parental care through the actions or omissions of the parent, guardian, or legal custodian —The child's environment is injurious to his or her welfare —The parent, guardian, or legal custodian fails or refuses to provide the child with proper or necessary subsistence, education, medical care, or any other necessary care

(continued)

Table 8-2. Variations in State Definitions of Neglect *(continued)*

State	Definition
Detailed	
Colorado	— The child is homeless, without proper care, or not domiciled with his or her parent, guardian, or legal custodian through no fault of such parent, guardian, or legal custodian. — The child has run away from home or is otherwise beyond the control of his or her parent, guardian, or legal custodian. — The child tests positive at birth for either a schedule I or schedule II controlled substance, unless the child tests positive for a schedule II controlled substance as a result of the mother's lawful intake of such substance as prescribed. *EXCEPTIONS* **Citation: Rev Stat §§ 19-1-103; 19-3-103** Those investigating cases of child abuse shall take into account child-rearing practices of the culture in which the child participates, including the work-related practices of agricultural communities. The reasonable exercise of parental discipline is not considered abuse. No child who, in lieu of medical treatment, is under treatment solely by spiritual means through prayer in accordance with a recognized method of religious healing shall, for that reason only, be considered neglected. The religious rights of the parent shall not limit the access of a child to medical care in a life-threatening situation.
New York	**Citation: Soc Serv Law § 371** "Neglected child" means a child younger than age 18 whose physical, mental, or emotional condition has been impaired or is in imminent danger of becoming impaired as a result of the failure of his or her parent or other person legally responsible for his or her care to exercise a minimum degree of care: — In supplying the child with adequate food, clothing, shelter, education, or medical or surgical care, although financially able to do so or offered financial or other reasonable means to do so — In providing the child with proper supervision or guardianship — By unreasonably inflicting or allowing harm to be inflicted, or a substantial risk thereof, including the infliction of excessive corporal punishment — By misusing drugs or alcoholic beverages to the extent that he or she loses self-control of his or her actions — By any other acts of a similarly serious nature requiring the aid of the court

(continued)

Table 8-2. Variations in State Definitions of Neglect *(continued)*

State	Definition
Detailed	
New York	**Citation: Soc Serv Law § 371** "Neglected child" means a child younger than age 18 whose physical, mental, or emotional condition has been impaired or is in imminent danger of becoming impaired as a result of the failure of his or her parent or other person legally responsible for his or her care to exercise a minimum degree of care: — In supplying the child with adequate food, clothing, shelter, education, or medical or surgical care, although financially able to do so or offered financial or other reasonable means to do so — In providing the child with proper supervision or guardianship — By unreasonably inflicting or allowing harm to be inflicted, or a substantial risk thereof, including the infliction of excessive corporal punishment — By misusing drugs or alcoholic beverages to the extent that he or she loses self-control of his or her actions — By any other acts of a similarly serious nature requiring the aid of the court
West Virginia	**Citation: Ann Code § 49-1-3** "Neglected child" means a child: — Whose physical or mental health is harmed or threatened by a present refusal, failure, or inability of the child's parent, guardian, or custodian to supply the child with necessary food, clothing, shelter, supervision, medical care, or education — Who is presently without necessary food, clothing, shelter, medical care, education, or supervision because of the disappearance or absence of the child's parent or custodian "Child abuse and neglect" or "child abuse or neglect" means negligent treatment or maltreatment of a child by a parent, guardian, or custodian who is responsible for the child's welfare under circumstances that harm or threaten the health and welfare of the child. "Imminent danger to the physical well-being of the child" means an emergency situation in which the welfare or the life of the child is threatened. Such emergency situations may include: — Nutritional deprivation — Inadequate treatment of serious illness or disease

(continued)

Table 8-2. Variations in State Definitions of Neglect *(continued)*

State	Definition
Moderate	
Idaho	**Citation: Idaho Code § 16-1602** "Neglected" means a child: — Who is without proper parental care and control, subsistence, medical, or other care necessary for his or her well-being because of the conduct or omission of his or her parents, guardian, or other custodian, or their neglect or refusal to provide them — Whose parents, guardian, or other custodian is unable to discharge his or her responsibilities to and for the child and, as a result of such inability, the child lacks the parental care necessary for his or her health, safety, or well-being — Who has been placed for care or adoption in violation of the law — Who is without proper education because of the failure to comply with § 33-202
Iowa	**Citation: Ann Stat § 232.68** The terms "child abuse" or "abuse" include: — The failure on the part of a person responsible for the care of a child to provide adequate food, shelter, clothing, or other care necessary for the child's health and welfare when financially able to do so or when offered financial or other reasonable means to do so — The presence of an illegal drug in a child's body as a direct and foreseeable consequence of the acts or omissions of the person responsible for the care of the child — That the person responsible for the care of a child has, in the presence of the child, manufactured a dangerous substance or possesses a product containing ephedrine, its salts, optical isomers, salts of optical isomers, or pseudoephedrine, its salts, optical isomers, or salts of optical isomers, with the intent to use the product as a precursor or an intermediary to a dangerous substance — Knowingly allowing a person to have custody or control of, or unsupervised access to a child after knowing the person is required to register or is on the sex offender registry
Kansas	**Citation: Ann Stat § 38-2202** "Neglect" means acts or omissions by a parent, guardian, or person responsible for the care of a child that results in harm to a child or presents a likelihood of harm, and the acts or omissions are not due solely to the lack of financial means of the child's parents or other custodian. Neglect may include but shall not be limited to: — Failure to provide the child with food, clothing, or shelter necessary to sustain life or health — Failure to provide adequate supervision of a child or to remove a child from a situation that requires judgment or actions beyond the child's level of maturity, physical condition, or mental abilities and that results in bodily injury or a likelihood of harm to the child — Failure to use resources available to treat a diagnosed medical condition if such treatment will make a child substantially more comfortable, reduce pain and suffering, or correct or substantially diminish a crippling condition from worsening

(continued)

Table 8-2. Variations in State Definitions of Neglect *(continued)*

State	Definition
Moderate	
Montana	**Citation: Ann Code § 41-3-10** "Physical neglect" means: —Failure to provide basic necessities, including but not limited to appropriate and adequate nutrition, protective shelter from the elements, and appropriate clothing related to weather conditions —Failure to provide cleanliness and general supervision —Exposing or allowing the child to be exposed to an unreasonable physical or psychological risk to the child "Physical or psychological harm to a child" means the harm that occurs whenever the parent or other person responsible for the child's welfare: —Causes malnutrition, failure to thrive, or otherwise fails to supply the child with adequate food; fails to supply clothing, shelter, education, or adequate health care, though financially able to do so or when offered financial or other reasonable means to do so —Exposes the child, or allows the child to be exposed, to an unreasonable risk to the child's health or welfare by failing to intervene or eliminate the risk "Withholding of medically indicated treatment" means failure to respond to an infant's life-threatening conditions by not providing treatment, including appropriate nutrition, hydration, and medication, that in the treating physician's or physicians' reasonable medical judgment is most likely to be effective in ameliorating or correcting the conditions.
Minimal	
Georgia	**Citation: Ann Code § 19-7-5(b)** The term "child abuse" includes neglect or exploitation of a child by a parent or caregiver *Physical Abuse* "Abused or neglected child" means a child whose physical health, psychological growth and development, or welfare is harmed or is at substantial risk of harm by the acts or omissions of his or her parent or other person responsible for the child's welfare. "Harm" can occur by physical injury. "Physical injury" means death, permanent or temporary disfigurement, or impairment of any bodily organ or function by other than accidental means. *Neglect*
Vermont	**Citation: Ann Stat Tit 33, § 4912** "Harm" can occur by failure to supply the child with adequate food, clothing, shelter, or health care.

(continued)

Table 8-2. Variations in State Definitions of Neglect *(continued)*

State	Definition
Minimal	
Washington	**Citation: Rev Code § 26.44.020; 9A.42.100** "Negligent treatment or maltreatment" means an act or a failure to act, or the cumulative effects of a pattern of conduct, behavior, or inaction, that evidences a serious disregard of consequences of such magnitude as to constitute a clear and present danger to a child's health, welfare, or safety, including but not limited to conduct prohibited under § 9A.42.100—endangerment with a controlled substance. When considering whether a clear and present danger exists, evidence of a parent's substance abuse as a contributing factor to negligent treatment or maltreatment shall be given great weight. It is "endangerment with a controlled substance" if the person knowingly or intentionally permits a dependent child to be exposed to, ingest, inhale, or have contact with methamphetamine or ephedrine, pseudoephedrine, or anhydrous ammonia, including their salts, isomers, and salts of isomers, that are being used in the manufacture of methamphetamine, including its salts, isomers, and salts of isomers.

Adapted from Child Welfare Information Gateway. Definitions of child abuse and neglect. Child Welfare Information Gateway Web site. https://www.childwelfare.gov/systemwide/laws_policies/statutes/define.pdf#Page=7&view=Fit. Published February 2011. Accessed June 23, 2013.

Epidemiology of Neglect

Despite year-to-year variation in child maltreatment rates, occurrences of neglect consistently exceed those of physical and sexual abuse. Data from 2009 show 78.3% of reported maltreatment cases were for neglect, 17.8% for physical abuse; and 9.5% for sexual abuse.[1] Despite its prevalence, neglect generally receives less attention in research literature and the public policy arena compared to physical and sexual abuse. This prompts some to criticize the neglect of neglect,[13] which may result from its relationship to poverty, indolent and insidious nature, generally low-tech management, and relationship to a host of other associated social problems.[14,15]

The *Fourth National Incidence Study (NIS-4)* aggregated child maltreatment data from child protective services (CPS), social services, and law enforcement agencies during 3-month periods in 2005 and 2006.[16] The NIS-4 used 2 standards known as the harm standard and the endangerment standard to categorize child abuse and neglect. Under the harm standard, 1 in every 58 children experience child abuse or neglect, while under the endangered standard, 1 in every 25 children experience child abuse or neglect. Regardless, neglect is the prevalent form of child maltreatment as defined by either standard.

The harm standard considered a child to be neglected if he or she had obviously experienced an act of omission that clearly resulted in demonstrable harm. Using the stringent harm standard, an estimated 61% of 1.25 million maltreated children experienced neglect (approximately 771 700 children). Almost one-half of these children experienced educational neglect (360 500 children), one-third physically neglect (295 300 children), and one-quarter emotional neglected (193 400children). Using the harm standard, there has been no overall change in physical, emotional, or educational neglect between the *Third National Incidence Study (NIS-3)* completed in 1993 and the NIS-4[16] **(Table 8-3)**.

Table 8-3. National Incidence of Harm Standard Maltreatment in the NIS-4 (2005-2006) and Comparison with the NIS-3 (1993) and the NIS-2 (1986) Harm Standard Estimates

Harm Standard Maltreatment Category	NIS-4 Estimates 2005–2006		Comparisons with Earlier Studies			
			NIS-3 Estimates 1993		NIS-2 Estimates 1986	
	Total No. of Children	Rate per 1000 Children	Total No. of Children	Rate per 1000 Children	Total No. of Children	Rate per 1000 Children
All Maltreatment	1 256 600	17.1	1 553 800	23.1 m	931 000	14.8 ns
Abuse:						
All abuse	553 300	7.5	743 200	11.1*	507 700	8.1 ns
Physical Abuse	323 000	4.4	381 700	5.7 m	269 700	4.3 ns
Sexual Abuse	135 300	1.8	217 700	3.2*	119 200	1.9 ns
Emotional Abuse	148 500	2.0	204 500	3.0 m	155 200	2.5 ns
Neglect:						
All Neglect	771 700	10.5	879 000	13.1 ns	474 800	7.5 m
Physical Neglect	295 300	4.0	338 900	5.0 ns	167 800	2.7 m
Emotional Neglect	193 400	2.6	212 800	3.2 ns	49 200	0.8*
Educational Neglect‡	360 500	4.9	397 300	5.9 ns	284 800	4.5 ns

* *The difference between this and the NIS–4 incidence rate is significant at p<.05.*
m The difference between this and the NIS–4 incidence rate is statistically marginal (ie, .10>p>.05).
ns The difference between this and the NIS–4 incidence rate is neither significant nor marginal (p>.10).
‡*Educational neglect is identical under the Harm and Endangerment Standards. It is included in both tables because it is in the summary categories in both standards: All Neglect and All Maltreatment*
Note: Estimated totals are rounded to the nearest 100.
Reprinted from Sedlak AJ, Mettenburg J, Basena M, et al. Fourth National Incidence Study of Child Abuse and Neglect (NIS-4). *Washington, DC: United States Department of Health and Human Services; 2010.*

The endangerment standard identified an estimated 77% of nearly 3 million children (approximately 2 251 600 children) who either: (1) met the harm standard for neglect, (2) had not yet been harmed but were thought to be endangered by neglect by sentinel reporters, or (3) had experienced neglect substantiated by CPS. Slightly more than one-half of the children were physically neglected (1 192 200 children), with a similar number estimated to be emotionally neglected (1 173 800 children). Approximately 16% experienced educational neglect (360 500 children). Under the endangerment standard, the estimated number of emotionally neglected children significantly increased from 584 100 in 1993 to 1 173 800 in 2005-2006.

Fatal Child Neglect

Between 2008 and 2009, an estimated 1770 children are known to have died from child maltreatment,[1] with 66.7% of the children either victims of neglect exclusively or a combination of neglect and other forms of maltreatment. More than one-third (35.8%) of the 2008-2009 fatalities were exclusively due to neglect while less than one-third (23.2%) of the fatalities resulted exclusively from physical abuse. Each year more children die from neglect than from physical abuse.[17] Fatal child neglect typically occurs in the context of lack of physical or supervisional neglect. For example, a lapse in supervision may result in drowning or death in a fire. In rare cases, severe nutritional neglect may result in death.[18]

Risk and Protective Factors for Neglect

No theory fully explains or predicts neglectful behavior, but research has identified associated risks for neglect. Researchers and clinicians agree that for neglect to occur, the caregiving inadequacy or omission must result in some observable disruption in the general well-being of the child.[10,19] In clinical practice, disruption spans a wide continuum of observations ranging from minor disruptions in the child's care to cases so severe that a lack of provision for the child's basic needs leads to disability or death.[20,21]

Epidemiologically, predictors for substantiated child maltreatment and neglect include male caregiver, poverty, and a high child care burden.[2] Socioeconomic status is inversely correlated with neglect.[1] It is unclear whether minority race is related to neglect or whether the increased representation of minorities compared with their population is due to lower socioeconomic circumstance. Protective factors which lower risk of substantiated child maltreatment include higher levels of family support, married status, support from friends, higher income, and a high school diploma, at least.[2]

Ecological Models of Neglect: Child, Family, and Community Characteristics

Parental depression, parental substance abuse, and intimate partner violence (IPV) have historically been associated with child neglect. However, definitions that focus exclusively on the parent's deficits have proven to be of little value in designing interventions and have been criticized for reinforcing negative images of some societal groups, such as the poor or young parents.[22] The professional view of neglect has evolved over time, and the field has moved from psychopathological models focused on blaming deficient parents to ***ecological models*** focused more on contributing factors that cause those in a given environment to inadequately meet a child's basic needs.[19,23] In the ecological approach, parents in specific communities and the larger community in general each have a role to play in making sure that the child's basic needs are met. Rather than absolving parents from the responsibility of nurturing and protecting their children, ecologically-based models seek to define a shared responsibility that identifies social factors that influence their ability to provide that care.[8]

Garbarino[24] applied ecological concepts initially developed by Hawley[25] and Bonfenbrenner[26] to the problem of child maltreatment and neglect. In the ecological model, neglect arises from a mismatch between child and family as well as a mismatch between family and neighborhood or community. This ecological asynchrony manifests itself in that neglectful families are consistently unable to access basic family support systems within their environments. The notion of neglectful families being essentially isolated has given rise to the conceptualization of social impoverishment as a risk factor for child neglect. An impoverished environment often lacks the consistent supportive relationships that are a source of nurturance and feedback to the family and provide a protective barrier against neglectful behavior.[3,4] There is also a relationship between socially impoverished neighborhoods and neglectful parents who do not seem to have the social or interpersonal connections with others that generally characterize the non-neglectful parents who experience and describe a healthier and more supportive environment.[22,27]

Research studies have shown that neglectful parents tend to perceive their neighborhoods and communities as more socially cold and isolated than do non-neglectful parents.[3,4,28] Neglectful parents may manifest a self-fulfilling prophecy of sorts in that their perception of a socially impoverished environment leads to behavioral patterns that further isolate them. This self-fulfilling prophecy may be realized because the neglectful parents' neighbors perceive that neglectful parents will not appreciate or reciprocate positive interchanges when extended in social situations. This results in a vicious cycle in which the parents' perceptions of isolation lead to further isolation. The etiology of child neglect depends on several complex factors and interactions. However, in the neglect scenario, there seems to be a fairly consistent component of social isolation or impoverishment, whether actual or perceived.[28]

Burke et al[22] define neglect as a characteristic pattern of parental behavior sustained by problematic parent capacities to use knowledge, support, and resources in carrying out the parental role. This definition describes a general pattern of parenting performance that would be amenable to nursing approaches to health promotion discussed by various nursing theorists, including Virginia Henderson. Viewing this in the context of a shared responsibility paradigm as advocated by Dubowitz et al[8] ideally speaks to the strengths that the nursing profession brings to dealing with child neglect. Intervention strategies are best designed with attention to shared contributions that the individual caregiver, family, community, and society can each make toward the solution.[29] This takes into account that parents and other caregivers remain ultimately responsible and are accountable for the well-being of their children despite challenging environmental conditions.[8]

The preceding discussion of the ecological approaches to the issue of neglect demonstrates the systems nature of this model and makes clear the interrelatedness of the participants and their social and physical environment.[19,30-33] The "eco" in each of these approaches comes from the belief that maltreatment or neglect is the end result of complex interactions among potential risk factors within the abuser (eg, depression), his or her family (eg, single-parent family), and the environment (eg, social isolation). To understand prevention and treatment of neglect, ecological theorists focus on interactions between a large number of risk and resilience factors present among the child, parents, and sociocultural environment. The ecological model ensures a broad approach to the study of neglect and is concordant with the health promotion role that underpins the role and function of nurses and nursing in the health care setting.

Basic Needs of Children

Dubowitz[34] notes that clinicians are often tasked with diagnosing neglect in the context of varying definitions of neglect, state laws, and child welfare mandates. He eloquently frames neglect as centered on the needs or rights of children and the circumstances that indicate the child's needs or rights are not being meet,[8,34] rather than defining neglect in the context of parental blame. This is a very useful framework for nurses striving for a consistent, child-centered approach to the identification and management of neglect.

The basic needs of children vary at different ages and developmental levels. A 2-month-old infant's total dependence on the responses of caregivers for all of his or her needs is starkly contrasted with the needs of a 17-year-old high school senior. Hobbs et al[35] describe a clinical viewpoint that addresses the positive needs of children and includes the following:

— Food

— Warmth

— Clothing

— Shelter and protection

— Grooming and hygiene

— Fresh air and sunlight

— Activity and rest

— Prevention from illness and accidents

— Affection

— Continuity of care

— Security of belonging

— Self-esteem

— Opportunity to learn

— Opportunity to achieve independence and success

Further, Ludwig and Rostain[36] developed a useful description of neglect based on family functioning and dysfunction that contrast too much and too little attention to a child's basic needs. **Table 8-4** juxtaposes the excess and inadequate provision of the child's needs.

Table 8-4. Family Dysfunction

Task	Dysfunctional Inadequacy	Dysfunctional Excess
Providing for physical needs		
— Protection — Food — Housing — Health care	— Failure to protect — Child abuse — Underfeeding — Homelessness — Medical neglect	— Overprotection and overanxiety — Overfeeding and obesity — Multiple residences — "Yo-yo"/vagabond children — Excessive medical care — Medical child abuse
Providing for developmental, behavioral, and emotional needs		
Stimulation	*Understimulation*	*Overstimulation*
— Developmental and cognitive — Guidance (approval and discipline) — Affection (acceptance, intimacy)	— Neglect — Inadequate approval — Overcriticism — Psychological abuse — Inadequate affection — Emotional neglect — Rejection — Hostility	— "Hothousing" — Parental perfectionism — Overindulgence — Spoiled child — Sexual abuse — Incest
Socialization		
— Intrafamilial relationship — Extrafamilial community relationships	— Attenuated family relationships — Distanced parents — Boundaryless families — Deficiency in training in extrafamilial relationships	— Parenting enmeshment — Overinvolved relationships — Insular families — Excessive restriction from extrafamilial relationships

Reprinted with permission from Ludwig S, Rostain A. Family function and dysfunction. In: Levine MD, Carey WB, Crocker AC, eds. Developmental-Behavioral Pediatrics. *2nd ed. Philadelphia, PA: WB Saunders; 1992:147-159.*

Perceptions about Neglect

The results of studies comparing the perceptions of both parents and professionals about the presence or absence of child neglect vary, but suggest that differences do exist between professional and laypeople's views of neglect.[12,37] In general, there is broad agreement among laypeople, CPS professionals, and people of different ethnic, socioeconomic, and geographic groups about situations that place children at risk of harm.[38] However, modest differences exist with respect to views about specific forms of neglect. In general, CPS professionals tended to have a higher threshold than mothers for physical and psychological neglect.[38] Interestingly, CPS workers differed amongst themselves, with investigative CPS workers more likely to see physical, medical, nutritional, and psychological neglect as more serious than service-providing CPS workers.[37] In addition to these varying perceptions among parents and professionals, there are other modest differences among ethnic and socioeconomic groups concerning the physical care and neglect of a child.[12,37,38] Lower- and middle-class African American parents may be more concerned than their middle-class white counterparts about physical care, such as maintenance of household furnishings, availability of utilities, physical safety of the home, and sanitation.[38] Middle-income African American and white parents may be more concerned about psychological care than unemployed welfare-dependent caregivers.[38]

Neglect in the Health Care Setting

The health care setting demonstrates a focus on anticipatory guidance concerning environmental safety and child development, physical assessments, and medical treatment for acute and chronic diseases, and as a result, physical, medical, and nutritional neglect are more likely to come to the health care provider's attention.

Physical Neglect

Presentation

Physical neglect involves a caregiver's failure to provide adequate shelter, personal hygiene opportunities, clothing, nutrition, or other forms of disregard for a child's basic needs and safety. The NIS-4[16] also includes abandonment, illegal transfer of custody, and unstable custody arrangements in the definition of physical neglect. Physical neglect may come to light either from a single episode that points to a serious breach in acceptable parenting or from multiple episodes that suggest a lack of reasonable supervision or little attention or ability to create and maintain a safe environment. Young children with mental health diagnoses, behavioral problems, and chronic medical illnesses are at increased risk for child maltreatment, including neglect.[39]

Possible indicators of physical neglect in the health care setting are as follows:

- A hungry child who reports having to prepare his or her own meals or reports frequently missing meals
- Improper clothing for seasonal or environmental conditions; clothing that is too small
- Unkempt appearance with dirty, excessively soiled clothing; filth in skin creases
- Multiple bruises or abrasions attributed to frequent falls

Findings indicating that a child is unwashed will be obvious during a visit. Such findings may indicate that the child's living environment is unsanitary or even that the child is homeless. Conversely, custody-related forms of physical neglect are varied and more nuanced. The child may be brought in for care by a caregiver who reports the child as abandoned or endangered by a second caregiver. This should raise concern for physical neglect. However, the more subtle forms of physical or custody-related neglect may elude the health care provider, especially if the parent does not provide accurate information about the child's caregiving and living situation.

Epidemiology

An estimated 295 300 children (4 per 1000)[16] experienced harm-standard physical neglect from 2005 to 2006. To be included in the harm standard for physical neglect, a parent or parent-substitute must have been responsible for demonstrable injury to or impairment in the child that was serious or fatal. Using the more inclusive endangerment standard, 1 1922000 children (16.2 per 1000 or 1 in every 62 children) were physically neglected in the United States. Those counted under the endangerment standard included any adult caregiver who failed to provide appropriate care, thus not meeting the child's basic needs, or who demonstrated disregard for the child's safety. The rate of endangerment standard physical neglect was highest among children aged 3 to 8 years (15.3 per 1000), reflecting their greater needs for physical care and supervision than older children. Black children had more than 1.5 times the rate of both harm standard and endangerment standard physical neglect compared with Hispanic and white children.[16]

Finally, there were marked differences in the rate of physical neglect for various family income levels using both standards. The highest rates were for children in families earning less than $15000 per year followed by those in families earning between $15 000 and $29 999 per year. The lowest rate of physical neglect was in families earning $30 000 or more.[40] Professional literature debates whether or not the income relationship is real or merely an artifact of how the data are reported and collected.

History

Even the most diligent caregiver may make an omission that results in actual or potential harm to a child. More often, the types of physical neglect that may come to light in the health care setting revolve around eliciting a history of behaviors or decisions that demonstrate inattention to avoidable risks to the child. Obtaining a history of physical neglect often depends on the history provided by the caregiver and the presence of other responsible adults in the child's environment who may fill in the gaps for the child. Depending on the setting and reason for seeking care, custody-related issues may or may not come to light during history taking.

The health care provider may use open-ended screening questions or comments directed at the caregiver or child to identify whether the child's basic needs are being addressed:

- Hygiene
    - What access do you have to bathing and laundry facilities?
    - Who helps you (child) take a bath or brush your teeth?
    - Clothing or shelter (for a child who is inappropriately dressed for the season)
    - How did you decide what to wear today?
- Shelter or housing
    - How is your home kept clean?
    - What do you dislike or wish you could change about where you live?
    - Have you (caregiver) made any changes to your home because of your children?

— Custody or supervision

— Who cares for children when you (caregiver) need a break or have to run an errand?

— Have you (child) ever been at home without a grownup?

— What would you (child) do in case of an emergency?

The health care provider may also ask specific questions about well-known environmental hazards. Examples include:

— How do you heat your home in the winter?

— Are you able to adjust your water heater to a safe setting?

— Where are the smoke alarms installed in your home?

— How is your child restrained when traveling in an automobile?

— Do you (child) use a bicycle helmet?

— Is the gun in your home stored separately from the bullets?

— Do you have the phone number for the Poison Center (1-800-222-1222) in more than one location?

Physical Examination

It is important to assess the physical appearance of the child. Poor hygiene and inappropriate dress may become apparent on examination. The health care provider should note general appearance, including degree of cleanliness, infestations with parasites such as scabies and pediculosis capitis, and appropriateness of dress for weather conditions. If clothing is inappropriate for the external climate, the health care provider should look for any evidence of environmental exposure, such as frostbite on the fingers or toes. Lack of gloves or inappropriate foot coverings in cold weather should be noted. Additionally, the health care provider should look for evidence of acute or healed skin injuries and check the child's medical records to determine the history that the caregiver provided for prior injuries.

Clinical Observations of Caregiver-Child Interactions

In observing the caregiver-child interaction, the health care provider should note whether the caregiver responds to the child's natural curiosity about the environment in a supportive manner and then redirects the child to safer activities. For example, if the child touches the electric receptacle, does the caregiver redirect the child to a more appropriate activity? If the child climbs on a chair, does the caregiver move into a position to offer assistance and protection, or does it appear that the child is ignored?

Laboratory Assessment

The clinician should order laboratory studies according to diagnostic considerations suggested by the clinical information. For example, a toxicology screen may be indicated if there is concern about ingestion, or parental drug use is strongly suspected.

Failure to Thrive

Presentation

A child who fails to grow as expected, compared to peers of the same age, gender, and ethnicity is traditionally referred to as having a failure to thrive. When there is reasonable evidence that a child's nutritional needs are not being met by the child's primary caregiver(s), concern about nutritional neglect should be raised. Nutritional neglect may manifest as FTT; however, FTT is a symptom rather than a diagnosis.[41]

Although some professionals suggest more appropriate terms, such as *growth failure* or *growth faltering*, these have not taken root in the health care setting and FTT remains entrenched in the lexicon of most pediatric clinicians.[42]

FTT was classically described as either organic or nonorganic. Organic FTT was initially seen as a failure to grow adequately based on the presence of an underlying medical condition that could be evaluated and diagnosed. Several medical conditions may be associated with FTT (see *Chapter 7, Differential Diagnosis: Conditions That Mimic Child Maltreatment*). Nonorganic FTT, on the other hand, was traditionally seen as a failure to grow according to expectations secondary to underlying psychosocial dysfunction unfavorably affected by the parenting received by the child. Adverse psychosocial factors that may contribute to nonorganic FTT include many of the sequelae of poverty along with parental strife, parental medical or mental health diagnoses, social isolation, substance abuse, parents focused on activities external to the home, and lack of knowledge about normal growth and formula or food preparation.[43] This polarity between organic and nonorganic FTT was eventually seen to be less than complete. Taking a more holistic approach, Homer and Ludwig[5] described many cases of FTT as mixed FTT. Ultimately, FTT is inadequate intake of calories relative to a child's need to maintain normal growth. FTT can, therefore, occur across all segments of society. The evaluation of a child's growth pattern involves a history, physical examination, and laboratory evaluations as well as observations of parent-child interactions, especially regarding feeding. Possible indicators of FTT in the health care setting are as follows:

— Weight or height below the 5th percentile for age and sex on more than one occasion

— Weight crossing at least 2 major percentiles over time (eg, from 75th to 25th) from a previously established curve

— No weight gain for age after addressing issues with the caregivers regarding feeding and provision of appropriate calories

History

The history in an FTT evaluation focuses on several key issues:

— Prenatal history

— Multiple miscarriages, suggesting a genetic disorder

— Use of tobacco, alcohol, or illicit substances during pregnancy

— Use of prescribed medications during pregnancy

— Birth history

— Preterm or full term infant

— Asphyxia, infection, or other perinatal complications

— Birth weight, length, and head circumference

— Maternal perception of feeding difficulties

— Medical history

— Availability of newborn screening report available[44]

— Vomiting or excessive spitting up

— Frequent, large, or oily stools

— Difficulty or pain with sucking, chewing, or swallowing

— Recurrent respiratory infections

— Medical diagnoses: cardiac disease, obstructive sleep apnea, urinary tract infections (UTIs)

— Hospitalizations, surgeries, and emergency room (ER) visits

— Developmental milestones

— Loss of previously acquired milestones

— Previous medical workups and results of previous interventions

— Eczema or urticaria exacerbating by select foods

— Family history

— Weight and height of biological parents and siblings

— Parental history of growth delay in childhood

— Current and past medical and mental health diagnoses of parents and siblings

— Maternal postpartum depression

— Social history

— Difficulty purchasing or preparing formula or food

— Structure of feedings or meal times

— Caregiver typically responsibly for feeding the child

— Perception of child's behaviors and interactions around meal times

— Dietary history

— Breastfeeding frequency and duration of active suck at each breast

— Formula-frequency, type and preparation, quantity of each typical feed

— Change in feeding patterns overnight

— Water, juices, and sodas in a typical 24-hour period

— Food allergies, intolerances or food restrictions

Physical Examination

When considering FTT, accurate measurement of growth parameters and trends over time is essential. General appearance should be assessed for symptoms and signs of other forms of neglect or maltreatment, such as severe diaper rash or widespread dental decay. The clinician should complete a head-to-toe physical examination, focusing on any findings that suggest a primary pathophysiological condition of the various systems examined. Wheezing and decreased breath sounds on lung examination suggest pulmonary disease, whereas a non-innocent murmur suggests cardiac disease as a contributor to abnormal weight gain. It is important to assess skin integrity and evaluate muscle mass to determine the child's general nutritional status. The neurological and musculoskeletal examination also helps to assess coordination and developmental level (see *Chapter 7, Differential Diagnosis: Conditions That Mimic Child Maltreatment*). The physical examination in a FTT evaluation focuses on several key issues:

— Vital signs

— Normal or abnormal

— Presence or absence of pain

— General appearance

— Dysmorphisms

— Activity level (lethargic infant, hyperactive toddler)

— Engagement with caregiver (eye contact, physical approximation, checking)[45]

— Oral-motor difficulties with feeding

— Hygiene (skin, nails, clothes)

— Head, eyes, ears, nose, throat (HEENT)

— Dry, dull hair, or hair loss

— Fontanel size

— Absent red reflex

— Otitis

— Mucus membrane abnormalities

— Glossitis

— Thrush

— Delayed dental eruption

— Dental caries or abscesses

— Enlarged tonsils

— Neck

— Cervical lymphadenopathy

— Torticollis

— Cardiovascular

— Murmur

— Abnormal femoral pulses

— Chest and lungs

— Retractions

— Wheezing, crackles, or both

— Abdomen

— Abdominal masses

— Hepatomegaly

— Genitalia

— Severe diaper rashes

— Anal fissures or hemorrhoids

— Extremities

— Edema

— Decreased muscle mass

— Skin

— Loss of subcutaneous tissue

— Thrush

— Bruises or scars

— Hygiene, including nails and hair

— Neurologic

— Hypotonia or hypertonia

Clinical Observations of Caregiver-Child Interactions

As with any evaluation for child neglect, careful observation of how the caregiver interacts with the child is valuable. In the FTT evaluation, special attention is given to how the parent addresses the child's hunger and thirst, how food is provided, and the observable care given in responding to the child's cues.[46] Additionally, the response of the child to the caregiver is important to note. The health care provider should consider the following:

— Are there problems with ease of feeding the infant during the encounter?

— Does the infant or parent appear frustrated or satisfied?

— Are the parental perceptions that are verbalized consistent with what is being observed?

Similarly, the manner in which a parent responds to a young child's behavior during a clinical encounter may offer valuable insight into some of the dynamics of a feeding session that takes place at the child's home. A parent who, during an office encounter, verbalizes inappropriate expectations of how a young child should behave during the physical examination may also have inappropriate expectations about the child's ability to carefully self-feed and remain focused during meals. Health care providers should engage and partner with parents, a process that involves understanding parents' expectations and concerns about food, weight, and child behavior; addressing parents' concerns respectfully; educating parents about the adverse outcomes following undernutrition; and reinforcing the positive parent-child interactions noted during, what will likely be, multiple encounters.

Laboratory Assessment

The laboratory assessment in the FTT workup is focused and directed by the history and physical examination.[47] A basic screening set of laboratory tests should be sufficient initially and should include a complete blood count (CBC), lead, urinalysis (UA), electrolytes, and a purified protein derivative (PPD) skin test. More involved or invasive laboratory or diagnostic studies may follow the basic screening set as suggested by the historical and physical examination data.

Children with severe FTT might benefit from assessment of protein status as determined by laboratory testing of prealbumin and albumin. A child with less severe FTT and a history of classroom behavioral disturbances, snoring, and enlarged tonsils likely needs a sleep study to assess for obstructive sleep apnea.[48] Testing for food allergies should be considered if a child with FTT also has atopic dermatitis along with urticaria and gastrointestinal symptoms after ingesting certain foods. Gastrointestinal symptoms in combination with history of travel might prompt screening for intestinal parasites. Selected screens such as human immunodeficiency virus (HIV) antibody testing and sweat testing may also be considered for selected, high-risk populations. In some circumstances, endoscopic studies and bone age x-ray studies may complement the laboratory assessment.

Case Study 8-1

The following case study presents a case of suspected neglect, noting possible findings and outlining guidance for evaluation.

JH, a 9-month-old former preterm infant boy, was brought to the clinic by his mother and a CPS social worker. The CPS social worker made JH's appointment and asked that the boy be evaluated 1 week after his 2-year-old sister was removed from the home because of multiple unexplained fractures. JH lived with his biological parents and his 3-year-old brother at the time he was brought to the clinic for care. CPS was considering whether or not to take JH into custody.

JH's mother noted that he was healthy with a good appetite. She stated he was smaller than his older siblings were at his age. JH's mother noted all of her children were born prematurely at around 30 to 32 weeks. She reported that JH stayed in the neonatal intensive care unit (NICU) for 4 weeks. The boy's mom was unable to remember his birth weight, stating "Possibly 3 lb." Per mom, JH had multiple visits to his pediatric nurse practitioner (PNP) since birth. He was noted to be up-to-date with vaccines. JH's mom provided the telephone number of the PNP. The PNP noted she last saw JH 3 weeks before the visit to the clinic. The PNP provided the boy's weights, heights, and head circumferences from previous well-child examinations and sick visits. It was noted that JH had only gained 300 grams since he was aged 4 months. Per JH's PNP, the boy had never been referred for subspecialty consultations.

On physical examination at the clinic, JH was found to be a severely emaciated and lying still in a supine position on the examination table. There were small healing abrasions on his face and anterior trunk, which his mom said were self-inflicted. Otherwise, his examination was within normal limits. JH's mother made no effort to engage him or pick him up during the first 20 minutes of the encounter. At one point, she removed a bottle from her purse, placed the nipple in his mouth, and wrapped his hands around the bottle. JH attempted to drink while supine on the examination table. When the bottle fell from the boy's hands the mother picked it up and placed it into her purse.

JH's mom noted he self-feeds 6 oz to 8 oz of formula every 3 to 4 hours. JH's mom stated she supplements his formula by adding either applesauce or rice cereal to each bottle. She was unable to describe how much of either solid she "pours in" to each bottle of formula. JH's mom stated he occasionally spits up, but does not vomit, and has normally formed bowel movements.

Consider the following questions regarding JH's presentation:

— Is this nutritional neglect?

— Is there concern for more than one form of neglect?

— What nursing skills and interventions might benefit to JH and his mother?

— Did JH's PNP overlook important aspects of the boy's care?

— What knowledge about diet and development should be shared to help create a more optimal environment for JH?

Consider the following questions that may be asked of JH's mother regarding the boy's home care:

— Do you perceive JH to have difficulty with sucking and swallowing?

— Has JH ever been prescribed a high-calorie or other specialized formula?

— Are you able to purchase adequate formula and food throughout the month for JH and other household members?

— Does anyone else help you care for and feed JH?

Consider the following questions that may be asked of the boy's mother regarding availability or prior utilization of community resources:

— Are you enrolled in the Special Supplemental Nutrition Program for Women, Infants, and Children (WIC) or the Supplemental Nutrition Assistance Program ([SNAP]; formerly known as food stamps)?

— How do you feel about the possibility of home visiting nurses?

Reflection about the answers to these questions will help determine how to proceed in engaging and partnering with JH's mother and CPS. At minimum, most providers would call this neglect because a mother who had prior experience with preterm infants and a PNP failed to adequately address JH's abnormally low weight gain over an approximately 5-month period.

Medical Neglect

Presentation

Medical neglect is a broad term that, at times, is included under physical neglect.[20] However, it is best to separate medical from physical neglect to highlight the unique expertise that health care providers have in identifying this form of neglect and fashioning specific interventions. Medical neglect involves a caregiver's failure to recognize obvious signs of physical injury, medical illnesses or mental health concerns or follow through on a health care provider's reasonable plan of care. In medical neglect, the child is brought in to the health care setting only after the clinical situation is well beyond what would be considered reasonable or when the child has deteriorated to the point of being seriously ill or perhaps near death.

Delay in seeking health care assistance at a reasonable point in an acute illness may be a sign of medical neglect. Additionally, medical neglect may be seen in families with a child who has a chronic illness where medical therapies are not followed as prescribed, resulting in serious consequences to the child's health. Not seeking assistance for obvious developmental delays or mental health illnesses may also qualify as medical neglect. Finally, refusing appropriate medical care for treatable illnesses that place the child at risk for serious complications is also a form of medical neglect.[35]

These commonly accepted definitions and indicators of medical neglect might conflict with religious or cultural beliefs that restrict multiple forms of traditional medical care, including potentially lifesaving medical and surgical care and preventative pediatric care.[49] Jehovah's Witnesses prohibit transfusion, including auto-transfusion, of most blood products. Christian Scientists may rely solely on prayer to promote healing unless a dispensation has been granted by church leaders. Scientologists may refuse psychiatric care. Routine vaccines may also be refused by parents for religious or philosophical reasons. When religious or philosophical conflicts place a child at risk of serious harm or cause a child to experience preventable pain or suffering and in cases where mainstream medical care would result in a high likelihood of normalcy or survival, consultation with an ethicist and legal consultation may be in the child's best interests.[49]

Epidemiology

Approximately 763 000 children experienced substantiated child maltreatment in 2009; of those children, 2.4% experienced medical neglect.[1] Possible indicators of medical neglect in the health care setting are as follows:

— Failure to immunize a child who is at increased risk for a vaccine-preventable disease such as pneumococcal prophylaxis in a patient with sickle cell disease

— Many missed school days secondary to lack of appropriate treatment of a chronic illness, such as asthma or diabetes

— Infected burns that have not been seen by a primary care provider

— Medications that are not being taken as prescribed or prescriptions that have not been filled

— Brain tumor that cannot be treated with surgery and chemotherapy because parents intend to work only with a spiritual healer

— Rampant dental caries in obvious locations

The American Academy of Pediatrics (AAP) notes factors that result in a child experiencing medical neglect[50]:

— Child and parental factors

— Poverty

— Lack of access to care

— Family chaos

— Lack of awareness, knowledge, or skills

— Lack of trust in health care professionals

— Impairment of caregivers

— Caregiver's belief systems

— The child's attitudes and behavior

— Clinician factors

— Misunderstanding of different cultures

— Lack of parental health literacy and lack of communication in the health care setting

Similarly, the American Academy of Pediatric Dentistry (AAPD) has emphasized factors that might affect dental care[51]:

— Poverty

— Family isolation

— Parental ignorance about the ramifications of extensive caries, infections, and dental trauma

The AAPD noted that concern for dental neglect should be raised when a parent has failed to follow through with dental care despite previous education in the following areas:

— Extent of carious lesions

— Specific treatment needed

— Manner in which dental care can be accessed

History

When assessing a child for possible medical neglect, the provider should first determine the appropriateness of the caregiver's response to the child, given the illness. This involves the following aspects:

— Timeliness for routine care

— Response to presence of symptoms and signs

— Adherence to regimens (pharmacy records of filling prescriptions, corroboration of visits to other providers)

— Whether there is caregiver concern and interest in the evaluation

— Whether caregiver asks appropriate questions about possible causes of the problem and treatments

If there is a concern for dental neglect, the health care provider should attempt to ascertain whether a parent has sought care for their child's dental needs in a manner commiserate with their financial and community resources.

The health care provider may also use open-ended screening questions or comments to identify whether the child's basic needs are being addressed:

— What happens when you are in pain?

— Who gives you medicine when you are sick?

— How many times has the child missed school in the previous week or month because of the medical concern?

Physical Examination

Evaluation of the child's condition in cases of medical neglect should be guided by the presenting symptoms and history provided as well as information gleaned from the medical record. The following should be assessed:

— General appearance for signs of neglect; specific signs that point to a clinical condition

— Assessment findings; overt nature of findings

— Obvious dental caries of the anterior teeth

— Delay in seeking treatment in the context of new or acute symptoms

— Obvious nature of findings to a reasonable non-clinician

— Current state of disease control for ongoing care of chronic conditions compared to health care provider's expectations (eg, if the prescribed treatment was followed as planned)

— Degree of severity or distress when a patient with a chronic concern presents for treatment

— Routine care

— Child's overall appearance of wellness

— Concordance of child's development with chronological age

Laboratory Assessment

Laboratory studies requested usually depend on the child's clinical condition. If there is delay in the caregiver seeking treatment for care, some laboratory tests may give information about diagnostic possibilities. In dehydration, an electrolyte panel may reveal the severity or chronicity of the situation. For certain chronic conditions, laboratory tests help determine the child's current clinical state. The hemoglobin $A1_C$ test for diabetes management may indicate prior blood glucose control. Overall, wide-ranging laboratory panels are generally not useful.

Medical Neglect versus Noncompliance (Nonadherence)

Failure to follow through with a reasonable plan of care and failure or refusal to obtain health care may result in actual or potential harm. However, noncompliance, or nonadherence, is not automatically medical neglect, in large part because there may not be readily apparent negative outcomes. In pediatrics, compliance rates vary from 7% to 89% for short-term medical regimens and 11% to 83% for long-term regimens.[52] Specifically, in treating acute otitis media, approximately 7% of children completed the entire therapy and 53% took less than half the prescribed antibiotics. Compliance figures are not much better for chronic conditions such as asthma and cystic fibrosis (CF).[52]

Assessing the impact of the noncompliance on the child as well as the pattern of noncompliance with health care recommendations by the caregivers is paramount in distinguishing noncompliance from medical neglect. In attempting to determine whether noncompliance constitutes medical neglect, the health care provider may have to decide whether the clinical condition or subsequent negative outcome is likely due to failure to comply with a reasonable and otherwise effective plan of care. For example, a variety of reasons have been offered by caregivers to account for medication administration noncompliance, including forgetting to take the medication, stopping because of symptom improvement, misunderstanding instructions, child resistance, perceived ineffectiveness, fears about adverse effects, onset of side effects, and lack of medical insurance. The health care provider's ability to communicate with the family in a clear and empathetic fashion about these factors and to follow-up with the family is critical.

Of note, failure to follow-up with routine, well-child care is generally not considered medical neglect, especially when the child remains healthy. As previously noted, such noncompliance should be addressed with caregivers. The health care provider should strive to determine the caregiver's perceptions about the need for well- and ill-child care.

Case Study 8-2

SG, an 18-month-old infant girl, was brought to her health care provider's office for a sick visit. Her mother was concerned about her pulling on her right ear and her increased crying during the night. SG had a history of one previous ear infection that started the same way, according to her mother. It was noted that SG lived with her mother, aged 16 years; her maternal grandmother, aged 34 years, who has just started to work as part of a new state initiative; her aunt, aged 18 years; and her 2 cousins, aged 2 years and 3 years. The girl's mother was a junior in the neighborhood high school, and the aunt provided childcare for the 3 children. SG's mother stated that the ear pulling started 2 nights before the visit to the provider's office and was slightly relieved with 2 droppers full of acetaminophen infant drops every 4 hours. The mother wanted an antibiotic for the ear pain.

A history revealed bowel and bladder function, sleep, and nutrition within normal limits. Immunizations were not up-to-date; the child was missing booster diphtheria, tetanus, acellular pertussis (DtaP). There were no allergies, ER visits, hospitalizations, or other illnesses since the last visit at age 12 months.

On doing the physical examination a bright red, bulging tympanic membrane with a diffuse light reflex and no mobility was assessed. Her nose had boggy red turbinates and a yellow mucous discharging from both nostrils. Her throat was normal.

On the left side of the forehead, a healing scab measuring 3 cm by 0.5 cm was noted in addition to and 2 additional healing scabs on her right thigh. When asked about these scabs, the girl's mother said SG got burned with a hair-curling iron that the mother left on the floor of her room while getting ready for school. The mother described how the blisters formed and how, after they broke, she applied some medicine the aunt used on the cousins for minor burns.

After the physical assessment, the health care provider sat down to talk to Susan about leaving small appliances that get hot, like a curling iron, plugged in and within a child's reach. The health care provider also asked SG's mother about a safe place for the girl to play while the mother is getting ready for school. The mother noted that there was no playpen or gate to keep any of the children confined to a safe space while an adult prepares for school or work or answers a ringing phone or doorbell.

Consider the following questions regarding the injury, delay in seeking medical care, and administering someone else's medicine:

— Is this a case of neglect?

— Should it be reported to CPS?

A practical definition of neglect looks at the role responsibility and intent of the child's caregiver.[20]

— Was SG's mother extraordinarily inattentive?

— What was the degree of avoidable suffering or actual harm (the burns)?

— Did the girl's mother respond in a reasonable way?

— How serious is it that SG is not up-to-date on her immunizations and was not brought for medical care?

— If this were the second or third occurrence of burns, how would the plan of care change?

Now for concerns based on community resources:

— What role does the primary care setting play if the last appointment for immunizations is 3:00 PM and there are no evening or Saturday hours?

— Can no one other than a parent sign permission for the immunizations?

— Does the mother's high school have a school-based clinic?

— Does the mother's high school provide childcare for young children?

— Is there an immunization clinic open on Saturdays or evenings at the public health center?

— Did the primary care center notify the mother of the inadequate level of SG's immunizations?

Concerning other supervisors or caregiver, the following can be addressed:

— What responsibility, if any, does the maternal grandmother have in this issue?

— What responsibility, if any, does the aunt have?

— Have the aunt's young children been burned by a curling iron?

— Is the household overcrowded?

Concerning SG's temperament, or more importantly, the mother's perception of the girl:

— Does the mother describe SG as a difficult child?

— Is the girls' mother feeling more stress associated with parenting as SG gets older?

Answers to these questions can help decide how to proceed in working with SG and her mother and whether a report about suspected neglect is warranted. Most providers would call this neglectful behavior but not neglect.

Obesity as a Manifestation of Medical Neglect

When a child is obese or has multiple comorbid medical conditions, family intervention is critical to mitigate or prevent the sequelae of obesity. Health care providers should begin by engaging the child's family in lifestyle interventions such as appropriate nutrition and exercise and referring the family to specialty clinics. Structured, multidisciplinary interventions in the child's home, school, and community should be facilitated to the extent possible. These interventions can be driven by the health care provider or be facilitated by CPS.

Varness et al[53] offer guidelines on when and how to involve CPS when it is suspected that a child's parents are not reasonably adhering to a weight-reduction plan of care and the child is at risk of comorbid conditions related to obesity.[53] The guidelines are based on the presence, severity, and reversibility of comorbid medical conditions. CPS will invariably work to ensure the child's family structure remain intact. However, Varness et al[53] propose that the child should undergo a trial period of removal from the home when there is (1) a high likelihood that serious harm will occur in the absence of weight management, (2) a reasonable likelihood that coercive state intervention will result in weight loss, and (3) an absence of alternatives for addressing the child's obesity and comorbidities.

Nursing as a Basis for the Prevention, Identification, Evaluation, and Management of Neglect

To this point, this chapter has defined neglect, described its presentations in the health care setting, and discussed how health care providers can identify caregiving that meets the diagnostic criteria for neglect. To reach an end point (eg, the diagnosis of a specific form of neglect, such as physical, nutritional or medical), prevention efforts may have been less than successful, assuming that the health care provider applied both generic and screening techniques to reach the diagnosis. Nurses and nurse practitioners in both traditional and nontraditional roles may play a significant role in preventing, identifying, evaluating, and managing child neglect as discussed in the following sections.

Primary, Secondary, and Tertiary Prevention of Neglect

The prevention of neglect requires establishing a relationship with the caregivers that provides a fair degree of parental education and close clinical follow-up.[54] Nurses are ideal participants on the health care team to provide a comprehensive, longitudinal approach to intervention. Indeed, nurses have historically played significant roles in the prevention of child maltreatment, including neglect.[55] Nurse home visiting programs have been shown to be effective in preventing child abuse and neglect for at least 15 years after the intervention.[56] Research findings on these programs show that the nurse's intervention contributes to changing the mother's life course.[57] The ability of nursing intervention to persuade mothers to make better decisions for their children and themselves in terms of education, employment, and health relationships has been validated (see *Chapter 17, Prevention of Child Maltreatment*).

Identification of Neglect

Health care providers should consider both generic and specific screens for neglect because of the many manifestations of neglect. Generic screens are broadly applicable and seek to find any pattern of caregiving or symptoms or signs that suggest the need to further explore the possibility of neglect. Building on the generic screens, a set of specific screens can then be done for particular forms of neglect that may be suspected.

During primary care visits, health care providers should generically and in an open-ended fashion, ask screening questions about child safety in the home, playground, and car as a generic screen for possible physical neglect. Similarly, open-ended questions should be asked about prior medical care, immunization status, and dietary habits. More direct questions and specific screens related to the possible form of neglect should be undertaken when the generic screen or clinical situation causes the health care provider to suspect a particular form of neglect. Obtaining additional information from parents gives the health care provider a place to begin to assist them in performing the parental role, which will contribute to the child's health.

In seeking to identify factors indicative of child neglect, ecological models suggest adding questions to the family history during a well-child or newborn visit such as the following:

— Were you (mother or father) abused or neglected as a child?

— Do you have a supportive, close relationship with someone?

— Have you ever been in therapy or used social support services?

— What was your experience with therapy or social services?

When possible, verbal patients and their siblings should be allowed to answer questions that may help substantiate the health care provider's concerns about neglect. Questions directed at children should be as open-ended as possible and asked in a nonthreatening fashion. The health care provider should make eye-level contact with a child and use developmentally appropriate words to ensure that the child understands the questions being asked.

Irrespective of verbal abilities of a child, the nurse can utilize ***observation skills*** to help identify neglect. Neglectful mothers may interact minimally with their children and may offer lower rates of verbal instructions to their children compared to controls.[58] Abused and neglected female children are less likely to move towards the caregiver, reach for or touch the caregiver, sustain gaze with the caretaker, check to see what the caregiver is doing, or check to see where the caregiver is looking compared with their non-maltreated peers.[45] Conversely, abused and neglected boys are more likely to reach and touch than non-maltreated boys.[45]

Generic Screening for Neglect

The generic screening includes attention to the following 6 core issues that apply globally to any child suspected of having experienced neglect[11]:

— Indications that basic needs are not being met: general appearance, signs of actual harm, risk of harm based on clinical situation, and child's past medical history

— Pattern of care-giving that suggests the presence of neglect: lack of adherence to routine health care recommendations, past episodes of neglect, and previous CPS involvement

— Assessment of potential contributing factors: Parental coping strategies and presence of domestic violence in family

— Assessment of strengths and possible resources available to the child and family: parental interest in child's well-being, other involved family members who are genuinely helpful, and access to community-based family support programs

— Past successes and failures with previous interventions: what did and did not work before; who was involved; reasons for success or failure

— Prognostic information related to family motivation, capacity to change, and access to resources: family track record of accepting help and achieving goals, record of resistance to recommendations, and resources available to the family in the community

After the generic assessment of the core issues described, the health care provider can move into a more specific, directed assessment of issues that need attention based on the type or form of neglect suspected (**Table 8-5**).

Specific Screening

Specific screening for particular forms of neglect such as physical neglect, medical neglect, and FTT have been emphasized in this chapter in terms of the health care evaluation. It is also important to incorporate reports by other disciplines, especially professionals who visit the child at home, into the health care assessment. Overall, though, the health care evaluation should include a medical history, physical examination, possible laboratory and diagnostic studies, and careful observation of the caregiver-child interaction during the office visit(s). Every child assessed by a health care provider should be screened for general appearance, hygiene and grooming, height and weight, and, if aged younger than 2 years, head circumference (**Figures 8-1** to **8-4**).

Evaluation

Health care providers often participate with multidisciplinary teams (MDT) in a variety of ways when evaluating neglect. Participation ranges from the office-based nursing professional who collects growth parameters and performs a nursing assessment to the advanced practice nurse (APN) who delivers a full range of primary care services. Regardless of the role, nursing's focus on the holistic evaluation of both the child and adult caregivers and on restoring health and well-being makes the nurse ideally suited for to play an important part in dealing with child neglect.

Management

Once neglect has been identified, health care providers may deliver ongoing education to families and non-health care providers, such as social workers, about child develop-

Table 8-5. United States Department of Health and Human Services Assessment of Neglect

Type of Neglect	— Specific indicators of neglect — Chronicity
Problems	— Identified by referral source — Identified by parent — Identified by helper

Factors Affecting Provision of Adequate Care	— Individual personality
	  — Strengths
	  — Mental status (intelligence)
	  — Parenting knowledge and skills
	  — Interpersonal skills
	  — Physical health
	  — Cooperation, motivation
	— Family system
	  — Strengths
	  — Family size and composition
	  — Income
	  — Marital relationship
	  — Special needs of children
	  — Stability of family composition (membership)
	  — Structure, organization, and communication (interaction) patterns
	  — Family boundaries

Environmental and Community Stressors and Resources	— Housing — Job (employment) — Neighborhood — Informal social networks — Cultural factors — Availability and responsiveness of formally organized services
Setting Priorities	— Break goals into manageable, achievable subgoals.
Structured Assessment Measures	— Learn about neglect characteristics. — Provide focus for interventions. — Provide a means for assessing intervention outcomes.

Adapted from Gaudin JM Jr. Child Neglect: A Guide for Intervention. *Washington, DC: United States Department of Health and Human Services, Administration for Children and Families, Westover Consultants (Contract No HHS-105-89-1730); 1993.*

ment and the basic needs of the associated stage. Additionally, the nurse specifically may be the provider responsible for monitoring the child's progress, either in the office or in the child's home, and may be part of the support team that encourages the family to meet the challenges they face. This type of ongoing intervention is essential and contributes to secondary and tertiary prevention efforts while providing treatment to the involved child in the manner described below.

Generic Treatment

The treatment of child neglect begins with a clear assessment of the types(s) of neglect, determination of the family's strengths, and evaluation of challenges that will face the family. Positive first steps in constructing a treatment plan include communicating concern for the child; showing an interest in helping the parents and family meet the child's needs; and understanding that, in the majority of cases, the family cares about what is best for the child. It is essential to explain the seriousness of the situation and to clearly communicate that actions are being taken to ensure that the child's needs are being met. Ideally, the health care provider should have other disciplines available to assist in treatment planning, and have a working knowledge of what programs and resources are available in the community to help support the child and family.

The goal of treatment is to have the child's basic needs met in a manner that fosters the child's ongoing health and well-being and is a positive experience for the child and family. It is ideal to engage the caregiver about how to understand and then meet the child's needs. Unless the child is in immediate danger, efforts should be made to work with the parent or caregiver to optimize their potential for success in meeting the child's basic needs. At any point in the nurse's evaluation, if the child is believed to be in imminent danger of sustaining harm, immediate actions must be taken to ensure safety, including reporting the child's presentation to CPS.

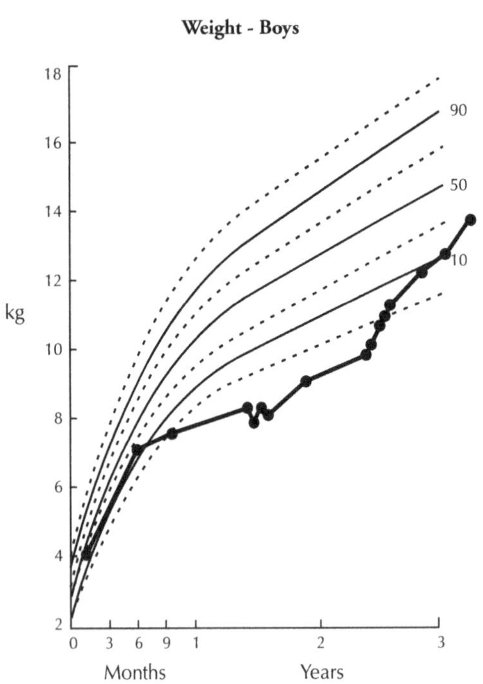

Figure 8-1. *Weight chart showing catch-up growth from age 2½ years when a diagnosis of neglect was made and conveyed to the parents. The child remained at home showing that his normal growth potential could be reached. Reprinted from Hobbs CJ, Hanks HGI, Wynne JM. In: Hobbs CJ, Hanks HGI, Wynne JM, eds.* Child Abuse and Neglect: A Clinician's Handbook. *New York, NY: Churchill Livingstone; 1993:89-105. © 1993, with permission from Elsevier.*

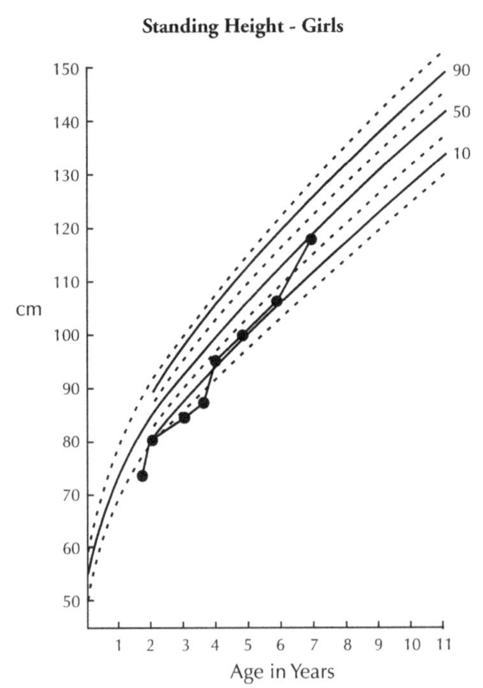

Figure 8-2. *Height chart demonstrating gradual catch-up of height to 50th percentile at age 7 years in an emotionally abused child (same case as Figure 8-4). Reprinted from Hobbs CJ, Hanks HGI, Wynne JM. In: Hobbs CJ, Hanks HGI, Wynne JM, eds.* Child Abuse and Neglect: A Clinician's Handbook. *New York, NY: Churchill Livingstone; 1993:89-105. © 1993, with permission from Elsevier.*

Figure 8-3-a. *Height chart of index child failing to thrive who shows 2 episodes of catch-up growth. Reprinted from Hobbs CJ, Hanks HGI, Wynne JM. In: Hobbs CJ, Hanks HGI, Wynne JM, eds.* Child Abuse and Neglect: A Clinician's Handbook. *New York, NY: Churchill Livingstone; 1993:89-105. © 1993, with permission from Elsevier.*

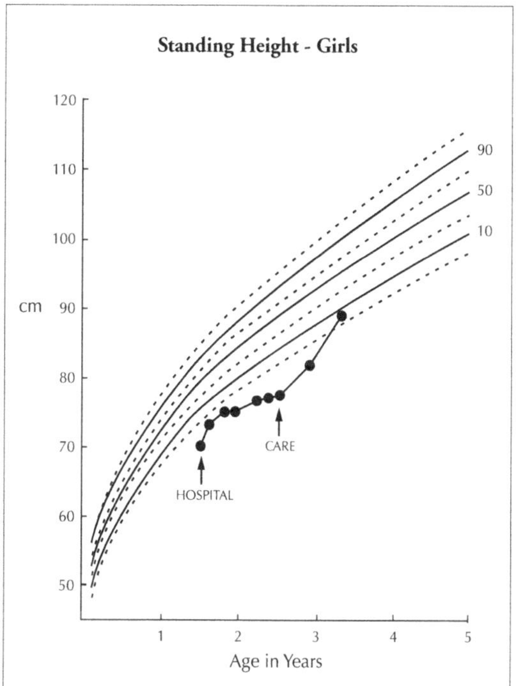

Figure 8-3-a

Figure 8-3-b. *Weight chart of the same child. Reprinted from Hobbs CJ, Hanks HGI, Wynne JM. In: Hobbs CJ, Hanks HGI, Wynne JM, eds.* Child Abuse and Neglect: A Clinician's Handbook. *New York, NY: Churchill Livingstone; 1993:89-105. © 1993, with permission from Elsevier.*

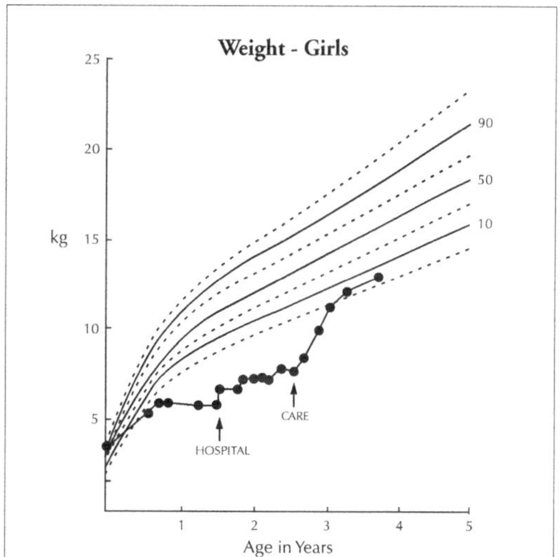

Figure 8-3-b

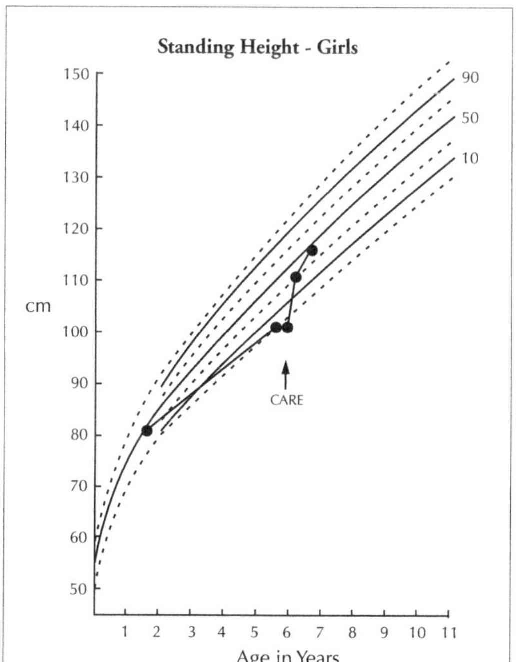

Figure 8-3-c

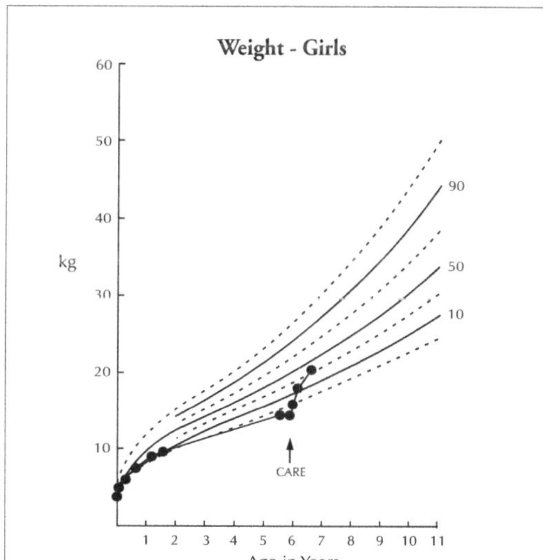

Figure 8-3-d

Figure 8-3-c. *Height chart of older sibling whose FTT was unrecognized before admission to foster care but recognized only retrospectively when she showed accelerated growth. Reprinted from Hobbs CJ, Hanks HGI, Wynne JM. In: Hobbs CJ, Hanks HGI, Wynne JM, eds.* Child Abuse and Neglect: A Clinician's Handbook. *New York, NY: Churchill Livingstone; 1993:89-105. © 1993, with permission from Elsevier.*

Figure 8-3-d. *Weight chart of the same older sibling. Reprinted from Hobbs CJ, Hanks HGI, Wynne JM. In: Hobbs CJ, Hanks HGI, Wynne JM, eds.* Child Abuse and Neglect: A Clinician's Handbook. *New York, NY: Churchill Livingstone; 1993:89-105. © 1993, with permission from Elsevier.*

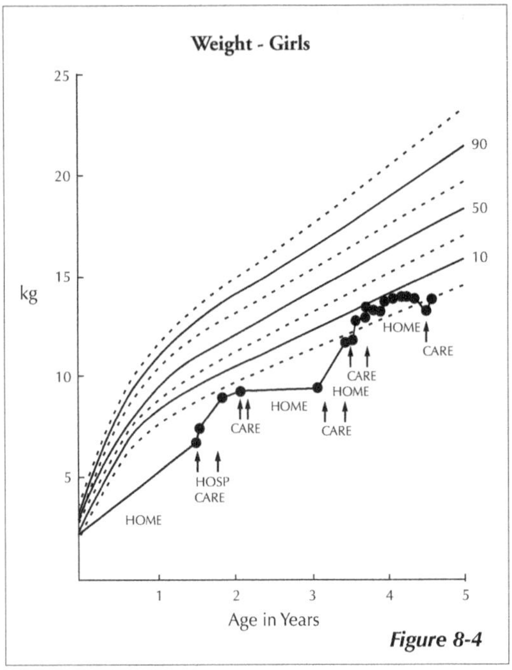

Figure 8-4. *Weight chart demonstrating the use of weights and life events to chart progress in a child with severe emotional abuse and FTT. Prolonged efforts of rehabilitation to parents' care had failed while the child repeatedly showed catch-up growth in substitute care. Reprinted from Hobbs CJ, Hanks HGI, Wynne JM. In: Hobbs CJ, Hanks HGI, Wynne JM, eds.* Child Abuse and Neglect: A Clinician's Handbook. *New York, NY: Churchill Livingstone; 1993:89-105. © 1993, with permission from Elsevier.*

Specific Treatment

Specific interventions for neglect depend on several factors, including the type of neglect, the amount of risk to the child, the developmental level of the child, the abilities of the caregivers, and the types of services available in the community. In assessing the types of community services that may be of benefit to the child and family, psychological assessments and therapy for parents and children should not be overlooked. Play therapy has been shown to improve peer interaction and decrease aggression in neglected children.[59]

Treatment for physical neglect involves parental education concerning child safety and avoidable environmental hazards along with follow-up office visits to reinforce the anticipatory guidance. Assessment of the child's well-being and provision of additional age-appropriate information as the child grows should also be included. Home services, such as social work and nursing visits, are essential to ensure that the topics discussed in the office setting are carried through once the parent and child return home.

Treatment for FTT depends on identifying the underlying, organic, inorganic, or both, causes of FTT. Health care providers can share responsibility for helping to determine the child's appropriate nutritional intake and for offering dietary counseling in addition to reviewing the records of what the child is offered and consumes. Caregiver education concerning food preparation, presentation, and assistance is also important.[60] When nutritional supplements are used, the health care provider should support the family by ensuring the family knows how to obtain prescribed resources or suitable alternatives. When technological interventions such as nasogastric feedings are suggested, parent training and ongoing home support is essential because sophisticated medical interventions can be challenging to the most motivated of parents and caregivers. Home nursing visits during which the child's growth parameters are measured and discussed with the family are a critical adjunct to scheduled office visits.[61] When possible and clinically warranted, home visits provide valuable insight for the health care provider into what is actually happening regarding meal time and nutritional intake.[62]

Treatment for medical neglect hinges on the identity of the particular medical condition. Caregiver education, once again, is central, and should focus on what symptoms and signs the caregiver needs to know and address. The caregiver must learn the following in order to appropriately care for a medically compromised or neglected child:

— How and when to contact the health care provider

— What constitutes an emergency

— Importance of adhering to the treatment plan as outlined

— How to connect to helpful community resources

— Components of routine care that cannot be ignored

Routine and follow-up visits should be scheduled, ideally at times that are mutually agreeable to caregivers and clinicians. Failure to attend planned, mutually agreed upon visits should be viewed as a sentinel indicator of the family not being able to optimally care for the child. Finally, some level of case management is essential if the child's medical condition is complex and requires the input of several different health care providers. Nurses can play an important role in helping the child's team of caregivers understand the child's needs in a holistic manner.

Parental Responses to Nursing Interventions for Child Neglect

When working with neglectful parents, valuable resources include home visitors, whether nurses or laypeople, to determine the state of the home and community-sponsored support groups for parents. In addition, communicating with parents using the term *neglectful* can cement an observation and give the parent an opportunity to respond. The health care provider might expect a range of responses from total outrage to total passivity from a parent. However, the health care provider must share the fact that he or she is worried about the child's condition and then determine where the parents are with regard to behavioral change and preventing a repeat event. Based on Henderson's[8] definition of nursing and stages of behavioral change discussed by Prochaska et al,[63] the health care provider could define caregivers' need for services and education based on a categorization of willing, willing but unable, or unwilling to change.

Parents willing to change who describe a chaotic home life, but do not live in unsafe conditions (eg, little food, garbage and excrement in living space, exposed wiring, drugs and poisons within reach of children) are most often open to a change in their behavior to prevent an injury, such as a curling iron burn. Such a parent often states a need for more money or may need to be given ideas on ways to purchase safety gates or a playpen for their young child. Parents who are willing to change often benefit from a resourceful health care provider who knows the area lending closets, second-hand stores, and inexpensive large chain stores that carry such safety devices. This correlates with the preparation or action stage of behavioral change.[63]

Willing but unable neglectful parents often describe how they do not have the money for safety items or do not have a lending closet in their community. These parents may abuse alcohol or marijuana, have a flat affect, have little education, and have little experience with real-life success. They want the best for their children, but are ambivalent about change. They do not see a way to accomplish any change in the next month, but they may see the possibility in the next 6 months. This behavior corresponds to the contemplation stage of behavioral change.[63]

Unwilling neglectful parents are often outraged at the implication that a minor injury such as a burn could be considered neglectful on their part. They describe having many emotional needs that were not met by their parents. Their overall tendency is to react with passivity, but they become outraged if called neglectful and have little motivation or skill to effect change in their lives. In fact, they are usually impulsive and seek immediate gratification without regard for long-term consequences. Therefore, saving for a future purchase of safety equipment is beyond their comprehension. They do not anticipate any change in their parenting in the next 6 months. This behaviors correlates with the precontemplation stage of behavioral change.[63]

Nursing Leadership in the Multidisciplinary Evaluation of Neglect

As noted, nurses have the opportunity to participate in, and in some cases lead, the multidisciplinary efforts directed at prevention, identification, evaluation, and management of the health care–related aspects of neglect. In order to fully determine the extent to which a caregiver fails to meet a child's basic needs, health care considerations regarding neglect must be paired with legal definitions of neglect. Medicolegal discussions should occur with multidisciplinary professionals who each bring a variety of perspectives to the evaluation process.

Organizations serving children and the professionals operating within them must then operationalize legal definitions and mandates to determine acceptable practice.[64] Professionals should familiarize themselves with policies and procedures of the organization and jurisdiction within which they practice. Finally, both professionals and laypeople within a community need to personally interpret what constitutes adequate caregiving or parenting. A person's own definition of neglect is the most prone to variation because many factors influence an individual's view of providing care to children, including upbringing, training, knowledge, and other life experiences over time.[64]

Professionals working in the child maltreatment area rely on legal definitions of what constitutes neglect to guide practice and intervention decisions.[64] Law enforcement and prosecution use legal definitions to determine if they should become involved in a case. Involvement of the criminal justice system usually requires a level of seriousness that places the child at significant risk for severe bodily harm. The less severe forms of maltreatment tend to be handled by CPS agencies without police or prosecutor involvement.[65] The health care provider may see a pattern of neglect emerge early on in the care of the child and report the situation to CPS. Identified patterns of neglect may include a failure to meet the child's basic needs despite reasonable health care interventions, such as parent education, more frequent office-based health-supervision visits, or the use of home nursing.[66]

Nurses as Mandated Reporters: Reporting Neglect to Child Protective Services

Once a reasonable treatment plan is designed and the caregiver is engaged and educated about the treatment plan, ongoing follow-up is necessary. Health care providers should reinforce parents' efforts to fulfill each component of the treatment plan. The treatment plan should also clearly identify what would constitute failure because caregivers may make multiple attempts to meet the child's needs and fail consistently. After a caregiver demonstrates a number of failed attempts to meet the child's needs, CPS may need to consider more disruptive solutions, including out-of-home placement.

Neglect should be reported when parental omission is a major contributor to a child's basic needs or rights not being met.[34] Utilizing the framework generally outlined by Dubowitz,[34] the following questions should be reflected upon when deciding to report reasonable suspicion of neglect:

- How much parental care or supervision is reasonably needed given the child's age, health status, or other unique circumstances?
- Has the child's behavior or emotional status been impaired and, if so, to what extent?
- Is there potential for the child to be harmed because a basic need (right) is not being met?

— Is there actual, demonstrable harm that has resulted from a basic need (right) not being met?

— Is the actual or potential harm minor or life-threatening?

— Is the omission reasonably a single event?

— Does the omission represent a pattern that may reoccur in the future without intervention?

— Can meaningful interventions and monitoring be offered in the office setting?

— What is the goal in contacting CPS?

At times, following a report to CPS, the child may need to be hospitalized to receive appropriate medical services and or allow a CPS investigation to proceed. In such extreme circumstances, actual custody of the child may need to be taken from the parents or caregivers with the assistance of the courts. In this situation, CPS determines to whom the child should be discharged when leaving the hospital. This determination is made as the investigation unfolds. In less critical situations, a report to CPS may be followed by office-based interventions in the outpatient setting, which may include home nursing visits along with other community-based services.

Outcomes Following Neglect

Neglect has far-reaching effects on children that can influence physical health and psychological adjustment as well as intellectual, social, behavioral, and affective development.[67] The impact of neglect on an individual child depends on many factors, including developmental level at the time of the neglect and the type, severity, and chronicity of the neglectful behavior.[68] One can conceptualize the consequences of neglect as having acute, short-term, and long-term effects in the realms of physical and psychological functioning.

Acute consequences of neglect may range from exposure to environmental hazards to hunger and unidentified or untreated medical problems to death. Over the short-term period, Hildyard et al[6] note that preschool- and school-aged survivors of physical and emotional neglect have more severe cognitive, language, and academic deficits and experience more attachment disorders, social isolation, and internalizing behavior compared with their physically abused peers.[6] School-aged children who experience abuse or neglect are also at increased risk for behavioral problems as adults.[69]

The effects of FTT seem to be mitigated by young age if FTT is not experienced in combination with another form of neglect. Children aged younger than 6 months who were diagnosed with FTT demonstrated good catch up growth by age 4 years with no significant difference in cognition at age 11 years.[70] Eight years after home intervention for nonorganic FTT, children were taller and heavier with better arithmetic scores compared to controls.[71] Conversely, cumulative effects are seen among children who have FTT and experience neglect, demonstrating less academic success and more behavioral problems compared to children with either one or neither diagnosis.[72] Of interest, maternal self-report of child neglect is associated with obesity in preschoolers.[73] Neglected children aged 9 to 10 years followed longitudinally in a prospective population-based study also had a greater risk of adult obesity independent of age, childhood body mass index (BMI), and sex.[74]

The overall impact of neglect on a child's life is likely immeasurable. Additionally, neglect has societal effects, especially when considered in light of the impact on child health and well-being and social programs needed to deal with long term effects of maltreatment. A 2007 Prevent Child Abuse America report estimated the societal cost of child maltreatment to be $103.8 billion.[75] Neglect consistently accounts for two-thirds of the cases of child maltreatment. Social impacts are seen in law enforcement and the courts as well as the juvenile and adult criminal justice systems.

Conclusion

Wodarski's[76] early literature review identified that treatment approaches to neglect must address the multifactorial nature of the problem. Nurses are ideally suited to offer a holistic approach to such a comprehensive, ideally multidisciplinary, undertaking. Policies from professional organizations can give additional guidance to the practice of the nursing professional. The National Association of Pediatric Nurse Associates and Practitioners (NAPNAP) has issued multiple position statements on child abuse and neglect. In 1992 NAPNAP noted that child abuse and neglect was a national emergency.[77] In 2007, NAPNAP affirmed support principles to guide nurses in prevention, identification, and intervention in cases of suspected child maltreatment, including the education and empowerment of children, clinicians, and the community; use of child maltreatment protocols during clinical care; recognition of nurse practitioners as members of child protection teams; support of efforts to decrease violence and increase primary prevention; and emphasis on the importance of mental health care.[78] Ells[79] further challenges nurses to form multidisciplinary teams and to marshal community resources to favorably affect children and families in the area of child maltreatment.

Appendix 8-1: Report of Suspected Neglect Form

(Contributed by Texas Children's Hospital; Houston, TX.)

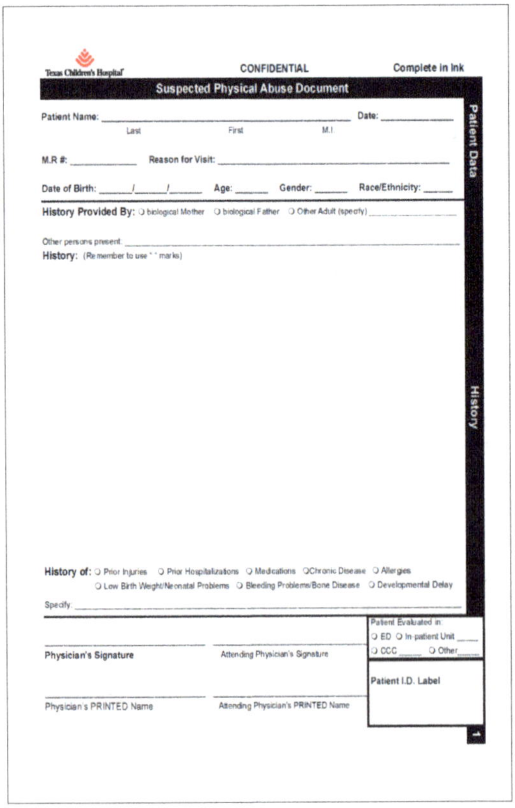

Texas Children's Hospital CONFIDENTIAL Complete in Ink

Suspected Physical Abuse Document

Patient Data

Patient Name: ______ Last First M.I. Date: ______

M.R #: ______ Reason for Visit: ______

Date of Birth: ___/___/___ Age: ___ Gender: ___ Race/Ethnicity: ___

History Provided By: ❍ biological Mother ❍ biological Father ❍ Other Adult (specify) ______

Other persons present: ______

History

History: (Remember to use " " marks)

History of: ❍ Prior Injuries ❍ Prior Hospitalizations ❍ Medications ❍ Chronic Disease ❍ Allergies ❍ Low Birth Weight/Neonatal Problems ❍ Bleeding Problems/Bone Disease ❍ Developmental Delay

Specify: ______

Physician's Signature ______ Attending Physician's Signature ______

Physician's PRINTED Name ______ Attending Physician's PRINTED Name ______

Patient Evaluated in: ❍ ED ❍ In-patient Unit ___ ❍ CCC ___ ❍ Other ___

Patient I.D. Label

1

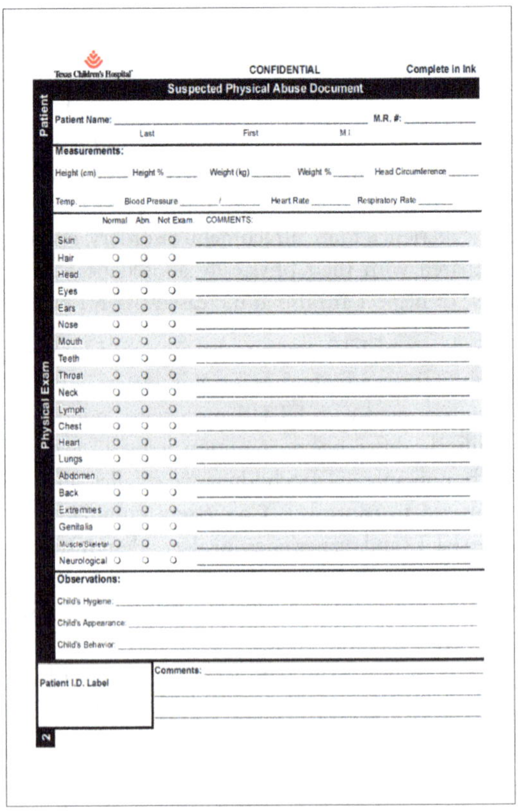

Texas Children's Hospital CONFIDENTIAL Complete in Ink

Suspected Physical Abuse Document

Patient

Patient Name: ______ Last First M.I. M.R. #: ______

Measurements:

Height (cm) ___ Height % ___ Weight (kg) ___ Weight % ___ Head Circumference ___

Temp. ___ Blood Pressure ___/___ Heart Rate ___ Respiratory Rate ___

Physical Exam

	Normal	Abn.	Not Exam.	COMMENTS:
Skin	❍	❍	❍	
Hair	❍	❍	❍	
Head	❍	❍	❍	
Eyes	❍	❍	❍	
Ears	❍	❍	❍	
Nose	❍	❍	❍	
Mouth	❍	❍	❍	
Teeth	❍	❍	❍	
Throat	❍	❍	❍	
Neck	❍	❍	❍	
Lymph	❍	❍	❍	
Chest	❍	❍	❍	
Heart	❍	❍	❍	
Lungs	❍	❍	❍	
Abdomen	❍	❍	❍	
Back	❍	❍	❍	
Extremities	❍	❍	❍	
Genitalia	❍	❍	❍	
Muscle/Skeletal	❍	❍	❍	
Neurological	❍	❍	❍	

Observations:

Child's Hygiene: ______

Child's Appearance: ______

Child's Behavior: ______

Patient I.D. Label

Comments: ______

2

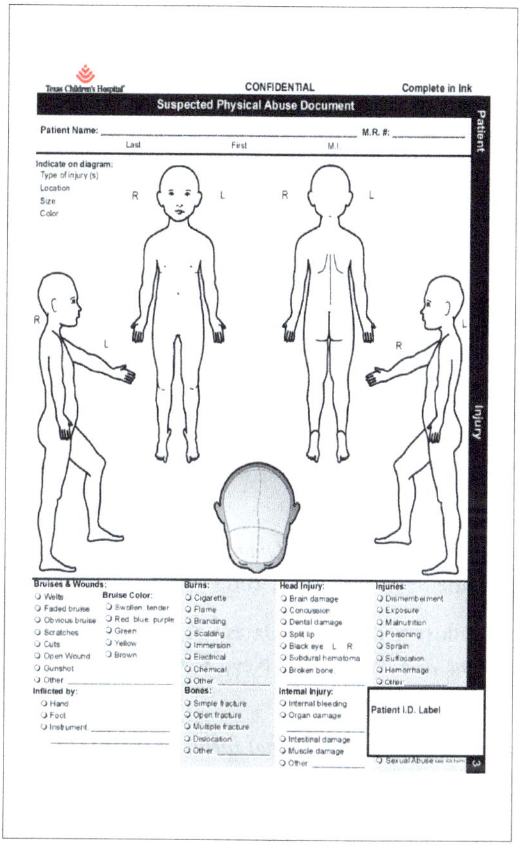

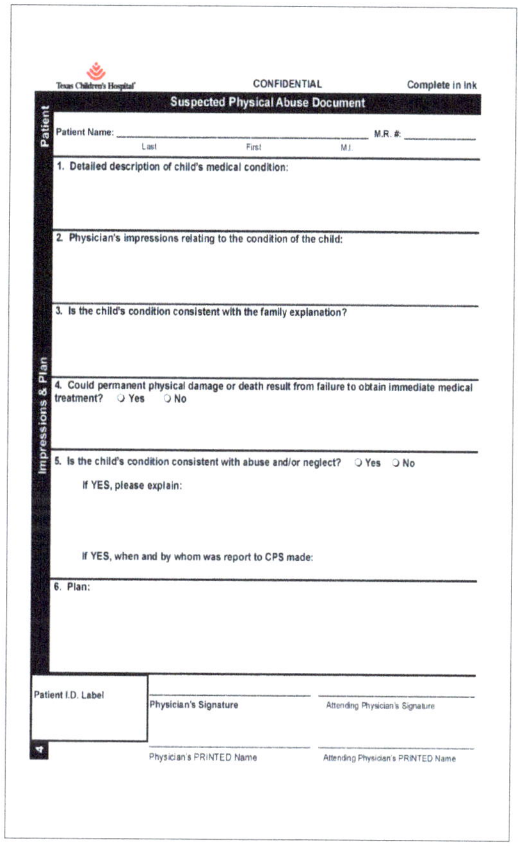

References

1. United States Department of Health and Human Services. *Child Maltreatment 2009*. Washington, DC: United States Department of Health and Human Services, Administration for Children and Families, Administration on Children, Youth and Families Children's Bureau; 2010.

2. Merritt DH. Child abuse potential: correlates with child maltreatment rates and structural measures of neighborhoods. *Child Youth Serv Rev*. 2009:31(8): 927-934.

3. Garbarino J, Crouter A. Defining the community context for parent-child relations: the correlates of child maltreatment. *Child Dev.* 1978;49(3):604-615.

4. Garbarino J, Sherman D. High-risk neighborhoods and high-risk families: the human ecology of child maltreatment. *Child Dev.* 1980;51(1):188-198.

5. Homer C, Ludwig S. Categorization of etiology of failure to thrive. *Am J Dis Child.* 1981;135:848-51.

6. Hildyard KL, Wolfe DA. Child neglect: developmental issues and outcomes. *Child Abuse Negl.* 2002;26(6-7):679-695.

7. Henderson V. *The Nature of Nursing: A Definition and Its Implications for Practice, Research and Education.* New York, NY: The Macmillan Company; 1966:15.

8. Dubowitz H, Black M, Starr RH, Zuravin S. A conceptual definition of child neglect. *Crim Justice Behav.* 1993;20(1):8-26.

9. Zuravin SJ. Child neglect: A review of definitions and measurement research. In: Dubowitz H, ed. *Neglected Children: Research, Practice, and Policy.* Thousand Oaks, CA: Sage Publications Inc;1999:24-46.

10. DePanfilis D. *Child Neglect: A Guide for Prevention, Assessment, and Intervention.* Washington, DC; United States Department of Health and Human Services, Administration for Children and Families, Administration for Children, Youth, and Families, Children's Bureau, Office on Child Abuse and Neglect; 2006.

11. Dubowitz H, Giardino A, Gustavson E. Child neglect: guidance for pediatricians. *Pediatr Rev.* 2000;21(4):111-116.

12. Rose SJ. Reaching consensus on child neglect: African American mothers and child welfare workers. *Child Youth Serv Rev.* 1999;21:463-479.

13. Cantwell HB. The neglect of child neglect. In: Helfer ME, Kempe RS, Krugman RD, eds. *The Battered Child.* 5th ed. Chicago, IL: University of Chicago Press; 1997:347-373.

14. Reece RM, Christian CW, eds. *Child Abuse: Medical Diagnosis and Management.* 3rd ed. Elk Grove, IL: American Academy of Pediatrics; 2009.

15. Oates RK. Neglect and nonorganic failure to thrive. In: Oates RK, ed. *The Spectrum of Child Abuse: Assessment, Treatment and Prevention.* New York, NY: Brunner/Mazel, Inc; 1996:15-19.

16. Sedlak AJ, Mettenburg J, Basena M, et al. *Fourth National Incidence Study of Child Abuse and Neglect (NIS-4).* Washington, DC: United States Department of Health and Human Services; 2010.

17. Brown J, Cohen P, Johnson JG, Salzinger S. A longitudinal analysis of risk factors for child maltreatment: findings of a 17-year prospective study of officially recorded and self-reported child abuse and neglect. *Child Abuse Negl.* 1998;22(11):1065-1078.

18. Piercecchi-Marti M, Louis-Borrione C, Bartoli C, et al. Malnutrition, a rare form of child abuse: diagnostic criteria. *J Forensic Sci.* 2006;51(3):670-673.

19. Dubowitz H, ed. *Neglected Children: Research, Practice, and Policy.* Thousand Oaks, CA: Sage Publications, Inc; 1999.

20. Johnson CF, Coury DL. Child neglect: general concepts and medical neglect. In: Ludwig S, Kornberg AE, eds. *Child Abuse: A Medical Reference.* 2nd ed. New York, NY: Churchill Livingstone; 1992:321-331.

21. Ludwig S. Failure-to-thrive/starvation. In: Ludwig, S, Kornberg AE, eds. *Child Abuse: A Medical Reference.* 2nd ed. New York, NY: Churchill Livingstone; 1992:303-319.

22. Burke J, Chandy J, Dannerbeck A, Watt JW. The parental environment cluster model of child neglect: an integrative conceptual model. *Child Welfare.* 1998;77(4):389-405.

23. Crittenden PM. Child neglect: causes and contributors. In: Dubowitz H. *Neglected Children: Research, Practice, and Policy.* Thousand Oaks, CA: Sage Publications, Inc; 1999:47-68.

24. Garbarino J. The human ecology of child maltreatment: a conceptual model for research. *J Marriage Fam.* 1977;39(4):721-736.

25. Hawley A. *Human Ecology: A Theory of Community Structure.* New York, NY: Ronald Press; 1950.

26. Bonfenbrenner U. Toward an experimental ecology of human development. *Am Psychol.* 1977;32:512-531.

27. Polansky NA, Gaudin JM, Ammons PW, Davis KB. The psychological ecology of the neglectful mother. *Child Abuse Negl.* 1985;9(2):265-275.

28. Garbarino J. The price of privacy in the social dynamics of child abuse. *Child Welfare.* 1977;56(9):565-575.

29. Runyan DK, Hunter WM, Everson MD, et al. *Longitudinal Studies of Child Abuse and Neglect, LONGSCAN: The First Five Years at the Coordinating Center, North Carolina and Seattle Site, 1991-1996.* Washington, DC: National Center on Child Abuse and Neglect, Department of Health and Human Services; 1997.

30. Belsky J. Etiology of child maltreatment: a developmental-ecological analysis. *Psychol Bull.* 1993;114(1):413-434.

31. Garbarino J, Barry F. The community context of child abuse and neglect. In: Garbarino J, Eckenrode J, eds. *Understanding Abusive Families: An Ecological Approach to Theory and Practice.* San Francisco, CA: Jossey-Bass Publishers; 1997:56-85.

32. Kaplan SJ. Child and adolescent abuse and neglect research: a review of the past 10 years. part I: physical and emotional abuse and neglect. *J Am Acad Child Adolesc Psychiatry.* 1999;38(10):1214-1222.

33. Lutzker JR, Bigelow KM, Doctor RM, Gershater RM, Greene BF. An ecobehavioral model for the prevention and treatment of child abuse and neglect: history and applications. In: Lutzker JR, ed. *Handbook of Child Abuse Research and Treatment.* New York, NY: Plenum Press; 1998:239-266.

34. Dubowitz H. Tackling child neglect: a role for pediatricians. *Pediatr Clin N Am.* 2009;56(2):363-378.

35. Hobbs CJ, Hanks HGI, Wynne JM. Neglect. In: Hobbs CJ, Hanks HGI, Wynne, JM, eds. *Child Abuse and Neglect: A Clinician's Handbook.* New York, NY: Churchill Livingstone; 1993:89-105.

36. Ludwig S, Rostain A. Family function and dysfunction. In: Levine MD, Carey WB, Crocker AC, eds. *Developmental-Behavioral Pediatrics.* 2nd ed. Philadelphia, PA: WB Saunders; 1992:147-159.

37. Rose SJ, Meezan W. Variations in perceptions of child neglect. *Child Welfare.* 1996;75(2):139-160.

38. Dubowitz H, Klockner A, Starr RH, Black MM. Community and professional definitions of child neglect. *Child Maltreat.* 1998;3(3):235-243.

39. Jaudes PK, Mackey-Bilaver L. Do chronic conditions increase young children's risk of being maltreated? *Child Abuse Negl.* 2008;32(7):671-681.

40. Sedlak AJ, Broadhurst DD. *Third National Incidence Study of Child Abuse and Neglect (NIS-3).* Washington, DC: United States Department of Health and Human Services; 1996.

41. Oates K, Kempe RS. Growth failure in infants. In: Helfer ME, Kempe RS, Krugman RD. *The Battered Child.* 5th ed. Chicago, IL: The University of Chicago Press; 1997:374-391.

42. Wright CM, Parkinson KN, Drewett RF. How does maternal and child feeding behavior relate to weight gain and failure to thrive?: data from a prospective birth cohort. *Pediatrics*. 2006;117(4):1262-1269.

43. Block RW, Krebs NF; American Academy of Pediatrics Committee on Child Abuse and Neglect, American Academy of Pediatrics Committee on Nutrition. Failure to thrive as a manifestation of child neglect. *Pediatrics*. 2005;116(5):1234-1237.

44. Ficicioglu C, an Haack K. Failure to thrive: when to suspect inborn errors of metabolism. *Pediatrics*. 2009;124(3):972-979

45. Hecht M, Foster SH, Dunn DJ, Williams JK, Anderson DR, Pulbratek D. Nonverbal behavior of young abused and neglected children. *Communication Education*. 1986;35(2):134-142.

46. Chatoor I, Schaefer S, Dickson L, Egan J. Non-organic failure to thrive: a developmental perspective. *Pediatr Ann*. 1984;13(11):829-835,838,840-842.

47. Zenel JA Jr. Failure to thrive: a general pediatrician's perspective. *Pediatr Rev.* 1997;18(11):371-378.

48. Bourke RS, Anderson V, Yang JS. Neurodevelopmental function is impaired in children with all severities of sleep disordered breathing. *Sleep Med.* 2011;12(3):222-229.

49. Linnard-Palmer L, Kools S. Parents' refusal of medical treatment based on religious and/or cultural beliefs: the law, ethical principles, and clinical implications. *J Pediatr Nurs* 2004;19(5):351-356.

50. Jenny C. Recognizing and responding to medical neglect. *Pediatrics*. 2007;120(6): 1385-1389.

51. American Academy of Pediatrics Committee on Child Abuse and Neglect, The American Academy of Pediatric Dentistry. Guidelines on oral and dental aspects of child abuse and neglect. *AAPD Clinical Guidelines*. 2010;34(6):158-161. http://www.aapd.org/media/Policies_Guidelines/G_Childabuse.pdf. Accessed March 28, 2011.

52. Matsui DM. Drug compliance in pediatrics. clinical and research issues. *Pediatr Clin North Am*. 1997;44:1-14.

53. Varness T, Allen DB, Carrel AL, Fost N. Childhood obesity and medical neglect. *Pediatrics*. 2009;123(1):399-406.

54. Wolfe DA. Child abuse prevention: blending research and practice. *Child Abuse Rev*. 1993;2(3):153-165.

55. Olds D, Hill PL, Mihalic SF, O'Brien RA. Nurse-family partnership. *Blueprints for Violence Prevention*. Denver, CO: C&M Press; 1998:3-96.

56. Olds D, Eckenrode J, Henderson CR, et al. Long-term effects of home visitation on maternal life course and child abuse and neglect. *JAMA*. 1997;278:637-643.

57. Olds D, Kitzman H. Review of research on home visiting for pregnant women and parents of young children. *Future Child.* 1993;3:53-92.

58. Bousha DM, Twentyman CT. Mother-child interactional style in abuse, neglect, and control groups: naturalistic observations in the home. *J Abnorm Psychol.* 1984;93(1):106-114.

59. Allin H, Wathen CN, MacMillan H. Treatment of child neglect: a systematic review. *Can J Psychiatry*. 2005;50(8):497-504.

60. Layzer JI, Goodson BD. *Parenting Education and Support: A Review of Research and Recommendations for Practice.* Philadelphia, PA: Department of Human Services, Division of Community-Based Prevention Services; 2001:1-28.

61. Raynor P, Rudolf MC, Cooper K, Marchant P, Cottrell D. A randomised controlled trial of specialist health visitor intervention for failure to thrive. *Arch Dis Child.* 1999;80(6):500-506.

62. Black MM, Dubowitz H, Hutcheson J, Berenson-Howard J, Starr RH. A randomized clinical trial of home intervention for children with failure to thrive. *Pediatrics.* 1995;95(6):807-814.

63. Prochaska JO, Johnson S, Lee P. The transtheoretical model of behavior change. In: Shumaker SA, Schron EB, Ockene JK, McBee WL, eds. *The Handbook of Health Behavior Change.* 2nd ed. New York, NY: Springs Publishing Company; 1998:59-84.

64. Ludwig S. Defining child abuse: clinical mandate—evolving concepts. In: Ludwig S, Kornberg AE, eds. *Child Abuse: A Medical Reference.* 2nd ed. New York, NY: Churchill Livingstone; 1992:1-12.

65. Pence D, Wilson C. *Team Investigation of Child Sexual Abuse: The Uneasy Alliance.* Thousand Oaks, CA: Sage Publications, Inc; 1994.

66. English D. Evaluation and risk assessment of child neglect in public child protection services. In: Dubowitz H, ed. *Neglected Children: Research, Practice, and Policy.* Thousand Oaks, CA: Sage Publications, Inc; 1999:191-210.

67. Crouch JL, Milner JS. Effects of child neglect on children. *Crim Justice Behav.* 1993;20(1):49-65.

68. Gaudin JM Jr. Child neglect: short-term and long-term outcomes. In: Dubowitz H, ed. *Neglected Children: Research, Practice, and Policy.* Thousand Oaks; CA: Sage Publications, Inc; 1999:89-108.

69. Kaplow JB, Widom CS. Age of onset of child maltreatment predicts long-term mental health outcomes. *J Abnorm Psychol.* 2007;116(1):176-187.

70. Beckett C, Maughan B, Rutter M, et al. Do the effects of early severe deprivation on cognition persist into early adolescence? findings from the English and Romanian adoptees study. *Child Dev.* 2006;77(3):696-711.

71. Black MM, Dubowitz H, Krishnakumar A, Starr RH. Early intervention and recovery among children with failure to thrive: follow-up at 8 years. *Pediatrics.* 2007;120:59-69

72. Kerr MA, Black MM, Krishnakumar A. Failure-to-thrive, maltreatment and the behavior and development of 6-year-old children from low-income urban families: a cumulative risk model. *Child Abuse Negl.* 2000;24(5):587-598.

73. Whitaker RC, Phillips SM, Orzol SM, Burdette HL. The association between maltreatment and obesity among preschool children. *Child Abuse Negl.* 2007;31(11-12):1187-1199.

74. Lissau I, Sørensen TI. Parental neglect during childhood and increased risk of obesity in young adulthood. *Lancet.* 1994:343(8893):324-327.

75. Wang CT, Holton J; Prevent Child Abuse America. Total estimated cost of child abuse and neglect in the United States. Prevent Child Abuse America Web site. http://www.preventchildabuse.org/about_us/media_releases/pcaa_pew_economic_impact_study_final.pdf. Accessed March 28, 2011.

76. Wodarski JS. Treatment of parents who abuse their children: a literature review and implications for professionals. *Child Abuse Negl.* 1981;5:351-360.

77. National Association of Pediatric Nurse Practitioners. Position statements. *J Pediatr Health Care.* 1992;6(4):226.

78. National Association of Pediatric Nurse Practitioners. Position statements. *J Pediatr Health Care.* 2007;21(1):25A-26A.

79. Ells M. Forming a multidisciplinary team to investigate child abuse. In: *Portable Guides to Investigating Child Abuse.* Washington, DC: United States Department of Justice; 1998:1-23.

Chapter 9

Documenting the Evaluation of Suspected Child Maltreatment Cases

Angelo P. Giardino, MD, PhD
Eileen R. Giardino, PhD, RN, FNP, ANP
Jennifer Pierce-Weeks, RN, CEN

Key Points

1. Findings for the assessment of child maltreatment should be recorded legibly, accurately, and completely.
2. The health care provider should never rely on his or her memory to reconstruct the details of the history and physical findings.
3. The health care provider should not record personal opinions regarding the caregiver or the situation because such information undermines the credibility of the professional and the medical record.
4. In reference to the record, it is best that the health care provider avoid medical terms that may be misunderstood by nonmedical professionals who may access and use the findings of the medical evaluation. As an alternative, the health care provider may include nonmedical explanations of medical terms in parentheses to clarify certain findings. For example, for finding of "...subdural hematoma, one could put in parentheses (a collection of blood inside the skull, around the brain...)."[1]
5. The issue of obtaining consent to authorize an examination of the child in cases of suspected abuse and neglect is complicated and may vary from state-to-state. The health care provider must be aware of the consent laws and regulations under which he or she operates.
6. The health care provider should document the specific questions as well as the child's verbatim answers,[2] nonverbal behaviors, and emotional responses.

Introduction

The medical evaluation of a suspected victim of child abuse or neglect is an essential component of the multidisciplinary approach to the overall evaluation. The findings of the medical evaluation are important to the investigation of suspected child maltreatment and may be included as evidence in judicial or legal proceedings. The findings of the medical evaluation may also play a central part in the ongoing process of the emotional and physical healing and well-being of the child who has been abused or mistreated.

In cases where a child is suspected of having been the victim of maltreatment, documentation of the history, physical findings, and laboratory assessment preserves evaluation data.[3] Accurate documentation of the history, physical examination, laboratory findings, and formulation of diagnostic impression is important because the medical record stands as a legal document and is used by law enforcement, district attorneys, and child protective services (CPS) to make decisions concerning the child's welfare.[1,4] The health care provider can expect that the medical chart will be scrutinized in legal procedures for decisions regarding the child's welfare or a perpetrator's fate.[5]

The medical evaluation of a child in cases of suspected abuse or neglect requires skill to perform a sensitive and developmentally appropriate history and physical examination. Thorough documentation of appropriate data is a learned skill that requires the health care provider to incorporate legal implications surrounding abuse situations with the components of a complete medical evaluation. A complete record is composed of data, including a developmental history for younger children, documentation of specific history questions and answers, sketches and photographs of physical injuries, genital examination findings, and witnesses to injury (see *Chapter 4, The Physical Examination in the Evaluation of Suspected Child Maltreatment: Physical Abuse and Sexual Abuse Examinations; Chapter 5, Laboratory Findings, Diagnostic Testing, and Forensic Specimens in Cases of Child Sexual Abuse;* and *Chapter 14, Legal Issues*).

General Considerations for the History and Physical Examination

Meticulous documentation of the findings of the medical evaluation is essential in cases of suspected child abuse. Findings should be recorded legibly, accurately, and completely.[6] The health care provider should never rely on his or her memory to reconstruct the details of the history and physical findings.[7] The purpose of the medical history is multifaceted and accomplishes the following specific goals.

— Gather information that leads to a diagnosis.

— Evaluate the physical safety of the child.

— Determine if medical treatment is necessary.[8]

Accurate documentation of the child's history, questions asked, and answers given is critical because the record is a legal document, and the data may be admitted as evidence in court trials. When court testimony is necessary, a well-documented chart serves to refresh the clinician's memory and, as a result, possibly decrease the time taken for court proceedings.[1,9] It is less likely that the health care provider may need to testify in civil court proceedings when the documents reflect detailed reports of the evaluation and explicit opinions of the findings.[10] Furthermore, CPS uses the record to make decisions regarding the child's placement in protective care with parents, caregivers, or foster care.[1]

Documentation Guidelines

The medical record should reflect the health care provider's knowledge of specific aspects of child abuse and neglect as well as an understanding of growth and development.[8] With child sexual abuse, the history is a critical component of the evaluation[11] because the physical examination findings are usually within normal limits or nonspecific. Studies have shown that the documentation of child abuse findings from medical evaluations is suboptimal in that the documentation may not support what was actually seen or heard. The way to decrease the incidence of poor documentation and charting of abuse findings is through an educational process aimed to improve the knowledge and skills base of clinicians in the area of child abuse.[12-14]

The health care provider should begin the history-taking process by asking questions of the appropriate person(s), typically the child and the child's caregivers, who have knowledge of the details of the case. The goal of the history-taking process is to obtain subjective data that provides background information regarding the abuse and the health status of the child. In sexual abuse evaluations where physical findings are rare, the history often provides the only data of the actual abuse. As much as possible, the health care provider should document the patient's subjective statements using quotations rather than paraphrasing the statements. This allows the reader, jury, attorney, or CPS worker to get a sense of the child's own words. By using quotations, the health care provider makes a clear distinction between the questions that he or she asked the child and the child's answers, This documentation process proves helpful in legal proceedings.[15] The interpretation of a statement can change dramatically depending on the context and question(s) asked. Additionally, some states have enacted hearsay exceptions that may allow health care providers to present the child's descriptions in court on behalf of the child. As permitted by state law, the hearsay process is enhanced if documentation included in the record is completed carefully and accurately.[5] The health care provider should follow the standards set for the questioning process by asking non-leading question and avoid coercing the child into answering.[1] The court is always concerned about the possibility of improper or suggestive questioning methods that could lead the respondent's answers. When leading is suspected or determined, the court may request a pretrial taint hearing to determine how information was obtained and if information was obtained appropriately. The court may challenge the admissibility of the child's history if it is determined that questioning was not conducted appropriately.[16] The health care provider should not record personal opinions regarding the caregiver or the situation because such information undermines the credibility of the professional and of the medical record.[17]

Because the medical record is a legal document that can be subpoenaed for any court proceeding, it is important that the handwriting be legible; data comprehensive; and, when necessary, events documented chronologically.[1,5] Any corrections that the health care provider makes to the notes should be inserted as addenda and marked as such. The health care provider should write a clear signature for the correction, followed by his or her printed name. For the record, it is best that the health care provider avoid medical terms that may be misunderstood by nonmedical professionals who access and use the findings of the medical evaluation. As an alternative, the health care provider may include nonmedical explanations of medical terms in parentheses to clarify certain findings. For example, for the finding of "...subdural hematoma, one could put in parentheses (a collection of blood inside the skull, around the brain...)."[1]

General information regarding the context of the health care evaluation should be entered into the record. It is recommended that the health care provider document that: (1) the child was informed that the purpose of questioning was for medical diagnosis and treatment and (2) the child was told of the importance of providing accurate information.[18] The following general information should be documented in the medical evaluation[1,17]:

— Qualifications of the person completing the medical evaluation

— Name of the person making a given statement or demonstrating a given behavior and that person's relationship to the child

— Name(s) of accompanying adult(s) and their relationship to the child

— Date and time of the assessment

— Referral source

— Reason for referral or chief complaint

— Names of people present at the time a given statement was made or given behavior was observed

— Name and phone number, when possible, of the person making the entry into the record or chart

Documentation of Consent

The issue of obtaining consent to authorize an examination of a child in cases of suspected abuse and neglect is complicated and may vary from state-to-state. The health care provider must be aware of the consent laws and regulations under which he or she operates on both the institution and state level. For example, an emergency health care situation in which the child arrives at the emergency room (ER) for care often implies consent for urgent care. In less urgent situations, parental consent is essential. However, when child maltreatment is suspected, the health care provider is obligated to act upon suspicions and may need to pursue other avenues for obtaining consent to protect the interests of the child and keep him or her safe should the parents deny permission for an examination.

The authorizing party usually prints and signs his or her name in the medical record and provides a statement that he or she consents to the evaluation. The status of the consenting party may be complicated and depends on the details of the child's case. In child maltreatment settings, the child may be brought to the health care facility for medical evaluation at the request of a parent or caregiver, CPS or law enforcement personnel, or the agency that was assigned physical custody of the child from the court (see *Chapter 14, Legal Issues*).

Format of Assessment Documentation

Studies looking at the quality of documentation resulting from child physical and sexual abuse examinations have found that clinicians do not always document the history and physical examination findings in the clearest or most complete manner.[4,19] Health care providers can benefit from training in all aspects of documentation because of the complexity of specific abuse-related data. In reviewing child abuse records, the quality of documentation was shown to be improved by using structured records to aid in the documentation process.[20] Checklists can serve to remind the health care providers what details should be documented in the medical record. Structured forms have long been used to help to increase the amount of collected information included in the medical records, particularly in the area of dates and times and the illustration of physical injuries on provided diagrams.[4]

Documentation of Taped Interviews

The guidelines put forth by the American Professional Society on the Abuse of Children (APSAC) suggest that the use of videotapes or audiotapes should be determined by clinical considerations, logistics, and professional preference.[21] Documentation of a taped interview requires careful notation of what occurred, including information that makes it clear who was doing what and who was present during the taping. When using taped recordings, the health care provider should provide explicit information regarding the following[2]:

— Name of the child in question

— Name of the interviewer

— Date, time, and location of the interview

— Other person(s) present during the taping and history-taking

By videotaping an interview and allowing other investigators to view the recorded statements and responses, the health care provider can decrease the number of interviews a child must undergo during the investigative process. Taping allows the practitioner to give the patient full attention without concern for writing anything during the session. The tape can be used to show the child's affect during the interview and may enable other professionals to evaluate the strengths of the case.[21] Taping also allows for later review of the record and critique of the methods with colleagues.[16,22]

Guidelines for audiotaping and videotaping the history-taking process in child abuse evaluations continue to be controversial and lack apparent consensus among professionals. Such documentation techniques are of particular concern for prosecutors because the recordings highlight any deficiencies that the interviewer might have and provides evidence to flawed techniques, such as misphrased or leading questions. Additionally, such documentation allows defense experts the opportunity to critique the tape and characterize the actions and interactions of the interviewer in a negative perspective to favor the alleged perpetrator.[23] The use of videotape testimony is not permitted in certain states and jurisdictions, so it is imperative that the health care provider be knowledgeable of the specific state guidelines under which he or she operates. It is recommended that clinicians who decide to use audio and video technology to aid in documentation efforts follow accepted practice guidelines for taping, storing, and releasing of information.[23,24]

Documentation of the History

Documentation of the history findings should be detailed and complete. The health care provider should include the specific questions asked along with the child's verbatim answers,[2] nonverbal behaviors, and emotional responses. Any drawings made by the child should be labeled with an appropriate heading that describes what the diagram is and should then be dated and signed by the health care provider and child and made a part of the permanent record.[2] Additionally, it is especially important that the health care provider include a statement indicating that he or she asked the child to state the words he or she uses to name body parts. For example, the record may include a statement similar to the following: "Words describing body parts are the words used by the child."[25] When an interpreter is used, it is important to document the name of the professional providing translation and the language interpreted.[26]

In cases of physical abuse, the health care provider should document specific information in the medical record regarding what the caregiver stated about how the injury occurred to determine whether the reasons provided for the injury seem plausible or reasonable given the type and degree of the injury sustained. Because the child's recollection of the circumstances that resulted in his or her injury as obtained by the health care provider can be admitted as evidence in court trials, it is critical the health care provider thoroughly document questions and answers during the evaluation.[15] The clinician should document any information gathered from the caregiver or child that raises his or her suspicion of abuse. The following are such areas of suspicion that should be documented in the record[7,27,28]:

— Caregiver's explanation for injury

— History of injury that changes with time or is vague

— No reasonable explanation of injury

— Inappropriate history for observed injury

— Developmentally incompatible history

— Incongruous or implausible trauma history compared with physical examination

— Inappropriate caregiver concerns for severe injury

— Nonspecific behavioral indicators from child or caregiver

— Caregiver without explanation for injury

— Claim of sibling-inflicted injury

— Delay in seeking medical care for life-threatening or serious injury

History from the Caregiver

It is common practice for the health care provider to first take a medical history from the child's caregiver before speaking with the child. The caregiver's information forms the initial basis for the examination of the child. This history should be obtained from the caregiver without the child present whenever possible.[29,30] In cases where the child to be interviewed is an infant, young child, or developmentally delayed, the primary history is usually obtained from the caregiver.

The documentation of the history should reflect that the interviewer did not use blaming or accusatory statements or make assumptions or speculations. Documentation of the history should include the following information:

— When and how injury occurred

— Whether injury was witnessed; if so, by whom

— Person responsible for the child at time of injury

— If the injury was not witnessed by the caregiver, how the caregiver came to know of the incident

— General health of the child

— Child's previous surgeries and hospitalizations

— Child's significant medical history

— Whether the child previously has been evaluated for this complaint; if so, where

Documentation of Neglect: A Longer View

When documenting cases of neglect, the health care provider should record the clues that raise his or her suspicion for neglect as they become evident during the history-taking and observation process. The health care provider should note aspects of the child's basic needs such as shelter, food, clothing, and medical care. Neglect that stems from a caregiver's lack of knowledge or developmental or psychological deficits still must be documented and reported. It is appropriate to note observations of the child's appearance, physical or developmental concerns, and home environment concerns.[31] Generally, neglect becomes apparent over time; therefore, the medical record should contain the history, physical examination, laboratory, and diagnostic information that confirm a pattern of care that has failed to meet the child's basic needs.

Documentation of Parent-Child Interactions

It can be especially important that the health care provider document the child's demeanor during the history and examination as well as his or her interactions with the accompanying caregiver. Such data not only serves as a record of parent-child rapport as observed during the evaluation process, but also to trigger the health care provider's memory during testimony. The interactions and relationships between and among the people who are part of the history and physical examination may have bearing on the overall investigation of suspected child abuse and maltreatment.[1] When describing particular interactions noted during the assessment, either between the caregiver and healthcare provider or the caregiver and child, the following guidelines should be employed[1,17]:

— Describe health care provider's actions or questions that immediately preceded the caregiver's or child's behavior or statement.

— Detail the demeanor of the person making the statement or exhibiting the behavior.

— Include exact words of the person using quotation marks.

— Describe behavior the child or adult exhibited.

— Note caregiver's concern over, knowledge of, and support for child.

— Note caregiver's indifference or hostility toward child, if applicable.

Documentation of Physical Findings

Documentation of the physical examination should include descriptions of the physical findings and the specifics of each injury observed and evaluated. The medical chart should reflect documentation of any signs of trauma using detailed diagrams as well as photographic documentation, whenever possible. Photographs are an excellent evidence source and add credibility to written and verbal statements; however, it should be noted that photos serve to augment documentation of findings and cannot be used in place of accurate written documentation.[6] Due to the possibility of civil or criminal court action, all records, drawings, or photographs must be kept as part of the chart record.[10]

In cases of physical abuse, the health care provider should carefully and legibly record descriptions of each injury. A chart is helpful for documenting the type, size, shape, color, and age of each injury[32] (**Table 9-1**). Included in the documentation of injuries should be an explanation for how the injury occurred as stated by both the child and the caregiver(s). Any incompatibilities between the history of how the injury occurred and its physical manifestations should be recorded in the medical record. Inconsistencies in the caregiver's statements regarding how an injury occurred are a major reason for filing a report of abuse to CPS agencies. Detailed information concerning injuries is essential when the examiner must appear in court.

Pediatric sexual assault nurse examiners (SANEs) are nurses trained specifically in the physical, emotional, and intellectual development of adolescents and children. Their physical examination skills and interview training enables them to prepare the child for the examination, conduct a thorough examination, and document findings in a way that holds up under legal scrutiny.[2] A study comparing evidence collected by SANE nurses and non-SANE-trained nurse and physician colleagues found that evidence collection kits prepared by SANE nurses were more accurate and complete than those kits prepared by clinicians who were not SANEs. Study findings may speak to the fact that education and preparation in the area of physical examination and evidence collection does improve a clinician's ability to accurately collect, prepare, and document evidence findings.[33,34]

Table 9-1. Chart for Documenting Injuries

Injury Number	Type of Injury	Size	Shape	Object	Color	Observed Age of Injury	Stated Age of Injury	Explanation Given by Mother, Father, Child or Other	Is Injury Consistent with History?		
									Yes	No	Uncertain

Reprinted with permission from Johnson CF. Inflicted injury versus accidental injury. Pediatr Clin North Am. *1990;37(4):791-814.*

Photographic Documentation of Findings

All traumatic injuries, whether new or old, should be photographed as an adjunct to written, descriptive documentation. Visual findings are valuable in influencing court proceedings and for peer review and teaching efforts.[6,35] Photographs of injuries may save the child from the need for reevaluation when there is the need for the injury to be evaluated for a second opinion. Pictures communicate quickly and effectively to all who see them and add credibility to patient statements. Medical providers are usually responsible for determining whether all appropriate areas of the child's body are photodocumented properly, even when other professionals such as law enforcement or CPS workers may have taken the photographs.[35] Photographic documentation becomes a permanent part of the medical record and can last indefinitely when stored properly.

There is much discussion about the types of camera equipment that can and should be used to photograph injuries. Camera equipment should require the need for minimal training and provide true color balance to document injuries. The camera should be able to photograph the subject from a comfortable distance and be able to produce life-size reproductions of trauma sites. It is ideal to photograph both small and large body areas and the mechanism or device believed to have caused injury(s).[36]

The role of digital photography in photodocumentation in child maltreatment continues to evolve. Initial criticism revolved around the ability to manipulate the images; however, this is rarely a concern when the digital images are properly identified and supported in the medical record. It is true that digital cameras do compress and enhance images, but these concerns need not exclude the images forensically. Modern digital cameras automatically compress images into something like a JPEG (**J**oint **P**hotographic **E**xperts **G**roup) format, resulting in unavoidable loss of information; however, the cameras used for forensic photographs remove only redundant and irrelevant information. When there is a concern that important image content may be lost, the degree of compression is typically lowered before storing images. Enhancement and restoration techniques are commonly used to improve the appearance of an image and to remove motion artifacts. Specific documentation is usually not required when enhancement techniques involve processes that are comparable to traditional darkroom methods, such as brightness adjustment, contrast adjustment, color balancing, and cropping.

Another common misconception is that image files should be left on the camera's flash drive and made available to the court if requested. Because temporary storage on a flash drive is susceptible to corruption by improper handling and storage over time, it is not recommended that it be used for permanent storage. Duplicate images stored on a hard drive, compact disc (CD), or digital versatile disc (DVD) are generally admissible as original images in court proceedings. Written protocols regarding the process for producing photographic evidence and standardized documentation can help child abuse teams minimize errors that can lead to questions regarding the reliability, reproducibility, security of the images, or all 3.

The composition of the photograph should reflect proper arrangement of significant injuries and body part elements to document the patient's condition (**Table 9-2**). The picture should realistically show injuries without overly exaggerating trauma.[35] Before-and-after pictures are helpful to show the change in condition of the skin and injuries over a stated timeframe. Photographs taken before wounds are cleaned show the original condition of the child, while photographs taken after the wounds are cleaned show the child at a different stage. Photographing a bruise from different angles may help to show the amount of bruising or swelling present compared to the natural structures of the body. Such angles provide perspective within the photograph to show the relationship

Table 9-2. Photographing the Injuries

— Photograph all injuries with and without a color and measure standard.

— Label each photograph with the patient's name, medical record number, date and time taken, and name of photographer.

— If close-up photographs are taken, also indicate the location of injury on the patient's body.

— Take follow-up photographs if injuries have not fully developed, usually several hours to days later.

— Do not throw away any photographs in a series, regardless of how well or poorly they develop.

— Make certain the entire injury is viewed in the photograph.

— Respect the patient's modesty by draping any uninvolved breast or genital areas.

— Check photographs before discharging patient.

of the bruises to the anatomical structures. Proper perspective helps to accurately depict the full impact of the injuries or bruises.[35,36]

Despite their value, photographs remain supplemental to the written record. Written descriptions of all injuries or abnormalities must accompany the pictures and must include the location, type, size, and color of the injury. It is appropriate to include descriptive text and hand-drawn diagrams with each photograph, because the quality of the photograph cannot be guaranteed.[17] The written record should never be in conflict with the photographs. Proper documentation of all photographic evidence should include a form with the child's name, case number, and date and time the photographs were taken.[17,36] It is helpful to include any outline drawings of the child's body to show the specific photographed areas. A measuring device should be positioned above or below the injury to clearly depict the size of the injury.[29,35]

It is a challenge to capture injuries that have not yet bruised or those in which the bruise is clearing.[16] Ultraviolet and infrared photography are the best approaches to obtaining visual documentation of such findings. However, the equipment is technologically advanced and expensive and requires a level of photographic skill that most people do not have.[16]

For photographic documentation of injuries to be used as court evidence, the photographs must show proper verification, meaning that a medical evaluator can verify that the pictures are an accurate portrayal of original findings, and be relevant to the issue.[28] Additionally, the photographs must accurately portray a complete and fair representation of the scene. During court proceedings, it is important that the health care provider who examined the child, if other than the photographer, is able to verify that the photographs accurately represent the actual findings of the child's injuries.[16,36] Proper verification of photographs is essential, so they can be shown to be relevant to the case; it is also important when reconstructing the case for court purposes. Verification involves keeping meticulous records of photographic data, including date, time, location, case number, camera, lens, aperture, light source, subject distance, and macro lens magnification.[35] Also, the record should include documentation that proper chain of custody procedures were followed according to state and local law enforcement procedures.[6,26] Finally, photographs and negatives should be carefully stored and preserved because the prosecution may depend on the medical photographs when arguing the case in court[17] (see *Chapter 4, The Physical Examination in the Evaluation of Suspected Child Maltreatment: Physical Abuse and Sexual Abuse Examinations*).

Obtaining Consent for Photodocumentation

Most state laws regarding child abuse evaluations do not require the health care provider to obtain permission from the guardian to photograph the child. The health care provider should be aware of the specific state laws under which he or she practices and should, in some situations, request consent even if it is not required.[28] The health care provider should also ask permission of the child to be photographed. It is not recommended to take photographs if the child does not consent or assent.[6]

It is important to inform the child of the need to photodocument his or her body and attempt to engage him or her in the process. The age of the child should dictate his or her sensitivity to the procedures. In order to gain clear and accurate photos, it may be necessary to have an assistant help by distracting the child or stabilizing needed limbs or body areas.[6]

Use of Colposcope

In cases of child sexual abuse, the colposcope or a fiberoptic scope enables the health care provider to visualize anal and genital anatomy to a much greater degree than with the eye alone. The advantage of the colposcope is its ability to photograph the anatomy and findings and then share those findings with others in the medical and legal systems.[37] The colposcope enables illumination and magnification of the field of vision and allows the health care provider to simultaneously conduct the examination and document the findings using video technology.[35] Standard colposcopies include a digital adaptation that allows the health care provider to achieve greater visibility by viewing the examination on a computer monitor.[6,16] Some colposcopes are equipped with mounted cameras enabled with computer software that stores text and findings. For some children, being able to view the examination decreases their anxiety because it takes away some of the fear of the unknown; therefore, the health care provider may elect to use a computer monitor with the colposcope to allow the child to view the examination.[16]

Forensic Evidence Collection

Although most examiners of child maltreatment focus on the medical examination and treatment, the forensic evidence collection component cannot be separated, eliminated, or forgotten. Forensic evidence collection is a component of the complete examination whenever child maltreatment is suspected. Proper documentation of the evidence collected is important in maintaining the integrity of the process in the event of legal proceedings. The following data should be recorded in the medical record[26]:

— Names of the person(s) completing the examination

— License number, signature, credential, and telephone number of the clinician(s)

— Description of all evidence sent to the forensic laboratory (see *Chapter 5, Laboratory Findings, Diagnostic Testing, and Forensic Specimens in Cases of Child Sexual Abuse*)

— Distribution of the evidence, including name of persons accepting the evidence, date, and time

— Name and signature of person who receives the evidence

— Distribution of the medicolegal report; to whom the report has been given

— Name and telephone number of the person to whom the child was discharged

Documenting Conclusions, Opinions, or Diagnoses from the Medical Evaluation

It is the norm of practice for health care professionals to form conclusions from the data gathered during the history, physical examination, and laboratory assessment of a patient. In suspected abuse, it is appropriate to form a conclusion and document whether the physical findings are consistent or inconsistent with a given history.[17] The examiner should be as definitive as possible in stating a diagnosis or formulation of opinion.[3] When findings are conclusive for physical abuse, it is acceptable to diagnose child abuse and state that injuries are consistent with a specific situation, such as battered child syndrome. When the findings are not clear, it is acceptable to use words such as possible or probable.[1]

In many types of abuse, especially child sexual abuse, there are few to no physical examination findings that support the allegation. Most victims of child sexual abuse have nonspecific or normal genital and anogenital findings; therefore, it is appropriate to state the conclusions of the history and objective findings in a way that does not negate the possibility that sexual abuse did occur. In cases of neglect in which physical findings are absent, the health care provider should provide a description of findings for each system, so they can be compared to former or future examinations of the child. The following are examples of how to formulate diagnostic assessments in the presence or absence of physical findings[37]:

— The history or behavior is descriptive of inappropriate sexual contact; however, no diagnostic residual is evident.

— The history or observations are limited, and although the behaviors observed by the parents have raised concern, there are insufficient historical or behavioral details to support a concern of inappropriate sexual contact.

The health care provider should avoid using statements such as "no evidence of abuse" or "evidence confirms abuse" when documenting assessment findings because such statements may be used to support an opposite conclusion in legal proceedings.[17] Both examples stress the importance of the history and the findings. The health care provider may document normal examination findings while still asserting his or her concern for potential sexual abuse by saying, "The results of the examination were normal but this does not rule out the possibility of sexual abuse."[1] When the history and physical examination findings do not support each other, it is appropriate to document that "the examination is inconsistent with the history and an alternative explanation should be sought."[37]

Documentation of the Treatment and Plan

The complete plan of treatment and recommendations for follow-up are an important part of the medical record. Careful documentation of the specific health care needs of the child and the prognosis are important as well. The health care provider should include reports to public agencies, such as CPS or law enforcement, and recommended consultations.[1]

Mandated Reporting Requirements

All states require nurses to report cases of suspected child abuse or neglect. Many also grant immunity from liability when such a report is made in good faith. The health care provider can be held accountable in many states for failure to report; therefore, when the clinician makes a report to law enforcement or CPS, the record should reflect why the report was made and to whom the report was given. Although it is important to follow institutional policies and procedures, it is equally important to know the reporting requirements of the state in which the health care provider practices. Of course, state and federal law override institutional policy, and those policies should be in accordance with governmental laws.[38]

Court Testimony and Documentation

The prospect of testifying in court about a case often elicits stress and concern among health care professionals. Testifying can certainly be a stressful experience; however, the health care provider should always keep in mind that he or she is not expected to be an attorney, judge, or juror, but rather a professional who is being asked to tell the truth. The health care provider must review all written documentation of the case and be familiar with the details and conclusions of the examination on specific cases. Relying on one's memory of a case can be detrimental to the process. It is the health care provider's responsibility to be clear about the details of the case. Whether expert or fact witness, nervous or calm, remaining professional at all times is the most important component of testifying effectively (see *Chapter 14, Legal Issues*).

Conclusion

The implications of an abuse allegation for the child, child's family, alleged perpetrator, and community are profound. The health care provider evaluating suspected cases of child maltreatment must make documentation a priority. The goal of documentation is to preserve the valuable information uncovered during the health care evaluation for use during the investigation and possible judicial process.

Appendix 9-1: Child Abuse Evaluation Form

Children's Medical Center of Dallas Child Abuse Form

(Contributed by Benjamin Retta, LMSW; Children's Hospital of Dallas; Dallas, TX.)

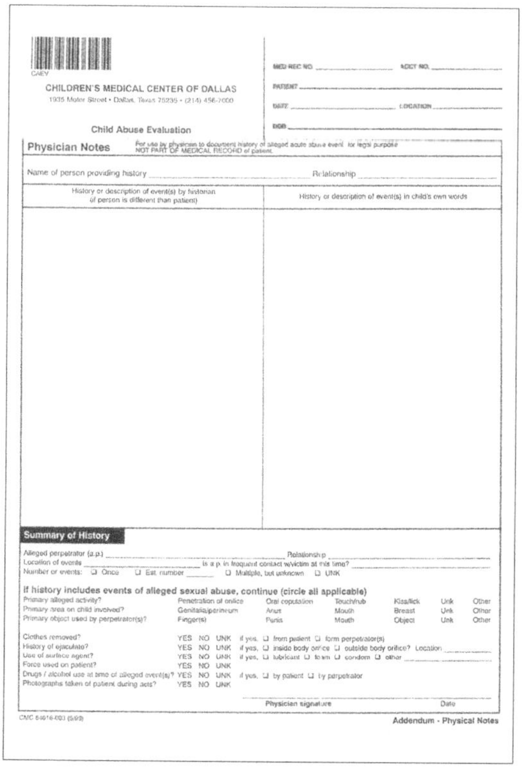

CAEV

CHILDREN'S MEDICAL CENTER OF DALLAS

1935 Motor Street • Dallas, Texas 75235 • (214) 456-7000

Child Abuse Evaluation

MED REC NO. ______ ACCT NO. ______

PATIENT ______

DATE ______ LOCATION ______

DOB ______

Physician Notes For use by physician to document history of alleged acute abuse event for legal purpose NOT PART OF MEDICAL RECORD of patient

Name of person providing history ______ Relationship ______

History or description of event(s) by historian (if person is different than patient)	History or description of event(s) in child's own words

Summary of History

Alleged perpetrator (a.p.) ______ Relationship ______

Location of events ______ Is a.p. in frequent contact w/victim at this time? ______

Number or events: ☐ Once ☐ Est. number ______ ☐ Multiple, but unknown ☐ UNK

If history includes events of alleged sexual abuse, continue (circle all applicable)

Primary alleged activity?	Penetration of orifice	Oral copulation	Touch/rub	Kiss/lick	Unk	Other
Primary area on child involved?	Genitalia/perineum	Anus	Mouth	Breast	Unk	Other
Primary object used by perpetrator(s)?	Finger(s)	Penis	Mouth	Object	Unk	Other

Clothes removed? YES NO UNK if yes, ☐ from patient ☐ form perpetrator(s)

History of ejaculate? YES NO UNK if yes, ☐ inside body orifice ☐ outside body orifice? Location ______

Use of surface agent? YES NO UNK if yes, ☐ lubricant ☐ foam ☐ condom ☐ other ______

Force used on patient? YES NO UNK

Drugs / alcohol use at time of alleged event(s)? YES NO UNK if yes, ☐ by patient ☐ by perpetrator

Photographs taken of patient during acts? YES NO UNK

Physician signature ______ Date ______

CMC 64016-003 (5/93)

Addendum - Physical Notes

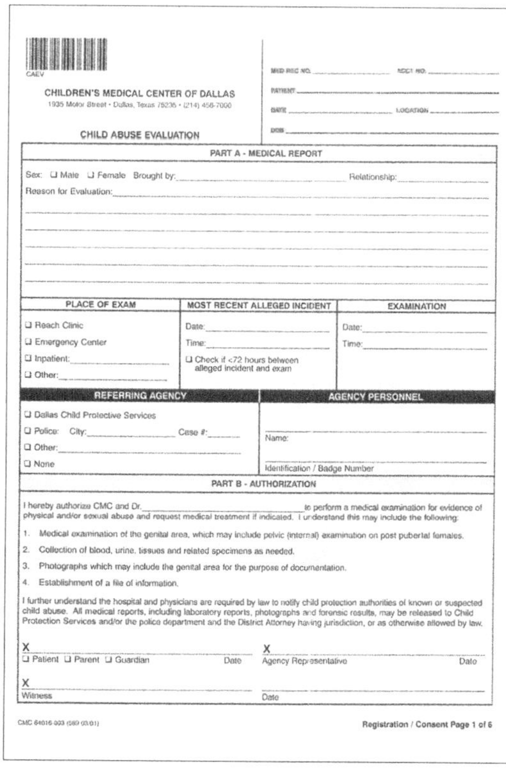

CAEV

CHILDREN'S MEDICAL CENTER OF DALLAS

1935 Motor Street • Dallas, Texas 75235 • (214) 456-7000

CHILD ABUSE EVALUATION

MED REC NO. ______ ACCT NO. ______

PATIENT ______

DATE ______ LOCATION ______

DOB ______

PART A - MEDICAL REPORT

Sex: ☐ Male ☐ Female Brought by: ______ Relationship: ______

Reason for Evaluation: ______

PLACE OF EXAM	MOST RECENT ALLEGED INCIDENT	EXAMINATION
☐ Reach Clinic ☐ Emergency Center ☐ Inpatient: ______ ☐ Other: ______	Date: ______ Time: ______ ☐ Check if <72 hours between alleged incident and exam	Date: ______ Time: ______

REFERRING AGENCY	AGENCY PERSONNEL
☐ Dallas Child Protective Services ☐ Police: City: ______ Case #: ______ ☐ Other: ______ ☐ None	Name: ______ Identification / Badge Number ______

PART B - AUTHORIZATION

I hereby authorize CMC and Dr. ______ to perform a medical examination for evidence of physical and/or sexual abuse and request medical treatment if indicated. I understand this may include the following:

1. Medical examination of the genital area, which may include pelvic (internal) examination on post pubertal females.
2. Collection of blood, urine, tissues and related specimens as needed.
3. Photographs which may include the genital area for the purpose of documentation.
4. Establishment of a file of information.

I further understand the hospital and physicians are required by law to notify child protection authorities of known or suspected child abuse. All medical reports, including laboratory reports, photographs and forensic results, may be released to Child Protection Services and/or the police department and the District Attorney having jurisdiction, or as otherwise allowed by law.

X ______ ☐ Patient ☐ Parent ☐ Guardian Date

X ______ Agency Representative Date

X ______ Witness

______ Date

CMC 64016-003 (5/93 03/01)

Registration / Consent Page 1 of 6

CAEV

CHILDREN'S MEDICAL CENTER OF DALLAS
1935 Motor Street • Dallas, Texas 75235 • (214) 456-7000

CHILD ABUSE EVALUATION

MED REC NO. ______ ACCT NO. ______
PATIENT ______
DATE ______ LOCATION ______
DOB ______

PART C - SOCIAL INFORMATION

PATIENT (VICTIM)		AGE (Years)	SEX (M / F)	RACE
❑ Mother ❑ Stepmother ❑ Guardian				
❑ Father ❑ Stepfather ❑ Guardian				
Siblings				

Previous involvement of family with child protection authorities? ❑ Yes ❑ No ❑ Unknown

DATE	TIME	SOCIAL NOTES

Signature: X

Social Page 2 of 6

CAEV

CHILDREN'S MEDICAL CENTER OF DALLAS
1935 Motor Street • Dallas, Texas 75235 • (214) 456-7000

CHILD ABUSE EVALUATION

MED REC NO. ______ ACCT NO. ______
PATIENT ______
DATE ______ LOCATION ______
DOB ______

PART D - MEDICAL HISTORY

PAST HISTORY

Usual Health Provider: ______
Hospitalization / Surgery / Trauma: ______
Birth / Development: ______
Past Health Problems: ______
Medicines: ______

SEXUAL HISTORY (❑ Check if Not Applicable to Patient)

Hx of voluntary sexual intercourse? ❑ Yes ❑ No
Use of contraception? ❑ Yes ❑ No
Hx of prior STD? ❑ Yes ❑ No

FEMALE:
Menarche? ❑ Yes ❑ No
Age menses: ______ Date LMP: ______
Use of tampons? ❑ Yes ❑ No
Hx vaginitis? ❑ Yes ❑ No
Hx pregnancy(s)? ❑ Yes ❑ No

BEHAVIOR / EMOTIONAL SYMPTOMS

Sleep Disturbances ❑ Yes ❑ No ❑ Unknown
Eating Problems ❑ Yes ❑ No ❑ Unknown
School Problems ❑ Yes ❑ No ❑ Unknown
Sexual Acting Out ❑ Yes ❑ No ❑ Unknown
Fear ❑ Yes ❑ No ❑ Unknown
Anger ❑ Yes ❑ No ❑ Unknown
Signs of Depression ❑ Yes ❑ No ❑ Unknown
Other Symptoms (Describe) ❑ Yes ❑ No ❑ Unknown

PHYSICAL SYMPTOMS / HISTORY

Abdominal / Pelvic Pain ❑ Yes ❑ No ❑ Unknown
Vomiting ❑ Yes ❑ No ❑ Unknown
Genital Discomfort or Pain ❑ Yes ❑ No ❑ Unknown
Dysuria ❑ Yes ❑ No ❑ Unknown
Urinary Tract Infection ❑ Yes ❑ No ❑ Unknown
Enuresis ❑ Yes ❑ No ❑ Unknown
Vaginal Itching or Penile Irritation ❑ Yes ❑ No ❑ Unknown
Vaginal Discharge or Penile Discharge ❑ Yes ❑ No ❑ Unknown
Vaginal Bleeding or Penile Bleeding ❑ Yes ❑ No ❑ Unknown
Rectal Pain ❑ Yes ❑ No ❑ Unknown
Rectal Bleeding ❑ Yes ❑ No ❑ Unknown
Constipation ❑ Yes ❑ No ❑ Unknown
Stool Incontinence ❑ Yes ❑ No ❑ Unknown

FURTHER HISTORY

Medical History Page 3 of 6

CAEV

CHILDREN'S MEDICAL CENTER OF DALLAS
1935 Motor Street • Dallas, Texas 75235 • (214) 456-7000

CHILD ABUSE EVALUATION

MED REC NO. ______ ACCT NO. ______
PATIENT ______
DATE ______ LOCATION ______
DOB ______

PART E - GENERAL PHYSICAL EXAMINATION

Immunizations: ______
Allergies: ______
Pulse ______ /min **Respirations** ______ /min **Temperature:** ______ **Blood Pressure** ______ / ______
include percentiles of children under age six
Height: ______ ______ %tile Weight: ______ ______ %tile FOC (< age 3): ______ ______ %tile

EXAM	NORMAL	ABNORMAL	COMMENTS
General			
HEENT			
Lungs			
CV			
Abdomen			
GU			
Neurologic			

SKIN

Record any injuries and findings on diagrams: Erythema, Abrasions, Bruises, Contusions, Induration, Lacerations, Fractures, Bites, Burns. Record Size, Appearance and Color of Injuries / findings.

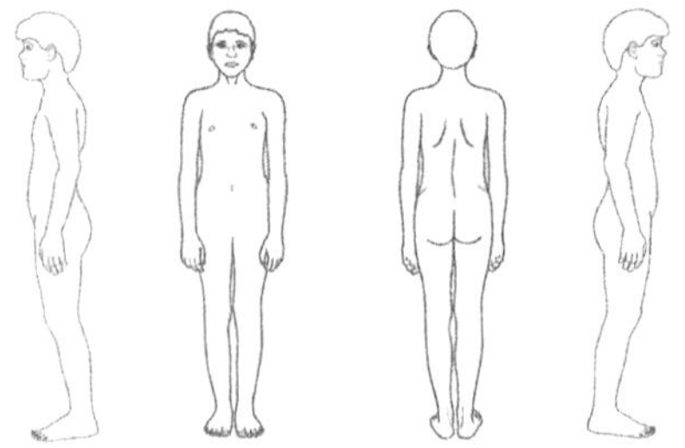

Examination Page 4 of 6

CAEV

CHILDREN'S MEDICAL CENTER OF DALLAS
1935 Motor Street • Dallas, Texas 75235 • (214) 456-7000

CHILD ABUSE EVALUATION

MED REC NO. ______ ACCT NO. ______
PATIENT ______
DATE ______ LOCATION ______
DOB ______

ADDITIONAL HISTORY, DESCRIPTION OF EXAM, ASSESSMENT NOTES OR TREATMENT RECOMMENDATIONS

ATTACH ANY APPROPRIATE DOCUMENTATION TO THIS FORM

Addendum - Additional Documentation

CAEV

CHILDREN'S MEDICAL CENTER OF DALLAS
1935 Motor Street • Dallas, Texas 75235 • (214) 456-7000

CHILD ABUSE EVALUATION

MED REC NO. ______ ACCT NO. ______
PATIENT ______
DATE ______ LOCATION ______
DOB ______

PART F - GENITAL EXAM (Describe all abnormal findings in spaces. Use illustrations when appropriate).

GENITAL EXAM DONE BY	PATIENT DEMEANOR	TANNER STAGING
❑ Direct visualization only ❑ Colposcopy ❑ Hand held magnifier	❑ Full cooperation ❑ Partial cooperation ❑ Uncooperative ❑ Other	Breast 1 2 3 4 5 N/A Genitals 1 2 3 4 5

GENITAL (Female / Male)

SKIN FINDINGS:
Thighs ❑ Normal ❑ Abnormal
Perineum ❑ Normal ❑ Abnormal
Buttocks ❑ Normal ❑ Abnormal

OTHER:
Genital Warts ❑ Yes ❑ No
Other abnormalities ❑ Yes ❑ No
If yes, explain: ______

ANAL EXAM (Female / Male)

Exam position used: ❑ Supine ❑ Prone ❑ Lateral ❑ Knee-chest

EXTERNAL FINDINGS:
Perianal Skin ❑ Normal ❑ Abnormal
Anal verge / folds / rugae ❑ Normal ❑ Abnormal

ANAL TONE:
Anal spasm ❑ Yes ❑ No
Anal laxity ❑ Yes ❑ No
Anal dilation > 20 mm ❑ Yes ❑ No
If yes, stool present? ______
Anal wink ❑ Yes ❑ No
Assessment of tone as normal ❑ Yes ❑ No
Exam method for anal tone: ❑ Observation ❑ Digital exam

GENITAL - FEMALE

(Draw shape of hymen, note any lesions)

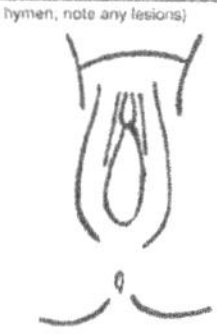

Exam position used: ❑ Supine ❑ Knee-chest ❑ Both
Labia majora ❑ Normal ❑ Abnormal
Clitoris ❑ Normal ❑ Abnormal
Labia minora ❑ Normal ❑ Abnormal
Periurethral tissue / urethral meatus ❑ Normal ❑ Abnormal
Hymen ❑ Normal ❑ Abnormal
Describe: ______

Orifice measurement: Vertical ______ mm
Horizontal ______ mm
How measured ❑ Visual ❑ Other: ______
Vagina ❑ Normal ❑ Abnormal
Fossa Navicularis ❑ Normal ❑ Abnormal
Posterior Fourchette
Other abnormalities: ______
Discharge? ❑ Yes ❑ No If yes, describe: ______
Pelvic exam done ❑ Yes ❑ No

GENITAL - MALE

(Draw any lesions)

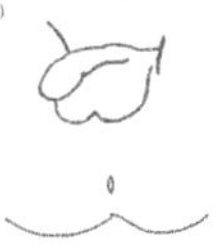

Penis ❑ Normal ❑ Abnormal
Circumcised ❑ Yes ❑ No
Urethral meatus ❑ Normal ❑ Abnormal
Urethral discharge ❑ Yes ❑ No
If yes, describe: ______
Scrotum ❑ Normal ❑ Abnormal
Testes ❑ Normal ❑ Abnormal
Other ❑ Normal ❑ Abnormal

CMC64016-003 (9/98) **Examination Page 5 of 6**

CAEV

CHILDREN'S MEDICAL CENTER OF DALLAS
1935 Motor Street • Dallas, Texas 75235 • (214) 456-7000

CHILD ABUSE EVALUATION

MED REC NO. ______ ACCT NO. ______
PATIENT ______
DATE ______ LOCATION ______
DOB ______

PART G - EVALUATION

❑ **PHYSICIAN NOTES** (Check if history of acute event(s) recorded by physician and filed in REACH office)
❑ **FORENSIC COLLECTION** (Check if samples collected for forensic evaluation; complete Forensic form)
❑ **LABORATORY COLLECTION** (Check if samples collected. Document results when available)

GC CULTURES:	CHLAMYDIA CULTURE:			
❑ Cervical / Vaginal	❑ Cervical / Vaginal	❑ Urinalysis	❑ VDRL	❑ Pregnancy: ❑ Urine ❑ Blood
❑ Urethral	❑ Urethral	❑ Urine Culture	❑ Hep B	❑ Other: ______
❑ Rectal	❑ Rectal	❑ KOH prep	❑ HIV (Consent)	
❑ Oral		❑ Wet mount	❑ CBC	
			❑ PT / PTT	

❑ X-RAYS: ❑ Skeletal Survey ❑ Other: ______
Preliminary Results: ______

PART H - IMPRESSIONS FROM EXAM (All positive findings should be further described in non-medical terms)

❑ No physical findings suggestive of abuse at this time. A normal genital exam does not rule out sexual abuse.
❑ Nonspecific findings: Could be consistent with physical abuse or sexual abuse, but also seen in non-abused children.
❑ Specific physical findings consistent with physical abuse or sexual abuse.

X ______ Physician Signature ______ Printed last name of physician

Other Medical Diagnoses: ______
Agencies Notified: ❑ Child Protective Service ❑ Law Enforcement ❑ Other: ______

PART I - TREATMENT AND FOLLOW UP

PRESCRIBED TREATMENTS	MEDICAL FOLLOW UP	NOTARIZATION
	❑ Hospitalization ❑ F/U Appointment (REACH Office 640-6134) ❑ Return to primary care system ❑ Other: ______	*(Optional, only if requested)* **I have personal knowledge of the above and I swear it is true and just.** Affiant Date Notary Public in and for the State of Texas

CMC64016-003 (9/98) **Summary Page 6 of 6**

CAEV

CHILDREN'S MEDICAL CENTER OF DALLAS
1935 Motor Street • Dallas, Texas 75235 • (214) 456-7000

Child Abuse Evaluation

MED REC NO. ______ ACCT NO. ______
PATIENT ______
DATE ______ LOCATION ______
DOB ______

Forensic Evaluation For use by Southwestern Institute of Forensic Sciences if alleged assault <72 hours and if forensic specimens obtained. Not part of medical record of patient.

Estimate number of hours since incident: ______

History of Ejaculate? (circle one): YES Probable/Possible NO UNK

Condom used? (circle one): YES NO

Since the assault has the patient:

Wiped / washed off	YES	NO	UNK
Bathed / showered	YES	NO	UNK
Urinated	YES	NO	UNK
Defecated	YES	NO	UNK
Rinsed mouth / brushed teeth	YES	NO	UNK
Eaten / drank	YES	NO	UNK
Changed clothes	YES	NO	UNK

Evidentiary Collection

Specimen Collected?	Step	Evidence to Crime Lab	Taken by (signature or name)
YES NO	4	Outer clothing	
YES NO	5	Underwear	
YES NO	6	Debris (mark source on drawing) ❑ Fingernail scraping ❑ Blood on body ❑ Dried secretions on body ❑ Dirt ❑ Other (fibers, hair, ect.)	
YES NO	8	Pubic hair combings	
YES NO	9	Cut pubic hair	
YES NO	10	Known blood sample on patient (optional)	
YES NO	11	Pelvic swabs and smears	
YES NO	12	Vaginal swabs and smears	
YES NO	13	Sperm motility (optional on children)	
		OPTIONAL	
YES NO	15a	Oral rinse	
YES NO	15b	Rectal smears	

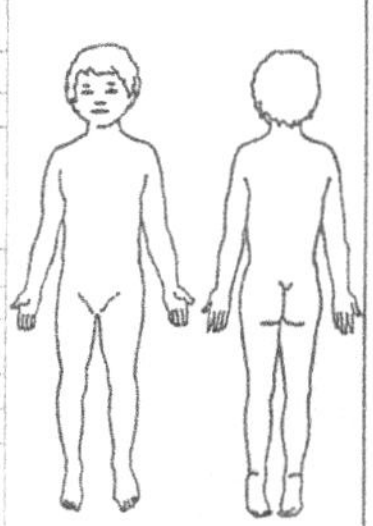

I certify that this is a true and correct record concerning examination of the patient ______ (name)
The completed sexual assault kit was placed in the evidence lock box on ______ at ______ am-pm.

______ Nurse present during examination Date ______ Examiner's signature Date

______ Examiner's name (printed)

CMC 64016-003 (9/98) **Addendum - Forensic Evaluation**

References

1. Dubowitz H, Bross DC. The pediatrician's documentation of child maltreatment. *Am J Dis Child.* 1992;146(5):596-599.
2. Ledray LE. *Sexual Assault Nurse Examiner (SANE) Development & Operation Guide.* Washington, DC: United States Department of Justice, Office of Justice Programs, Office for Victims of Crime; 1999.
3. Lyden C. Uncovering child abuse. *Nurs Crit Care.* 2010;5(3):18-24.
4. Limbos MA, Berkowitz CD. Documentation of child physical abuse: how far have we come? *Pediatrics.* 1998;102(1):53-58.
5. Jenny C. *Medical Evaluation of Physically and Sexually Abused Children: The APSAC Study Guides 3.* Thousand Oaks, CA: Sage Publications, Inc; 1996.
6. Botash A. Child abuse evaluation and treatment for medical providers SUNY upstate medical university pediatric department, Syracuse. Child Abuse MD Web site. http://childabusemd.com/index.shtml. Accessed 2012.
7. Giardino AP, Lyn MA, Giardino E, eds. *A Practical Guide to the Evaluation of Child Physical Abuse and Neglect.* 2nd ed. New York, NY: Springer; 2010.
8. Barnes M. Child abuse histories: what you need to know. *Patient Care Nurs Pract.* 2001;4:17-18,21,25-27.
9. Bar-on ME, Zanga JR. Child abuse: a model for the use of structured clinical forms. *Pediatrics.* 1996;98(3, pt 1):429-433.
10. American Academy of Pediatrics Committee on Child Abuse and Neglect and Committee on Community Health Services. Investigation and review of unexpected infant and child deaths. *Pediatrics.* 1999;104(5):1158-1160.
11. Heger AM, Emans SJ, Muram D. *Evaluation of the Sexually Abused Child: A Medical Textbook and Photographic Atlas.* New York, NY: Oxford University Press, USA; 2000.
12. Christian, CW. Professional education in child abuse and neglect. *Pediatrics.* 2008;122(supp 1):S13-S17.
13. Reece RM, Jenny C. Medical training in child maltreatment. *Am J Prev Med.* 2005;29(5 suppl 2):266-271.
14. Guenther E, Olsen C, Keenan H, et al. Randomized prospective study to evaluate child abuse documentation in the emergency department. *Acad Emerg Med.* 2009;16(3):249-257.
15. Lahoti SL, McClain N, Girardet R, McNeese M, Cheung K. Evaluating the child for sexual abuse. *Am Fam Physician.* 2001;63(5):883-892.
16. Finkel MA, Ricci LR. Documentation and preservation of visual evidence in child abuse. *Child Maltreat.* 1997;2(4):322-330.
17. Marx S. Legal issues and documentation. In: Giardino AP, Christian CW, Giardino E, eds. *A Practical Guide to the Evaluation of Child Physical Abuse and Neglect.* Thousand Oaks, CA: Sage Publications, Inc; 1997:247-273.
18. Myers J. Expert testimony. In: Briere J, Berliner L, Bulkley J, Jenny C, Reid T, eds. *The APSAC Handbook on Child Maltreatment.* Thousand Oaks, CA: Sage Publications; 1996:319-340.

19. Parra JM, Huston RL, Foulds DM. Resident documentation of diagnostic impression in sexual abuse evaluations. *Clin Pediatr (Phila)*. 1997;36(12):691-694.

20. Socolar RR, Champion M, Green C. Physicians' documentation of sexual abuse of children. *Arch Pediatr Adolesc Med*. 1996;150(2):191-196.

21. Faller KC. *Evaluating Children Suspected of Having Been Sexually Abused: The APSAC Study Guides 2*. Thousand Oaks, CA: Sage Publications, Inc; 1996.

22. Pence D, Wilson C. Team Investigation of Child Sexual Abuse: The Uneasy Alliance. Thousand Oaks, CA: Sage Publications, Inc; 1994.

23. Pence D, Wilson C, Broadhurst D; United States Department of Health and Human Services. *The Role of Law Enforcement in the Response to Child Abuse and Neglect*. Washington, DC: United States Department of Health and Human Services, National Center on Child Abuse and Neglect; 1992.

24. Monteleone JA, Brodeur AE. *Child Maltreatment: A Clinical Guide and Reference*. 2nd ed. St. Louis, MO: GW Medical Publishing, Inc; 1998.

25. Turman K, Poyer K. *Child Victims and Witnesses: A Handbook for Criminal Justice Professionals*. Washington, DC: United States Department of Justice, United States Attorney's Office; 1998.

26. American College of Emergency Physicians. *Evaluation and Management of the Sexually Assaulted or Sexually Abused Patient*. Dallas, TX: United States Department of Health and Human Services, Health Resources and Services Administration, Maternal and Child Health Bureau; 1999.

27. Cheung KK. Identifying and documenting findings of physical child abuse and neglect. *J Pediatr Health Care*. 1999;13(3, pt 1):142-143.

28. Myers JEB. Legal aspects of child abuse. In: Reece RM, Christian CW, eds. *Child Abuse: Medical Diagnosis and Management*. 3rd ed. Elk Grove, IL: American Academy of Pediatrics Publications; 2008.

29. McDonald KC. Child abuse: approach and management. *Am Fam Physician*. 2007;75(2):221-228

30. Sorenson E, Bottoms B, Perona A; The National Children's Alliance. *Handbook on Intake and Forensic Interviewing in the Children's Advocacy Center Setting, 2002*. Washington, DC: Office of Juvenile Justice and Delinquency Prevention, Office of Justice Programs, United States Department of Justice; 1997.

31. Chiocca EM. Documenting suspected child abuse, part II. *Nursing*. 1998;28(9):25.

32. Johnson CF. Inflicted injury versus accidental injury. *Pediatr Clin North Am*. 1990;37(4):791-814.

33. Sievers V, Murphy S, Miller JJ. Sexual assault evidence collection more accurate when completed by sexual assault nurse examiners: Colorado's experience. *J Emerg Nurs*. 2003;29(6):511-514.

34. Stokowski LA. Forensic nursing: part 2, inside forensic nursing. Medscape Today News Web site. http://www.medscape.com/viewarticle/571555. Accessed August 18, 2008.

35. Ricci L. Photodocumentation of the abused child. In: Reece RM, Ludwig S, eds. *Child Abuse: Medical Diagnosis and Management*. 2nd ed. Philadelphia, PA: Lippincott Williams & Wilkins; 2001:385-404.

36. Ricci LR, Smistek BS. Photodocumentation in the investigation of child abuse. United States Department of Justice, Office of Justice Programs, Office of Juvenile Justice and Delinquency Prevention Web site. https://www.ncjrs.gov/pdffiles1/ojjdp/160939.pdf. Published 1996. Updated 2000. Accessed January 8, 2014.

37. Finkel M, Dejong A. Medical findings in child sexual abuse. In: Reece RM, Ludwig S, eds. *Child Abuse: Medical Diagnosis and Management.* 2nd ed. Philadelphia, PA: Lippincott Williams & Wilkins; 2001:207-286.

38. Sullivan GH, Mattera M. *RN's Legally Speaking: How to Protect Your Patients and Your License.* Montvale, NJ: Medical Economics; 1997.

Chapter 10

Mental Health Aspects of Child Survivors of Abuse and Neglect

Paul Thomas Clements, PhD, RN
Karyn E. Holt, CNM, PhD
Kathleen M. Benasutti, MCAT, ATR-BC, LPC

Key Points

1. An effective discipline system must contain 3 vital elements: (1) a learning environment characterized by positive, supportive parent-child relationships, (2) a strategy of systematic teaching and strengthening of desired behaviors (proactive), and (3) a strategy for decreasing or eliminating undesired or ineffective behaviors (reactive).
2. Although incidents of child abuse and neglect can frequently be found in today's literature and media, child abuse is not a new phenomenon. Many societies, both past and present and motivated by both spiritual and political factors, have practiced infanticide with the intent to control the population and eliminate children with birth defects.
3. It is imperative that health care providers confront their own perceptions and beliefs regarding child abuse because such beliefs may ultimately have an impact on the level of care provided to abused and neglected children.
4. Clinicians must protect against the throwaway child syndrome, which leads one toward the belief that some children are so damaged that they cannot be helped. Competent health care providers must be in touch with their own issues and perceptions in order to provide compassion and understanding regarding the nature of abuse.
5. The perception of a child as a being intrinsically problematic, special, or different from other children or siblings is often seen when assessing the family system in cases of abuse and neglect. This may be related to a caregiver's negative attitude toward the child or inadequate knowledge of child development that encourages unrealistic expectations of behavioral, emotional, and psychological needs.
6. Although most parents do not intend to abuse their child, it is a typical cycle that reflects a counterintuitive situation wherein positive behaviors displayed by the child do not meet his or her emotional needs, resulting in the child behaving in a proactive manner in order to have those needs met and risking painful contact rather than feeling ignored.
7. A tremendous amount of pressure can be put on a family system when there are limited financial resources or a poor distribution of social and family responsibility.

A caregiver in the family system may experience a sense of failure that may lead to low self-esteem and poor emotional control. This can result in poor frustration tolerance and anger management during overwhelming crises, which can easily result in abusive episodes.

8. According to the Diagnostic and Statistical Manual of Mental Disorders, Fourth Edition: DSM-IV-TR, a child is at risk for posttraumatic stress disorder (PTSD) (Diagnostic Category 309.81) after there has been exposure to a traumatic event in which both of the following are present: (1) the child experienced, witnessed, or was confronted with an event or events that involved actual or threatened death or serious injury, or a threat to the physical integrity of others, and (2) the child's response involved intense fear, helplessness, or horror.[1]
9. Characteristics of PTSD have been identified as common in children who have experienced sexual or physical abuse. Typical responses include misperceptions of the duration and sequencing of time and events; premonition formation; reenactment or the unknowing performance of act similar to the traumatic occurrence; marked and enduring personality alterations; and changes in the recognition and tolerance of the affective response of fear, contributing to inhibition or counter-phobic behaviors.[2]
10. The optimal response pattern after a traumatic event is no resultant PTSD and the subsequent integration of the traumatic event into the victim's life experience. In the integrated pattern, the child is able to acknowledge the traumatic event but is not compelled to dwell on it or avoid it through psychological defenses.
11. Depending on the length of treatment, the child may face dealing with the past trauma while simultaneously facing the challenges inherent in the next development level.

Introduction

On any given day, people are able to pick up a newspaper or turn on a television set and hear yet another report of a battered or otherwise abused or neglected child. One of the greatest challenges for child survivors of abuse, their families, their health care providers and the community at large is grappling with the perception of the abused child as damaged goods.[3,4] Because survivors of child abuse must learn to cope with the issues of growth and development within an altered context of safety and appropriate adult behavior, they can experience role confusion and problems determining typical developmental tasks; specifically, compounded by fear and additional threats to their physical and emotional integrity, they may embrace the concept of believing that they can never be like other kids.[5]

Although significant advances have been made in the process of identifying and treating child abuse, providers are still attempting to grasp the extent of the psychological impact of child maltreatment. One of the largest issues confronting health care providers in addressing the psychological impact of child abuse and maltreatment is consistent identification, terminology, and definition.[6] Historically, a wavering line has been drawn between appropriate physical punishment and abuse. Typically, spanking a child with a hand has not been defined to be abusive. Spanking or whipping a child with a belt or paddle may also be viewed within the realm of parental discipline. However, either of the same actions that leave marks on bare skin might be legally prosecuted as child abuse in some jurisdictions. This change in culturally, as well as legally, acceptable definitions of abuse over the past decades, and even centuries, makes the handling of child abuse from discovery to intervention, treatment to posttreatment care a complex and difficult problem.[7]

The seminal works of Ludwig et al[8,9] have continued to be used to address the complexity of the concepts and definitions of child abuse, categorizing these into legal, institutional, and personal definitions **Table 10-1**. Child abuse, regardless of the actual mechanism, is typically a result of either the inappropriate use of power and control over a child as driven by anger from various issues and dynamics, or insufficient and ineffective parenting stemming from poor parenting skills or a lack of commitment to parenting and ensuring the well-being of the child.[10-13]

Table 10-1. Definitions of Child Abuse

Definition of Abuse	Overview	Indicators
Physical	Serious bodily injury creates a substantial risk of death or causes serious, permanent disfigurement or protracted loss or impairment of the function of a body member or organ.	Causes the child severe pain, significantly impairs the child's physical functioning, whether temporarily or permanently, and is accompanied by physical evidence of a continuous pattern of separate, unexplained injuries to the child.
Sexual	Defined based on associated indicators listed in this table when committed on a child by a perpetrator.	— Statutory rape: sexual intercourse with a child who is aged 14 years and younger by a person aged 18 years or older — Involuntary or voluntary deviate sexual intercourse: intercourse by mouth, rectum, or animal — Sexual assault: sexual involvement, including the touching or exposing of sexual or other intimate parts of a person for the purpose of arousing or gratifying sexual desire in either the perpetrator or the subject child — Incest: sexual intercourse with an ancestor or descendent by blood or adoption — Promoting prostitution: inducing or encouraging a child to engage in prostitution — Rape: sexual intercourse by force or compulsion — Pornography: includes the obscene photographing, filming, or depiction of children for commercial purposes or for arousal of self, subject child, or viewing audience
Neglect	Serious physical neglect	A physical condition caused by the acts or omissions of a perpetrator that endanger the child's life or development or impair physical functioning, serious physical neglect is the result of prolonged or repeated lack of supervision or failure to provide essentials of life, including adequate medical care

(continued)

Table 10-1. Definitions of Child Abuse *(continued)*

Definition of Abuse	Overview	Indicators
Emotional or Psychological	Serious mental injury is a psychological condition diagnosed by a physician or licensed psychologist.	Emotional abuse and neglect are defined as a relationship between child and adult that is characterized by patterns of harmful interactions; none include physical contact with the child. Motivation to harm the child is not necessary for the definition. Caused by the acts or omissions, including the refusal of appropriate treatment, of the perpetrator that render the child chronologically and severely anxious, agitated, depressed, socially withdrawn, psychotic, or in reasonable fear that his or her life or safety are threatened or seriously interfere with the child's ability to accomplish age-appropriate developmental and social tasks.
Institutional	Beyond legal definitions, clinicians are also subject to institutional or operational definitions. Although all institutions are bound to state laws, the practical interpretation of that legality may vary among institutions.	These definitions are determined by institutional policy or procedure. This may include community policies regarding the procedure for reporting suspected and actual child abuse. What one institution may determine to be abuse may not be defined as such by another institution.
Personal	The definitions for abuse, especially determining when to file a report, may have varying levels of individual and acceptable parental behaviors.	Definitions may vary based on family background, child-rearing history, socioeconomic status, religious background, racial background, cultural beliefs, the surrounding environment, and other subjective factors.
Terrorizing	The child is exposed to terrorizing behaviors during episodes of intimate partner violence (IVP).	Such acts can immediately or ultimately result in behavioral, cognitive, or affective damage to the child.
Medical	Medical child abuse (MCA) has been known by many names over the years, including Munchausen syndrome by proxy (MSBP), factitious disorder by proxy (FDBP), and, most recently, pediatric condition falsification (PCF).	By definition, MCA occurs when a child undergoes or receives unwarranted medical care at the hands of a caregiver.

Adapted from Ludwig S. Defining child abuse: clinical mandate—evolving concepts. In: Ludwig S, Kornberg AE, eds. Child Abuse: A Medical Reference. *2nd ed. New York, NY: Churchill Livingstone; 1992:1-12. Adapted from Ludwig S. Child abuse. In: Fleisher GR, Ludwig S, Bachur R, et al, eds.* Textbook of Pediatric Emergency Medicine. *6th ed. Philadelphia, PA: Lippincott Williams & Wilkins; 2010. Adapted from Myers JEB, Berliner L, Briere J, eds.* The American Professional Society on Abuse of Children (APSAC) Handbook on Child Maltreatment. *2nd ed. Thousand Oaks, CA: Sage Publications, Inc; 2002. Adapted from Glaser D. Emotional abuse and neglect (psychological maltreatment): a conceptual framework.* Child Abuse Negl. *2002;26(6-7):697-714.*

It is inherently against all social expectations to purposefully injure a child, which suggests that the dynamics that lead to abusive situations are powerful enough to make the perpetrator override and disregard social and moral safeguards set forth to avoid such situations. According to Anda et al,[14] studies on adverse child events (ACE) in children exposed to intimate partner violence (IPV) support the assertion of negative long-term impacts on health and mental health that can interfere with expected goals and tasks of normal growth and development. Additionally, treatment for survivors of childhood abuse includes a higher usage of mental health comprehensive services. This higher usage of mental health comprehensive services needs to be planned for, as the childhood abuse survivor continues to grow socially, psychologically, and mentally away from their former position as a victim of childhood abuse or neglect. Disclosing abuse is done at a pace and time set by the survivor. Sometimes verbal accounting is fraught with shame, fear, mistrust, and even feelings of deserved abuse. Feelings of abandonment and betrayal are common and, often, later develop into rage. The increased need for comprehensive mental health services is evident for these survivors of childhood abuse.

This chapter explores the dynamics that may potentially result in child abuse, provides a theoretical framework for understanding the cycle of violence, and describes select indicators that should guide health care providers during patient interviews to screen for potentially abusive situations and the need for additional mental health assessment and referral.

Historical Perceptions

Just the word child can evoke strong emotional responses, including an instantaneous smile at the innocence and joy associated with childhood or fond memories of one's own childhood days. Additionally, laughter may result from the funny things that children sometimes say and do as they work their way toward understanding and exerting social appropriateness. Parents, probably more than anyone, can easily connect with these strong associations.

It is a worldwide normative expectation that parents are in the best position to provide for the welfare and well-being of their children in all aspects as they navigate through the years defined as childhood. It is a commonly held belief in society that parents have an obligation to raise their children until they reach adulthood. Included in this authority and responsibility is the use of discipline as a teaching method of instilling morals, understanding cultural and societal mores, making choices, and developing a consciousness of self, family, and community.

Although discipline is an expected facet of raising children and although this discipline may include a parental belief that physical punishment is required to reinforce certain tenets of emotional and behavioral discipline, most parents do not intend to purposefully inflict permanent injury on their children. Commonly, it is when parents overexert the basic tenets of effective child discipline that abusive situations arise. According to the American Academy of Pediatrics (AAP) Policy Statement,[15] An effective discipline system must contain 3 vital elements: (1) a learning environment characterized by positive, supportive parent-child relationships, (2) a strategy of systematic teaching and strengthening of desired behaviors (proactive), and (3) a strategy for decreasing or eliminating undesired or ineffective behaviors (reactive). Each of these components needs to be functioning adequately to result in improved child behavior.[15]

Although incidents of child abuse and neglect can frequently be found in today's literature and media, child abuse is not a new phenomenon. Many societies, both past and present and motivated by both spiritual and political factors, have practiced infanticide with the intent to control the population and eliminate children with birth defects.[16,17] In the past, abandonment, smothering, and drowning were common forms of terminating the lives of children. Some societies continue to engage in certain forms of abuse, such as tattooing, genital mutilation, exaggeration of certain body parts, or piercing of body parts with sharp objects. These forms of abuse are still debated worldwide in terms of perpetuating and upholding religious and cultural heritage versus purposeful infliction of pain and suffering on children.[18-22] Further, history has revealed that children were seen as chattel and considered property, particularly by the typically male head of the household.[23]

American society still struggles with the parental rights and control of children versus the rights of the child, especially in regard to seemingly abusive practices. As a health conscious society, significant efforts have been made to solidify unilateral definitions of abuse: physical, sexual, emotional, and neglect.[24] At times, however, in light of the strong respect for family rights and a stance of cautious noninterference, it is conceivable that many children suffer the consequences of abuse on a regular basis and receive little or no treatment because they do not tell or clues to the abuse are undiscovered, overlooked or dismissed during assessment.[25]

Stereotypical Beliefs

It is imperative that health care providers confront their own perceptions and beliefs regarding child abuse because such beliefs may ultimately have an impact on the level of care provided to abused and neglected children. There are many myths and stereotypes regarding child abuse that must be challenged, explored, and understood by the health care providers who are in a position to uncover abuse and provide effective care (**Table 10-2**).

Table 10-2. Myths and Realities About Child Abuse

Myth	Reality
Child abuse is a recent phenomenon that, as evidenced by the media, has occurred much more often in the past 10 years.	Child abuse has occurred at all points in the historical continuum. The difference in this past decade has been an increase in reporting, education and understanding, not necessarily an increase in abuse. Historically, victims do not report for fear that no one will believe them, fear of threats (to hurt or kill someone they love if they tell), or fear of physical reprisal by the perpetrator.
Child abuse typically occurs with strangers.	Various people can abuse children. Whoever has repeated access to a child can be a potential perpetrator. Adult perpetrators may include parents, neighbors, babysitters, schoolteachers, bus drivers, or strangers at a playground. Typically, physical abuse, sexual abuse, emotional abuse, and neglect occur by persons in a caregiving role. If the perpetrator is a stranger, it is a criminal assault. Children and adolescents can also be perpetrators, including older children or even same-age peers. Much to the surprise of many professionals, the abuser may even be a businessman, clergy person, schoolteacher, or health care professional, which adds to the difficulty of assessment and treatment of child victims who face disbelief and fear of false accusation by care providers that any abuse could have occurred from such an upstanding member of society.[26-28]

(continued)

Table 10-2. Myths and Realities About Child Abuse *(continued)*

Myth	Reality
Child abuse happens in unusual places.	Children are abused in obvious places. Although there are attempts to maintain the secrecy of the abuse, the abuse itself typically occurs in a place where it is not unusual for the child to be. Although this seems counterintuitive, most parents or other caregiving adults would have their suspicions aroused or become fearful if the child was not where he or she is supposed to be, which, in turn, would potentiate the likelihood of discovering the perpetrator in the act of abuse. Because this is exactly what the perpetrator does not want to happen, he or she will make attempts to merge the abuse into the child's typical environment or schedule, thereby promoting an illusion of normalcy and decreasing the chance of discovery. This situation is typically compounded by secrecy imposed on the child by the perpetrator through threats of reprisal or harm if the child reveals the abuse.
Perpetrators of child abuse are mentally ill or have fantasies about hurting children.	There is no typical child abuser. Most are ordinary people who come from all economic, ethnic, and social groups. The presence of a mental health disorder is not a prerequisite for abuse. Actually, child abuse is a very complex and organized system of behaviors and secrecy that may make it difficult for mentally ill people to proceed without detection.[4,28] There is a small segment of sexual predators who are classifiable as mentally ill; however, their behaviors typically result in more significant damage or death to the child, including any combination of sexual, physical, or emotional abuse of a severe nature.[29]
Some children behave in such a way that they provoke child abuse.	Any type of abuse is the sole responsibility of the perpetrator. Children do not ask for abuse, and they do not deserve abuse.[30]
Most victims of child abuse are female.	Although it is true that the majority of reported cases of abuse are female, this may be a result of the social barometer that projects an ongoing stigma for males who fear shame and questions regarding their masculinity and sexual orientation if the secret is revealed.[27,31]
Children with emotional or physical challenges or deformities are not typically targets of abuse.	Statistical data may still reflect a significant level of underreporting of children with developmental, physical, or emotional disability. These children may be unaware that the abuse is wrong, unable to communicate the abuse, or fearful for their own safety because they are already in an ongoing position of dependence for their safety and security needs.[32-34]
It cannot be considered abuse if a child consents to sexual intercourse or if the child says he or she deserves to be beaten because of being bad.	First and foremost, a child cannot consent to any sexual acts, because this contradicts the age of consent laws in the United States.[35] This is compounded by the fact that children, although experiencing sexual urges and drives, do not possess the emotional and cognitive tools to completely encompass the dynamics involved in sexual relationships with others. Physical abuse, such as beating, is never acceptable or justified. Children may truly believe and may say that the beating was deserved; however, such a statement is a significant warning sign that the child has now embraced the position of inequity, and, as a result, may even purposefully provoke additional abusive episodes.[36]

The Evaluation of Survivors of Abuse

Issues to Consider before Beginning Treatment

Multifaceted and complex issues arise in survivors of child abuse; each of these issues is seemingly monumental and ominous. Issues typically experienced by child survivors include an impaired ability to trust, blurred role boundary and role confusion, and pseudomaturity coupled with failure to accomplish developmental tasks, self-mastery, and control. Each survivor's experience with these issues may vary depending on whether he or she represses the abuse, immediate intervention and therapy is provided after abuse or an assault, and therapy continues as mediated by existing support systems and understanding.[37] It is critical to understand that all victims of child abuse and neglect benefit from having a clinician focus on these issues during assessment and treatment. Additionally, health care providers must protect against the throwaway child syndrome, which leads one toward the belief that some children are so damaged that they cannot be helped. Competent clinicians must be in touch with their own issues and perceptions in order to provide compassion and understanding regarding the nature of abuse. They should strive to provide a neutral, yet supportive environment to start the process of undoing the child's sense of self-blame, avoiding the perception of the child as damaged goods.[4] All survivors require and deserve treatment and the opportunity to heal emotionally and physically.

It is important to diminish the child's anxiety and engender trust as a first step in the treatment process.[38] The abused child should sense the health care provider's belief that there is a possibility for future orientation and hope for a normal life. The clinician should focus on teaching empowerment and boundary-setting skills to survivors of childhood abuse.[39] In addition, the health care provider should encourage and guide the child to communicate his or her feelings because the child may be hesitant to express those feelings of fear and loss by virtue of age and position within the family. Without these basic tenets, the therapeutic relationship is immediately in jeopardy, and all attempts at assessment and intervention are at risk for failure.[40]

Mental Health Principles to Keep in Mind During the Abuse Evaluation

Points to Remember During the History Taking Process

Mental health aspects of the health care evaluation of child maltreatment begin with the actual health care encounter and may be viewed as parallel to the medical and physical health care aspects. The following discussion highlights several areas the clinician should consider during the health care evaluation.

The abused or neglected child is often in a position of significant inequity of control. Someone, typically a "grownup," has exerted his or her power and control to the disadvantage of the child. Additionally, the child has probably been told that he or she can never tell anyone about what is happening or else something more terrible will occur. It is important to use the knowledge of this inequity of control as a guide for clinical assessment. The supportive environment of the history and physical examination or other clinical assessment can provide a conduit for children to reveal abuse and to seek an anchor for safety.[4,13] It is also critical to remember that information gleaned from the assessment may be used to prosecute an alleged abuser. This means that the techniques used to gain the most accurate and reliable information as well as detailed documentation, may be among the most important things that the health care provider can do for the child. The suggestions in **Table 10-3** can enhance the assessment interview and maximize the potential for gaining pertinent data from a suspected victim of child abuse.

The contemporary era of health care has increased focus on issues related to cultural awareness, including those related to the assessment of child abuse. Fontes[41] notes that

Table 10-3. Dos and Don'ts for the Assessment Interview

Do's	Don'ts
— Get out from behind the desk.	— Stay behind the desk in the adult power position.
— Get down to the child's physical level.	— Act as if this situation has ruined the child's chances for a normal life.
— Be casual and matter of fact. Talk about other things first that are developmentally appropriate (eg, school, friends, hobbies).	— Use clinical terminology that might cause confusion and create a sense of anxiety in the child. Remember, children often want to please the therapist or provider and may provide answers that are seemingly positive or OK.
— Play, laugh, and create an environment that is age-appropriate.	— Act as if the child is damaged, sick, or different.
— Treat the child as you would any child in any health care setting.	— Jump to the conclusion that the child hates the perpetrator.
— Treat the subject with a matter-of-fact approach. Maintain a calm and steady stream of tone and conversation. Take a break if needed.	— React negatively to the words or subject matter.
— Take the lead in asking questions, but avoid leading questions. Obtain as much detail as the child is willing to provide.	— Neglect or disregard the interviews of the entire family. Collateral interviews can provide unique perspectives for the assessment.
— Assure the child that this is not his or her fault.	— Give up if there is some initial resistance and become angry if the child tests your limits or tries to push your buttons.
— Believe what the child tells you, even when seemingly inconsistent. Remember, children perceive the world differently than adults based on their repertoire of life experience.	Doubt a small child who tells you he or she been abused.
— Be aware of your body language since children are just as savvy at interpreting what is not said.	

Adapted from Butler-Smith S. Children's Story: Sexually Molested Children in Criminal Court. *Walnut Creek, CA: Launch Press; 1985.*

people affected by child abuse are often nestled within a variety of social domains that are highly interconnected and interactive. These can be described as a set of concentric circles with the innermost circle being the abused child; the second being the child's home and family; the third being the child's ethnic culture, which includes not only ethnicity, but also religious beliefs; the fourth being the child's proximal social systems, which includes the child's neighborhood, peers, schools and treatment providers; and the fifth being the child's wider social systems, which is comprised of state and national policies which impact all the other systems (**Figure 10-1**).

Points to Remember During the Physical Evaluation

The health care provider may experience a certain level of discomfort while assessing a child who is suspected of having been the victim of abuse. There may be hesitation to provide a thorough physical assessment for fear of creating additional stress and trauma; this becomes more readily evident during the assessment of the child who has been sexually abused. However, a thorough assessment, performed in a matter-of-fact, nonreactive

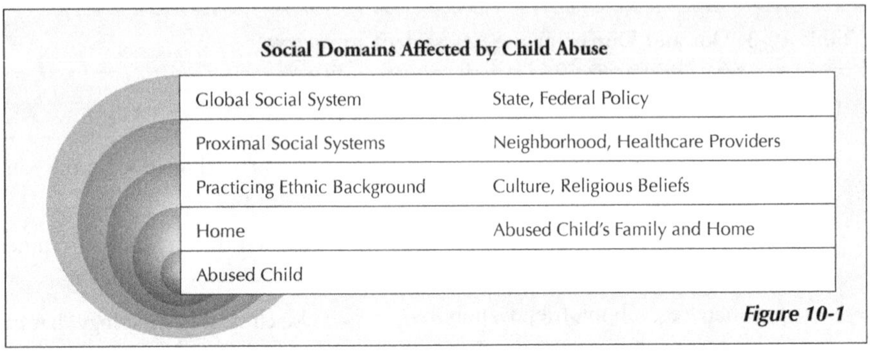

Figure 10-1. *Social domains of those affected by child abuse. Data from Fontes LA.* Child Abuse and Culture: Working with Diverse Families. *New York, NY: The Guilford Press; 2005.*

manner can assess the level of physical trauma related to the abuse, check for additional physiological and psychological issues that require intervention, and promote the therapeutic relationship while building the child's self-esteem. The health care provider should communicate his or her concern and respect for the child's rights as an individual, keeping in mind that such an approach is beneficial to the child who has been abused.

Children watch adults for behavioral and verbal cues to self-assess the seriousness of the situation. It is imperative that the assessment be completed in a safe, secure, and neutral environment, and that the attitude be one that reflects an expectation of attainment of both complete and eventual healing. This is best accomplished when the health care provider maintains a neutral but supportive stance during the conversation, reinforces that the child can indeed live a normal life, and discusses age-appropriate behaviors and activities as part of the interaction.

Developmental Level

Children change rapidly during their 18 years of development, so the health care provider should assess and intervene at a level that matches the child's cognitive and emotional abilities. Communication with and education of the child should be geared toward instilling skills and tools for self-preservation, self-esteem, and communication. Approaches to this interaction vary greatly across the childhood developmental continuum and may include play for younger children and group therapy or journaling for adolescents. It is optimal if children can identify activities that they enjoy and also that the health care provider believes to be conduits toward building self-esteem, safety, and communication. Health care providers should also educate children regarding the need to avoid maladaptive methods of coping, such as fighting, sibling violence, cigarettes, drugs, or alcohol, and instruct them to seek adult guidance and support when impulses toward these behaviors arise.

Family Structure

Because all children are inherently members of a larger family system, it is imperative that the health care provider explores dynamics that may increase the likelihood for abusive situations. The perception of a child as being intrinsically problematic, special, or different from other children or siblings is often seen when assessing the family system in cases of abuse and neglect. This may be related to a caregiver's negative attitude toward the child or inadequate knowledge of child development that encourages unrealistic expectations of behavioral, emotional, and psychological needs. Additionally, parents may experience intense difficulty with unconditional acceptance of a child who may have been of low birth weight, premature, handicapped, or illegitimate.

Although most parents do not intend to abuse their child, it is a typical cycle that reflects a counterintuitive situation wherein positive behaviors displayed by the child do not meet his or her emotional needs, resulting in the child behaving in a proactive manner in order to have those needs met and risking painful contact rather than feeling ignored.[42]

Certain situational factors and parental behaviors should indicate to the nurse that additional assessment for abuse or neglect is warranted, including the following:

— Chaotic household

— Marital discord

— Minimal interaction and attachment between parent and child

— Inappropriately leaving the child at home alone

— Apparent or expressed disregard for the child's needs or safety

— Exaggerated anger response to child behavior (eg, extreme and unrealistic approaches at discipline)

— Unilateral negativity when speaking about or referring to the child

— Anger regarding the inconvenience that the child's legitimate needs creates in the parent's life (eg, getting sick, going to therapy, driving the child to school)

— Poor understanding of childhood developmental tasks and behaviors

— Overtly protective of the child

— Exhibited or expressed jealousy over all the attention the child is getting

Lack of Resources

There are common factors in cases of abuse and neglect of children that are related to financial stressors and lack of emotional and social support. A tremendous amount of pressure can be put on a family system when there are limited financial resources or a poor distribution of social and family responsibility. A caregiver in this family system may experience a sense of failure that may lead to low self-esteem and poor emotional control. This can result in poor frustration tolerance and anger management during overwhelming crises, which can easily result in abusive episodes. Unless there is an alleviation of the financial and social stressors, or there is education and intervention regarding anger management and impulse control, a destructive circuit is created that can be used as relief during conflicts. This circuit includes a charged emotional atmosphere in the adult that seeks an outlet for the negative energy. The conduit for the release of energy is the act of abuse, and the outlet is the child.[43]

Social isolation can also promote abusive situations. Many families live in a paucity of knowledge regarding resources available to them within the community. Families who are accused of child abuse may be unaware of the myriad social services that could have alleviated the potential for abuse. Additionally, they may admit that they were too ashamed to ask for help for fear that they would be perceived as parental failures.

Trauma Response Patterns

van der Kolk[44] cites 5 major characteristics of human responses to trauma, as follows:

— A persistence of startle response and irritability

— Proclivity toward explosive outbursts of aggression

— Fixation on the trauma

— Generally constricted level of personality function

— An atypical dream life

These symptoms represent a few of the multitude of traumatic presentations and behaviors exhibited by victims of abuse and violence across the childhood continuum.

Emotional and Behavioral Aspects: Attempts at Mastery and the Compulsion to Repeat the Trauma

Posttraumatic Stress Disorder

The DSM-IV-TR classifies PTSD as an anxiety disorder characterized by a cluster of symptoms that result from the impact of a significantly traumatic experience.[1] These symptoms are disruptive and disturbing to the survivor of the trauma and can derail his or her usual developmental trajectory and ability to complete the activities required in daily life.

Children who have been exposed to abuse or violence are at significant risk for developing PTSD-related symptoms. "Within the first hours after the event a child may crystallize an altered and restricted view of his or her personal future."[45] Such a response requires treatment to reduce the symptom intensity and to potentially integrate the event into the child's life history.

According to the DSM-IV-TR, a child is at risk for PTSD (Diagnostic Category 309.81)[2] after there has been exposure to a traumatic event in which both of the following are present: (1) the child experienced, witnessed, or was confronted with an event or events that involved actual or threatened death or serious injury or a threat to the physical integrity of others, and (2) the child's response involved intense fear, helplessness, or horror. In children, PTSD may be expressed by disorganized or agitated behaviors.

In addition to the existence of the recognizable stressor, the traumatic event is persistently re-experienced as described in one or more of the groups of symptoms listed in **Table 10-4**. The first group of symptoms involves the re-experiencing of the event through recurrent and intrusive distressing memories of the event as images, thoughts, or perceptions. In children, this may manifest itself in repetitive play during which themes of the trauma are expressed. The child may have recurrent dreams without recognizable content that he or she describes as frightening. Additionally, a child may act or feel as if the traumatic event was recurring again, which can include a sense of reliving the experience, illusions, hallucinations, and dissociative flashback episodes. There may be intense psychological or physiological distress at exposure to internal or external cues that symbolize or resemble an aspect of the traumatic event.

Persistent avoidance of associated stimuli and a numbing of responsiveness in thought and activity characterize the second group of symptoms. This may present as difficulty with memory retrieval, affective and cognitive blunting, interpersonal detachment, and a pessimistic outlook on the future. Efforts are made to avoid all thoughts and feelings or conversations associated with the traumatic event as well as activities, places, or people that arouse recollection of the trauma. The child may display an inability to recall an important aspect of the traumatic event or a markedly diminished interest and participation in significant activities. The child may express and display feelings of detachment and estrangement from others. Additionally, the child may display a restricted range of affect and may express a sense of a foreshortened future.

The third group of symptoms is manifested by an increased level of arousal not present before the traumatic event. These symptoms may include sleep pattern disturbances (eg, difficulty falling asleep or staying asleep), irritability, or outbursts of anger, hypervigilance, difficulty concentrating, and exaggerated startle response.[2,46,47] The startle response is a critical indicator of PTSD. This primitive response to noise is evident as early as 24 to 36 hours after birth and typically disappears by age 4 months.[48] Children with PTSD have demonstrated an autonomic arousal related to a traumatic event, with the salient feature being absence of an extinction of a symptomatic response

Table 10-4. PTSD Diagnostic Criteria

One or more of the following re-experiencing symptoms:	— Involuntary intrusive thoughts related to the event — Recurrent upsetting dreams — Flashbacks of the event — Distressing psychological reactions to trauma cues — Physiological reactions to trauma cues
At least 3 of the following avoidant symptoms:	— Avoids thoughts, feelings, or talk related to the traumatic event — Avoids activities, persons, or places associated with the event — Fails to remember significant portions of the event — Has decreased interest in activities — Feels estranged from others — Has difficulty feeling emotions — Has difficulty trusting others — Has feelings of impending doom or lack of future orientation
At least 2 symptoms of increased arousal:	— Sleep disturbance — Irritability or mood swings — Difficulty with concentration — Hypervigilance to surroundings — Pronounced startle response

Adapted from American Psychiatric Association. Diagnostic criteria for PTSD (309.81). In: Diagnostic and Statistical Manual of Mental Disorders: DSM-IV-TR. *4th ed. Text revision. Washington, DC: American Psychiatric Association Publications; 2000.*

to traumatic cues; specifically, there is a reflex, exaggerated startle response to auditory, visual, tactile, or olfactory cues that are reminders of the traumatic event.[49]

Characteristics of PTSD have been identified as common in children who have experienced sexual or physical abuse. Typical responses include increased misperception of the duration and sequencing of time and events; premonition formation; reenactment or the unknowing performance of acts similar to the traumatic occurrence; marked and enduring personality alterations; and changes in the recognition and tolerance of the affective response of fear, contributing to inhibition or counterphobic behaviors.[1] A diagnosis of PTSD must be considered for abused children. This disorder is a physiological and psychological response pattern to overwhelming trauma. Child abuse is clearly classifiable as such an overwhelming trauma. In fact, historically, child abuse has inevitably raised the impact of the issue of human accountability, which supports the statement that the risk for PTSD is apparently more severe and longer lasting when the stressor is of human design.[1]

If a child is unable to integrate the traumatic event into his or her life history, then an acute PTSD response may ensue. This is identified by a display of intrusive or avoidant behaviors. Exposure to stimuli may induce a state of hyperarousal and numbing, which may cause the child to experience highly emotional states with lower levels of thinking. In many cases, the ego cannot adapt to the trauma and becomes disorganized, flooded, and overwhelmed.[50] Rainey et al[51] described visual and motoric reliving of traumatic events with nightmares and flashbacks that are generally preceded by physiological arousal. The disruptions may also impact sensory, perceptual or cognitive, and interpersonal performance levels. Symptoms of sensory disruption may include hyperactivity, headaches, stomachaches, back pain, genitourinary distress, and nightmares.[52] Perceptual and cognitive disruptions may include both internal and external cues that produce intrusions of images and auditory and kinesthetic information associated with the trauma. These may be related to future concerns about repeated danger. Symptoms of interpersonal disruption include avoidant behaviors, such as an excessive fear of others and an inability to assert or protect oneself. Other disruptions may be masked as aggressive behaviors, including aggression toward peers, family members, and pets.

The patterns of acute PTSD symptoms are typically noted by the child's caregiver or other adults who interface with the child on a regular basis, such as schoolteachers, daycare workers, and grandparents. The avoidant pattern of PTSD is characterized by denial of the event. This child appears distant and alienated and demonstrates a lack of energy for learning and living. Often there is a preoccupied daydreaming quality to the behavior. These children may turn to substance abuse, display phobic behavior, encounter adjustment problems at home and school, display affect and behaviors of depression, and exhibit conduct disorders.

The aggressive pattern of PTSD is characterized by externalized and, typically, angry behavioral displays. This acting out may be bold or secretive, with testing and breaking of rules. Impulsivity is increased, and there may be fighting with peers and siblings or overt defiance toward adults.

Eventually, when the body and mind become overwhelmed with the traumatic event and can no longer successfully manage the impact that it has on the child's daily life, trauma learning may occur. Trauma learning emphasizes the repetition of behavior, which Freud[53] discussed in Moses and Monotheism, exploring the positive and negative effects of trauma. This repetition can be observed in traumatized children in several presentations, including reenactment of the trauma, repetition of the trauma as either victim or victimizer, or displacement of the aggression.[37,54-56]

Emotional and Behavioral Presentations

Burgess and Hartman's[54] conceptual framework describes information processing of traumatic events and a suggested path of symptom responses. This anatomy of trauma is predicated on neuropsychosocial concepts of information processing and the role of the neuromodulatory systems on cognition and memory.[56] Burgess et al[37] developed a framework based on the work of Hartman and Burgess[54] to look at information processing of traumatic events in children. This framework suggests the progression of patient symptom responses as sequelae to a traumatic event. This framework is congruent with the tenets currently set forth in the DSM-IV-TR for a diagnosis of PTSD and provides a continuum for the emotional and behavioral responses after a traumatic event. It can provide a model for assessing the psychological and behavioral aftermath for children who have been victims of abuse.

The model represents a continuum of responses that a child may have after a traumatic event. This spectrum ranges from ***integration***, no subsequent sequelae, to displacement, psychotic reactions.

Integration

The optimal response pattern after a traumatic event is no resultant PTSD and the subsequent integration of the traumatic event into the victim's life experience. In the integrated pattern, the child is able to acknowledge the traumatic event but is not compelled to dwell on it or avoid it through psychological defenses. Rutter[57] speculated that a child's ability to incorporate a traumatic event into his or her belief system depends on several factors, including appraisal of the situation and his or her capacity to process the life event. It is unclear how many children can readily integrate trauma without experiencing PTSD. Clinically, these children are typically not encountered for therapeutic intervention because it is usually the disruptive behaviors and emotional responses and not necessarily the traumatic event itself that lead caregivers to bring children to health care professionals for evaluation and treatment.

Reenactment

Literature suggests that an abused child may be driven to compulsively reenact the traumatic event. Johnson[58] wrote, "Victims of trauma often find themselves repeatedly re-enacting abusive relationships throughout their lives. It was in the study of such disorders that Freud[59] first described 'repetition compulsion.'"[58] Reenactment is experienced by children as recollections of the traumatic event. This may occur as flashbacks, which may contain fragmented detail and an intense sensory experience. In young children, there may be repetitive themes and aspects of the traumatic event expressed through play.[37,60] There may be frightening dreams that have unrecognizable content. The verbal or play behaviors demonstrate that the child is acting as if the trauma is happening again. During this stage, the child continues to identify with the role of the victim. The child may fear that the perpetrator will come and get him or her just as the person did before.

Repetition

During the repetition stage of the trauma learning process, behavior patterns are generally noted in the child's play with others. The behavioral repetition of the trauma may be played out in either the role of the trauma victim or the role of the victimizer. Repetition of the trauma in the role of the victimizer is a major cause of aggression and violence. The traumatized child may attempt to act out the dynamics of the event on other children, who are usually smaller and weaker, in an attempt to gain a sense of control or mastery over the trauma that originally happened to him or her.

Displacement

During the displacement stage, behaviors and thoughts of the trauma are elaborated symbolically. The elaboration may manifest as a dream or fantasy and include symbolic representations of the violent act. Ultimately, this symbolic elaboration may lead to psychotic reactions that have patterns of the original trauma embedded in them.

When a child is unable to link ongoing, self-defeating, disrupting behaviors to the original trauma, there is no resolution or integration, and the underlying fear persists. This leads to an inability to use new experiences to develop and grow. Instead, the flexibility of the child to discriminate new information may be lost, and the child is either numb or hyperalert to the new information, or he or she may perceive it as dangerous.

The Issue of Belief

The role of the health care provider is to assess and evaluate the need for intervention. It is not the clinician's role to determine the veracity of the child's allegation. It is far more dangerous to not believe a child and send him or her home to the abuser than to investigate the child's allegations and have the result of an exoneration of the alleged abuser. It is critical to understand that, for an abused child, telling may represent the most difficult and daring act of his or her entire existence. In this light, if the child tells and is indeed telling the truth but no additional assessment occurs, the health care provider has potentially reinforced the child's belief that the situation is without hope of rescue.

Interventions

There are myriad interventions for working with children who have experienced abuse. Traditional talk therapy is appropriate, although not necessarily the modality of choice or preference, especially for children. Options for intervention should include consideration of the child's developmental level and trauma-related behaviors. For example, having alternative experiential approaches for communication, such as art therapy, play therapy, storytelling, doll play, and, more recently, computer-based technology play, are significantly important.[61,62]

It has been said that the work of children is play. In this light, approaching children on their level can provide a valuable conduit toward gleaning pertinent information or tailoring effective interventions. Additionally, it can promote an exchange of significant information and allow an opportunity for children to ask questions of the health care provider. This alone can be substantial in establishing a sense of trust while strengthening the therapeutic alliance.

Abused, neglected, or emotionally abused children are frequently overstimulated or understimulated; therefore, they may lack the ability to explore, experiment, and even play. The caregiver must facilitate these natural and now constricted or disorganized tendencies. Expressive therapies can be used to discover and resolve problems and are best used for nonpsychotic children. The expressive approach combines both directed and nondirected expression to facilitate communication concerning traumatic issues.

Short-term Goals

The short-term goals of age-appropriate and expressive therapies include establishment and promotion of therapeutic rapport between the health care provider and the child and creation of an anchor for safety.[4] By communicating to the child, either verbally or through collaborative expressive methods (eg, drawing pictures, play therapy, storytelling, etc.), that the clinician is interested in what the child has to say about anything traumatic that has happened, the child is more likely to reveal relevant information for assessment and intervention[61] (**Figure 10-2**). Violation of trust is one of the basic tenets to all abuse; therefore, dealing with it is the first and most critical step in providing effective treatment. Children can learn from the provider that adults can be trusted

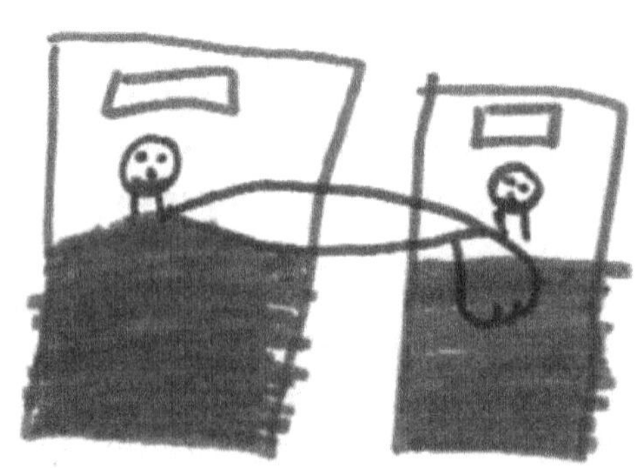

Figure 10-2

Figure 10-2. *Drawing by an 11-year-old boy during a therapeutic session with a nurse revealing an episode of sexual abuse by a male relative who was spending the night at his house.*

and that their words and actions are performed within an environment of honesty and with a display of healthy interpersonal boundaries. Strategies for attaining this trust includethe following:

— Telling the child what you are going to do before you do it

— Clarifying that the child understands what you are going to do

— Checking in with the child during the process to assess the level of anxiety and understanding

— Providing the opportunity for the child to control the therapeutic environment whenever feasible

Regardless of the expressive modality, it is important to remember that the child has encountered a real or perceived lack or loss of control and that allowing the child to regain a sense of some control can only enhance trust and communication.

With assistance and guidance, goals for treating abused and neglected children are to integrate the traumatic event into their life history and to facilitate the ability to reinvest in mastering age-appropriate developmental tasks and goals. Although there may be some early evidence of this in the short-term in behaviors such as improved affect, increased play and verbalizations and improved levels of trust, there is probably no other kind of therapy that requires ongoing assessment to monitor for these, sometimes, subtle changes. Additionally, children may unfold during therapeutic interactions and share their emotions more freely as they begin to trust. This requires the care provider to continue to assess the perceptions of the child regarding his or her level of autonomy, empowerment, and safety.

Long-term Goals

Unlike the adult patient, the child experiences more developmental changes and expected tasks as therapeutic interventions progress. Depending on the child's age, inherent developmental tasks and expectations may provide additional dynamics that can make integration of the trauma more problematic. This can include things such as peer pressure, establishment of identity and role perceptions, ongoing expansion of ego structure, and moral development. Depending on the length of treatment, the child may face dealing with the past trauma while simultaneously facing the challenges inherent in the next development level.

The length of treatment varies among children relative to the nature, severity, and duration of the abuse and to the child's methods of coping before the abuse. The goal of integration can be easily conveyed by the clinician to the child if expressed in everyday language such as the following:

— "It was a terrible thing that happened to you."

— "You didn't ask for it to happen to you."

— "It wasn't your fault that it happened to you."

— "Sometimes adults make bad decisions and do things that are wrong."

— "Now it is time to focus on yourself and to figure out how to get back to your everyday life."

— "Trying to forget what happened isn't really the answer. Remembering what happened may be scary at first, but thinking about it in a new way can help you learn to live with it and continue to do the things that other children do."

Conclusion

Maltreatment and abuse are words that clinicians may hear daily. One of the greatest challenges is to provide comprehensive assessment, intervention, and referral to the child survivors of abuse and their families. Survivors of child abuse must learn to adaptively cope with their own growth and development within the context of the loss of power and control with which they had to previously contend. This can lend itself to role confusion and lack of clarity regarding what are typical developmental tasks encountered by most children and what are misperceptions of additional threats to their integrity.

Children benefit from assessment strategies and interventions that can help promote adaptive coping and healing. As mental health professionals expand and then apply their understanding of the identification and treatment of child abuse, they potentially prevent the derailment of a child's emotional growth and development and minimize the extent of the psychological impact of the maltreatment.

This chapter provided an overview of the basic tenets necessary for the psychological assessment and guidance required in planning interventions for children who survive abusive situations. Ultimately, it is the therapeutic relationship between the child, the child's family, and the clinician that can be the strongest intervention of all. Trust facilitates assessment, successful intervention, and ultimately healing.

Appendix 10-1: Additional Resources

Appendix 10-1. Additional Resources

Organization	Resources	Web site
Rape, Abuse and Incest National Network (RAINN)	Victim services, prevention information, and abuse education	http://www.rainn.org
Child Welfare Information Gateway (State Statutes Search)	Information, resources, and tools that cover child welfare issues; accessible to child welfare, adoption, and related professionals as well as the general public; promotes the safety and well-being of children, adolescents, and families	http://www.childwelfare.gov/systemwide/laws_policies/state/can/
Office for Victims of Crime (OVC)	General information about child abuse, resources, and referrals	http://www.ojp.usdoj.gov/ovc/help/index.html
The National Child Traumatic Stress Network (NCTSN)	Educational resources for providers, families, and military-related services	http://www.nctsn.org/nccts/nav.do?pid=hom_main

References

1. American Psychiatric Association. Diagnostic criteria for PTSD (309.81). In: *Diagnostic and Statistical Manual of Mental Disorders: DSM-IV-TR.* 4th ed. Text revision. Washington, DC: American Psychiatric Association Publications; 2000.
2. American Psychiatric Association. *Diagnostic and Statistical Manual of Mental Disorders: DSM-IV-TR.* 4th ed. Text revision. Washington, DC: American Psychiatric Association Publications; 2000.
3. American Humane Association. Guidelines for helping children experiencing abuse or neglect. American Humane Association Web site. http://www.americanhumane.org/children/stop-child-abuse/fact-sheets/guidelines-for-helping.html. Accessed June 12, 2013.
4. Burgess AW, Clements PT. Child and adolescent victimization. In: Burgess AW, Regehr C, Roberts AR, eds. *Victimology: Theories and Applications.* Sudbury, MA: Jones & Bartlett Publishers; 2009.
5. Braiker HB. *Who's Pulling Your Strings?: How to Break the Cycle of Manipulation and Regain Control of Your Life.* New York, NY: McGraw Hill; 2004.
6. United States Department of Health and Human Services. Definitions of child abuse and neglect. Child Welfare Information Gateway Web site. httdp://www.childwelfare.gov/systemwide/laws_policies/statutes/define.cfm. Accessed 2012.
7. Child Welfare Information Gateway. Laws and policies. Child Welfare Information Gateway Web site. https://www.childwelfare.gov/systemwide/laws_policies/. Accessed March 29, 2013.
8. Ludwig S. Defining child abuse: clinical mandate—evolving concepts. In: Ludwig S, Kornberg AE, eds. *Child Abuse: A Medical Reference.* 2nd ed. New York, NY: Churchill Livingstone; 1992:1-12.
9. Ludwig S. Child abuse. In: Fleisher GR, Ludwig S, Bachur R, et al, eds. *Textbook of Pediatric Emergency Medicine.* 6th ed. Philadelphia, PA: Lippincott Williams & Wilkins; 2010.
10. Myers JEB, Berliner L, Briere J, eds. *The American Professional Society on Abuse of Children (APSAC) Handbook on Child Maltreatment.* 2nd ed. Thousand Oaks, CA: Sage Publications, Inc; 2002.
11. Glaser D. Emotional abuse and neglect (psychological maltreatment): a conceptual framework. *Child Abuse Negl.* 2002;26(6-7):697-714.
12. National Council on Child Abuse and Family Violence. Child abuse information. National Council on Child Abuse and Family Violence Web site. http://www.nccafv.org/child.htm. Accessed June 12, 2013.
13. McDonald KC. Child abuse: approach and management. *Am Fam Physician* 2007;75(2):221-228.
14. Anda RF, Felitti VJ, Brown DW, et al. Insights into intimate partner violence from the adverse childhood experiences (ACE) study. In: Salber PR, Taliaferro E, eds. *Physician's Guide to Intimate Partner Violence and Abuse.* Volcano, CA: Volcano Press; 2006.
15. American Academy of Pediatrics Committee on Psychosocial Aspects of Child and Family Health. Guidance for effective discipline. *Pediatrics.* 1998;4(1):723-728.

16. Friedman SH, Resnick P. Child murder by mothers: patterns and prevention. *World Psychiatr.* 2007:6(3):137-141.

17. Radbill S. Children in a world of violence: a history of child abuse. In: Helfer R, Kempe R, eds. *The Battered Child.* Chicago, IL: University of Chicago Press; 1987:3-22.

18. Annas C. Irreversible error: the power and prejudice of female genital mutilation. *J Contemp Health Law Policy.* 1996;12(2):325-353.

19. Lagaipa SJ. Suffer the little children: the ancient practice of infanticide as a modern moral dilemma. *Issues Compr Pediatr Nurs.* 1990;13(4):241-251.

20. Milner LS. *Hardness of Heart, Hardness of Life: The Stain of Human Infanticide.* Kearney, NB: Morris Publishing; 1998.

21. Toubia N. Female circumcision as a public health issue. *New Engl J Med.* 1994;331(11):712-716.

22. United Nation's International Children's Emergency Fund. Female genital mutilation/cutting. United Nation's International Children's Emergency Fund Web site. http://www.unicef.org/protection/index_genitalmutilation.html. Accessed June 12, 2013.

23. Maillard KN. Rethinking children as property: the transitive family. *Cardozo Law Rev.* 2010;32(1):225-263.

24. United Nation's International Children's Emergency Fund. Children's protection and civil rights. United Nation's International Children's Emergency Fund Web site. http://www.unicef.org/specialsession/about/sgreport-pdf/sgrep_adapt_part2c_eng.pdf. Accessed 2000.

25. Asher JB. Moving beyond a don't-ask-don't-tell approach. In: Giardino AP, Datner E, Asher JB, et al. *Sexual Assault Victimization Across the Life Span: A Clinical Guide and Color Atlas.* St. Louis, MO: STM Learning, Inc; 2003:447-547.

26. American Prosecutors Research Institute. *Investigation and Prosecution of Child Abuse.* Thousand Oaks, CA: Sage Publications, Inc; 2003.

27. United States Department of Health and Human Services, Administration for Children and Families. *Child Maltreatment 2008.* Washington, DC: United States Department of Health and Human Services, Administration for Children and Families, Administration on Children, Youth and Families; 2008. http://archive.acf.hhs.gov/programs/cb/pubs/cm08/cm08.pdf. Accessed January 9, 2014.

28. van Dam C. *The Socially Skilled Child Molester: Differentiating the Guilty from the Falsely Accused.* Binghamton, NY: Hawthorne Press; 2006.

29. Salter A. *Predators: Pedophiles, Rapists and Other Sex Offenders: Who They Are, How They Operate, and How We Can Protect Ourselves and Our Children.* New York, NY: Basic Books; 2003.

30. Fontes LA. *Child Abuse and Culture: Working with Diverse Families.* New York, NY: The Guildford Press; 2008.

31. Male sexual victimization myths & facts. Male Survivor Web site. http://www.malesurvivor.org/myths.html. Accessed 2007.

32. Focht-New G, Clements PT, Barol B, Faulkner M, Service KP. Persons with developmental disabilities exposed to interpersonal violence and crime strategies and guidance for assessment. *J Adv Pract Psychiatr Nurs.* 2008;44(1):3-13.

33. Hardman ML, Drew CJ, Egan MW. *Human Exceptionality: School, Community and Family*. 8th ed. Boston, MA: Allyn & Bacon; 2004.

34. Mitchell LM, Buchele-Ash A. Abuse and neglect of individuals with disabilities: building protective supports through public policy. *J Disability Policy Stud.* 2000;10(2):225-243.

35. United States Sentencing Commission. Report of the United States sentencing commission to the judicial conference of the United States, September 1999. United States Sentencing Commission Web site. http://www.ussc.gov/Research/Research_Projects/Miscellaneous/199909_Judicial_Conference_Report.pdf. Accessed June 12, 2013.

36. Filipas HH, Ullman SE. Child sexual abuse, coping responses, self-blame, posttraumatic stress disorder, and adult sexual revictimization. *J Interpers Violence.* 2006;21(5):652-672.

37. Burgess AW, Hartman CR, Clements PT Jr. Biology of memory and childhood trauma. *J Psychosoc Nurs Ment Health Serv.* 1995; 33(3):16-26.

38. Substance Abuse and Mental Health Services Administration, Center for Substance Abuse Treatment. *Treatment Improvement Protocols: Substance Abuse Treatment for Persons with Child Abuse and Neglect Issues, Series 36.* Rockville, MD: SAMHSA; 2000.

39. Briere J, Elliott DM. Prevalence and psychological sequelae of self-reported childhood physical and sexual abuse in a general population sample of men and women. *Child Abuse Negl.* 2003;27(10):1205-1222.

40. Clements PT, Benasutti KM, Henry GC. Drawing from experience: utilizing drawings to facilitate communication and understanding with children exposed to sudden traumatic deaths. *J Psychosoc Nurs Ment Health Serv.* 2001;39:12-20.

41. Fontes LA. *Child Abuse and Culture: Working with Diverse Families.* New York, NY: The Guilford Press; 2005.

42. Englander EK. Child abuse and physical punishment. In Englander, EK. *Understanding Violence.* 3rd ed. Mahwah, NJ: Lawrence Erlbaum Associates; 2006.

43. Kerr ME, Bowen M. *Family Evaluation.* New York, NY: WW Norton & Company, Inc; 1988.

44. van der Kolk BA. *Psychological Trauma.* Washington, DC: American Psychiatric Press; 1987.

45. Eth S, Pynoos R. Children who witness the homicide of a parent. *Psychiatry.* 1994;57(4):287-306.

46. Cohen JA, Bukstein O, Walter H, et al. Practice parameter for the assessment and treatment of children and adolescents with posttraumatic stress disorder. *J Am Acad Child Adolesc Psychiatry.* 2010;49(4):414-430.

47. United States Department of Veterans Affairs, National Center for PTSD. Child sexual abuse. United States Department of Veterans Affairs Web site. http://www.ptsd.va.gov/public/pages/child-sexual-abuse.asp. Accessed June 12, 2013.

48. Zafeiriou DI. Primitive reflexes and postural reactions in the neurodevelopmental examination. *Pediatr Neurol.* 2004;31(1):1-8.

49. Understanding child traumatic stress. The National Child Traumatic Stress Network Web site. http://www.nctsn.org/nccts/nav.do?pid=ctr_aud_prnt_under#q12. Accessed June 12, 2013.

50. Giardino AP. Postraumatic stress disorder due to child abuse and neglect. Medscape Reference Web site. http://emedicine.medscape.com/article/916007-overview. Accessed June 12, 2013.

51. Rainey JM, Aleem A, Ortiz A, et al. A laboratory procedure for the inducement of flashbacks. *Am J Psychiatry.* 1987;144(10):1317-1319.

52. Kendall-Tackett KA. Physiological correlates of childhood abuse: chronic hyperarousal in PTSD, depression, and irritable bowel syndrome. *Child Abuse Negl.* 2000;24(6):799-810.

53. Freud S. Moses and monotheism. In: Strachey J, ed. *The Standard Edition of the Complete Psychological Works of Sigmund Freud.* London: Hogarth Press; 1939:3-137.

54. Hartman CR, Burgess AW. Information processing of trauma: case application of a model. *J Interpers Violence.* 1988;3(4):443-457.

55. Goldman L. *Raising Our Children to Be Resilient: A Guide to Helping Children Cope with Trauma in Today's World.* New York, NY: Brunner-Routledge; 2004.

56. van der Kolk BA. The compulsion to repeat the trauma: re-enactment, revictimization, and masochism. *Psychiatr Clin North Am.* 1989;12(2):389-411.

57. Rutter M. Resilience in the face of adversity: protective factors and resistance to psychiatric disorder. *Br J Psychiatry.* 1985;147:598-611.

58. Johnson DR. The role of creative arts therapies in the diagnosis and treatment of psychological trauma. *Arts Psychother.* 1987;14:7-13.

59. Freud S. Constructions in analysis. In: Jones E, ed; Riviere J, trans. *Collected Papers.* New York, NY: Basic Books; 1959(5):358-371.

60. Court Appointed Special Advocates (CASA) for Children. How children and adolescents respond to trauma. CASA of Baltimore Web site. http://www.casabalt.org/pgs/trauma.htm. Accessed 2006.

61. Malchiodi C, ed. *Creative Interventions with Traumatized Children.* New York, NY: The Guilford Press; 2008.

Chapter 11

Sexual Abuse of Adolescents

Michelle Clayton, MD, MPH, FAAP
Suzanne P. Starling, MD, FAAP
Barbara Speller-Brown, RN, MSN

Key Points

1. Adolescent females have a higher rate of sexual assault than any other age group.[1]
2. Despite the variety of drugs that can facilitate assault, alcohol is the most commonly used drug during date rapes or other types of assaults perpetrated against adolescents.
3. There are common associated features present in cases of drug-facilitated sexual assault (DFSA), including sudden intoxication; intoxication or hangover out of proportion to alcohol consumed, especially after leaving a beverage unattended; witness reports that the victim was incapacitated; waking in an unexpected location, with an unexpected person, or with clothing removed or in disarray.
4. Since examination findings alone cannot distinguish between injury resulting from consensual intercourse and injury resulting from assault, asking about previous or concurrent consensual intercourse and the time frame in which it occurred is helpful in making assessments regarding the etiology of any injury found on examination.
5. Before the interview, the practitioner should inform the adolescent that information related to his or her safety must be disclosed to appropriate authorities and that some private information may also need to be shared, such as information about consensual sexual activities.
6. Since a sexually transmitted infection (STI) could have been acquired before the assault, some centers do not test adolescent assault victims for forensic purposes. However, this is not a recommended practice because a substantial proportion of infections could remain undetected.
7. It is important for medical providers to know that rape is a legal term and not a medical diagnosis. Therefore, when evidence of penetrating trauma is noted on examination (eg, ecchymosis, edema, abrasions, lacerations, or transections of the hymen or external genitals), the findings should be considered diagnostic of blunt force trauma (or blunt force penetrating trauma) to the genitals, rather than diagnostic of rape.

Sexual abuse is a serious problem effecting adolescents in our society. Awareness of sexual abuse has increased over the past few decades, and medical providers are frequently asked to evaluate adolescents with abuse allegations. Sexual assault nurse examiners (SANEs) are professionals who are trained to provide care to victims of sexual assault and sexual abuse and collect forensic evidence to aid in the prosecution of sexual crimes.[2] SANEs have been shown to have a positive impact on the care of sexually assaulted patients. Patients evaluated by SANEs are more likely have evidence collected, and to receive prophylaxis for pregnancy and STIs.[3,4] The sexual abuse of adolescents presents unique challenges for the examiner because of the adolescent's distinctive psychological, emotional, and physical makeup. This chapter explores the special issues surrounding sexual abuse of adolescents and the examination of adolescents suspected of having been sexually abused.

Epidemiology

Adolescents have a higher rate of sexual assault than any other age group. Data collected by the National Child Abuse and Neglect Data System (NCANDS)[5] in 2009 reveals that 9.5% of the 702 000 cases of child abuse substantiated by child protective services (CPS) involved sexual abuse. In 2009, the CDC's Workgroup on Adolescent Sexual and Reproductive Health[6] reported rates of sexual assault among adolescents and young adults aged 10 through 24 years based on information reported in multiple surveys, surveillance systems, and vital record systems. The rates of emergency room (ER) visits for nonfatal sexual assaults were substantially higher for adolescents than for young adults, with 90.0 per 100 000 for adolescent aged 10 through 14 years, 152.6 per 100 000 for adolescents aged 15 through 17 years, 163.7 per 100 000 for adolescents aged 18 through 19 years, and 97.1 per 100 000 for persons aged 20 through 24 years.[6] Other national data also reveals similar trends, with the highest rates of sexual assault among victims aged 12 through 15 years.[7]

The prevalence of child sexual abuse is surprisingly difficult to determine. Numerous factors contribute to the difficulty of ascertaining a precise assessment of sexual abuse prevalence in the population. Many estimates rely on information gathered about reported cases of abuse; however, it is widely believed that sexual abuse is underreported, with estimates that less than one-third of child sexual abuse cases are captured in incidence calculations.[8] For example, a random digit dial telephone survey in Quebec revealed that only 21.2% of adults reported disclosing abuse within a month after the event occurred and over 57% delayed disclosure for more than 5 years after the abuse occurred.[9] Among an ethnically diverse sample of adolescents and young women, rates of reported rape to investigative agencies was extremely low (less than 2%).[1] Self-reported data may give more accurate estimates of the frequency of child sexual abuse since so many cases remain unreported. Prevalence figures founded on population-based surveys range from 17.2 % to 35% in females[10,11] and 6.7% to 10% in males.[10,9] The reported prevalence of child sexual abuse differs because of the diverse populations, varying numbers of participants, and different methods seen in each study.

Although significantly more abuse is reported among females in the United States, sexual abuse of boys is especially underreported and underdiagnosed.[12,13] A classic study of sexual abuse in men found that 16% of men aged older than 18 years reported sexual abuse at some point in their lives.[14] Most assaults of adolescent boys are committed by extrafamilial offenders who are known by, but not related, to the victims.[12,15] Although male perpetrators are identified more often in cases involving boys living in 2-parent homes, female perpetrators are implicated more often in cases involving adolescent male victims living in 1-parent homes.[16] Other studies report a high number of male perpetrators among younger age groups and an overall male predominance in perpetration of abuse.[17,18] Being kissed and touched without intercourse is the most frequently described act among incarcerated males who were sexually abused as children. Most of the perpetrators of sexual abuse (90%) identified by this population of incarcerated males were female friends or family members.[19]

Research has identified several factors associated with an increased risk of sexual abuse. Regardless of socioeconomic status, the risk of adolescent sexual abuse increases in families that are less cohesive, more disorganized, or dysfunctional. Living in a single-parent home also increases the likelihood of childhood sexual abuse for both males and females, an effect that persists even if socioeconomic status is factored into the analysis.[16,20] Children with behavioral or mental health problems are abused nearly twice as often as children without such problems.[21] Based on reported cases, deaf females experience twice the rate of contact childhood sexual abuse as females without hearing impairments.[22] Additionally, children and adolescents with a physical disability or long-term health problem are more likely to have experienced sexual violence than those without a disability.[23,24] This increased risk of sexual assault continues into adulthood; women with disabilities have over 4 times the risk of sexual assault, compared to women without disabilities.[25]

Sexual Maturity

Adolescence is the transitional stage between childhood and adulthood during which boys and girls undergo a series of pubertal changes. Providers must be able to proficiently and accurately evaluate stages of sexual maturation when examining adolescents for sexual abuse. The most widespread method of assessing sexual maturity employs the use of the sexual maturity ratings (SMR) stages. In the 1960s, James M. Tanner conducted longitudinal studies to collect detailed information about sexual maturation in males and females which he then used to develop the SMR stages. The stages of pubertal changes for each secondary sexual characteristic are outlined in **Table 11-1**. According to Tanner, sexual maturation is classified into 5 stages, with SMR stage 1 referring to children without any evidence of pubertal development, SMR stages 2 through 4 referencing intermediate stages of growth, and SMR stage 5 referring to adolescents with completed physical maturation. Breast and pubic hair development is evaluated in girls, and genital and pubic hair development is evaluated in boys. It is important to stage the different elements separately because it is common for an adolescent to have a different SMR for each evaluated area. For example, a child can be SMR stage 3 for breasts and SMR stage 2 for pubic hair. When assessing physical maturation in females, the health care provider should stage the breasts and pubic hair (Table 11-1). In **Figure 11-1**, Breast development and menarche are primarily controlled by estrogen production, whereas the growth of pubic hair is stimulated by androgens. Secondary sexual development in girls involves the enlargement of the ovaries, uterus, vagina, labia, and breast and the growth of pubic hair. With the onset of puberty, estrogen causes changes in breast tissue and the hymen in most girls. Breast development is usually the first manifestation of puberty in girls with the duration of puberty most often ranging from 2 to 3 years.[26] Breast budding (thelarche)

Figure 11-1. *Female and male stages of pubertal changes. Reprinted with permission from Giardino AP, Datner EM, Asher JB, et al.* Sexual Assault: Victimization Across the Life Span. *STM Learning, Inc: St. Louis, MO; 2003.*

Stages of Pubertal Changes

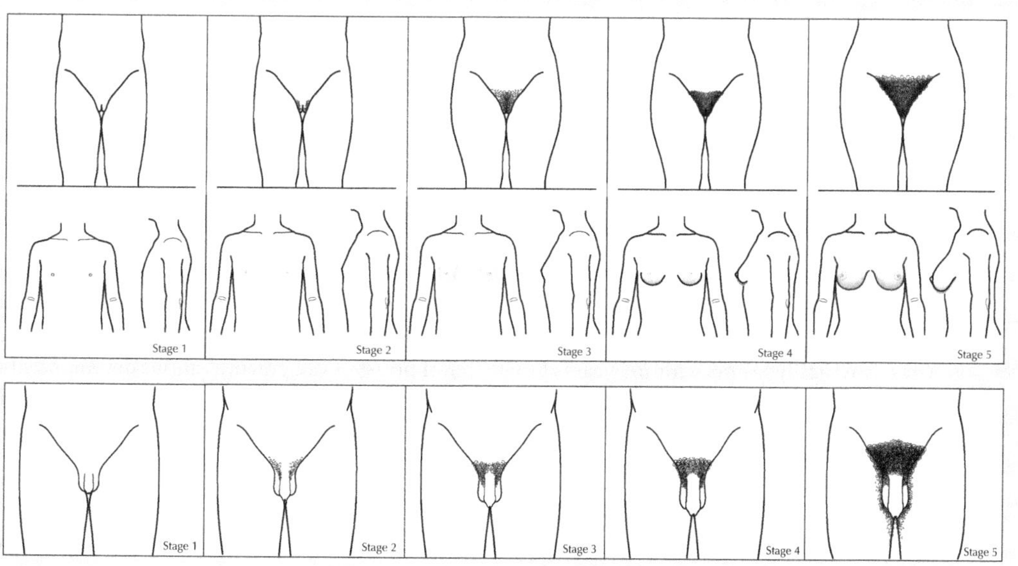

Figure 11-1

Table 11-1. Tanner Stages of Maturity

Breast Sexual Maturity Rating (SMR)	
Stage 1 (prepubertal)	Elevation of the papilla
Stage 2	Breast budding with areolar enlargement and later tenderness Enlargement with no separation of breast/nipple contour
Stage 3	Enlargement with no separation of breast/nipple contour
Stage 4	Projection of the areola and papilla to form a clear mound (nipple)
Stage 5	The nature stage with areolar recession
Pubic Maturity Rating	
Stage 1 (preadolescent)	Only vellus over the pubes, no pubic hair
Stage 2 (pubarche)	Sparse growth downy hair, straight, little curl, hairs easily counted
Stage 3	Hair darker, coarser, curlier, mainly over the pubes, still countable
Stage 4	Adult type hair over the mons and labia, counting now requires compulsive behavior
Stage 5	Mature stage spreads to medial thighs and forms the female escutcheon (inverted triangle)
Boys SMR	
Stage G1 (preadolescent)	Infantile, no enlargement of penis, testicular volume 1.5mL
Stage G2	Testes enlarge (volume 1.6-mL), early sparse pubic hair
Stage G3	Hair increases, both testes (volume 6-12mL) and penis grow
Stage G4	Hair now thickened, scrotum more rugated, volume of testes 12-20mL
Stage G5	Adult male hair on the thighs; penis and testes (volume >20mL) full size; male escutcheon is triangular shaped

Reprinted with permission from Giardino AP, Datner EM, Asher JB, et al. Sexual Assault: Victimization Across the Life Span. *STM Learning, Inc: St. Louis, MO; 2003.*

signifies the onset of SMR stage 2.[27,28] Breast development usually occurs before pubic hair appears.[26-28] Menarche generally does not happen before breast SMR stage 3 or 4, and typically occurs within 2 years of the onset of breast development. Various developmental events are tied to certain SMR stages. In females, menarche usually does not occur until at least SMR stage 3; peak growth velocity in females occurs during SMR stage 2, so by the time a girl's first period occurs, more than 98% of adult height has been attained.[29]

The same increase in estrogen that causes breast changes also causes the hymen to become elastic, thickened, and redundant, therefore allowing the hymen to stretch during vaginal penetration without causing injury in many cases. This is why it is possible for adolescents to have a normal hymenal examination after a history of vaginal penetration.[29-34]

When assessing development in males, the genitalia (testes, scrotum, and penis) and pubic hair should be staged. Similar to the pubertal development of females, the development of male genitals is controlled by testosterones, with pubic hair development being stimulated by androgens. On average, male pubertal development begins a year later than female pubertal development.[35] Development of secondary sexual characteristics in boys involves genital development and pubic hair growth. A change in genital development usually precedes the appearance of pubic hair, which often does not appear until 18 to 24 months after the onset of testicular growth. Enlargement of the scrotum and testes defines the onset of SMR stage 2, with little or no enlargement of the penis. Ejaculation generally first occurs in SMR stage 3, with semen appearing between SMR stage 3 and 4. Spermarche and nocturnal emissions begin in SMR stage 3. In SMR stage 4, peak height velocity in males occurs, along with the growth of facial and body hair and changes in voice depth. In SMR stage 5, males develop the ability to grow a beard.[36]

Timing of early versus late maturation in males and females has been associated with lasting psychosocial effects in some individuals. In females, early physical maturation has been associated with increased risk of behavioral problems or emotional difficulties, such as depression or lower self-image, and higher rates of anxiety and disordered eating.[37,38] Early-maturing girls spend more time with older peers and are often popular but have increased parental conflict.[37-39] Early-maturing girls are also more likely to engage in risky behaviors, including early sexual intercourse and drug and alcohol use.[37]

In contrast, the effects of early maturation on boys are more positive. Early-maturing boys, like early-maturing girls, tend to be popular but without the difficulties encountered by their female counterparts. Early-maturing boys tend to have increased confidence, athletic involvement, and achievement and a positive self-image, compared with late maturing boys.[37-39] However, they are at risk for aggression or delinquent behaviors, including drug and alcohol use, truancy, and early sexual activity.[37,39,40] On the other hand, late-maturing boys have relatively lower self-esteem, a feeling of inadequacy, and decreased achievement, compared to early-maturing boys.[37,39]

Finally, there is evidence that the rate of pubertal maturation in both males and females may have profound psychosocial influences on adolescents. Rapid pubertal tempo, rapid progression through puberty, may lead to increased depressive symptoms in males but not females, particularly when there is early onset of puberty. This was not the case among males with a later and slower rate of physical maturation.[35]

Adolescent Risk-Taking Behaviors

Adolescence is a period of rapid physical, emotional, and cognitive growth. It is a time associated with a spike in risk-taking behaviors. Several biopsychosocial factors contribute to participation in or refrainment from risk-taking behavior among adolescents. Decision-making capability is thought to be dependent on the prefrontal cortex, which continues to develop into young adulthood.[41] This feature results in variability in decision-making capability among teenagers. There is evidence that different rates of maturation of various brain regions can give rise to risk-taking behavior in adolescents. More rapid maturation of the striatal regions, which are sensitive to novelty and reward, may interact with the slower-maturing prefrontal cortex in influencing risky behavior.[41] Individual factors are also involved; for example, an extremely positive emotional state is associated with an increase in risk behavior.[42] In addition, genetic factors have been identified that moderate adolescent sexual risk behaviors with substance use.[43] Additionally, environmental factors are also involved; for example, households in which the mother works more nightshifts are associated with a poorer quality home environment and less time spent with children.[44] As stated earlier, teenagers who mature early are more likely to experiment with drugs and other substances than teenagers who do not mature early.[45] There are demonstrated protective factors that can reduce risky behavior among adolescents. Natural mentoring relationships (mentoring that occurs outside of a formal mentoring program) and school attachment were inversely correlated with adolescent risk behaviors, such as cigarette, alcohol, and other substance use and dating violence victimization or perpetration.[46] Particularly among teenagers with the early onset of puberty, a high level of parental monitoring reduced substance initiation and use, and also reduced exposure to deviant peers.[45]

Dating Violence

Dating violence is defined as physical, sexual, psychological, or emotional violence within a dating relationship.[47] Surveys of adolescents reveal that both males and females report perpetrating dating violence. Forty-seven percent to 65% of physically aggressive couples report mutual violence. Girls are more likely than boys to be the sole perpetrator of dating violence.[48] According to the 2009 Youth Risk Behavior Surveillance produced by the Centers for Disease Control and Prevention (CDC),[49] approximately 10% of teenagers reported they had been hit, slapped, or physically hurt on purpose by a dating partner in the previous 12 months. The prevalence of self-reported dating violence is higher among black (14.3%) and Hispanic (11.8%) adolescents, compared to white (8.0%) adolescents. Dating violence perpetrated against males is also a significant problem, with approximately 10% of males reporting physical aggression with male or female dating partners. Feeling sad or hopeless and engaging in risky sexual behavior, such as having multiple sexual partners or unprotected sex, has been associated with dating violence victimization independent of gender. However, among males, being a victim of physical dating violence is also associated with getting into physical fights, and carrying guns.[50] Among adolescent victims of dating violence, there are associations with having tried alcohol, having ridden in a car with a partner who was doing alcohol or drugs, fighting with peers, and a history of STIs.[51]

With rapid growth in the number of adolescents having access to electronic devices such as computers and smart phones, electronic aggression has become a serious health concern. It is difficult to estimate the number of adolescents affected by electronic aggression because population-based surveys have not been conducted to determine its prevalence. The occurrence appears to be rising rapidly because adolescents have reported that electronic devices are used to monitor, control, or perpetrate aggression against a dating partner.[52]

Individual factors and community-based interventions can predispose adolescents to dating violence or dating victimization or facilitate resilience against it. For example, a history of emotional abuse is associated with increased dating violence victimization.[53] On the other hand, educational programs about healthy relationships have been shown to reduce physical dating violence among adolescent males.[54] Given the high prevalence of dating violence among adolescents and the large proportion of female perpetrators, both boys and girls should be targeted for dating violence prevention programs.

Sexual abuse is a type of intimate partner violence (IPV) and occurs within adolescent relationships. Nationally, 7.4% of adolescents reported being physically forced to have sexual intercourse when they did not want to. The reported prevalence is significantly higher among female (10.5%) than male (4.5%) students.[49] Adolescents with partners of both sexes were more likely than adolescents having only opposite-sex or same-sex partners to have experienced IPV and forced sex.[55] Approximately 80% of female sexual assault victims know the perpetrator; when this situation occurs, it is often referred to as *date rape* or *acquaintance rape*.[7] Factors associated with early rather than delayed disclosure of date or acquaintance rape among adolescent and young adult women include fewer than 5 dates with the perpetrator, alcohol use by the perpetrator, and lack of a current dating relationship with the perpetrator.[1]

Attitudes about sexual violence by adolescents appear to be grounded in gender role experiences and persist into adulthood. Among males in middle school, exposure to professional wrestling and music videos was associated with acceptance of date rape.[56] Acceptance of rape is more common among those with traditional attitudes toward gender roles than those with more liberal views toward gender roles. Females are also less likely to have accepting attitudes toward rape than males. In addition, those who know a survivor of sexual violence are less likely to be accepting of rape.[57] Video games featuring sexual exploitation and violence against women have resulted in a significant increase in rape myth acceptance for male (but not female) study participants.[58] Television programming that influences a propensity toward violence, such as professional wrestling and music videos, is prevalent in American society. Given the wide availability of such programs, broad-based societal interventions are needed to change attitudes toward sexual violence.

Similar psychosocial factors influence the attitudes of young adults about rape. Female behavior, female responsibility, peer pressure, acceptance of use of alcohol or drugs for coercion, and gender role acceptance are among the powerful factors that influence attitudes toward rape among college men.[59] According to one study, college-aged males believe that intercourse is more acceptable if a male paid for an expensive date.[60] Males are more likely to have attitudes accepting rape and also tend to have a more traditional view of gender roles. In a different study of college students, this attitude was believed to have an association with victim blaming in cases of sexual assault.[57] Therefore, interventions aimed at preventing sexual violence need to target these beliefs and misperceptions.

Drug-Facilitated Sexual Assault

Alcohol and drugs have been identified as contributing factors in the date and acquaintance rape of adolescents. Nearly two-thirds (64.9%) of victims of alleged sexual assault reported voluntary use of alcohol immediately before the event in a study of consecutive victims reporting to hospital-based sexual assault treatment centers.[61] The prevalence of DFSA varies widely, with reports of 20.4% in a population presenting to sexual assault centers with a complaint of sexual assault[62] to 54% in patients presenting to an ER for care after a sexual assault.[63] Commonly used substances include alcohol; cocaine or crack; heroin or opiates, such as codeine or morphine; gamma hydroxybutyrate (GHB); benzodiazepines; cannabis; stimulants, such as amphetamine, ecstasy, and related substances; and miscellaneous substances, including ketamine and chloral hydrate.[63,64]

It is estimated that fewer than 2% of DFSAs are the result of surreptitious administration of sedating substances; most occur due to use of substances that are taken voluntarily.[64] Alcohol is by far the most commonly used substance in drug-facilitated sexual assaults, found in an estimated 34.8% to 46.4% of such assaults. Cannabis is second in frequency to alcohol and is used in an estimated 17.4% to 34.9% of DFSA.[64] College women with a history of binge drinking falsely perceived themselves to be more successful at resisting rape while intoxicated.[65] Chemical substance use lowers inhibitions, decreases mental capacity, and may decrease the person's ability to defend against any unwanted advances. The date rape drugs, such as flunitrazepam (Rohypnol, also called forget-me-pill, roofenol, roofies, or ruffies) or GHB (G, Georgia home boy, grievous bodily harm, or liquid ecstasy) have received a great deal of media attention. These drugs are sedative hypnotics that are generally mixed in beverages and can cause somnolence, decreased anxiety, or profound sedation; they can be associated with amnesia during the period of drug action.[66] Flunitrazepam is infrequently found (0.5% to 0.6% of the time) when urine or blood testing is performed in cases of sexual assault. This low prevalence is most likely because it is not prescribed in many and illegal in some countries. Even in countries where it is outlawed, it is used recreationally.[64] GHB is also infrequently found (0.2% to 4.4% of the time) when drug testing is performed in alleged sexual assault; in part, this may occur because it is rapidly eliminated from the body and may be missed with testing.[63] Benzodiazepines other than flunitrazepam are used with a frequency ranging from 9.5% to 77.1%; most prevalence estimates range from 8% to 14%.[63] Street drugs, such as methamphetamines (crank, crystal, glass, meth, speed, white cross, ice), ecstasy (Adam, E, methylenedioxymethamphetamine [MDMA], X, XTC), or lysergic acid diethylamide (LSD) (acid, hits, microdot, sugar cubes, tabs, trips) have also been found with testing of sexual assault victims.[66] Despite the variety of drugs that can facilitate assault, alcohol is the most commonly used drug during date rapes or other types of assaults perpetrated against adolescents.

Symptoms

A wide range of symptoms may be associated with DFSA, including nausea, vomiting, headache, confusion, slurred speech, dizziness, and drowsiness. Total or partial amnesia is often reported. Disinhibition, in addition to impaired judgment, motor skills, and concentration, is also commonly seen. Less commonly reported symptoms include conscious paralysis and delirium or hallucinations. In addition to these reported symptoms, there are common associated features present in cases of DFSA, including sudden intoxication; intoxication or hangover out of proportion to alcohol consumed, especially after leaving a beverage unattended; witness reports that the victim was incapacitated; or waking in an unexpected location, waking with an unexpected person, or waking to find clothing removed or in disarray. Unexplained genital or rectal injury, unexplained bodily injuries, or clothing stained with bodily fluids are also common features of drug-facilitated sexual assault. In patients with these symptoms or with these patterns noted, urine testing, blood testing, or both should be obtained to assess for the presence of substances.[61,67] Health care providers must be alert to the possibility of DFSA in patients who arrive for evaluation of sexual assault with ataxia, muscle incoordination, loss of consciousness, hypotension, bradycardia, or respiratory depression.

When an adolescent presents with symptoms or common features of DFSA, it is recommended that the health care provider immediately collect of a sample of blood or urine as soon as possible while taking care to document chain of custody. Collected blood samples should be tested for blood alcohol levels while urine samples should undergo drug screening, with confirmation of positive results using quantitative levels. Gas chromatography-mass spectrometry can be used on urine to detect a variety of substances, including opioids, amphetamines, GHB, hallucinogens, benzodiazepines, antihistamines, antidepressants, selective serotonin reuptake inhibitors (SSRIs), antipsychotics, barbiturates, muscle relaxants, and other drugs.[68] Discovering a substance not voluntarily ingested by or prescribed to the patient becomes of particular importance when the patient's memory is impaired because discovery of such substances may become important evidence.

Medical Evaluation of Acute Sexual Assault

Acute sexual assault is typically defined as an assault occurring within 72 hours of the evaluation. While some adolescents immediately report the assault and seek medical attention, many do not disclose the event for days or weeks. If too much time has passed since the assault, an acute assault examination may not be possible. Adult protocols typically indicate that a forensic evidence kit is not necessary after 72 hours, based on the length of time seminal products could be collected from the victim's body orifices after the assault. However, advances in the DNA amplification technology used for identification of seminal products are increasing the length of time the forensic evidence kit may be useful. Therefore, adolescents who arrive at a health care facility for care more than 72 hours after an assault occurs may still benefit from evidence collection. Decisions should be made on a case-by-case basis for evaluation as an acute or nonacute sexual abuse victim. **Table 11-2** contains an overview of acute assault protocols.

Table 11-2. Acute Examination Protocol

Identifying information	— Patient's name, date of birth, address, parents' names — Alleged perpetrator's name, age, address (if known)
History of present event (Obtain separate histories from patient and parent or caregiver.)	— Description of the event: sexual acts, exact place and time — Physical complaints: discharge, bleeding, pain — Other injuries sustained in event: cuts, bruises, fractures, bite marks — Behavioral concerns: nightmares, anorexia, school failure, runaway behavior
Past medical history	— Previous illnesses: include surgeries, previous STIs — Medications, including birth control — Onset of menarche and last menstruation — Allergies and immunizations, including tetanus and hepatitis B — History of previous sexual abuse or assault — History of consensual sexual activity
Social history	— Names or relationships of people in the patient's home — Education level, including any developmental delay or special classes — Support of friends and family members (Obtain separate histories.)
General physical examination	— Thorough general examination including vital signs, height and weight — Special attention to skin, mucous membranes, hair — Photographs of nongenital injuries

(continued)

Table 11-2. Acute Examination Protocol *(continued)*

Genital examination	— For females: — SMR stage of breasts and genitals — Indicate position for examination and use of any instrumentation — Describe labia majora and minora, urethra, clitoris, periurethral and perihymenal tissue — Describe hymen: configuration, margins, evidence of trauma — Describe posterior fourchette and fossa navicularis — Internal speculum examination, if needed, to describe injury to vaginal walls and cervix — For males, describe penis and scrotum — Collection of specimens for STIs — Forensic evidence kit — Photographs: digital photography or video, 35mm, or other image capture
Anal Examination	— Indicate examination position and any instrumentation. — Describe buttocks and surrounding skin. — Document anal tone, tags, tears, fissures, lesions, or other evidence of trauma. — Photographs: digital photography or video, 35-mm photography, or other image capture
STI Testing and Prophylaxis	— (see *"Laboratory Evaluation"* and Table 11-3)
Pregnancy prophylaxis	— 2 tablets of 50 mcg ethinyl estradiol 0.5 mg dl-norgestrel (Ovral®) within 72 hours of assault — 2 tablets 12 hours after first dose — Consider antiemetic before both doses *or* — 1.5 mg levonorgestrel administered 1 time (Plan B One-Step®, Next Choice™) within 72 hours *or* — 30 mg ulipristal acetate (Ella®) administered within 5 days of assault
Follow-up	— Follow-up for acute assault with injury to assess healing. — Repeat rapid plasma reagin (RPR), human immunodeficiency virus (HIV), hepatitis B antibodies at recommended intervals. — Mental health counseling for patient and family members — Provide detailed, written follow-up instructions.

Drug dosage recommendations listed herein are those of the authors and are not endorsed by the United States Public Health Service or the United States Department of Health and Human Services.

History and Interview

As with all evaluations for sexual abuse, obtaining a thorough history of the event is paramount. The patient interview is important with adolescents because the teen may be the only witness to the event. He or she may be able to give details that were not previously disclosed to parents or investigators. As with all forensic interviews, adolescents should be interviewed alone and questions should be open-ended and nonleading. Initial history from the adolescent should include the timing and chronology of the assault. The health care provider should determine whether the assault has been reported to the authorities. Additional information such as timing of menstrual cycle, painful urination, and genital bleeding or discharge should be obtained from the patient as well. Other information that the health provider should obtain at this time includes any type of sexual contacts, including consensual acts; use of contraceptives; use of tampons; and pertinent history of anogenital injuries, surgeries, or diagnostic procedures. Since examination findings alone cannot distinguish between injury resulting from consensual intercourse and injury resulting from assault, asking about previous or concurrent consensual intercourse, and the time frame in which it occurred, is helpful in making assessments regarding the etiology of any injury found on examination. In many cases, the examiner can only conclude that injuries are present, not which activity may have resulted in the injuries. The court best decides legal issues of consent in sexual assault.

Laws pertaining to adolescent confidentiality and reproductive health vary from state-to-state. In many medical situations, adolescents have a right to confidentiality when seeking health care, particularly when care is related to reproductive health and contraception issues. However, when sexual abuse is being investigated, the health care provider should inform the adolescent that the same confidentiality right does not apply. Before the interview, the practitioner should inform the adolescent that if a concern regarding the teenager's safety is raised, this information must be shared with appropriate authorities. The adolescent should also be made aware that other information indirectly related to the assault, such as consensual sexual activity, might also be shared with investigators.

The interview of the adolescent may give the examiner a clue to the adolescent's state of mind and his or her ability to tolerate the examination procedures. Assault victims may be suffering from acute traumatic stress and may display a variety of emotional behaviors; some cry hysterically or giggle, while others may appear calm and in control. Every effort should be made to be sensitive to the victim's mental state. Male victims may be embarrassed by their inability to prevent the assault or may harbor fears of homosexuality.

Parental or guardian interviews should also be conducted whenever an adolescent is suspected of having been sexually abused. During the caregiver interview, the health care provider should obtain information regarding the adolescent's past medical and family history. The health care provider should be aware that parents are often able to offer insight and observations not elicited from the adolescent patient. Although the parent may wish to be present during the examination, adolescents should be allowed to choose who accompanies them during their examinations. Some adolescents may be embarrassed while others may be comforted by the presence of parents in such examinations. Modifications to the setup of the examination room may accommodate the wish of an adolescent to have his or her parent present while still preserving the teenager's privacy. For example, the examining table could be moved to shield the adolescent's genitals from the parent's view while enabling the parent to be present for support.

Physical Examination

The health care provider should explain the procedures of the examination to the adolescent. Additionally, the health care provider should make sure that the adolescent understands the need for instruments, such as the colposcope attached to a digital camera, which may be used during the examination. The health care provider may need to explain examination techniques and the use of the vaginal speculum to the adolescent girl who has not experienced a gynecologic examination. The health care provider should also explain the use of any culture swabs and forensic-kit evidence collection that may occur in the examination. The adolescent should be encouraged to ask questions, so any misconceptions may be clarified before the examination.

Once the health care provider has prepared the adolescent for the examination, a head-to-toe examination, assessment, and review of systems may commence. During the acute evaluation, the health care provider should examine the skin for areas of abrasions, bruising, or bite marks that may have occurred during the assault. Bite marks can prove to be valuable forensic evidence (see *Chapter 5, Laboratory Findings, Diagnostic Testing, and Forensic Specimens in Cases of Child Sexual Abuse*). The health care provider should also examine the neck for linear bruising or ligature marks that may indicate strangulation injuries. Other areas that should be considered for evaluation include the oropharynx for petechiae or lacerations; the breasts for bruising or sucking wounds; and the hands, forearms, and knees for abrasions. The gluteal cleft should be swabbed, since semen and other fluids often flow inferiorly and posteriorly along the body's contour (see *Chapter 4, The Physical Examination in the Evaluation of Suspected Child Maltreatment: Physical Abuse and Sexual Abuse Examination*).

As part of the genital examination, the health care provider should inspect the thighs and external genitalia for injury. Common injuries resulting from the sexual assault of adolescent females include abrasions or lacerations of the fossa navicularis and posterior fourchette, bruising or petechiae of the hymen, and injury to the perineal body or labia. Acute transections of the hymen may also be seen. Although less frequent, injury of the cervix, such as ecchymosis, lacerations, and petechiae, may also be visualized.[69] The elasticity of the adolescent hymen allows a great deal of manipulation without injury; as a result, the hymen often does not have visible injuries. Although use of instrumentation, such as cotton swabs and Foley catheters, in prepubertal children is not recommended, the adolescent hymen often has significant redundancy and thickening due to the effects of estrogen, which makes it more difficult to examine and requires that health care providers use specialized techniques during examination. Cotton swabs may be used to examine the rim of the adolescent hymen. The health care provider should carefully move the swab over the entire rim to look for transections or other acute injuries.[70] Some examiners have found that inserting a Foley catheter into the vaginal vault and inflating the balloon of the catheter with air or water to explore the leaflets of the hymenal rim permits a thorough and gentle hymenal examination.[71-73] A speculum examination may be performed in adolescents to rule out injury to the vaginal vault or cervix and is always indicated when unexplained bleeding is present. Speculum examination should also be used to obtain necessary forensic, evidentiary swabs from the cervix. To avoid disturbance in evidence collection, the speculum examination should be performed after the external examination has taken place and external swabs have been collected.

Many examiners value the use of toluidine blue, an agent that stains nucleated cells, as a method for diagnosing latent abrasions and tears resulting from sexual assault. While this technique may identify abrasions, it cannot determine whether or not the abrasions were sustained before the sexual assault or if they resulted from generalized skin irritation or maceration. For this reason, use of toluidine blue for diagnostic purposes is not recommended because the findings are nonspecific for assault. However, use of the dye for the purposes of photodocumentation may be warranted to highlight the injuries present and capture the images more clearly.

A thorough anal examination is required for both female and male victims. The health care provider should examine the anus for signs of injury or infection, such as bruises and abrasions, tears, edema, inflammation, and discharge. Normal elasticity of the anus can allow penetration without injury; therefore, many anal examinations result in normal findings after sexual assault. As with genital examinations, the closer to the time of the assault that the adolescent is examined, the more likely that acute injury will be noted on examination. With males, the health care provider should carefully inspect the penis and scrotum for signs of acute injury or infection, such as bite marks, bruising, lesions, foul odor, soreness, focal sensitivity, pain on urination, or discharge.

Often, evidence is collected during the acute sexual assault examination using a forensic evidence kit, which is afterward sent to the state crime laboratory for analysis. STI testing of the vagina, anus, and oral cavity should be considered in all acute assaults. The health care provider should obtain swabs for a vaginal wet mount, which is useful for identifying sperm and various infections. Since an STI could have been acquired before the assault, some centers do not test adolescent assault victims for forensic purposes. However, this is not a recommended practice because a substantial proportion of infections could remain undetected.

Documentation

Careful documentation of the history and examination is imperative. Statements made by the patient should be differentiated from those made by the parent and by other witnesses to the events surrounding the actual assault. It may be helpful to have separate documentation sections to distinguish the patient history from that of the parent and collateral witnesses. The health care provider should use direct quotes as much as possible when documenting. The physical examination should include both the nongenital and genital portions of the examination. Documentation of the genital examination should include descriptions of all the genital structures as well as detailed descriptions of any injuries. Use of such nonspecific terminology as "intact hymen" is insufficient. Use of specific descriptions, such as "an estrogenized hymen without transections, abrasions, lacerations, edema, or ecchymosis," is more appropriate. Photographic documentation of injuries is standard of care in sexual assault centers but is not mandatory for legal purposes. Use of photodocumentation improves assessment of injury by allowing both magnification and illumination of potential injuries as well as providing the ability to document the examination. Photodocumentation also permits peer review of images, which is an important part of quality assurance. Use of digital video, digital photography, or less frequently, 35-mm photography is practiced in most centers. For those centers using digital imaging, regular data backup procedures, or server maintenance of patient images, are necessary to maintain the data files.

The medical provider's assessment should reflect whether the examination results are consistent with the history. A normal examination does not exclude the possibility of sexual assault given the elasticity of the hymen and anus. It is important for medical providers to know that rape is a legal term and not a medical diagnosis; therefore, when evidence of penetrating trauma, such as ecchymosis, edema, abrasions, lacerations, or transections of the hymen or external genitals, is noted on examination, the findings should be considered diagnostic of blunt force trauma (or blunt force penetrating trauma) to the genitals, rather than diagnostic of rape.

Laboratory Evaluation

Given the high prevalence of STIs in younger age groups, it is strongly recommended that adolescents and young adults receive STI testing. The prevalence of STIs among sexually experienced girls aged 14 to 19 years was found to be 37.7% according to a national study.[74] Female adolescents (aged 15 to 19 years) and young adult females (aged 20 to 24 years) had the highest rates of gonorrhea and *Chlamydia* in 2009, while young adult males (aged 20 to 24 years) had the highest rates of primary and secondary syphilis.[75] STI testing should be performed even for adolescents who deny sexual activity because they may be hesitant to discuss symptoms or sexual history. Failure to perform testing could lead to undetected disease. A detailed history of the assault, including the areas of the body involved, is essential to appropriate testing.

Adolescents with allegations of sexual assault should be tested for STIs, including *Neisseria gonorrhoeae* (GC), *Chlamydia trachomatis, Trichomonas vaginalis,* human immunodeficiency virus (HIV), and syphilis. Such testing permits proper medical and psychological management of the teenaged sexual assault victim. Culture, nucleic acid hybridization tests, and nucleic acid amplification tests, which use amplification of DNA or ribonucleic acid (RNA), are all available options for testing of *C. trachomatis*. Culture and hybridization tests require the health care provider to use urethral swabs to collect samples, but NAATs can be obtained using urine. The United States Food and Drug Administration (FDA) has approved the use of NAATs for the testing of *Chlamydia* in urine; some NAATs are also approved for testing of *Chlamydia* on vaginal swabs.[76] NAATs for *Chlamydia* have shown greater sensitivity and specificity than culture for rectal, oropharyngeal, endocervical, and urethral specimens. In addition, there is evidence that NAATs are more sensitive than culture for rectal chlamydial and gonococcal infections as well as for gonococcal oropharyngeal infections (excepting Polymerase chain reaction [PCR]).[77-80] The use of NAATs is preferred for testing of *C. trachomatis* given the higher sensitivity of NAATs compared to culture, provided clinicians are aware of the limitations of testing in low prevalence populations.[81] Concern exists about the use of these tests in prepubertal children because there is a possibility of a false-positive result given the low prevalence of STIs in children; however, use in adolescents is widely accepted. Routine confirmation of positive NAATs in prepubertal children can be accomplished using NAATs with an alternate target; use of a second NAAT using an alternate technology; or sending specimens to a separate lab. Urine specimens are a reliable alternative to culture and other invasive methods of specimen collection that provide a high specificity and sensitivity for chlamydial infections.[82]

Testing for *N. gonorrhoeae* can be performed using endocervical, vaginal, urethral (males only), or urine specimens. For diagnosis of gonorrheal infections in both men and women, NAATs are recognized as the best option for detecting *N. gonorrhoeae* and are, therefore, recommended for testing in both men and women.[81] Culture and nucleic acid hybridization tests require female endocervical or male urethral swabs. The FDA has cleared performance of NAATs using endocervical swabs, vaginal swabs, urethral swabs (in males), and urine. The FDA has not approved the use of NAATs on specimens from rectal, pharyngeal, or conjunctival sites; however, some laboratories have established standards for using NAATs from these sites. Similar to chlamydial infections, the sensitivity of NAATs is superior to that of cultures, even for rectal and pharyngeal sites.[77-80] Overall, the sensitivity of NAATs for detecting gonorrhea in genital and nongenital sites is superior to culture.

Swabs of vaginal secretions and a urine sample should be collected for identification of *T. vaginalis*. Some centers use microscopic examination of secretions for diagnosis of trichomoniasis; however, vaginal wet mount has a low sensitivity for *T. vaginalis*, ranging from 60% to 70%.[76,83,84] Several culture techniques are available for the diagnosis of trichomoniasis with 95% sensitivity[84]; however, these tests are time consuming. Nucleic acid probes, rapid antigen tests, and immunochromatography are also in use as point of care diagnostic tests that can detect twice as many positives as vaginal wet mounts. These techniques are not as sensitive as NAATs.[85] NAATs using transcription-mediated amplification (TMA) with swabs or urine detect trichomoniasis 3 times as often as vaginal wet mount.[86] Polymerase chain reaction (PCR) and TMA testing can use specimens from a variety of sites, including urine or vaginal and endocervical swabs, with both tests having sensitivities ranging from 80% to 90% and specificities in the 90% range.[86] Similar to the testing of gonorrheal and chlamydial infections, false positives can occur with use of NAATs, particularly in low-prevalence populations. Therefore, use of multiple tests, duplicate tests and different labs, or alternate targets are needed to rule out false positive results. Care must be taken to distinguish *T. hominis*, an intestinal organism, from *T. vaginalis*, particularly if the adolescent has diarrhea or if there is a possibility of fecal contamination of the collected specimens.[87]

At the initial examination, the concentration of infectious agents acquired in the assault may not be sufficient to produce a positive test. If prophylactic antibiotics are not offered for STIs during the acute examination, adolescents should be retested with repeat NAATs for gonorrhea and Chlamydia 2 weeks postassault. In centers that do not culture for STIs in acute adolescent assault, the patients should be treated prophylactically with appropriate antibiotics. Screening for medication allergies should be performed before administration of any prophylactic treatment.

If there is a concern for contact with bodily fluids or penetrating genital or anal trauma, then testing for additional potential STIs, such as HIV or syphilis, should be performed using serologic tests such as HIV antibodies or rapid plasma regain (RPR). Other STIs, such as hepatitis C, should be tested for if there is a concern for recent exposure. Children are not routinely tested for hepatitis B (HBV) because universal immunization is practiced; however, if an adolescent has not been immunized, serologic testing for this pathogen should also be performed, and postexposure HBV vaccination should be administered. Serologic assessment requires repeated testing at 6 weeks, 3 months, and 6 months after the assault to rule out later seroconversion. The CDC provides guidelines for the testing, follow-up, and treatment of STIs in sexual assault.[76]

Prophylaxis of STIs

Since compliance with follow-up visits is poor among sexual assault victims, adolescents seen in acute examinations require prophylaxis for STIs. **Table 11-3** contains recommendations on testing and treatment. After acute assault, prophylaxis should be offered for gonorrhea, *Chlamydia*, and trichomoniasis. In cases where the assault places a nonimmune adolescent at risk for acquiring HBV, immunization must be considered. Prophylaxis for HIV infection is not routinely recommended by the CDC bacause the risk of HIV transmission is low (0.1% to 0.2%) during consensual vaginal intercourse. However, if there are known factors that place the patient at risk for contracting HIV infection, such as an assailant at risk for HIV infection, bleeding during event, occurrence of penetration, number of assailants, or presence of mucosal lesions, a consult with an infectious disease specialist may be warranted to determine the need for postexposure prophylaxis (PEP). In order for the effectiveness of HIV PEP to be maximized, it needs to be initiated as soon as possible after the assault. In more chronic sexual abuse evaluations, NAATs or cultures are generally performed and the child is treated only if positive.

Table 11-3. Testing and Prophylaxis for Sexually Transmitted Infections

Infectious Agent	Testing Methods or Sites	Recommended Prophylaxis
Neisseria gonorrhoeae	NAAT of endocervical, vaginal, urethral (in males), or urine specimens; rectal, oropharyngeal, conjunctival sites can only be tested with this method if laboratory has established standards for these specimens.	Ceftriaxone 250 mg IM in a single dose
Chlamydia trachomatis	NAAT of endocervical, vaginal, urethral (in males), or urine specimens; rectal, oropharyngeal, conjunctival sites can only be tested with this method if laboratory has established standards for these specimens.	Azithromycin 1 g orally in a single dose *or* Doxycycline 100 mg orally twice a day for 7 days
Trichomonas vaginalis	NAAT of endocervical, vaginal, urethral (in males), or urine specimens	Metronidazole 2 g orally in a single dose
Bacterial vaginosis	Vaginal wet mount of vaginal fluid	None recommended
Syphilis	Serum	None recommended
HIV	Serum	HIV prophylaxis recommended if exposure to infected secretions within 72 hours; specific prophylaxis to be given with guidance from expert in infectious diseases

Adapted from Centers for Disease Control and Prevention. Sexually transmitted diseases treatment guidelines, 2010. MMWR. *2010;59(No. RR-12):1-110.*
Adapted from Centers for Disease Control and Prevention. Update to CDC's Sexually transmitted diseases treatment guidelines, 2010: Oral cephalosporins no longer a recommended treatment for gonococcal infections. MMWR. *2012;6(31):590-594.*

Pregnancy Prophylaxis

Adolescent females are at risk for unwanted pregnancy resulting from assault. Adolescent menstrual cycles are often erratic and may be missed for several months. Adolescents who are SMR stage 3 or above but not yet reporting the onset of menarche may experience unrecognized menstrual cycles and should be tested for pregnancy. If the adolescent has a negative pregnancy test, prophylaxis can be offered. The contraceptive Ovral® (50 mcg ethinyl estradiol and 0.5 mg dl-norgestrel) may be given, with 2 pills administered when the adolescent arrives for care related to sexual assault and 2 more pills administered 12 hours after the initial dose. The primary mechanism of action for emergency contraception is to inhibit or delay ovulation through effects on follicular development.[88] When started within 72 hours of the assault, it is reported to be safe and effective, with reduction of pregnancy risk by 57% to 93%.[88,89] Levonorgestrel emergency contraceptive is a safe and effective method of emergency contraception and is the most widely used method across the globe. It was originally given as 0.75 mg of levonorgestrel followed by a second dose of levonorgestrel 12 hours later.[81] Recent studies have shown that a single dose of 1.5 mg is as effective as 2 divided doses.[88] Single-dose formulations include Plan B One-Step® and Next Choice One Dose™.

Both formulations are FDA-approved for nonprescription use in males and females aged 17 years and older.[90] A prescription is required for females aged 17 years and under even though there is evidence that use of Plan B in the younger age group is safe. Ulipristal acetate, another type of emergency contraception, is a selective progesterone receptor modulator that is available as a single 30-mg dose.[90,91] Ulipristal acetate is available under the name Ella® and can be taken up to 5 days after unprotected sexual intercourse.[90] A recent meta-analysis revealed that ulipristal acetate was more effective at pregnancy prevention than levonorgestrel, with a 42% lower risk of pregnancy when used within 72 hours of unprotected intercourse and a 65% lower risk of pregnancy when used in the first 24 hours. Ulipristal acetate is significantly more effective than levonorgestrel at pregnancy prevention beyond 72 hours.[88,91]

The decision to administer this prophylaxis must be discussed with the family since the ethical and moral beliefs of the parent or adolescent may factor into the decision. Occasionally, a situation will occur in which the adolescent and parent disagree on the administration of pregnancy prophylaxis. Although laws pertaining to adolescent confidentiality, reproductive health, and rights to contraception vary from state to state, mature minors in the United States have the right to obtain birth control without specific parental consent. Therefore in cases in which the adolescent's wishes do not correspond to the parents' wishes, the rights of the adolescent generally prevail. Prescribers are advised to know the laws of the state in which they practice before they evaluate their first sexual assault victim. Providers should not hesitate to consult their organization's legal counsel if medicolegal questions arise which are outside his or her area of expertise.

Medical Evaluation of Nonacute Sexual Abuse

Adolescents may delay disclosing sexual abuse or assault for a variety of reasons, including feelings of shame, helplessness, or fear of harm resulting from disclosure. An adolescent may make a spontaneous disclosure to a friend, relative, or counselor months or years after abuse occurs. Sexual abuse may manifest itself as depression or school failure, chronic vague medical complaints, or the onset of substance abuse. Still others may manifest feelings of helplessness, anger, and grief. **Table 11-4** lists common presenting complaints of sexually abused adolescents.

Table 11-4. Common Complaints of Sexually Abused Adolescents Upon Arrival for Care

Physical Signs and Symptoms	
— Genital discharge and bleeding	— Genital skin lesions
— Genital itching	— Genital or urethral trauma
— Pregnancy	— STIs
— Recurrent urinary tract infections (UTIs)	— Other genital infections
— Abdominal pain	— Fatigue or exhaustion
— Seizures	— Sleep disturbances
— Appetite disturbance	— Drug overdose

(continued)

Table 11-4. Common Complaints of Sexually Abused Adolescents Upon Arrival for Care

Psychosomatic Disorders	
— Diffuse somatic complaints	— Abdominal pain
— Anorexia	— Headaches
— Hysterical or conversion reactions	
Sexual Problems	
— Promiscuity or prostitution	— Sexual dysfunction
— Sexual perpetration on others	— Fear of intimacy
— Sexual revictimization	
Social or Behavioral Problems	
— School adjustment problems	— Family conflicts
— Mood swings	— Neurotic or conduct disorders
— Phobias, avoidance behaviors	— Social withdrawal
— Aggressive behavior	— Impulsive behavior
— Truancy or runaway behavior	— Substance abuse
— Self-mutilating behavior	— Suicidal ideation, gestures, or attempts
Psychosomatic Disorders	
— Anxiety	— Anxiety
— Depression	— Depression
— Self-hate, self-blame	— Self-hate, self-blame
— Mistrust	— Mistrust
— Hyperalertness	— Hyperalertness
— Terrified of rejection	— Terrified of rejection
— Flashbacks	— Flashbacks
— Dissociation	— Dissociation
Other	
— Asymptomatic sibling of a victim or association with a known perpetrator	

Adapted from Hunter RS, Kilstrom N, Loda F. Sexually abused children: identifying masked presentation in a medical setting. Child Abuse Negl. *1985;9(1):17-25.*

Providers should recognize this as a time of crisis for most adolescents and a multidisciplinary approach as optimal. Referral to a center that specializes in sexual abuse evaluation is preferable. If this is not an option, a social worker or child psychologist with experience in abuse dynamics should perform a mental health evaluation. Medical providers should be aware of referral resources for psychological intervention.

When the adolescent arrives for medical care, the health care provider should interview the adolescent and parents separately to determine the nature and extent of the abuse and to determine if CPS or law enforcement has been involved. Careful history taking may elicit a medical concern for STIs. The adolescent and his or her parents may harbor concerns regarding unwanted pregnancy, genital disfigurement, or future infertility, all of which should be addressed in a sensitive, age-appropriate manner.

The nonacute medical evaluation of sexual abuse is similar to the acute evaluation and should include a complete examination. Examination findings do not usually include acute injury such as bruising and abrasions but may include healing or healed transections of the hymen or other genital structures. Often, the examinations are normal, a finding which may be attributed to the complete healing of injury or the elasticity of the adolescent hymen and anus. The health care provider should complete STI testing for cases involving genital-genital, genital-anal, or genital-oral contact. However, some adolescents may not make a complete disclosure at the time they arrive for medical care, and only later make a disclosure involving contact with infected secretions. The ease and accuracy of NAATs simplifies the process of specimen collection. Many centers universally screen all adolescents who present with an allegation of sexual assault. In nonacute cases where a great deal of time has passed between the assault and the examination, the biochemical markers on the skin and in the anogenital area may have degraded. A forensic evidence collection kit is usually unnecessary when long periods of time have elapsed; however, the availability of DNA amplification technology has expanded the timeframe for the collection of forensic evidence, and individual consideration should be made for each case. If the clothing worn during the assault has not been laundered, this may have forensic value and should be collected as evidence for law enforcement.

Sequelae of Sexual Abuse

Adolescent sexual abuse and assault often result in severe psychological trauma that may continue into adulthood. Many adolescent victims experience feelings of embarrassment, guilt, grief, and fear. These feelings cause a reluctance to report the assault. A violation of trust may be experienced if the adolescent is a victim of date rape or had a social relationship with the assailant. They may blame themselves, especially if alcohol or drugs were involved or if they felt that they encouraged the act in any way with voluntary sexual play or provocative dress. Low self-esteem, anxiety, and depression can result from childhood sexual abuse.[92] Adolescents and adults who were abused as children are more likely to abuse tobacco and alcohol,[93] engage in risky sexual behavior,[92-94] and exhibit violent or criminal behavior. Those experiencing child sexual abuse have significant health consequences, as well. Children who have been physically abused, sexually abused, or neglected have a high risk of future victimization as adolescents and adults.[92,95] IPV is more likely to occur among survivors of childhood sexual abuse; this association is particularly strong among females.[96]

An abundance of literature exists regarding behavioral consequences of childhood sexual abuse. Victims of childhood sexual abuse are more likely to have multiple sexual partners and become pregnant as adolescents.[92] Table 11-4 identifies other nonspecific symptoms of sexual abuse. Physical and sexual abuse is significantly associated with initiation of drinking at or before 14 years of age.[97] Child sexual abuse also increases the risk of accidental fatal drug overdose.[98]

Adolescents with a history of childhood sexual abuse report significantly more psychological distress than peers without a history of abuse.[99] Mentally ill patients with a history of sexual abuse are more than twice as likely to attempt suicide compared to patients with severe mental illness and no abuse history.[100] A childhood history of sexual abuse also greatly increases the risk of suicide.[98] In a meta-analysis of 37 studies involving over 3 million participants, statistically significant associations were demonstrated between child sexual abuse and anxiety disorders, posttraumatic stress disorder (PTSD), depression, eating disorders, sleep disorders, and suicide attempts.[101]

Child sexual abuse also impacts the physical health of victims. Maltreated children have a 74% to 100% increased risk of hospital treatment by age 18 years compared to children who have not been maltreated.[102] Health effects can persist across the lifespan. Pregnancy complications, including premature contractions, cervical insufficiency, and premature birth are more likely among women with a history of child sexual abuse compared to pregnant women without such a history.[103] Women who have been physically abused, sexually abused, or both have increased health care use and increased health care costs compared to women without abuse histories.[104] When gynecologic, gastrointestinal, or cardiopulmonary systems were compared between those with a history of childhood sexual abuse and those with no such history, childhood sexual abuse was associated with a small to moderate increase in complaints involving these systems. When pain, general health, and obesity complaints were considered, childhood sexual abuse was also associated with a mild-to-moderate increase in such illnesses.[105] According to Wegman & Stetler,[106] child abuse is associated with poorer health in adulthood, with neurological and musculoskeletal conditions exhibiting the most significant effects.[106]

Consequences of adolescent sexual abuse or assault include promiscuity, pregnancy, prostitution, running away, and attempted suicide. Estimates of the number of children and adolescents who run away each year range from 1.7 million to 2.8 million.[107] Abuse and neglect is one of the leading issues runaway youth report to shelter staff as a contributing factor in their decision to leave home.[108] When studying the population of homeless children seeking services from youth shelters, those coming from homes in which a nonrelated adult was present had an elevated risk of physical and sexual abuse.[109] As many as 28% of adolescents living on the street and 10% of youth in shelters engage in "survival sex" as a way to get money, food, or drugs.[107] Homeless girls participating in survival sex are significantly more likely than nonparticipating girls to have been physically abused. Homeless girls who engage in survival sex are also more likely to have been sexually abused than girls who do not, but this difference was not significant.[110] Homeless teenagers may also engage in other illegal or dangerous activities such as theft, using and selling drugs, or engaging in pornography.[107] More than 1 out of 3 adolescent females who runs away initiates sexual activity within 12 months.[111] A history of childhood sexual abuse increases the likelihood that a homeless teenage girl will be forced or manipulated into sexual activity, which in turn increases the risk of acquiring an STI.[112] The risk of unprotected sex is apparent in increased rates of STIs and pregnancy in the homeless adolescent population.

The reaction of medical providers, law enforcement personnel, parents, and other adults can significantly impact the adolescent's experience of the sexual assault. If an adolescent discloses abuse and is blamed, disbelieved, or unprotected, they may recant their disclosures. This leaves them vulnerable to repeated abuse and prevents them from receiving necessary psychological intervention. Trauma to the adolescent victim can be minimized when medical and investigative personnel are trained to collect information and evidence in the case of sexual assault. These trained personnel can make the victim aware of the various steps in the process, act as a liaison and advocate for the victim, and limit redundancy by eliminating the need for the victim to repeatedly tell his or her story. PTSD, cognitive distortions, altered emotionality, dissociation, impaired self-reference, and avoidance are major types of psychological disturbances frequently found in adolescents who have been abused. PTSD refers to certain enduring psychological symptoms that occur in reaction to the abuse, with sudden and uncontrollable flashbacks being the most disturbing and intrusive symptom. The repetitive intrusive thoughts that include themes of danger, humiliation, sex, and guilt make it difficult to concentrate for extended periods or have a normal mental functioning. Adults with a history of childhood sexual abuse have a substantially increased risk of PTSD.[113]

Prevention and Anticipatory Guidance

Adolescent victims of sexual abuse may delay seeking health care because of embarrassment, shame, guilt, denial, and issues surrounding their right to confidentiality. The medical evaluation should not only include adolescent well care, but also an understanding of the dynamics of adolescent risk-taking behaviors. The practitioner should perform a complete health assessment to include analysis of physical and psychological growth; immunization history; sexual practices, including risk for HIV, STIs, and pregnancy; and assessment of the need for psychological intervention.

Medical providers treating adolescents are in a unique situation to provide preventive services. Health care providers should inform adolescents about normal growth and development; provide screening for behavioral and medical risks, including dating violence; and give guidance on how to avoid unhealthy behaviors and relationships. Providers should be aware of local community resources for the psychological treatment of sexually abused adolescents.

When discussing sexual abuse with adolescents, the health care provider should include prevention strategies for sexual assault. The adolescent should be made aware of the prevalence and nature of date and acquaintance rape. For example, a study of 100 adolescent, female rape victims revealed that most sexual assault occurred at night when the adolescent voluntarily agreed to go out with a young man she had known less than 24 hours, was impaired by drugs or alcohol, or was hitchhiking.[114] This information should be shared with adolescents. The health care provider should reinforce that the adolescent has the right to say no in any situation. Health care providers should emphasize the importance of the adolescent keeping him or herself safe and reducing risk of personal harm; avoiding the use of alcohol or drugs, which can interfere with judgment; and avoiding abusive or disrespectful partners. The health care provider should share that the adolescent is vulnerable to assault and advise him or her to try to avoid risky situations, such as walking alone at night, being alone in poorly lit areas, and using alcohol and other substances.

Conclusion

Health care providers possess the unique ability to provide education and intervention for adolescents in order to help treat and prevent sexual abuse. Still, adolescents pose a challenge for the medical provider in that adolescents present unique issues regarding confidentiality and have a say in their reproductive health concerns. The specifics of these issues vary from state-to-state; therefore, medical providers must ensure they are familiar with the applicable laws of the state within which they practice.

An understanding of an adolescent's evolving maturity level is necessary to provide the proper framework for the evaluation of sexual abuse and assault. Adolescents are known for risk-taking behavior, which can alter their perception of safety in various situations. The health care provider must take care to have a nonjudgmental approach to the adolescent that reflects an appropriate sensitivity based on the adolescent's mental state, emotional lability, or feelings of embarrassment or shame. After explaining examination procedures, a thorough medical examination, including testing for STIs and collection of evidence, should be conducted. Laboratory testing for documentation of drug use, including alcohol and prescription drugs, should also be performed. Careful documentation of examination findings should take place using appropriate anatomic terms and specific descriptions. Appropriate prophylaxis for pregnancy and infections should be administered after completion of the examination. Mental health evaluations should be conducted as needed.

References

1. Rickert VI, Wiemann CM, Vaughan RD. Disclosure of date/acquaintance rape: who reports and when. *J Pediatr Adolesc Gynecol.* 2005;18(1):17-24.
2. Murphy SB, Potter SJ, Stapleton JG, Wiesen-Martin D, Pierce-Weeks J. Findings from sexual assault nurse examiners (SANE): a case study of New Hampshire's pediatric SANE database. *J Forensic Nurs.* 2010;6(4):163-169.
3. Bechtel K, Ryan E, Gallagher D. Impact of sexual assault nurse examiners on the evaluation of sexual assault in a pediatric emergency department. *Pediatr Emerg Care.* 2008;24(7):442-447.
4. Sampsel K, Szobota L, Joyce D, Graham K, Pickett W. The impact of a sexual assault/domestic violence program on ED care. *J Emerg Nurs.* 2009;35(4):282-289.
5. United States Department of Health and Human Services. *Child Maltreatment 2009.* Washington, DC: United States Department of Health and Human Services, Administration for Children and Families, Administration on Children, Youth and Families, Children's Bureau; 2010.
6. Gavin L, MacKay AP, Brown K, et al. Sexual and reproductive health of persons aged 10-24 years—United States, 2002-2007. *MMWR Surveill Summ.* 2009;58(6):1-58.
7. Turman JL, Rand MR. *Criminal Victimization: 2009.* Rockville, MD: Justice Statistics Clearinghouse, NCJRS; 2010.
8. Palusci VJ. Epidemiology of sexual abuse. In: Jenny C, ed. *Child Abuse and Neglect: Diagnosis, Treatment, and Evidence.* St. Louis, MO: Elsevier Saunders; 2010:3.
9. Hëbert M, Tourigny M, Cyr M, McDuff P, Joly J. Prevalence of childhood sexual abuse and timing of disclosure in a representative sample of adults from Quebec. *Can J Psychiatry.* 2009;54(9):631-636.
10. Centers for Disease Control and Prevention. Adverse childhood experiences reported by adults—five states, 2009. *MMWR.* 2010;59(49):1609-1613.
11. Ulibarri MD, Ulloa EC, Camacho L. Prevalence of sexually abusive experiences in childhood and adolescence among a community sample of Latinas: a descriptive study. *J Child Sex Abue.* 18(4):405-421.
12. Holmes WC, Slap GB. Sexual abuse of boys: definition, prevalence, correlates, sequelae, and management. *JAMA.* 2007;280(21):1855-1862.
13. Stoltenborgh M, van IJzendoorn MH, Euser EM, Bakermans-Kranenburgd MJ. A global perspective on child sexual abuse: meta-analysis of prevalence around the world. *Child Maltreat.* 2011;16(2):79-101.
14. Finkelhor D, Hotaling G, Lewis IA, Smith C. Sexual abuse in a national survey of adult men and women: prevalence, characteristics, and risk factors. *Child Abuse Negl.* 1990;14(1):19-28.
15. Dubë R, Hëbert M. Sexual abuse of children under 12 years of age: a review of 511 cases. *Child Abuse Negl.* 1988;12(3):321-330.

16. Holmes WC. Men's childhood sexual abuse histories by one-parent versus two-parent status of childhood home. *J Epidemiol Community Health.* 2007;61(4):319-325.

17. Jenny C, Roesler TA, Poyer KL. Are children at risk for sexual abuse by homosexuals? *Pediatrics.* 1994;94(1):1-44.

18. Dube SR, Anda RF, Whitfield CL, et al. Long-term consequences of childhood sexual abuse by gender of victim. *Am J Prev Med.* 2005;28(5):430-438.

19. Johnson RJ, Ross MW, Taylor WC, et al. Prevalence of childhood sexual abuse among incarcerated males in county jail. *Child Abuse Negl.* 2006;30(1):75-86.

20. Amodeo M, Griffin ML, Fassler IR, Clay CM, Ellis MA. Childhood sexual abuse among "black" women and "white" women from two-parent families. *Child Maltreat.* 2006;11(3):237-246.

21. Jaudes PK, Mackey-Bilaver L. Do chronic conditions increase young children's risk of being maltreated? *Child Abuse Negl.* 2008;32(7):671-681.

22. Kvam MH. Sexual abuse of deaf children: a retrospective analysis of the prevalence and characteristics of childhood sexual abuse among deaf adults in Norway. *Child Abuse Negl.* 2004;28(3):241-251.

23. Alriksson-Schmidt AI, Armour BS, Thibadeau JK. Are adolescent girls with a physical disability at increased risk for sexual violence? *J Sch Health.* 2010;80(7):361-367.

24. Murphy NA, Elias ER; the Council on Children with Disabilities. Sexuality of children and adolescents with developmental disabilities. *Pediatrics.* 2006;118(1):398-403.

25. Martin SL, Ray N, Sotres-Alvarez D, et al. Physical and sexual assault of women with disabilities. *Violence Against Wom.* 2006;12(9):2006.

26. Christensen KY, Maisonet M, Rubin C, et al. Progression through puberty in girls enrolled in a contemporary British cohort. *J Adolesc Health.* 2010;47(3)282-289.

27. Aksglaede L, Sørensen K, Petersen JH, Skakkebæk NE, Juul A. Recent decline in age at breast development: the Copenhagen puberty study. *Pediatrics.* 2009;123(5):e932-e939.

28. Kashani HH, Kavosh MS, Keshteli AH, et al. Age of puberty in a representative sample of Iranian girls. *World J Pediatr.* 2009;5(2):132-135.

29. Kellogg ND, Parra JM, Menard S. Children with anogenital symptoms and signs referred for sexual abuse evaluations. *Arch Pediatr Adolesc Med.* 1998;152(7):634-641.

30. De Jong AR, Rose M. Frequency and significance of physical evidence in legally proven cases of child sexual abuse. *Pediatrics.* 1989;84(6):1022-1026.

31. Adams JA, Harper K, Knudson S, Revilla J. Examination findings in legally confirmed child sexual abuse: it's normal to be normal. *Pediatrics.* 1994;94(3):310-317.

32. Kellogg ND, Menard SW, Santos A. Genital anatomy in pregnant adolescents: "normal" does not mean "nothing happened". *Pediatrics.* 2004;113(1):e67-e69.

33. Heger A, Ticson L, Velasquez O, Bernier R. Children referred for possible sexual abuse: medical findings in 2384 children. *Child Abuse Negl.* 2002;26(6-7):645-659.

34. Hansen LA, Mikkelsen SJ, Sabroe S, Charles AV. Medical findings and legal outcomes in sexually abused children. *J Forensic Sci.* 2010;55(1):104-109.

35. Mendle J, Harden KP, Brooks-Gunn J, Graber JA. Development's tortoise and hare: pubertal timing, pubertal tempo, and depressive symptoms in boys and girls. *Dev Psychol.* 2010;46(5):1341-1353.

36. Tanner JM. *Growth at Adolescence.* Oxford : Blackwell Science Ltd; 1962.

37. Steinberg L, Morris AS. Adolescent development. *Ann Rev Psychol.* 2001;52:83-110.

38. Spear LP. The adolescent brain and age-related behavioral manifestations. *Neurosci Biobehav Rev.* 2000;24(4):417-463.

39. Waylen A, Wolke D. Sex 'n' drugs 'n' rock 'n' roll: the meaning and social consequences of pubertal timing. *Eur J Endocrincol.* 2004;151:I151-U159.

40. Lynne SD, Graber JA, Nichols TR, Brooks-Gunn J, Botvin GJ. Links between pubertal timing, peer influences, and externalizing behaviors among urban students followed through middle school. *J Adolesc Health.* 2007;40(2):181.13.

41. Casey BJ, Jones RM. Neurobiology of the adolescent brain and behavior: implications for substance use disorders. *J Am Acad Child Adolesc Psychiatry.* 2010;49(12):1189-1201.

42. Cyders MA, Zapolski TC, Combs JL, Settles RF, Filmore MT, Smith GT. Experimental effect of positive urgency on negative outcomes from risk taking and on increased alcohol consumption. *Psychol Addict Behav.* 2010;24(3):367-375.

43. Kogan SM, Beach SR, Philibert RA, et al. 5-HTTLPR status moderates the effect of early adolescent substance use on risky sexual behavior. *Health Psychol.* 2010;29(5):471-476.

44. Han WJ, Miller DP, Waldfogel J. Parental work schedules and adolescent risky behaviors. *Dev Psychol.* 2010;46(5):1245-1467.

45. Westling E, Andrews JA, Hampson SE, Peterson M. Pubertal timing and substance use: the effects of gender, parental monitoring and deviant peers. *J Adolesc Health.* 2008;42(6):555-563.

46. Black DS, Grenard JL, Sussman S, Rohrback LA. The influence of school-based natural mentoring relationships on school attachment and subsequent adolescent risk behaviors. *Health Educ Res.* 2010;25(5):892-902.

47. Centers for Disease Control and Prevention. Understanding teen dating violence fact sheet 2012. Centers for Disease Control and Prevention Web site. http://www.cdc.gov/ViolencePrevention/pdf/TeenDatingViolence2012-a.pdf. Accessed March 13, 2012.

48. Mulford C, Giordano PC. Teen dating violence: a closer look at adolescent romantic relationships. *NIJ J.* 2008;261:34-40.

49. Eaton DK, Kann L, Kinchen S, et al. Youth risk behavior surveillance—United States, 2009. *MMWR.* 2010;59(SS05):1-142.

50. Howard DE, Wang MQ, Yan F. Psychosocial factors associated with reports of physical dating violence victimization among U.S. adolescent males. *Adolescence.* 2008;43(171):449-460.

51. Erickson MJ, Gittelman MA, Dowd D. Risk factors for dating violence among adolescent females presenting to the pediatric emergency department. *J Trauma.* 2010;69(4 suppl):S227-S232.

52. Draucker CB, Martsolf DS. The role of electronic communication technology in adolescent dating violence. *J Child Adolesc Psychiatr Nurs.* 2010;23(3):133-142.

53. Wekerle C, Leung E, Wall AM, et al. The contribution of childhood emotional abuse to teen dating violence among child protective services-involved youth. *Child Abuse Negl.* 1009;33(1):45-58.

54. Moreno MA. Adolescents and dating violence. *Arch Pediatr Adolesc Med.* 2009;163(8):776.

55. Pathela P, Schillinger JA. Sexual behaviors and sexual violence: adolescents with opposite-, same-, or both-sex partners. *Pediatrics.* 2010;126(5):879-886.

56. Kaestle CE, Halpern CT, Brown JD. Music videos, pro wrestling, and acceptance of date rape among middle school males and females: an exploratory analysis. *J Adolesc Health.* 2007;40(2):185-187.

57. Talbot KK, Neill KS, Rankin LL. Rape-accepting attitudes of university undergraduate students. *J Forensic Nurs.* 2010;6(4):170-179.

58. Beck VS, Boys S, Rose C, Beck E. Violence against women in video games: a prequel or sequel to rape myth acceptance? *J Interpers Violence.* 2012;27(15):3016-3031.

59. Burgess GH. Assessment of rape-supportive attitudes and beliefs in college men: development, reliability, and validity of the rape attitudes and beliefs scale. *J Interpers Violence.* 2007;22(8):973-993.

60. Basow SA, Minieri A. "You owe me": effects of date cost, who pays, participant gender, and rape myth beliefs on perceptions of rape. *J Interpers Violence.* 2011;26(3):479-497.

61. Du Mont J, Macdonald S, Rotbard N, et al. Factors associated with suspected drug-facilitated sexual assault. *CMAJ.* 2009;180(5):513-519.

62. Du Mont J, Macdonald S, Rotbard N, et al. Drug-facilitated sexual assault in Ontario, Canada: toxicological and DNA findings. *J Forensic Leg Med.* 2010;17(6):333-338.

63. Avegno J, Mills TJ, Mills LD. Sexual assault victims in the emergency department: analysis by demographic and event characteristics. *J Emerg Med.* 2009;37(3):328-334.

64. Beynon CM, McVeigh C, McVeigh J, Leavey C, Bellis MA. The involvement of drugs and alcohol in drug-facilitated sexual assault: a systematic review of the evidence. *Trauma, Violence, Abuse.* 2008;9(3):173-188.

65. McCauley JL, Calhoun KS. Faulty perceptions?: the impact of binge drinking history on college women's perceived rape resistance efficacy. *Addictive Behav.* 2008;33(12):1540-1545.

66. Nicoletti A. Perspectives of the allied health professional: teens and drug facilitated sexual assault. *J Pediatr Adolesc Gynecol.* 2009;22(3):187.

67. Harper NS. Drug-facilitated sexual assault. In: Jenny C, ed. *Child Abuse and Neglect: Diagnosis, Treatment, and Evidence.* St. Louis: Elsevier Saunders; 2011:118-126.

68. Adamowicz P, Kala M. Simultaneous screening for and determination of 128 date-rape drugs in urine by gas chromatography-electron ionization-mass spectrometry. *Forensic Sci Int.* 2010;198(1-3):39-45.

69. Keller P, Nelson JP. Injuries to the cervix in sexual trauma. *J Forensic Nurs.* 2008;4(3):130-137.

70. McCann J, Voris J, Simon M. Genital injuries resulting from sexual abuse: a longitudinal study. *Pediatrics.* 1992;89(2):307-317.

71. Jones JS, Dunnuck C, Rossman L, Wynn BN, Genco M. Adolescent Foley catheter technique for visualizing hymenal injuries in adolescent sexual assault. *Acad Emerg Med.* 2003;10(9):1001-1004.

72. Ferrell J. Foley catheter balloon technique for visualizing the hymen in female adolescent sexual abuse victims. *J Emerg Nurs.* 1995;21(6):585-586.

73. Persaud DI, Squires JE, Rubin-Remer D. Use of Foley catheter to examine estrogenized hymens for evidence of sexual abuse. *J Pediatr Adolesc Gynecol.* 1997;10(2):83-85.

74. Forhan SE, Gottlied SL, Sternberg MR, et al. Prevalence of sexually transmitted infections among female adolescents aged 14 to 19 in the United States. *Pediatrics.* 2009;124(6):1505-1512.

75. Centers for Disease Control and Prevention. *Sexually Transmitted Disease Surveillance 2009.* Atlanta, GA: United States Department of Health and Human Services; 2010.

76. Centers for Disease Control and Prevention. Sexually transmitted diseases treatment guidelines, 2010. *MMWR.* 2010;59(No. RR-12):1-110.

77. Bachmann LH, Johnson RE, Cheng H, et al. Nucleic acid amplification tests for diagnosis of Neisseria gonorrhoeae and Chlamydia trachomatic rectal infections. *J Clin Microbiol.* 2010:48(5);1827-1832.

78. Bachmann LH, Johnson RE, Cheng H, Markowitz LE, Papp JR, Hook EW III. Nucleic acid amplification tests for diagnosis of *Neisseria gonorrhoeae* oropharyngeal infections. *J Clin Microbiol.* 2009;47(4):902-907.

79. Schachter J, Moncada J, Lisak S, Shayevich C, Klausner JD. Nucleic acid amplification tests in the diagnosis of chlamydial and gonococcal infections in the oropharynx and rectum in men who have sex with men. *Sex Tranm Dis.* 2008;35(7):637-642.

80. Mimiaga MJ, Mayer KH, Reisner SL, et al. Asymptomatic gonorrhea and chlamydial infections detected by nucleic acid amplification tests among Boston area men who have sex with men. *Sex Transm Dis.* 2008;35(5):495-498.

81. Association of Public Health Laboratories. Laboratory diagnostic testing for *Chlamydia trachomatis* and *Neisseria gonorrhoeae*. Association of Public Health Laboratories Web site. http://www.aphl.org/aphlprograms/infectious/std/Pages/stdtesting guidelines.aspx. Accessed June 3, 2011.

82. Black C, Driebe E, Howard L, et al. Multicenter study of nucleic acid amplification tests for detection of Chlamydia trachomatics and Neisseria gonorrhoeae in children being evaluated for sexual abuse. *Pediatr Infect Dis J.* 2009;28(7):608-613.

83. Gallion Hr, Dupree LJ, Scott TA, Arnold DH. Diagnosis of Trichomonas vaginalis in female children and adolescents evaluated for possible sexual abuse: a comparison of the InPouch TV culture method and wet mount microscopy. *J Pediatr Adolesc Gynecol.* 2009;22(5):300-305.

84. Nye MB, Schwebke JR, Body BA. Comparison of APTIMA Trichomonas vaginalis transcription-mediated amplification to wet mount microscopy, culture, and polymerase chain reaction for diagnosis of trichomoniasis in men and women. *Am J Obstet Gynecol.* 2009;200(2):188.e1-e7.

85. Huppert JS, Hesse E, Kim G, et al. Adolescent women can perform a point-of-care test for trichomoniasis as accurately as clinicians. *Sec Transm Infect.* 2010;86:514-519.

86. Hollman D, Coupey SM, Fox AS, Herold BC. Screening for Trichomonas vaginalis in high-risk adolescent females with a new transcription-mediated nucleic acid amplification test (NAAT): associations with ethnicity, symptoms, and prior and current STIs. *J Pediatr Adolesc Gynecol.* 2010;23(5):312-316.

87. Hammerschlag MR, Guillén C. Medical and legal implications of testing for sexually transmitted infections in children. *Clin Microbiol Rev.* 2010;23(3):493-506.

88. Gemzell-Danielsson K. Mechanism of action of emergency contraception. *Contraception.* 2010;82(5):404-409.

89. Raymond EG, Halpern V, Lopez LM. Pericoital oral contraception with levonorgestrel: a systematic review. *Obstet Gynecol.* 2011;117(3):673-681.

90. Fine PM. Update on emergency contraception. *Adv Ther.* 2011;28(2):87-90.

91. Fine PM. Ulipristal acetate: a new emergency contraceptive that is safe and more effective than levonorgestrel. *Women's Health (Lond Engl).* 2011:7(1):9-17.

92. Lalor K, McElvaney R. Child sexual abuse, links to later sexual exploitation/high-risk sexual behavior, and prevention/treatment programs. *Trauma Violence Abuse.* 2010;11(4):159-177.

93. Chaopricha S, Jirapramukpitak T. Child abuse and risky behaviors among youths. *J Med Assoc Thai.* 2010;93(suppl 7):S160-S165.

94. Senn TE, Carey MP. Child maltreatment and women's adult sexual risk behavior: childhood sexual abuse as a unique risk factor. *Child Maltreat.* 2010;15(4):324-335.

95. Widom CS, Czaja SJ, Dutton MA. Childhood victimization and lifetime revictimization. *Child Abuse Negl.* 2008;32(8):785-796.

96. Daigneault I, Hëbert M, McDuff. Men's and women's childhood sexual abuse and victimization in adult partner relationships: a study of risk factors. *Child Abuse Negl.* 2009;33(9):638-647.

97. Rothman EF, Edwards EM, Heeren T, Hingson RW. Adverse childhood experiences predict earlier age of drinking onset: results from a representative US sample of current or former drinkers. *Pediatrics.* 2008;122(2):e298-e304.

98. Cutajar MC, Mullen PE, Ogloff JR, et al. Suicide and fatal drug overdose in child sexual abuse victims: a historical cohort study. *Med J Aust.* 2010;192(4):184-187.

99. Newcomb MD, Munoz DT, Carmona JV. Child sexual abuse consequences in community samples of Latino and European American adolescents. *Child Abuse Negl.* 2009;33(8):533-544.

100. Alvarez MJ, Roura P, Osës A, et al. Prevalence and clinical impact of childhood trauma in patients with severe mental disorders. *J Nerv Ment Dis.* 2011;199(3):156-161.

101. Chen LP, Murad MH, Paras ML, et al. Sexual abuse and lifetime diagnosis of psychiatric disorders: systematic review and meta-analysis. *Mayo Clin Proc.* 2010;85(7):618-629.

102. Lanier P, Jonson-Reid M, Stahlschmidt MJ, Drake B, Constantino J. Child maltreatment and pediatric health outcomes: a longitudinal study of low-income children. *J Pediatr Psychol.* 2010;35(5):511-522.

103. Leeners B, Stiller R, Block E, Görres G, Rath W. Pregnancy complications in women with childhood sexual abuse experiences. *J Psychosom Res.* 2010;69(5):503-510.

104. Bonomi AE, Anderson ML, Rivara FP. Health care utilization and costs associated with childhood abuse. *J Gen Intern Med.* 2008;23(3):294-299.

105. Irish L, Kobayashi I, Delahanty DL. Long-term physical health consequences of childhood sexual abuse: a meta-analytic review. *J Pediatr Psychol.* 2010;35(5):450-461.

106. Wegman HL, Stetler C. A meta-analytic review of the effects of childhood abuse on medical outcomes in adulthood. *Psychosom Med.* 2009;71(8):805-812.

107. National Runaway Switchboard. National Runaway Switchboard 2010 Reporter's Source Book on Runaway and Homeless Youth. National Runaway Switchboard Web site. http://www.nrscrisisline.org/media/documents/2010ReportersSourceBookv07152010.pdf. Accessed 2012.

108. United States Department of Health and Human Services. Report to Congress on the Runaway and Homeless Youth Programs of the Family and Youth Services Bureau for Fiscal Years 2008 and 2009. United States Department of Health and Human Services, Administration for Children and Familes Web site. http://www.acf.hhs.gov/programs/fysb/content/docs/508-fysb-congress-0809.pdf. Accessed June 3, 2011.

109. McRee N. Child abuse in blended households: reports from runaway and homeless youth. *Child Abuse Negl.* 2008;32(4):449-453.

110. Warf C, Clark L, Desai M, Calvo R, Agahi G, Hoffman J. Coming of age on the streets: survival sex among homeless adolescent females in Hollywood. *J Adolesc Health.* 2010;46(suppl 1):S37-S38.

111. Thrane LE, Chen X. Impact of running away on girls' sexual onset. *J Adolesc Health.* 2010;46(1):32-36.

112. Noell J, Rohde P, Seeley J, Ochs L. Childhood sexual abuse, adolescent sexual coercion and sexually transmitted infection acquisition among homeless female adolescents. *Child Abuse Negl.* 2001;25(1):137-148.

113. Schoedl AF, Costa MCP, Mari JJ, et al. The clinical correlates of reported childhood sexual abuse: an association between age at trauma onset and severity of depression and PTSD in adults. *J Child Sex Abuse.* 2010;19(2):156-170.

114. Jenny C. Adolescent risk-taking behavior and the occurrence of sexual assault. *Am J Dis Child.* 1988;142(7):770-772.

Chapter 12

When the Medical System is Misused: The Condition Formerly Known as Munchausen Syndrome by Proxy

Marcella M. Donaruma-Kwoh, MD
Lisa C. Creamer, BSN, RN
Eileen R. Giardino, PhD, MSN, FNP, ANP
Angelo P. Giardino, MD, PhD
Julie Pape, CPNP

Key Points

1. When a health care provider encounters an example of the condition formerly known as Muchausen syndrome by proxy (MSBP), their focus should not be on the pathology of the offending parent but, instead, should be on the abuse suffered by the child at the hands of an abusive caregiver through misuse of the medical system. As a result, there is a movement within the medical community to rename this disease process child abuse in the medical setting, or ***medical child abuse (MCA)***. Pediatric condition falsification is another term that has made an appearance in recent literature.[1]

2. Belief that MCA occurs may be one of the most challenging dilemmas for health care providers. Bursch et al[2] found that although 95% of pediatric nurses felt that it is very important to know about MCA, only about half of the respondents had actually heard of MCA. Most pediatric nurses reported learning about MCA from direct experience (23.5%).

3. It is important to remember that a victim of MCA may have a valid underlying medical condition that is being exaggerated or misrepresented by the offending caregiver.

4. A plan for the evaluation of and interactions with the caregiver suspected of MCA should be developed and consistently followed by the entire health care team. If the caregiver is confronted too early about suspicion concerning the child's history, the caregiver will typically remove the child from that setting or practice or even the broader medical community to seek care elsewhere. MCA often takes months to years to diagnose accurately because caregivers frequently leave the health care setting when suspicion mounts.[3] Identification and diagnosis is often further complicated on account of the caregiver making particular efforts to ingratiate himself or herself with the bedside team. Maintaining professional boundaries is vital in such cases.

5. The multidisciplinary team (MDT) should be consulted as well as legal experts and forensic pediatricians before any plan for covert video surveillance (CVS) is put in place. Although CVS may be viewed as infringing on the civil liberties of the child and caregivers[4] and perhaps introducing a breach of trust with the child's caregivers, CVS can be used in appropriate circumstances in pediatric care to protect the child. There is a certain amount of discretionary latitude that health professionals can use to protect patients who are in life threatening situations. The following are common characteristics of the perpetrator of MCA:

— In more than 75% of cases the perpetrator is the mother.[5]

— Fathers represent the second largest group of perpetrators.[5]

— It is common for the perpetrator or offender to have in their history a career in the medical field, such as a nurse or medical assistant.[6]

— The perpetrator is often described as likeable, caring, attentive, friendly, and a model parent.

— While in some cases, the bedside nurse is first to identify the possibility of MCA due to the amount of contact he or she has with the child and family, in many cases the dynamic of multiple hospitalizations, primary nursing care, and a hyper-attentive parent make it difficult to believe that MCA is a possibility.

— Often MCA perpetrators suffer from personality disorders. Histrionic, borderline, narcissistic, and unspecified personality disorders and other psychiatric disorders have all been associated with MCA.

— Perpetrators have also been associated with past histories of abuse, parent-child symbiosis, and social disadvantages.

— Although there have been different psychological theories developed to attempt to explain MCA, it is essential that health care providers focus on the abuse inflicted on the child rather than the motivation for the abuse.[1]

— After dealing with MCA, the health care provider may find it difficult to take caregivers at their word when taking a patient history. Also, the perpetrator has oftentimes ingratiated him or herself with the hospital staff and may be perceived by the nursing staff as a caring and loving caregiver. It is sometimes difficult for the nurse to recognize that the caregiver's attentiveness to the child is an act, and the nurse may feel violated when it becomes apparent that the child is a victim of abuse.

Introduction

Known by many names, MCA is an abusive form of parenting that victimizes a child. MCA is a pediatric diagnosis that is made in situations where a caregiver, usually the mother, fabricates, exaggerates, or induces illness in his or her child. In such cases, the child presents for medical care with complaints that are so convincing that he or she is needlessly subjected to hospitalizations, diagnostic testing, medications, and even surgical interventions. The best-known term for this type of abuse is the now outdated nomenclature MSBP, a term that evokes a psychiatric diagnosis for an adult patient. The focus of this type of abuse should not be the pathology of the offending parent but, instead, the abuse suffered by the child at the hands of the abusive caregiver as manifested by a misuse of the medical system. As a result, there is a movement within the medical community to rename this disease process child abuse in the medical setting, or medical child abuse.[7] Pediatric condition falsification is another term that has made an appearance in recent literature.[1] This term clearly labels the caregiver who provides a false history on behalf of his or her child on presentation for medical care as the problem; however, using this term can make it difficult for nonmedical personnel, child protective services (CPS), law enforcement, and those involved with the judicial system to associate the term with child abuse.

For the purposes of this chapter, the disease formerly known as MSBP will be referred to as MCA. The majority of children involved in such cases are not yet school-aged; however, MCA may be seen in older children[8] as well as in other people in a dependent situation, such as adults with special needs. *The Diagnostic and Statistical Manual of Mental Disorders (DSM-IV-TR)*[9] lists MCA as Factitious Disorder by Proxy (FDP), though this may change when the next edition of this reference is reviewed and released. In any event, whatever the terminology used to denote the behavior, this phenomenon represents a serious health care emergency that requires careful evaluation and intervention by all members of the health care team.[1,10-12]

History

In 1951, Asher[13] described MSBP as a common syndrome in which a patient is admitted to a hospital with an apparent acute illness; provides a history mostly made up of falsehoods; and, on closer look, is found to have been successful in deceiving a number of hospitals and professionals as to the true nature of his or her health. The patient usually discharges himself or herself from the hospital against medical advice. The reality of the patient's condition is usually only discovered when someone recognizes the patient or the patient's story as having been witnessed at a different hospital. Asher[13] identified a desire to be the center of interest and attention as a possible motive for the patient's behavior.

Twenty-six years later, Meadow[14] described MCA as another expression of the dynamics seen in MSBP by highlighting 2 case reports. In both cases, the child's mother provided false stories to health care professionals and, even with close supervision, altered specimens, which resulted in unpleasant and serious consequences for the children. The children in both cases developed illness, and one of the children died. Meadow's[14] description of MCA recognized that the syndrome is a cluster of signs or symptoms that may have many different etiologies. The following aspects constitute the MCA cluster:

Illness in a child that is simulated (faked) or produced by a parent or someone who is *in loco parentis* (acting in the caregiving role of the parent):

— Child is brought to a health care facility for medical assessment and care, usually persistently, often resulting in multiple medical procedures.

— Perpetrator denies possessing knowledge as to the etiology of the child's illness.

— Acute symptoms and signs of the child abate when the child is separated from the perpetrator.

Meadow's[14] early descriptions of MCA continue to provide useful and necessary information regarding common characteristics of MCA and provide the basis for discussion of this mystifying disease process decades later.

The disbelief that MCA does occur may be one of the most challenging dilemmas for health care providers to overcome. Bursch et al[2] found that although 95% of pediatric nurses felt that it is very important to know about MCA, only about half of the respondents had actually heard of MCA. Most pediatric nurses reported learning about MCA from direct experience (23.5%). The challenge therein lies with the first case the nurse encounters. If recognition is most often based on past experience, this uphill battle presents a dynamic that must be factored in during the diagnostic process. Knowledgeable professionals must take time early on to discuss the dynamics of MCA with other members of the MDT involved in the patient's care to ensure that each member is able to determine that his or her approach is based on the most current information possible. As mandated reporters in all 50 states, nurses are required to notify the proper authorities when they encounter suspected victims of child abuse or neglect. In cases of MCA, it is critical that the health care provider recognize that for cases involving a complex history and perhaps no complex disease, all members of the health care team must be involved in a case assessment before preparing a well-informed and well-crafted referral to CPS in order to best protect the victimized child.

Differentiating Between the Accurate and Misleading Clinical History

One of the most difficult challenges in the diagnosis of MCA is the absence of an accurate history as given by the caregiver. The presenting history in cases of suspected MCA is often not accurate, just as the history may not be true or accurate in cases of child physical abuse. Many perpetrators of MCA are described as likeable, caring, knowledgeable, and attentive parents. It can be difficult for nurses and other health care providers to believe or recognize that the caregiver may be misrepresenting the child's history or inducing symptoms. It can be confusing to talk with the parent who may be the perpetrator of MCA because he or she reports information that is complicated to follow chronologically, difficult to corroborate, and simply atypical. Many of the children who suffer from MCA are represented as being seriously ill, chronically ill, or having special health care needs. Often, the caregiver latches on to diagnoses that are difficult to confirm or disprove with great enthusiasm.[11]

It can take a great deal of determination to obtain an accurate current and past medical history because the caregiver misrepresents or creates symptoms the child is not really experiencing naturally. As in any other diagnostic evaluation, the history is of paramount importance because it provides the foundation for appropriate testing and eventual diagnosis. When faced with a clinically confusing situation, the health care provider should consider the possibility that the given history may not be accurate. A caregiver's history can include over-reporting or under-reporting of signs and symptoms and falsehoods resulting from the caregiver's coaching of the victim or others in the child's environment to misrepresent the child as ill.

Conversely, it is also important to remember that a child victim of MCA may have a valid underlying medical condition that is being exaggerated or misrepresented by the offending caregiver. The caregiver may, for example, give a history for a child who has physical conditions such as allergies, seizures, apnea, and various gastrointestinal problems.[1] The child may be brought to the health care provider's attention for care with problems that are not backed up by the findings on physical examination or illnesses that do not have a typical presentation. Other conditions such as delayed healing, failure to thrive (FTT), or high infection rates also may be reported to the medical team.[1]

Primary providers should personally review the child's old medical records, as a review of the records may reveal that the caregiver has misrepresented the child's medical history. For example, a simple infection treated with intravenous (IV) antibiotics on a general care floor may be misrepresented by the caregiver as a 6-week admission in the intensive care unit (ICU) with septic shock. The old records may also reflect additional information that the caregiver neglected to disclose such as, negative test results, additional physicians and health care providers involved in the care of the child, and evaluations.

Perpetrators often "doctor shop" and have scattered preferred medical providers across a given geographic area or across a given specialty[11] (**Case Study 12-2**). The health care provider should interview other available family members and be mindful not to solely rely on the caregiver to reflect the contents of other records. A caregiver who reports records were lost should not be believed at face value; rather, members of the health care team should pursue the lost records, so they can be properly reviewed.[15]

When evaluating cases of suspected MCA, the health care provider should involve his or her institution's child abuse response team, or its equivalent response team when available. If no such team is available, the health care provider should contact the regional referral center in his or her community that has such a resource available. This team will typically offer guidance about the clinical facts being considered and likely suggest contacting other health care providers that have seen the child or even the insurance companies that have provided coverage to the child in the past in an effort to synthesize records that may have been created with multiple medical providers in the region and, sometimes, beyond.

The Multidisciplinary Team Approach

The approach taken to identify cases of suspected MCA is of utmost importance. In the hospital setting, it is often the bedside nurse who first begins to suspect MCA; therefore, it is imperative that the nurse voices those concerns to the child's health care team members. A plan evaluation must be developed and the entire health care team engaged. If the caregiver is confronted too early about suspicion concerning the child's history, the caregiver typically removes the child from that setting or practice, or even the broader medical community to seek care elsewhere. MCA often takes months to years to diagnose accurately because caregivers frequently leave the health care setting when suspicion mounts.[3] Identification and diagnosis is often further complicated on account of the caregiver making particular efforts to ingratiate himself or herself with the bedside team. Maintaining professional boundaries is vital in such cases.

The health care provider should take care and react with speed when suspected cases of MCA involve young children and the reported symptoms are significant. For example, the greatest risk for fatality typically occurs in settings where the child may suffer suffocation or poisoning. The greatest risk exists to the child's safety when symptoms are not only reported, or fabricated, but also induced. Schreier and Libow[16,17] estimate that nearly 10% of mothers who deliberately induce illness in their children ultimately kill them.

The greatest success in cases of MCA is met when all members of the MDT have reviewed the information relevant to the case. The health care provider should be especially observant of parent-child interactions; reports or manifestation of symptoms when the caregiver is with the child versus away; and the caregiver's reaction to good news, such as negative test results. It is imperative that the health care provider document and communicate observations to the team.

When the members of the MDT fail to communicate effectively, the offending parent is afforded the opportunity to assume control of the situation, and the child is often put at further risk. Even if a formal report has not been made to CPS or law enforcement, representatives from each of these agencies as well as prosecution, mental health care, and other members of the medical diagnostic team should collaborate to determine the best course of action for that particular case. In many cases, this should be done before the caregiver is confronted. The team must respond rapidly and plan quickly with regard to how the case should proceed. The immediate and long-term safety needs of a child must be discussed with all team members, in particular the floor nurse and charge nurse, because MCA cases are too complicated to have any one agency or professional acting in isolation. The child's safety may be jeopardized if an agency acts independently or another professional informs the family of the concern. Timing and collaboration of all team members may be the main tools a team can use to save the child's life.

Documentation

Documentation of a child's history and presenting physical symptoms is necessary to provide effective health care. In MCA, patterns regarding the manifestation of possible symptoms as well as the consistency of the child's physical presentation in relation to the history provide the necessary information to determine the reliability of the history.

Documentation must be as objective and specific as possible. For example: "Mother reports the child stopped breathing at home. Mother reports she provided rescue breathing until the paramedics arrived. Mother reports before incident, child was happy and playing on living room floor." Less specific documentation might be as such: "Child apparently stopped breathing at home. Paramedics responded." In cases of suspected suffocation, the health care provider should gather additional historical information about the child's condition, specifically when he or she began breathing (eg, choking, gasping, spontaneous breathing); who was with the child at the time of the event; and whether anyone else responded to or observed the event. The health care provider should document the caregiver's reactions and behaviors toward the health care team and parent-child interactions throughout the course of the hospitalization or visit. The clinician should also document his or her own assessment findings, making note of the developmental level of the child.

Considerations

As with any other diagnostic process, the list of differential diagnoses must be as complete as possible in order for the best possible diagnosis to be determined. For example, a differential diagnosis for apnea must include MCA. MCA must also be considered in cases of sudden onset of apnea, apnea that has only been documented by one caregiver, and apnea that occurs in children aged over 6 months with no documented underlying condition.

The role of the nurse is not to figure out how the caregiver could have created the symptoms; rather, it is to recognize when the history and symptoms do not fit. It is essential to entertain the possibility that MCA does happen and that it should be considered in the diagnostic process. Once the provider is well educated on MCA characteristics, methods of fabrication and corresponding diagnostic strategies prove to be useful resources[3] (**Table 12-1**). Ultimately, 3 questions must be answered to support the diagnosis of MCA:

— Are the history, signs, and symptoms of disease credible?

— Is the child receiving unnecessary and harmful or potentially harmful medical care?

— If care is proven unnecessary, harmful, or potentially harmful, who is instigating the evaluations and treatment?[11]

Hospitalization

In cases of suspected MCA, hospitalization during the diagnostic process has some benefits for the child and family. The medical diagnostic testing used to rule out organic disorders as the cause of the child's symptoms often requires, at least, a short hospital stay. Additionally, trained health care observers can provide a great deal of objective information to aid in the diagnostic process. The volume of information provided by hospitalization is favorable when compared with multiple office visits where concerns might be documented, but events unlikely, or where the child can be lost to follow-up.

Table 12-1. Medical Child Abuse: Methods of Fabrication and Corresponding Diagnostic Strategies

Presentation	Method of Simulation or Production	Method of Diagnosis
Bleeding	— Warfarin poisoning — Phenolphthalein poisoning — Exogenous blood applied — Exsanguination of child — Addition of other substances	— Toxicology screen — Diapers positive — Blood group typing (major and minor) — Cr labeling of erythrocytes — Single blind study — Mother caught in the act — Testing; washing (paint, cocoa, dyes)
Seizures	— Lying — Poisoning — Phenothiazines — Hydrocarbons — Salt — Imipramine — Suffocation, carotid sinus pressure, or both	— Other MCA features or retrospective — Analysis of blood, urine, IV fluid, milk — Witnessed — Forensic photos of pressure points
Central nervous system (CNS) depression	— Drugs — Lomotil — Insulin — Chloral hydrate — Barbiturates — Aspirin — Diphenhydramine — Tricyclic antidepressants — Acetaminophen — Hydrocarbons — Suffocation	— Assays blood, gastric contents, urine, IV fluid; analysis of insulin type (see "Apnea" and "Seizures")
Apnea	— Manual suffocation — Poisoning — Imipramine — Hydrocarbon — Lying	— Pinch marks on nose — CVS — Mother caught — Diagnosis of exclusion — Toxicology (gastric or blood) — Chromatography of IV fluid — Diagnostic process of elimination

(continued)

Table 12-1. Medical Child Abuse: Methods of Fabrication and Corresponding Diagnostic Strategies *(continued)*

Presentation	Method of Simulation or Production	Method of Diagnosis
Diarrhea	— Phenolphthalein or other laxative poisoning — Salt poisoning	— Stool, diaper, or both positive — Assay of formula, gastric content, or both
Vomiting	— Emetic poisoning — Lying	— Assay for drug — Admit to hospital
Fever	— Falsifying temperature — Falsifying chart	— Careful charting, rechecking — Duplicating temperature chart in nursing station
Rash	— Drug poisoning — Scratching — Caustic applied or painting skin	— Assay — Diagnosis of exclusion — Assay or wash off

Reprinted from Rosenberg D. Web of deceit: a literature review of Muchausen syndrome by proxy. Child Abuse Negl. *1987;11(4):547-563. ©1987, with permission from Elsevier.*

It is relatively common for the child's symptoms to persist throughout his or her hospital stay, and, sometimes, become exacerbated when plans for discharge draw near. In a classic review of MCA cases, 25% percent of cases reported involved simulation of symptoms only; in 72% of these cases, the simulation continued during hospitalization.[3] More dramatic were the cases of produced illness (50%) in which the production of symptoms occurred in 95% of the cases while the child was hospitalized. In 25% of the cases, simulation and production of illness were involved and continued at a rate of 84% while the child was hospitalized.[3]

Nursing staff has the most day-to-day interaction with the child and family during hospitalization. The child's immediate and long-term safety could be jeopardized if his or her caregiver hears of or supposes staff suspicions. An offender who is aware of suspicions may react by relocating the child and other family members. Nursing staff must be aware of the importance of their role in assisting in diagnosis by employing discretion as well as vigilant observation and documentation.

Separation Test

The separation test, which occurs when the child is separated from his or her caregiver, is often a telling sign of MCA because symptoms frequently disappear when the child is removed from the perpetrator. Separating the child from his or her caregiver may be a useful approach to begin the diagnostic process; however, when performed in the community setting, the separation test can leave the team with the knowledge that the caregiver may be harming the child without providing any concrete and specific information to support the suspicion.[18] The nurse is key to the diagnostic process during hospitalization and can provide the health care team with detailed observations, such as the caregivers response to the cessation of medications, his or her own objective descriptions of the child's signs and symptoms or lack thereof, and the child's own spontaneous statements about treatment as a well child. It is important for the separation test to occur in the hospital setting with the nurse providing the observation rather than in foster care placement. The nurse should provide a therapeutic environment for the child going through the trauma of parental separation and help the child deal with treatment as a well child. For example, a child who has been lead to believe that he or she cannot eat, has been using a gastrostomy tube (G-tube) for nutrition, and is receiving therapy to learn how to eat again may need a therapeutic setting with nursing interventions to include emotional support and encouragement.

Covert Video Surveillance

Since MCA is a form of abuse, nurses are obligated as mandated reporters to address concerns when there is reason to believe that the caregivers are harming the child. A nurse's failure to identify the disorder could increase morbidity and mortality.[19] One of the methods used to determine whether MCA is occurring is CVS. CVS is a unique intervention that presents ethical challenges for health care providers because it allows for the observation of what takes place in the child's hospital room when staff is not present. Although the nurse is not the one who makes the final decision to place a camera in a patient's room, the nurse should be informed that surveillance is in place and instructed to not tell the child's family or caregivers that they are under camera surveillance. CVS is at times a useful tool during the diagnostic process; however, its use should not be undertaken without careful thought and planning. Many arguments exist to dissuade the use of CVS, with the most compelling being that CVS essentially places the child in danger in order to make a diagnosis, an approach that is not taken when diagnosing any other type of child maltreatment.[7] The MDT should be consulted as well as legal experts and forensic pediatricians before CVS is put in place. Although CVS may be viewed as infringing on the civil liberties of the child and caregivers[4] and, perhaps, introducing a breach of trust with the child's caregivers, CVS may be used in appropriate circumstances in pediatric care to protect the child.[20] There is a certain amount of discretionary latitude that health providers can use to protect patients who are in life threatening situations.[20,21]

CVS should not replace careful history taking, thorough examination, or consultation and collaboration with the members of the entire MDT. Additionally, protocols must be in place for reviewing video documentation, determining the level of monitoring necessary for the child's safety, determining who should provide monitoring, and deciding how intervention will occur on a child's behalf if the situation becomes dangerous.

There is a question as to the ethic of a right to privacy in the hospital setting that health providers try to uphold to the best of their professional ability. Privacy in a hospital setting is often difficult to maintain and there is a limit on the amount of reasonable expectation of privacy in the inpatient setting. There is an ethical justification for breaches in confidentiality or privacy when potential harm to a third party is likely and preventable.[20] Nurses have an obligation to protect vulnerable patients and prevent them from experiencing harm. The use of surveillance helps to meet that goal by allowing prompt intervention and keeping the child from experiencing present and future harm.[20]

The health care provider is bound to uphold the ethical principles of beneficence and respect towards patients. As the caregiver is usually a person who suffers from a psychological impairment, the child's caregiver usually lacks an ability to make rational, informed decisions regarding what is in the child's best treatment and wellness interests. Therefore, intervention that may seem to go against usual ethical principles may in fact be beneficial and respectful for both the caregiver and the child victim.[20]

Although there are sound principles that support the use of CVS in appropriate situations, sound institutional guidelines should be in place to direct the use of CVS. Health care providers should understand the ethical and legal implications of using CVS whenever it is used as a tool to protect vulnerable patients. Shaw[22] recommended that an MDT assess a potential MCA case to ensure that an institutional framework is followed in order to protect the rights of all people involved. Evans[23] concluded that the best way to protect all people subjected to the CVS would be to have each individual situation reviewed by an independent committee for ethical assessment. The CVS process is one that needs stringent review to maintain the best ethical standards in its use.

Characteristics of the Caregiver

The perpetrator of MCA in more than 75% of cases is likely to be the mother, with fathers representing the second largest group of offenders.[5] Also, a career in the medical field is a common factor in the offender's history, most often nursing or medical students.[23] The perpetrator is often described as likeable, caring, attentive, friendly, and a model parent. While in some cases, the bedside nurse is first to identify the possibility of MCA due to the amount of contact he or she has with the child and family, in many cases the dynamic of multiple hospitalizations, primary nursing, and an attentive parent make the barrier of belief in the possibility of MCA difficult.

One common characteristic of the MCA perpetrator is that he or she suffers from personality disorders. Histrionic personality disorder, borderline personality disorder, narcissistic personality disorder, and unspecified personality disorder have been associated with MCA. Additionally, psychiatric illness, past histories of abuse, parent-child symbiosis, social disadvantage, and perpetrators who have studied or worked in the health care field are common elements. Many different psychological theories attempt to explain MCA, but it must be emphasized that it is more important to focus on the abuse inflicted on the child rather than the motivation for the abuse. For example, in child neglect there are many parental psychological factors that impede a parent's ability or desire to meet the child's needs, but there has been no effort to categorize the parent as having a syndrome known as child neglect.[7]

Management and Outcomes

In cases of suspected and confirmed MCA, many questions need to be addressed with input from the nursing staff most involved with the patient's care, namely:

— How and when should confrontation take place?

— What is the level of certainty that young children will be safe and older children will be able to cope and relearn how to be stable, productive members of society?

— What role should reunification play?

— If a child is placed in protective custody, how long will he or she remain there?

For example, it would be very dangerous to confront a child's mother by telling her that the health care team suspects she is attempting to smother her child and then to discharge the child to her care. Instead, a plan should be formulated during an MDT meeting so that everyone on the team is aware of his or her role. It may be decided that the hospital staff is in the best position to confront the mother; however, having CPS and law enforcement standing by is an essential element in a successful intervention. A perpetrator who becomes out of control may need to be removed from the premises. Additionally, the child may be placed in the custody of the courts until a safe environment can be determined. Hospital discharge should occur as soon as the child is medically ready and a safe environment can be secured.

Levin and Sheridan[24] originally described an approach based on the level of the team's concern for the child's safety if the child is exposed to the perpetrator that continues to be confirmed by Stirling.[11] A few points that are thought to project a more positive outcome for the child are whether the perpetrator confessed and if other adults involved are able to identify the risk to the child now that the true cause of the child's symptoms is known. Regardless, measures must be in place for trained professionals to monitor the home environment.

Connecting a family to services previously untapped may be a bridge for successful long-term placement for the child. In a now classic piece, Johnson[25] identified the following 4 elements for successful family preservation that continues to guide practice:

— Families have the potential and desire to change.

— The safety of the child is ensured.

— All recommended services are available.

— The plan is supported by professionals.

An ideal treatment for perpetrators of MCA has not yet emerged in clinical or research literature. Clinically, the short-term and long-term safety needs of the child are of utmost importance when determining future family continuity despite the potential benefits of family reunification; therefore, every case should be assessed independently and followed closely.

Conclusion

Health care providers play a vital role in the observation and confirmation of the profile of an MCA case. While MCA is a rare occurrence in light of other far more commonly encountered forms of child maltreatment, it often is an astute and knowledgeable health care provider who helps identify that a child who may be a victim of this type of abuse.

Cases of MCA may be among the most difficult cases of child abuse a health care provider will ever face in clinical practice owing to the dynamics at play in the typically safe health care setting. Mistrust, disbelief, and uncertainty are common elements identified by health care providers after working on these cases. After dealing with MCA, the nurse may find it difficult to take caregivers at their word when taking a patient history. Also, the perpetrator has oftentimes ingratiated himself or herself with the hospital staff and may be perceived by the health care provider as a very caring and loving caregiver. It is sometimes difficult for the health care provider to recognize that the caregiver's attentiveness to the child is an act, and the health care provider may feel violated when it becomes apparent that the child is a victim of child abuse. It is not uncommon for the nurse to feel a sense of guilt for unknowingly participating in the abuse by performing, what is now known to be, unnecessary nursing care, such as urinary or intravenous catheterizations, nasogastric tube insertion, or medication administration with uncomfortable or dangerous side effects. Whether the child's symptoms are inconsistent with known disease processes or the pathology only exists in the company of a single caregiver, the health care provider should keep an open and questioning approach to this form of child maltreatment.

Case Study 12-1.

Patient: DH, an 11-year-old boy

Major diagnoses: Developmental delay, seizure disorder, poor feeding, selective mutism, rectal bleeding

Status at time of diagnosis: Incontinent; unable to tie his shoes; multiple antiepileptic medications (AEDs); had never attended any form of formal school.

Intervention: Therapeutic hospitalization and separation test; initiated toilet training; evaluated for seizure disorder; assessed for developmental delay; referred to CPS agency; discharged to foster care; ultimate placement with a family member. While in therapy, DH disavowed his mother and has refused further visits with her. See **Table 12-2** for additional information regarding this case.

DH's case illustrates that a child with an underlying issue such as developmental delay or a neuropsychiatric disorder can also be a victim of symptom exaggeration and falsification. A complicated patient often presents the perpetrator with a golden opportunity to utilize the health care system to inflict abuse. In this case, the nurse, in both the role of the bedside nurse and case manager, would play a key part in diagnosing MCA by identifying the misrepresentation of the child's development, absence of a seizure disorder and rectal bleeding, and the nonexistent feeding disorder.

Table 12-2. Patient Follow-up

COMPLAINT	DOCUMENTATION
Developmental delay	DH had true developmental delay in several domains of neuropsychiatric assessment. Within several days of separation, he was out of diapers, learned how to tie his shoes within weeks of foster care, and demonstrated age-appropriate use of utensils at meals.
Seizure disorder	In 5 years of supervision in the same clinic, DH never had therapeutic blood levels of his various AEDs on outpatient assessments. This was attributed to his poor compliance with taking any oral medication as related to his poor feeding. While hospitalized for various complaints, blood concentrations of orally dosed medications within therapeutic range were achieved within days.
	No seizures were witnessed on multiple admissions with video-electroencephalographic (video-EEG) monitoring, despite the low, undetectable, or both levels of circulating AEDs. No medications were necessary to control any type of seizure activity in foster care.
	DH's mother would call in to the neurology clinic nurse with frantic reports that the boy had had a grand mal seizure and "hit his head so hard that he knocked out some of his teeth". Total estimate of the number of teeth lost during different episodes of violent seizure activity was 22. (Note: Adults have 32 teeth including 4 wisdom teeth.) DH still had all of his permanent teeth when assessed during a routine dental checkup.
Rectal bleeding	Multiple colonoscopies failed to reveal a source of bleeding. Complete blood count (CBC) did not demonstrate signs of chronic copious blood loss despite history of "clumps of blood" falling out of the boy's rectum. No rectal bleeding noted during hospital separation test; no reports after placement in foster care.
Poor feeding	During his separation test, DH ate carrot sticks, birthday cake, chicken nuggets, and other normal table food with gusto. He gained weight in foster care.
Selective mutism	After a year of foster care, special education classes at school, and gradual transition to the home of a family member, DH was able to conduct lively conversations about World Wrestling Federation (WWF) wrestling characters.

Case Study 12-2.

Patient: ST, a 3-year-old girl

Major diagnoses: Seizures, gastroesophageal reflux, episodic hypoglycemia, breathing problems, asthma, developmental delay, irritable bowel syndrome (IBS), possible familial dysautonomia (FD) or Riley-Day syndrome. History included prematurity, temperature instability, jaundice, hypotonia, feeding difficulties, apnea, and aspirations. ST reportedly spent several weeks in the NICU.

Status at time of diagnosis: Continuous G-tube feedings; intermittent oxygen; pulse oximetry, which mother reported as alarming several times a day; private-duty nursing for a total of 70 hours a week; 13 different medications daily; mother seeking confirmatory diagnosis of FD or Riley-Day syndrome; seen by 28 different physicians in 6 cities in 3 states; presentation at time of admission was one of an active, playful, energetic little girl, which was in direct contrast to the description provided by the mother.

Intervention: Reviewed all medical records from previous hospitalizations as well as medical appointments; evaluated for all reported diagnoses and need for multiple medications with subspecialty consults; involved psychology; developed timeline and reported to CPS. ST was discharged to foster care and CPS personnel contacted other care providers who did not know the extent of the mother's treatment-seeking behavior. See **Table 12-3** for additional information regarding this case.

ST's case demonstrates the ability of the perpetrator to use the complex medical system of hospitals, clinics, and subspecialists as well as the involved health care providers' reliance on the history that he or she provided instead of the results of diagnostic testing and observation. This case highlights the importance of a thorough review of medical records, verifying results of diagnostic tests rather than repeating them, and relying on objective data in making a diagnosis.

Table 12-3. Patient Follow-up

Complaint	Documentation
Possible FD or Riley-Day syndrome	Mother described symptoms such as lack of tears when crying, absence of pain sensation, and sweating, all of which are symptoms of FD or Riley-Day syndrome. Upon observation during hospitalization, ST was found to produce tears when crying; experience pain during procedures, such as IV starts; and sweat during periods of activity. Upon review of previous medical records it was noted that several physicians documented that ST "seems quite sensitive to pain."
Continuous G-tube feeds	ST was on continuous G-tube feeding at time of admission due to reported history of aspiration and inability to swallow, even though previous swallow studies had been normal. Swallow study conducted during hospitalization was normal; occupational therapy evaluation revealed no concerns for swallowing difficulties; upper gastrointestinal series was normal. ST started on regular diet without difficulties during hospitalization.
Use of intermittent oxygen and pulse oximetry	ST's mother had reported that she had episodes of "turning blue" resulting in a home apnea monitor, which she then reported as alarming "all the time." During hospitalization, ST had no instances of decreased oxygen levels, breathing or airway problems, or nocturnal apnea during hospitalization; use of oxygen and pulse oximetry discontinued.
Unsubstantiated history as provided by mother	Mother's history of ST's birth included a several-week stay in the NICU with prematurity, temperature instability, jaundice, hypotonia, feeding difficulties, apnea, and aspirations. Medical records of the birth revealed that ST was born at 36 weeks gestation, was in the newborn nursery, and was discharged 2 days after birth. Medical records reviewed also revealed additional providers or testing that the mother had not mentioned during history taking.

Case Study 12-3.

Patient: CM, a 9-year-old girl

Major Diagnoses: Precocious puberty, obstructive sleep apnea, new onset diabetes

Status at time of diagnosis: Child with precocious puberty brought to the hospital with a 2-week history of polyuria, polydipsia, 2-pound weight loss, double vision, dizziness, abdominal pain, nausea and vomiting, increased appetite, reports of high glucose levels by mother's home glucometer, episodes of severe hypoglycemia, and an 8-month absence from school due to mother's concerns that she was too sick to go to school.

Intervention: CM was brought to emergency room (ER) at the direction of her primary pediatrician after her mother reported that CM was diabetic and had blood glucose (blood sugar is considered colloquial), by her glucometer, of 400 to 450 mg/dL. During the first 12 hours of admission, CM had 2 episodes of severe hypoglycemia with blood glucose readings of 35 mg/dL and 38 mg/dL. Concerns were raised that the mother was injecting CM with insulin. Referral to CPS led to a separation test and discharge to foster care. See **Table 12-4** for additional information regarding this case.

The precarious position in which child victims of MCA are placed is highlighted by this case. Not only did her abuse result in physical deformity, but she experienced life-threatening hypoglycemic episodes. It is imperative to protect the child from further harm. Therapeutic separation not only ensures safety, but also allows for confirmation of diagnosis by allowing for a resolution of symptoms during separation.

Table 12-4. Patient Follow-up

Complaint	Documentation
Precocious puberty	CM had been followed by an endocrine specialist for several years. The mother, who is a diabetic, voiced concerns during every visit that CM would become diabetic and routinely requested hemoglobin A_{1c} ($HgbA_{1C}$) test to be done which always resulted in normal values.
Diabetes	During a visit with the endocrinologist, the mother reported that CM had $HgbA_{1C}$ level of 10.4. The physician suggested that the result was an error and repeated the test, which returned normal results. The physician reassured the mother that CM does not have diabetes. The next day, the mother called the primary care pediatrician to report that CM had been diagnosed with diabetes by the endocrinologist. Review of records revealed that the mother had sought care for CM at other hospitals for new onset diabetes and elevated blood glucose; all tests were normal.
Severe hypoglycemia	CM was brought to ER after her mother called CM's pediatrician to report that CM was having blood glucose of over 400 mg/dL. While in the ER, CM experienced a severe hypoglycemic episode and experienced another episode 1 hour after arriving at the general care unit. It was believed that the mother had given some of her own insulin to her daughter, though the mother denied giving insulin to CM. After CM was separated from her mother, her blood sugars were found to be normal while in the hospital as well as after discharge to foster care.
Sleep apnea	CM had been using a continuous positive airway pressure (CPAP) machine for several years and had developed a facial deformity as a result of the machine. Upon review of her records, no sleep study had been found that indicated a need for CPAP. A sleep study was done while in the hospital after separation from the mother, and it revealed no episodes of apnea. The CPAP was discontinued. The first night at bedtime, CM became very frightened when she was told that she would not be using her machine because her mother had always told her that she would die if she did not have it.

References

1. Ayoub CC, Alexander R. Definitional issues in Munchausen by proxy. *APSAC Adv.* 1998;11:7-10.
2. Bursch B, Weinberg HD, Shilkoff S. Nurses' knowledge of and experience with Munchausen syndrome by proxy. *Issues Compr Pediatr Nurs.* 1996;19(2):93-102.
3. Rosenberg DA. Web of deceit: a literature review of Munchausen syndrome by proxy. *Child Abuse Negl.* 1987;11(4):547-563.
4. Foreman DM. Detecting fabricated or induced illness in children: may now necessitate controversial surveillance tools. *BMJ.* 2005;331(7523):978-979.
5. Meadow R. Munchausen syndrome by proxy abuse perpetrated by men. *Arch Dis Child.* 1998;78(3):210-216.
6. Sheridan, MS. The deceit continues: an updated literature review of Munchausen syndrome by proxy. *Child Abuse Negl.* 2003;27(4):431-451.
7. Roesler TA, Jenny C. *Medical Child Abuse: Beyond Munchausen Syndrome by Proxy.* Elk Grove, IL: American Academy of Pediatrics; 2009.
8. Awadallah N, Vaughan A, Franco K, Munir F, Sharaby N, Goldfarb J. Munchausen by proxy: a case, chart series, and literature review of older victims. *Child Abuse Negl.* 2005:29(8):931-941.
9. American Psychiatric Association. *Diagnostic and Statistical Manual of Mental Disorders: DSM-IV-TR.* 4th Ed. Text Rev. Washington, DC; American Psychiatric Association; 2002:513-517.
10. Pasqualone G, Fitzgerald SM. Munchausen by proxy syndrome: the forensic challenge of recognition, diagnosis, and reporting. *Crit Care Nurs Q.* 1999;22(1):52-64.
11. Stirling J Jr; The American Academy of Pediatrics Committee on Child Abuse and Neglect. Beyond Munchausen syndrome by proxy: identification and treatment of child abuse in a medical setting. *Pediatrics.* 2007;119(5):1026-1030.
12. Galvin HK, Newton AW, Vendeven AM. Update on Munchausen syndrome by proxy. *Curr Opin Pediatr.* 2005;17(2):252-257.
13. Asher R. Munchausen's Syndrome. *Lancet.* 1951;257(6650):339-341.
14. Meadow R. Munchausen syndrome by proxy: the hinterland of child abuse. *Lancet.* 1977;2(8033):343-345.
15. Ayoub CC, Alexander R, Beck D, et al. Position paper: definitional issues in Munchausen by proxy. *Child Maltreat.* 2002;7:105-112.
16. Schreier HA, Libow JA. *Hurting for Love: Munchausen by Proxy Syndrome.* New York, NY: The Guilford Press; 1993.
17. Schreier HA, Libow JA. Munchausen syndrome by proxy: diagnosis and prevalence. *Am J Orthopsychiatry.* 1993;63(2):318-321.
18. Foreman DM, Farsides C. Ethical use of covert videoing techniques in detecting Munchausen syndrome by proxy. *BMJ.* 1993;307(6904):611-613.
19. Beard KV. Protect the children: be on the lookout for Munchausen syndrome by proxy. *RN.* 2007;70(12):33-36.

20. Vaught W, Fleetwood J. Covert video surveillance in pediatric care. *Hastings Center Report.* 2003;32:10-12.

21. Southall DP, Plunkett MC, Banks MW, Falkov AF, Samuels MP. Covert video recordings of life-threatening child abuse: lessons for child protection. *Pediatrics.* 1997;100(5):735-760.

22. Shaw S. The use of covert video surveillance: an inter-agency approach. In: Horwath J, Lawson B, eds. *Trust Betrayed: Munchausen Syndrome by Proxy, Inter-Agency Child Protection and Partnership with Families.* London: National Childrens Bureau; 1996:83-88.

23. Evans D. The investigation of life-threatening child abuse and Munchausen syndrome by proxy. *J Med Ethics.* 1995;21(1):9-13.

24. Levin AV, Sheridan MS, eds. *Munchausen Syndrome by Proxy: Issues in Diagnosis and Treatment.* New York, NY: Lexington Books; 1995.

25. Johnson MP. Patriarchal terrorism and common couple violence: 2 forms of violence against women. *J Marriage Fam.* 1995;57:283-294.

Chapter 13

Child Protective Services and Child Abuse

Elizabeth Henderson, RN, MSN, MS, EMT-P

Key Points

1. The focus of child protection is on reducing a child's risks for further maltreatment while trying to maintain family integrity as much as possible.
2. Preventative intervention is not generally the norm because of concerns regarding family integrity, confidentiality, and intrusiveness on the part of the state. Child protective services (CPS) agencies have a difficult task before them in that they have 2 major goals that are not always mutually obtainable, namely, protecting the child from further maltreatment and preserving the family in which the abuse or neglect occurred.
3. Children's advocacy centers (CACs) bring together a multidisciplinary team (MDT) to evaluate the child and coordinate services between CPS, law enforcement, and the family. This child-centered approach tries to coordinate needed interviews so a child does not have to tell his or her story multiple times to the different agencies involved in the investigation and prosecution of a case.
4. CPS determines that a case can close when risks to the child and within the family have been sufficiently reduced or eliminated so that the child is protected and his or her developmental needs are met sufficiently without societal intervention.
5. For persons who report potential abuse in good faith, reporting laws make provisions to protect such reporters from criminal prosecution and civil lawsuits resulting from filing a report. The law provides immunity to protect those who demonstrate concern for the child and family. State laws either presume that reports are filed in good faith or specify that reports must be made without malice.

Introduction

Child abuse and neglect remains a serious problem in the United States despite years of effort on the part of professionals and communities to prevent, investigate, and treat this problem. Child neglect composes the majority of reported cases, with physical abuse, sexual abuse, and emotional maltreatment following. A smaller number of cases involve other forms of abuse and exploitation.[1,2] Child abuse is a serious crime that not only violates the law but also carries with it social and moral implications. "The lasting effects of abuse on victims and society are far reaching. Victims of abuse are more likely to be arrested as juveniles and, as adults, for committing violent crimes. Abused children also have higher rates of adolescent suicide, depression, psychiatric disorders, violent behavior, drug and alcohol abuse, and developmental disabilities."[3] Furthermore, the nationwide cost of child abuse and neglect, most recently calculated for inflation and based on 2007 value estimated costs, is reported to be $103.8 billion. These total costs represent both direct and indirect costs, with direct costs referring to costs associated with the immediate needs of abused and neglected children and indirect costs referring to costs associated with long-term or secondary effects of child abuse and neglect.[4] The potential long-term social, emotional, and physical effects of child abuse are extensive and clearly could have a significant financial impact on society as a whole. Therefore, suspected and substantiated cases of child abuse "merit special attention by professionals trained in the evaluation and treatment of children and adolescents."[5]

The professionals who work with child abuse on a regular basis generally recognize that the reported incidence of abuse and neglect is an underestimate of the actual occurrence of the problem. Barriers to reporting abuse and neglect are plentiful and are further complicated by varying levels of comfort among professionals surrounding reporting in addition to varying degrees of knowledge deficits surrounding mandated reporting policies and procedures. Furthermore, child abuse and neglect is itself a complex social and health issue precipitated by a myriad of factors involving the individual, the family, and the community, all of which are subject to both circumstantial and environmental variations.

According to the National Child Abuse and Neglect Center, an estimated 763 000 children were determined to have been victims of abuse or neglect in 2009. The most common category of abuse was noted to be neglect (61.4%) followed by physical abuse (16%) and emotional and sexual abuse (10%). In 2009, nearly 80.9% of perpetrators of child maltreatment were parents and another 6.3% were other relatives of the victim. In 2009, an estimated 1770 children died due to child abuse or neglect. The overall rate of child fatalities was 2.34 deaths per 100 000 children. More than 40% of child fatalities were attributed to neglect; physical abuse was also a major contributor to child fatalities. More than three-fourths (80.8%) of the children who died due to child abuse and neglect were aged under 4 years.[6] In an ideal world, there are no statistical limits that are acceptable with regard to child abuse; certainly, fatalities are not acceptable. Unfortunately, violence and victimization exist in all aspects of society.

Despite the United States Advisory Board on Child Abuse and Neglect[7] declaring child maltreatment a national emergency, child abuse and neglect cases clearly continue to occur at a statistically significant rate leaving much work to be done to prevent child maltreatment.[8] However, with more aggressive preventative measures, this problem may be made a national initiative rather than its being relegated to the hands of professionals such as health care providers, social workers, or CPS, to name a few. Instead, in addition to educating individuals and families about the signs of and resolutions for abuse and neglect, education may also be provided at the community level because healthy families make healthy communities.

CPS serves to protect children and rehabilitate families in need of intervention or for which substantiated reports of child abuse and neglect exist.[9] The purpose of CPS is multifaceted. CPS is usually the agency that receives reports of suspected child abuse and neglect and then identifies those children who have been or are at risk for being abused or neglected. CPS also identifies services that may benefit the child and the child's family to reduce the occurrence of future incidences of abuse or neglect. The overall goal of CPS is to protect children and rehabilitate families to provide a safe environment that can appropriately address the safety and developmental needs of the child.[9] This chapter addresses the ways in which CPS interacts with families and other agencies to provide a safe environment for the child as well as the social context of child abuse and neglect. This chapter also addresses the ways in which communities and families can be strengthened to maximize the well-being of the child and the well-being of the family as a functional unit of the community.

The History of Child Abuse and Neglect Policy

Although child maltreatment is an old problem, efforts to address the problem in a consistent and meaningful way are a relatively recent phenomenon. The child welfare movement originated in 1875 with the founding of organizations such as the New York Society for the Prevention of Cruelty to Children and the American Humane Association, though at the time child abuse was of less concern than more pressing issues, such as infant mortality and maternal health.[10] The Social Security Act of 1935 provided the initial public funding for child welfare by offering financial support for the protection and care of homeless, dependent, and neglected children.[11] Later, in the 1940s, physicians published a series of clinical reports and the American Academy of Pediatrics (AAP) held a symposium to discuss combinations of injuries in infants that would later be seen as related to abuse, such as multiple fractures in the long bones and chronic subdural hematoma where diagnosis remains elusive, thereby providing the impetus for the development of reporting laws.

In 1962, Kempe et al[12] published the single most influential report on child maltreatment describing and giving name to the battered-child syndrome, thereby becoming the catalyst for the widespread recognition and identification of child abuse victims. Kempe et al[12] described this new medical diagnosis as "injury to soft tissue and skeleton" accompanied by "evidence of neglect, including poor skin hygiene, multiple soft tissue injuries, and malnutrition." In addition to recognizing detailed descriptions of trauma that were often in conflict with the available information from the case histories, Kempe et al[12] further speculated that physicians were unwilling to consider parents as the source of harm and were reluctant to report cases to the proper authorities. Kempe et al[12] also stated, "training and personality usually make it quite difficult for [a physician] to assume the role of policeman or district attorney, and start questioning patients as if he were investigating a crime."

Kempe's[13] 1977 address to the AAP identified the increasingly recognized problem of sexual abuse and raised the consciousness of pediatricians about the problem. Kempe's address identified the severe emotional problems a child faces as a result of incestuous relationships as both a major medical and social problem that health care providers needed to recognize and understand. Kempe[13] described the situation of child sexual abuse as a "hidden pediatric problem and a neglected area" in professional practice.[13]

The Children's Bureau drafted the first model reporting statute in 1963. Two other model statutes followed in 1965, drafted by the American Medical Association and the Program of State Governments. By 1966, legislation mandating physicians to report suspected child abuse appeared in every state except Hawaii. The first statutes specified, "Any physician...having reasonable cause to suspect that a child under the age of [the maximum age of juvenile court] brought to him or coming before him for examination, care or treatment has had serious physical injury or injuries inflicted upon him other than by accidental means by a parent or other person responsible for his care, shall report or cause a report to be made in accordance with the provisions of the Act."[14]

Every state constructed a system of CPS agencies to intervene in situations of alleged abuse. Individual state legislation broadened most aspects of the early statutes to expand the range of professionals required to report and the types of maltreatment to be reported. Definitions of abuse were expanded to include emotional abuse, sexual abuse, and exploitation, in addition to physical abuse. The Child Abuse Prevention and Treatment Act of 1974 (CAPTA) defined child abuse and neglect and set the standard for state mandatory reporting laws.[15] Essentially, CAPTA required designated personnel (eg, physicians, educators, social workers, law enforcement) in every state to report abuse.[3] This legislation provided funding to the states to establish the capacity in public child welfare agencies to receive and investigate reports of suspected abuse and neglect. It also promoted the establishment of statewide, central report receiving capabilities and central registry functions to ensure that situations would be investigated and that children could be protected from repeated instances of abuse and neglect. States were required to adopt similar definitions of abuse to qualify for federal child protection funding. The act defined abuse and neglect as "The physical or mental injury, sexual abuse, negligent treatment, or maltreatment of a child under the age of 18 by a person who is responsible for the child's welfare under circumstances which indicate the child's health or welfare is harmed or threatened thereby as determined in accordance with regulations prescribed."[16]

In 1997, Congress passed the first major reform of federal child welfare policy since 1980: the Adoption and Safe Families Act of 1997 (ASFA). The Guidelines for Public Policy and State Legislation Governing Permanence for Children were then developed as one of several steps undertaken by the federal government in response to Adoption 2002, President Clinton's initiative on adoption and foster care. Because the child protection and foster care system in the United States is primarily governed by state law and a state's implementation of their laws, the guidelines were meant to help states evaluate and modernize the laws that affect children and families who are having difficulties that require intervention by the child welfare system.[11]

Adoption 2002 addressed the problems associated with the long periods that America's foster children spend waiting for permanent and stable homes necessary for healthy development. Among the proposed action steps recommended in Adoption 2002 is that of developing model guidelines for state legislation to advance the goal of giving every child in the nation's public child welfare system a safe and permanent home and ensuring a timely decision-making process as to whom the permanent caregivers will be. Based on this recommendation, planning for the permanent home should begin when a child enters the foster care system because foster care is presumed to be a temporary setting. The purpose of this goal is to secure a permanent, safe, stable, custodial environment for the child and a lifelong relationship with a nurturing caregiver to help establish the foundation for the child's healthy development.[11] The law heightens the importance of providing quality services as quickly as possible to enable families in crisis to more quickly address their problems.[11]

While certainly a noble set of proposals, the practicality and attainability of the proposals asserted by Adoption 2002 is questionable. Approximately 491 000 children were reported to be in foster care nationally at the end of fiscal year (FY) 2007. In 2007, an estimated 293 000 children entered foster care, while roughly the same number of children exited foster care at the end of FY 2007. Those who exited foster care in FY 2007 were not necessarily discharged to a permanent foster care setting. Instead, 178000 were discharged to reunification, 51 000 were adopted; 17 000 were discharged with legal guardianship while approximately 27 000 children became emancipated from foster care. Effectively, based on these estimates, roughly 21% of children who exited foster care were adopted, 18% were discharged for others reasons, and 72% were reunited with the same families from which they were removed.[17]

While the large percentage of children who exited foster care for reunification purposes might at first seem the most ideal situation, at second glance this same statistic hints at possible flaws in the system. Several questions can be derived from these statistics: Is there consistency between reporters when deciding when and what to report? In what depth are cases being investigated? Are children being returned to their homes prematurely? Regardless of what variables in the system have resulted in these statistics, it is reasonable to conclude that there is a wide range in performance for measure across states that makes it near impossible to determine concrete factors that either prohibit or promote adoption.

Child Protective Services

The focus of CPS agencies is concern for the care of children as expressed through the established laws of every state. Mandated legal authority that evolved from child abuse laws provides a framework for CPS to take action when needed to protect children and work with families in need.[9] The focus of child protection is on reducing a child's risks of further maltreatment while trying to maintain family integrity as much as possible.[18,19]

CPS, as defined by most state legislation, exists as a reaction to the need to receive and investigate reports of suspected child abuse and neglect at the hands of parents or caregivers. Social and protective services are provided to the alleged offending parent(s) on a nonvoluntary basis as an alternative to the removal of their children for placement in protective care. Preventative intervention is not generally the norm, because of concerns regarding family integrity, confidentiality, and intrusiveness on the part of the state. CPS agencies have a difficult task before them in that they have 2 major goals that are not always mutually obtainable, namely protecting the child from further maltreatment and preserving the family in which the abuse or neglect occurred.[20,21] Although this may be possible in a large number of cases, it is not possible in all cases. CPS agencies and their caseworkers must constantly assess the risk of future abuse for children if they remain with the caregiver(s) who maltreated them, and this determination must be made with imperfect information. Tragic results may occur when misjudgments, in either direction, occur.[20,22]

Role of CPS in Investigations of Child Abuse

Allegations received by CPS are assessed for conformity with legal definitions of abuse; the relationship between the victim and perpetrator; the geographical location of the abused, abuser, and incident; and the level of severity. Many states have child abuse and neglect hotlines that receive reports and route them to local CPS offices for investigation. Generally, CPS receives reports and assigns them to a social worker or investigator who must begin an investigation immediately or within 24 hours, depending on the nature and severity of the allegations.

It is the responsibility of CPS to contact the child victim, parents, caregivers, and alleged perpetrator(s) and then visit them in person during the course of the investigation to determine whether abuse occurred. The investigation time frame varies by state and can be as short as 7 days and as long as 60 days. At the conclusion of the investigation period, the case is deemed substantiated, unsubstantiated, founded, or unfounded. If the findings are substantiated, the investigating agency may provide services to the child and family, whereas unsubstantiated claims warrant closure of the case.[9]

Many state legislatures took great pains to protect the confidentiality of the family and the freedom of the family from unnecessary state intrusion in their homes and lifestyles. For example, in the 1970s the confidentiality provisions of the CPS law in Pennsylvania prohibited the sharing of information about alleged child abuse cases between the CPS agency and local law enforcement personnel without the written consent of all of the parties involved. This was true even though many cases of child abuse rose to the level of criminal behavior, including homicide, aggravated assault, rape, and incest. These acts of violence were viewed differently because of the nature of the familial relationship between the alleged perpetrator and the victim. Consequently, law enforcement and child protection professionals frequently found themselves at odds in their separate investigations rather than able to work together on behalf of children and their families.

Collaboration in the Investigative Process

In more recent years, professionals who deal with child abuse and neglect and most state legislatures have come to recognize that the problem of child abuse and neglect is not the domain of a single agency or profession.[19] No single agency or profession has the resources or mandate to effectively intervene, treat, and prevent child abuse and neglect alone. Collaborative systems of intervention and treatment have developed, allowing for the sharing of information among professionals of various disciplines that can more effectively provide services and protect children. Multidisciplinary intervention teams, regional diagnostic centers, child assessment centers, and CACs are some innovative examples of coordinated systems of intervention and care that attempt to balance the rights of the family with the rights of children to be free from abuse and neglect.

The spectrum of individuals responsible for reporting suspected or actual cases of child maltreatment is broad and includes the professional as well as the layperson. Professionals, defined as persons who encounter an alleged victim as a part of their occupation, including, but not limited to, childcare providers, teachers, and health care providers, comprised approximately three-fifths of reporters, according to recent figures. Interestingly, the largest percentage of reports came from teachers (16.5%), followed by legal personnel (16.4%) and medical personnel (8.2%).[6] Health care providers did not rank among the top 3 professional sources of reporting. It is reasonable that teachers are the largest professional percentage of reporters, given that they interact with children on a daily basis. However, health care providers who should be somewhat familiar with issues surrounding child maltreatment are underrepresented in these statistics.

Models of Collaboration in Child Abuse Investigations

The investigation of child abuse is ideally a multidimensional process involving CPS, law enforcement, legal personnel, health care and mental health professionals, and other community agencies. In maltreatment cases, CPS often takes a lead role in organizing and overseeing collaborative relationships with potential referral sources and the agencies involved in the investigation. It requires coordinated efforts to include the broad range of services of individuals and organizations involved in the process. More importantly, it requires willingness across disciplines to not only coordinate, but also contribute resources, keeping in mind the shared goal of establishing healthy living environments for individuals that, in turn, foster healthy families that then lead to healthy communities.

When child abuse investigations take place in a fragmented manner, with CPS, law enforcement, health care providers, and the district attorney's office gathering information concerning the details of a case, the child may be subjected to numerous interviews at various times potentially creating confusion, clouding of details, and even secondary victimization.[23] Realizing that this situation is not ideal, models have been developed in which these agencies and disciplines work together to coordinate their respective mandated and professional responsibilities in a way that puts the interests of the child at the center of the child protection effort. In an effort to promote joint investigations, several government agencies convened a symposium to consider recommendations focused on fostering interdisciplinary work in child maltreatment investigations and treatment.[24] A coordinated response to child maltreatment was recommended based on the understanding that such an approach would lead to the following[24]:

— Reduction in the number of interviews that the child must endure

— Minimized number of people involved in the case

— Enhanced quality of the evidence that is discovered for both criminal prosecution and civil litigation

— Essential information provided to CPS and other family service organizations

— Decreased likelihood of conflicts between and among various involved agencies

Multidisciplinary and interdisciplinary work regarding the professional activity surrounding the evaluation and management of child maltreatment led to the development of the concept of the MDT. An MDT exists when a group of professionals agree to work together in a collaborative, coordinated manner to address the problems that arise as a result of child abuse and neglect. The MDT's goal is to ensure that the multidimensional needs of the child and family are addressed during the child maltreatment investigation and treatment interventions.[18,25,26] A variety of MDT models exist, with variations depending on need, locality, and setting.

Child Advocacy Center Joint Investigations

One model of collaborative agency involvement in the investigation of child sexual abuse that has evolved since the 1990s is that of the Child Advocacy Center, or CACs. CACs bring together an MDT to evaluate the child and coordinate services between CPS, law enforcement, and the family.[27] This child-centered approach tries to coordinate needed interviews so that a child does not have to tell his or her story multiple times to the different agencies involved in the investigation and prosecution of a case.[27]

The number of CACs in the United States is increasing as cities recognize the value of helping the child through the difficult process necessitated when child abuse is suspected. Many CACs employ specialists in forensic interviewing to assist the investigative process and help the agencies involved. It is ideal for the CAC to house both CPS and law enforcement to facilitate the investigative process.[27] The co-location of the agencies is not always possible, as a result of various constraints within the structures of some city governments.

According to the National Children's Alliance, CACs "...stress coordination of investigation and intervention services by bringing together professionals and agencies as a multidisciplinary team to create a child-focused approach to child abuse cases. The goal is to ensure that children are not re-victimized by the very system designed to protect them."[28] **(Table 13-1)**. In addition to the joint interviews of the suspected

Table 13-1. Description of National Children's Alliance and Member Child Advocacy Centers
The National Children's Alliance, formerly the National Network of Children's Advocacy Centers, is a not-for-profit organization whose mission is to provide training, technical assistance, and networking opportunities to communities seeking to plan, establish, and improve CACs. In 1987, the National Children's Alliance was founded by Congressman Bud Cramer, then District Attorney of Madison County Alabama, in response to the needs of a growing number of facility-based child abuse intervention programs and the demand for guidance from grassroots organizations working with child victims. Today, the Alliance is a membership organization providing services to CACs, multidisciplinary teams, and professionals across the country. *(continued)*

Table 13-1. Description of National Children's Alliance and Member Child Advocacy Centers *(continued)*

The purpose of CACs is to provide a comprehensive, culturally competent, MDT response to allegations of child abuse in a dedicated, child-friendly setting. A child-appropriate and child-friendly setting and an MDT are essential for accomplishment of the mission of CACs and for full membership in National Children's Alliance.

The team response to allegations of child abuse includes forensic interviews; medical evaluations; therapeutic interventions; victim support, victim advocacy, or both; case review; and case tracking. CAC staff or other members of the MDT may provide these components. To the maximum extent possible, components of the team response are provided at the CAC, to promote a sense of safety and consistency to the child and family.

The following program components are necessary for full membership in National Children's Alliance:

— **Child-appropriate and child-friendly facility:** A CAC provides a comfortable, private, child-friendly setting that is both physically and psychologically safe for clients.

— **MDT:** An MDT for response to child abuse allegations includes law enforcement, CPS, prosecution, mental health, medical, victim advocacy, and CAC representation.

— **Organizational capacity:** A designated legal entity responsible for program and fiscal operations has been established and implements basic sound administrative practices.

— **Cultural competency and diversity:** The CAC promotes policies, practices, and procedures that are culturally competent. Cultural competency is defined as the capacity to function in more than one culture, requiring the ability to appreciate, understand, and interact with members of diverse populations within the local community.

— **Forensic interviews:** Forensic interviews are conducted in a manner that is of a neutral, fact-finding nature and coordinated to avoid duplicative interviewing.

— **Medical evaluation:** Specialized medical evaluation and treatment are to be made available to CAC clients as part of the team response, either at the CAC or through coordination and referral with other specialized medical providers.

— **Therapeutic intervention:** Specialized mental health services are to be made available as part of the team response, either at the CAC or through coordination and referral with other appropriate treatment providers.

— **Victim support and advocacy:** Victim support and advocacy are to be made available as part of the team response, either at the CAC or through coordination with other providers, throughout the investigation and subsequent legal proceedings.

— **Case review:** Team discussion and information sharing regarding the investigation, case status, and services needed by the child and family are to occur on a routine basis.

(continued)

Table 13-1. Description of National Children's Alliance and Member Child Advocacy Centers *(continued)*
— **Case tracking:** CACs must develop and implement a system for monitoring case progress and tracking case outcomes for team components.
Adapted from National Children's Alliance. Standards for accredited members. National Children's Alliance Web site. http://www.nationalchildrensalliance.org/index.php?s=76. Accessed March 3, 2003.

child sexual abuse victim, most CACs provide the following formal processes to promote effective team functioning:

— Pre- and post-interview conferences that include the collaborating agencies

— Scheduled case reviews with the entire MDT

— Joint interdisciplinary training programs

— System of case tracking and follow-up that keeps each team member aware of case activities and outcome

Some communities are unable to create a formal organization such as a CAC but are still able to get agencies and disciplines to agree to conduct joint interviews. This initial collaboration may form the groundwork for a future CAC, should local factors be such that a more formal collaboration would be possible.

The benefits of effective joint investigations, including the ideal investigation performed within a CAC, are described as follows[29]:

— Less system-inflicted trauma to children and families

— Increased agency performance, including enhanced accuracy of investigations and more appropriate interventions

— Efficient use of limited community resources

— More capable professionals as they develop collaborative skills

— Recognition of the difficulty inherent in the maltreatment-related work and the opportunity to develop a professional network that decreases the sense of isolation and risk of professional burnout

Child Abuse Reports

The role of CPS in receiving reports of child abuse and neglect varies among the states ranging from being the sole receiver to sharing responsibility with law enforcement. Some states require notification of both CPS and law enforcement in certain forms of maltreatment, such as physical or sexual abuse.[9] Health care professionals must refer to local and state guidelines for specific reporting procedures.

CPS agencies receive referrals daily alleging that a child has been neglected or abused. After a referral has been screened in, the agency conducts an investigation to determine whether the child has been maltreated or is at risk for maltreatment. In 2009, CPS screened in and screened out an estimated 3.3 million reports in 2009. CPS agencies screened in an estimated 1.79 million family-based referrals from 50 states and screened out an estimated 1.17 million referrals. CPS agencies investigated approximately 61.9 % of the nearly 3 million referrals received, screened out approximately three-fourths of the referrals, and determined that at least 1 child was a victim of abuse and or neglect in a quarter of the cases.[6]

Reports to CPS of child abuse and neglect are commonly initiated by telephone contact from a variety of sources. Non-health-care-related sources might experience more fear related to retaliation on the part of the family or having to testify in court than mandatory reporters. In all cases, it is ideal for CPS staff to offer support and encouragement to all persons who decide to report[9] (**Table 13-2**). However, it is the very inconsistent nature of reporting that creates significant flaws in the system. Perhaps one of the largest barriers to reporting is the "enormous variability in how people define the threshold for mandated reporting of suspected child abuse."[23] This variability is further compounded by the various degrees of familiarity and exposure to child abuse, CPS, ethnic diversity, and attitudes towards discipline, all of which can affect an individual's comfort level with regard to reporting. While all 50 states have mandated reporting laws, the signs, symptoms, or explanations that should trigger reporting remain unclear and largely dominated by individual subjectivity.

Table 13-2. Typical Concerns of Mandated Reporter Regarding the Reporting of Suspected Child Abuse and Neglect

Concern	Response
"The parents seem like very angry people. What if the parents come after me?"	Although there may be a few exceptions, most abusive parents lack the social skills to face adults, especially those whom they perceive to be in authority positions. This inability to confront adults is one of the reasons why their children are vulnerable to being harmed. An occasional parent may yell or threaten, but that usually is as far as it goes.
"I have no right to intervene in a family's affairs."	The laws in your state give you the right to protect the child by reporting your suspicions of child abuse and neglect. It is the only way the child and family can begin receiving the help they need.
"Their cultural practices are different from mine. I have no right to impose my child-rearing beliefs on them."	The definitions of child abuse and neglect included in state laws apply to all families residing in a state or community. These laws do not provide for exceptions when, by legal standards, culturally accepted child-rearing practices are abusive or neglectful.
"I've worked for this director for 5 years. I just can't believe that she would sexually abuse the children. There must be some other explanation."	Adults who abuse or neglect children come from all kinds of backgrounds and are not always easy to identify. You must trust your observation skills and your knowledge of the physical and behavioral signs of child maltreatment. Also, remember that in your report you are not accusing any one person; you are reporting the condition of a child or children that you suspect was caused by child abuse or neglect.
"I just started at the center and don't want to be considered a troublemaker...but Mrs. Littleton is extremely rough with the children, and yesterday she left fingermarks on both of Carmen's arms."	Sometimes, your intervention with a colleague might prevent a child from getting seriously hurt. Most centers have administrative policies for how to report concerns about staff treatment of children.

(continued)

Table 13-2. Typical Concerns of Mandated Reporter Regarding the Reporting of Suspected Child Abuse and Neglect *(continued)*

Concern	Response
"The last time I reported, nothing happened. The child is still with his family, and the father is still abusing him. The CPS caseworker never even got in touch with me. I left lots of messages, but he never called me back. This time, I'm not going to bother reporting."	The facts and circumstances of each case are different, and you cannot assume that all cases will be handled in the same way or have the same results. Confidentially laws and policies often make it difficult for CPS to keep you informed. When you do not get the response you expect from a caseworker, ask to speak with his or her supervisor.
"I really don't think anything will get done, so what's the use of reporting."	It is true that filing the report does not guarantee that the child and family will get help. However, if you do not report, the children may continue to be at risk. At the very least, a record of the report will be made, your legal obligation fulfilled, and the investigative process begun. Abused and neglected children cannot be protected unless they are first identified, and the key is reporting.
"I might be sued by the parents for making a false report."	In every state, mandated reporters are immune from civil liability for making a report in good faith (where knowledge or reasonable suspicion exists), even if it is not substantiated by the investigator. Even if someone does sue you, the court will dismiss the case when they find out that you are a mandated reporter. Some states have provision to pay your legal fees if you must defend a lawsuit.

Reprinted from Koralek D. Caregivers of Young Children: Preventing and Responding to Child Maltreatment. *Washington, DC: United States Department of Health and Human Services; 1992.*

Reports from state-to-state include common information (**Table 13-3**). Detailed information regarding the condition and location of the child, the parents, the alleged abuser, details of the nature and character of the maltreatment, and information regarding the reporter are vital aspects of the formal report.[9] When potential maltreatment occurs in settings other than the home (eg, foster home, childcare center), specific information about that setting or facility is also included in the report.

Table 13-3. Content of Report to CPS

The report to CPS should include the following information:

— Name, age, sex, and address of the child(ren)

— Nature and extent of the child's injuries or condition

— Name and address of the parent or other person responsible for the child

Reprinted from DePanfilis D, Salus MK. Child Protective Services: A Guide for Caseworkers. *Washington, DC: United States Department of Health and Human Services; 2003.*

Table 13-4. Evaluating the Credibility of the Report

The following items should be considered when evaluating the credibility of the report:

— Is the reporter willing to give his or her name, address, and telephone number?

— What is the reporter's relationship to the victim and family?

— How well does the reporter know the family?

— If the reporter knew of previous abuse or neglect, why is he or she reporting now?

— How does the reporter know about the case?

— Does the reporter stand to gain anything for reporting or from the report being validated?

— Has the reporter made previous unfounded reports on this family?

— Is the reporter willing to meet with a caseworker in person if needed?

— Does the reporter appear to be intoxicated, extremely bitter, angry, or exhibiting behavior that that would make the caseworker question his or her competency?

— Can or will the reporter refer CPS to others who know about the situation?

— What does the reporter hope will happen as a result of the report?

Reprinted from DePanfilis D, Salus MK. Child Protective Services: A Guide for Caseworkers. *Washington, DC: United States Department of Health and Human Services; 2003.*

In the process of investigating maltreatment reports, CPS must ask questions to determine the credibility of the reported information, whether from professionals or lay people in the community. CPS must determine whether the complaint is valid and if the complaint should be accepted for an initial assessment and investigation (**Table 13-4**).

Sources of Reports

Professionals submitted the majority of the reports of child abuse and neglect in 1999 (**Figure 13-1**). A professional is someone who has contact with the alleged child victim as part of his or her job.[27] Education personnel (15.0%), legal or law enforcement personnel (13.6%), and social services personnel (13.2%) were the most common sources of reports. The remaining 45.3% of screened-in reports were from nonprofessional sources. The largest portion of reports in the nonprofessional category (12.2%) were from anonymous or unknown reporters.[27] Nonprofessional sources also included parents, relatives, neighbors, friends, alleged victims, alleged perpetrators, and other sources.[27]

Process of a CPS Case

Once a situation is reported to CPS, the caseworker follows steps in the process to intervene and treat the child and family (**Figure 13-2**). The steps are defined as follows:

— Intake

— Initial assessment

— Family assessment

— Case planning

— Case management and treatment

— Evaluation of family process

— Case closure

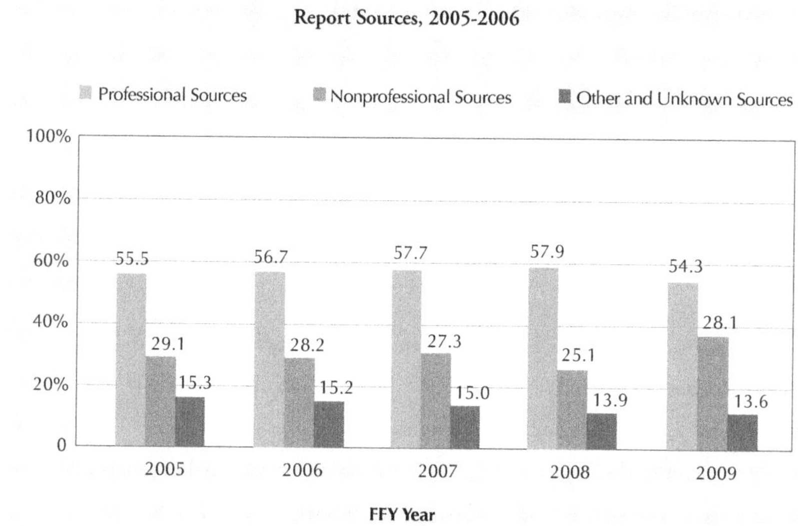

Figure 13-1

***Figure 13-1**. Reporters of child abuse and neglect. Reprinted from United States Department of Health and Human Services; Administration for Children and Families; Administration for Children and Families; Administration on Children, Youth, and Families; Children's Bureau.* Child Maltreatment 2009. *Washington, DC: United States Department of Health and Human Services; 2010.*

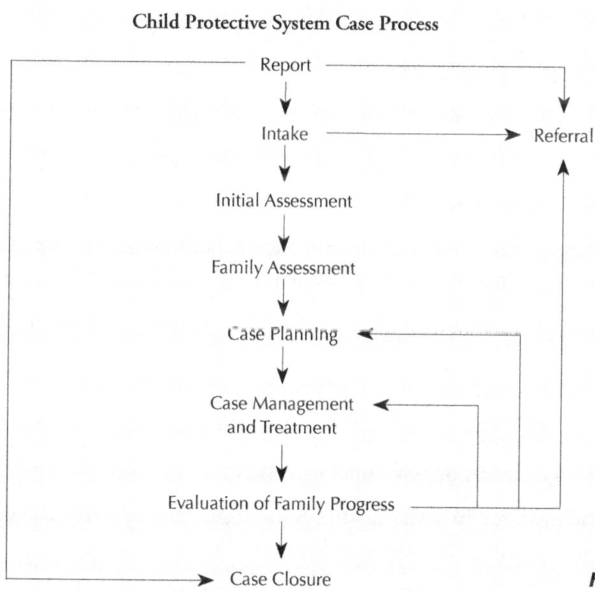

Figure 13-2

***Figure 13-2.** Child protective system case process. Reprinted from DePanfilis D, Salus MK.* Child Protective Services: A Guide for Caseworkers. *Washington, DC: United States Department of Health and Human Services; 2003.*

The essential decisions at intake concern 2 questions: (1) Does the reported information meet the agency guidelines for child maltreatment? (2) How urgent is the referral? CPS must consider many issues during the initial assessment of the investigative process because answers to questions may also involve input and collaboration with law enforcement (**Table 13-5**). Important decisions emerge from analyzing assessment data and talking with people who have information concerning the child, family, and agencies that are also involved in the process. Along with CPS, other systems involved in the assessment process include law enforcement, prosecutors, health care professionals, and mental health professionals.[18] The intricacies of the process are evidenced by the number of questions asked of, potentially, many people in the child's family system.

Table 13-5. CPS Process of Initial Assessment and Investigation

THE PRIMARY DECISIONS OR ISSUES TO CONSIDER AT THIS STAGE OF THE CHILD PROTECTION PROCESS ARE AS FOLLOWS:

— Did the child suffer maltreatment or is he or she threatened by harm as defined by the State reporting law? (CPS)

— Did a crime occur? (law enforcement)

— Is the parent(s) or caretaker(s) responsible for the maltreatment? (CPS)

— Who is the alleged offender? (law enforcement)

— Do sources of corroboration or witnesses exist? (CPS and law enforcement)

— Has all physical evidence been obtained or preserved? (CPS and law enforcement)

— Are there any other victims? (CPS and law enforcement)

— Is maltreatment likely to occur in the future? If so, what is the level of risk of maltreatment? (CPS)

— Is there evidence to arrest the alleged offender? (law enforcement)

— Is the child safe? If not, what measures are necessary to ensure the child's safety? (CPS)

— Should the child be taken into protective custody? (CPS and law enforcement)

— Does the family have emergency needs that must be met? (CPS)

— Are continuing agency services necessary to protect the child and reduce the risk of maltreatment occurring in the future? (CPS)

IN CASES INVOLVING OUT-OF-HOME CARE ABUSE, CONSIDER THE FOLLOWING:

— Are personnel actions indicated, and, if so, are they being initiated appropriately by the childcare facility? (licensing personnel)

— What responsibility do others in the facility have for any incident of maltreatment, and is a corrective action plan needed to prevent the likelihood of future incidents? (CPS and licensing personnel)

— Should the facilities or foster care or other childcare provider's license be revoked? (licensing)

IN ADDITION TO CPS AND LAW ENFORCEMENT,
OTHER DISCIPLINES HAVE A ROLE IN THE INITIAL ASSESSMENT PROCESS:

— Foster care, residential, or childcare licensing personnel may participate in the initial assessment if abuse is allegedly committed by an out-of-home caretaker.

— Medical personnel may be involved in assessing and responding to medical needs of a child or parent and perhaps in documenting the nature and extent of maltreatment.

— Mental health personnel may be involved in assessing the effects of any alleged maltreatment and in helping to determine the validity of specific allegations.

— Teachers may be involved in providing direct information about the effects of maltreatment and in describing information pertinent to risk assessment.

— Military family advocacy personnel may be directly involved by providing information when one of the members of the family is in the military.

— Other community service providers may have had past experience with the child or family and may be a resource in helping to address any emergency needs that the child or family may have.

Reprinted from DePanfilis D, Salus MK. Child Protective Services: A Guide for Caseworkers. *Washington, DC: United States Department of Health and Human Services; 2003.*

Family Assessment

CPS caseworkers and other professionals conduct a family assessment after the child's safety is determined and ensured. The goals of the family assessment are to determine the details of possible maltreatment, factors that contributed to the risk of maltreatment, and the effects of maltreatment on the child and family system. The family assessment should uncover personal and environmental factors that may have contributed to child maltreatment, as well as surrounding issues related to the abuse. The assessment should address the following[9]:

- Nature, extent, and causes of the factors contributing to the risk of maltreatment
- Effects of child's maltreatment and the treatment needs of all family members
- Individual and family strengths that can be identified in the intervention process.
- Conditions and behaviors that must change for the risk of maltreatment to be reduced
- Prognosis for family ability to change

Case Planning

The case planning process is ideally a collaborative effort, the plan of which is developed by the CPS caseworker and family and community professionals who are involved and may continue to be involved with the family. Case planning involves engaging family members in decisions regarding changes they need to make to reduce or eliminate the risk of maltreatment as well as agreement on what must be done to provide safe living conditions for the child. In some situations, the court orders the family to participate in services or complete certain actions that it deems necessary to provide a safe environment.[9]

After completing a family assessment, there is joint collaboration between CPS and other community service providers to determine strategies to change aspects of the family system that resulted in child abuse and neglect. Considerations in the case planning stage of the process include the identification of the following[9]:

- Goals that must be achieved to reduce the risk of maltreatment and meet the prescribed treatment plan
- Priorities among the goals
- Interventions or services that can be used to achieve the goals
- Steps or tasks that must be completed for goals to be achieved
- Designated responsibilities of the CPS caseworker
- Determination of the family members' responsibilities
- Responsibilities of other service providers
- Time frames for goal achievement
- How and when the case plan will be evaluated to determine goal accomplishment

The planning process seeks to engage family members in determining changes that should be made to reduce or eliminate maltreatment risks and to identify what client, caseworker, and other service providers can do to ensure that necessary changes occur.[9]

Case Management and Treatment

The case management and treatment stage of the process involves the implementation of the steps and services needed to accomplish the case plan. CPS often coordinates, arranges, and provides the delivery of services to the family. General procedures followed when child abuse or neglect is suspected include the following:

— Oral report given to the child abuse hotline or local CPS agency; if the child or the child's siblings are in immediate danger, this should be emphasized with other report information.

— In the case of serious bodily injury, sexual abuse, or death, a report is also made to the local police department.

— A physical examination is performed to determine condition, needed treatment, and possible evidence collection. In cases of sexual abuse, evidence of physical abuse and neglect is noted and efforts are made to minimize the psychological effects of a genital examination.

— All findings are recorded.

Evaluation of Family Process and Case Closure

CPS performs an ongoing assessment process that continues throughout the life of the case. CPS caseworkers evaluate family progress based on the following criteria[9]:

— The safety of the child

— Achievement of goals and tasks in the case plan

— Reduction of the risk of maltreatment

— Success in meeting the child's and other family members' needs resulting from the maltreatment

CPS determines that a case can close when risks to the child and within the family have been sufficiently reduced or eliminated so that the child is protected and his or her developmental needs are sufficiently met without societal intervention.[9] CPS caseworkers involve the child and the child's family in decisions regarding the welfare of the child and closure of the case. Caseworkers should apply specific principles to the case closure process to ensure the best possible outcome for the family and the child. The following are steps involved in the closure of a case[9]:

— Meet personally with the family to discuss the case closure.

— Together, establish timeframes for when the case should be closed.

— Acknowledge the family's and the caseworker's feelings about the case closure.

— Be prepared for a family-created crisis that may occur as a reaction to anticipated independence resulting from the planned closure.

— Review the progress made as a result of CPS involvement, emphasizing efforts that were essential for the resulting changes.

— Refer the family to any additional resources as needed.

— Leave the door open for services should they be needed in the future, including providing information to the family about how to contact the agency and who should be contacted in the future.

CPS and Mandatory Reporting

Mandatory reporting laws share several core components. Reporting laws define abusive situations; reportable circumstances; degree of certainty that reporters must attain before making a report, such as reason to suspect, reason to believe; and the age limits of reportable children. The laws define who must report, outline the sanctions for failing to report, and define immunity from civil and criminal liability for reports filed in good faith. However, state laws differ in important ways such as the definition and specificity of what constitutes abuse and under what conditions a report must be made. State CPS laws impose a penalty for failure to report suspected child abuse.

States have widely expanded the scope of the mandatory reporting requirements to include a broad range of human service providers, social workers, and teachers (**Table 13-6**). In some states, the requirement extends to commercial film processors who may see examples of sexually explicit photographs of children that may indicate possible abuse or exploitation. Animal humane officers may be included as well because of the association between cruelty to animals and child abuse. When all states are considered, there are approximately 40 different professions named in mandatory reporting laws.[30] Research has shown that various professions respond quite differently to reporting requirements. For example, psychiatric nurses were more likely to report abuse compared with non–medically trained mental health workers.[31] Nurses and ministers were found to be more likely to report abuse than family practice physicians and psychologists.[32] These results suggest differences in compliance with reporting laws among professions and service delivery settings.

Table 13-6. Mandated Health Care Reporters According to State Child Abuse Laws
— Physicians and surgeons
— Hospital residents and interns
— Physician's assistants
— Registered nurses (RN) and licensed practical nurses (LPN)
— Dentists
— Optometrists
— Chiropractors
— Podiatrists
— Psychologists
— Mental health practitioners
— Social workers
— Medical examiners or coroners

For people who report potential abuse in good faith, reporting laws make provisions to protect such reporters from criminal prosecution and civil lawsuits resulting from filing a report. The law provides immunity to protect those who demonstrate concern for the child and family.[9] State laws either presume that reports are filed in good faith or specify that reports must be made without malice. It is extremely rare for mandated reporters to be determined to have filed reports that are harassing or without just cause.[33] The immunity provision is designed to remove the hesitation to report based on uncertainty about whether abuse has occurred. Mandated reporters must only have reasonable cause to suspect that abuse has occurred. It is up to the investigators to make the determination that abuse occurred based on the evidence uncovered in a thorough investigation. A reporter can be sued, but the immunity component of the statute permits him or her to claim the immunity before the judge hears the case (see *Chapter 14, Legal Issues*).

A uniform application of reporting laws cannot account for particular circumstances, professional discretion, and judgment and can place mandated reporters in circumstances that conflict with basic professional values and ethical principles.[34,35] This can result in situations in which professionals do not follow the law. And in some instances, this can result in serious harm to children in need of protection.

The dilemma faced by many professionals about reporting requirements and when they are obligated to report can best be addressed by examining the explicit language of the child abuse law covering the jurisdiction involved. Reasonable grounds to report suspected abuse may exist if a child tells the professional that he or she has been physically or sexually abused; someone else, such as a relative, sibling, or friend, tells the professional that the child has been abused; or the professional's observations of the child's behavior or indicators of abuse leads to the belief that the child has been abused.

Some state laws require a report to be made only if mandated professionals have reason to suspect abuse has occurred based on a child's statement, the professional's observation of behavior, or signs or symptoms in a child they have directly examined. In general, health care providers should make a report to the appropriate CPS agency for investigation when they have reasonable cause to suspect that a child has been abused or neglected or is at imminent risk of harm. Typically, an oral report should be made immediately to the statewide child abuse hotline, followed by a written report, often completed using a standardized form provided for this purpose to the local CPS agency responsible for investigating such reports, within a time period established by state law. Most states have established a mechanism for receiving such reports, with a toll-free hotline number being the most common. State reporting laws are available on the Internet through various legal resource websites, including the Child Welfare Information Gateway (http://www.childwelfare.gov).

What to Report

Many states have standard report forms that help professionals determine what information is needed when contacting the hotline or local CPS agency. Information that is useful to the CPS agency includes the following[9]:

— Child's name, address, telephone number, and birth date

— Child's age and gender

— Parents' or caregivers' names, addresses, and phone numbers

— Name of the person or people suspected to have caused the child's injuries

— Nature and extent of the injury, maltreatment, or neglect

— Approximate date and time alleged abuse occurred

— Information about previous injuries, maltreatment, or neglect of the child or siblings

— How the information came to the attention of the reporter

— Any action taken to treat or help the child

— Any statements made by the child

— Any statements or explanation offered by the parent(s) or caregiver(s)

— Other information that would be useful, such as other individuals who live in the child's home or have caregiving responsibilities for the child who could then be potentially helpful in the investigation

The investigation of cases of sexual abuse requires considerable resources to identify and then assess the reported cases because the evidence is less clear-cut than in physical abuse and neglect, and there are rarely objective witnesses or physical findings.[9] Investigation of child sexual abuse cases is time–consuming because it involves skillful interviewing of people involved in the situation.[9] Likewise, emotional abuse substantiation rates are very low, and cases involving this type of abuse may be the most difficult to solve.

Legal definitions of abuse as outlined in state law may have a direct effect on whether cases are reported. A study conducted by Rycraft[36] found that states with broad and nonspecific definitions have the highest reporting and substantiation rates, while states with narrow and specific definitions of abuse have some of the lowest. He concluded that definitions of child abuse are a determining factor in both the decision to report and the dispositions of reported cases.

Benefits of Reporting

The reporting of suspected child abuse or neglect could be essential in protecting a child from further abuse or neglect and can lead to actions that assist the family in obtaining necessary services to improve parenting skills or living conditions. It can also help break the intergenerational cycle of child abuse and neglect by treating the child, reducing trauma, and preventing future abuse by that parent or that child victim. Even in the absence of services after a report, the very act of investigation and intervention can have positive consequences for the child and family. The child may experience the intervention by CPS professionals or law enforcement as evidence that someone will intervene on their behalf; parents may experience the intervention as evidence that their behavior is not acceptable and may cause further intervention in the future; and, of course, the report may result in the removal of the child from an abusive situation, effectively stopping the abuse.

Critics of mandatory reporting argue that, in many cases, the requirement to report has not had the desired outcome of protecting children and that mandated reporting may be immobilizing the very systems set up to deal with child abuse. By casting a broad net so as not to overlook an abused child, CPS agencies are swamped with reports that are in large part unsubstantiated, wasting limited resources. Also, mandated reporters can become frustrated with making reports that seem to generate little interest and intervention from CPS agencies. Some professionals believe that mandated reporting requires them to violate the confidentiality of their clients or patients, thereby undermining the therapeutic relationship. They believe this can endanger children by interfering with opportunities for effective treatment. Some believe that the investigation resulting from reporting can be destructive and harmful to children and families; therefore, reporting should only be pursued when there is compelling evidence that abuse is occurring. This is particularly problematic in states in which language and definitions of abuse laws are vague or overly broad. By focusing on the child and the child's safety first, mandated reporters can develop a framework for evaluating situations that come before them, knowing when and what to report, and determining how to assist the family in gaining maximum benefit and minimum trauma from the experience whenever possible.

There tends to be little, if any, training for mandated reporters with regard to handling suspected child abuse cases either during professional education, training, or continuing education courses. Most CPS agencies are charged with the responsibility of providing public education about child abuse and methods of reporting to mandated reporters and the larger community. However, most professionals learn from experience about making reports of suspected child abuse, and these experiences are not always positive.

Child abuse reporting sets in motion a chain of events that begins with the acceptance of the report by the hotline. The referral is screened according to the local laws and regulations governing the public child welfare system response. CPS conducts a risk assessment and, if warranted, initiates an investigation. The identity of the mandated reporter is generally kept confidential from the family. In many situations, the person or family can ascertain the identity of the reporting source based on the circumstances and nature of the reported allegations. In the case of a mandated reporter who is a medical provider, it can be beneficial for the family to be informed that a report is being made in accordance with the CPS law. A mandated reporter should be prepared to address the consequences of making a report. The mandated report should consider the following:

— How will the parents and child be informed that a report is being made?

— How will the mandated reporter interact with the family and with CPS personnel after making the report?

— What additional information must be collected?

— What information should be shared with CPS? What information should remain confidential between the health care provider and the family or child?

Many states have developed materials and publications for mandated reporters that outline local laws and regulations and provide information on responding to child abuse. It is most important for mandated reporters to educate themselves about the local community systems, learn about services available to children and families, and attend training on recognizing and responding to child abuse.

The mandated reporter is obligated to inform parents, caregivers, and the child that a report is being made. A report should be made out of care and concern for the child and family as well as the professional's ethical responsibility and legal mandate. Informing the family can help them know what to expect in response to the report and should actively involve the family in addressing the problem that led to reporting. Informing about the report can retain the family's trust in helping professionals who interact with them openly and honestly. Of course, there are instances when it would be counterproductive to inform the family before making a report to CPS or law enforcement. This would include situations in which doing so would put the child at risk for further abuse.[9]

Outcomes of CPS Interventions

The purpose of CPS is to protect children and strengthen the relationships between the child and caregivers. The greatest concern of CPS is to ensure child safety and make decisions regarding the dangers that a child faces and the appropriate services needed for the child and the family to make sure that a child is not abused again. The effectiveness of CPS interventions can be measured by the overall outcomes that the agencies achieve based on the goals they set. Child welfare agencies are generally held accountable for measuring, reporting, and tracking results for the children they serve.[6] An annual summary of child welfare data provides findings from the 30 states that kept the best outcome measures of the services provided.

The following are some of the performance data as determined by the 2009 annual report of child welfare outcomes, along with some practical implications of the data.[6]

— Eleven percent of child maltreatment victims were the victims of at least one additional incident of maltreatment within 12 months.

— In all cases, the CPS agency should evaluate the situation in a timely manner and evaluate the results of all interventions before deciding to close the case.

— Most children (86%) who exited foster care achieved permanency, but some children did not. Seventy-two percent of the children were reunified with their families, 21% were adopted, and 7% were adopted by a legal guardian.

— A goal of state child welfare agencies is to achieve permanency for all of the children under their placement and care and ensure that children grow up in safe and stable families.

— About four-fifths of all children leaving foster care exited to permanent settings, regardless of race or ethnicity.

— States can work to develop or reinforce community supports for families, address cultural differences, and increase parental child-rearing competencies to help parents overcome abusive behavior toward their children. It is important for state child welfare agencies to keep children safe and find them permanent placements as quickly as possible if they are removed from their homes.

— Approximately 11% of children exited foster care to emancipation. More than one-third of children were aged younger than 12 years when they entered the foster care system and had spent 6 or more years in care without finding a permanent home.

— The large number of children growing up in foster care supports the mandate of the Foster Care Independence Act of 1999 requiring states to provide independent living and supportive services to children who remain in foster care and to help them transition to self-sufficiency.

— Sixty-seven percent of children reunited with their parents or other relatives had been in foster care for less than 12 months.

— Although most children were reunited with their families within 12 months of entering foster care, many other reunifications took longer. The state child welfare agency should work for the child's return when it can be done safely. It is essential for the agency to identify needed family services for abused or neglected children and take steps to expedite the safe return of children to their families.

— Seventeen percent of the children who entered foster care in fiscal year 1998 had been in foster care previously.

— It is important that state child welfare agencies avoid reuniting children with their family without providing necessary support services to the families.

— Thirty-one percent of adoptions occurred after the children had been in foster care 4 years or more; 26% of adoptions occurred within 2 years of the child's entry into foster care.

— The time children wait to find permanent homes is too long. The Adoption and Safe Families Act strongly promotes timely adoption of children who cannot return to their own homes. Many state child welfare agencies work concurrently to reunite a family while planning for the possibility that reunification will not succeed. CPS needs to work on strategies to expedite adoption, such as listing the child with appropriate adoption exchanges or taking timely steps to complete home studies.

— Eighty-five percent of children in foster care fewer than 12 months had 2 or fewer placements; 31% of children in care at least 24 months or more had 2 or fewer placements.

— The longer a child remained in foster care, the less likely it was for that child to experience a stable placement. It is important that state child welfare agencies provide adequate supports to foster children and their foster parents to prevent the disruption of placements. Appropriate supports help reduce the number of placement settings experienced by children in foster care.

Statistical Resources

In order to be able to evaluate the prevalence and extent of reporting across the nation and the progress made across the decades, national databases must be carefully examined and interpreted. Reporting is an individual action that relies on personal integrity, ethics, and honesty. Databases and statistical measures are based on reported and investigated cases and do not represent the cases that individuals wanted to refer to CPS but didn't because it involved a friend, neighbor, or relative. It does not include the child who committed suicide because he or she couldn't survive one more day of the abuse and or neglect that characterized his or her world.

The National Child Abuse and Neglect Data System (NCANDS) is a federally sponsored initiative that analyzes data on child abuse and neglect. In 1988, CAPTA directed the United States Department of Health and Human Services (USDHHS) to establish the national program to collect and analyze data that continues today under the supervision of the Children's Bureau, a subsection of the USDHHS Administration on Children and Families.[9]

Conclusion

The role of CPS in the protection of children is essential. Children suspected of having been abused and neglected become part of the CPS system, and CPS is responsible for ensuring the safety and security of those children. The responsibility of CPS is to protect the victim of child maltreatment and help with the investigation of the alleged charges. CPS remains a part of the case until the best interests of the child are determined.

Most, if not all state CPS laws impose a penalty on those mandated reporters who fail to report suspected abuse. For those mandated reporters who do contact CPS with cases of suspected abuse, immunity from civil and criminal liability is provided in most instances. Reports of suspected child abuse submitted by mandated reporters, professionals, and laypeople set in motion a chain of events that begin with the acceptance of the report by, typically, a hotline and continues to include investigation and substantiation of the reports, arrangement of services for the child and family, and closure of the case or placement of the child in temporary or permanent alternative living arrangements. CPS strives to achieve permanency for all of the children under their placement and care and ensure that children grow up in safe and stable families

References

1. Sedlak AJ, Broadhurst DD. *Third National Incidence Study of Child Abuse and Neglect (NIS-3)*. Washington, DC: United States Department of Health and Human Services; 1996.

2. Wang CT, Daro D. *Current Trends in Child Abuse Reporting and Fatalities: The Results of the 1997 Annual Fifty State Survey.* Chicago, IL: Prevent Child Abuse America; 1998.

3. Jain AM. Emergency department evaluation of child abuse. *Emerg Med Clin North Am.* 1999;17(3):575-593.

4. Wang CT, Holton J. Total estimated costs of child abuse and neglect in the United States. Prevent Child Abuse America Web site. http://www.chhs.ca.gov/initiatives/CAChildWelfareCouncil/Documents/PCA%20A%20cost_analysis.pdf. Published September 2007. Accessed August 19, 2013.

5. Laraque D, DeMattia A, Low C. Forensic child abuse evaluation: a review. *Mt Sinai J Med.* 2006;73(8):1138-1147.

6. United States Department of Health and Human Services; Administration for Children and Families; Administration for Children and Families; Administration on Children, Youth, and Families; Children's Bureau. *Child Maltreatment 2009.* Washington, DC: United States Department of Health and Human Services; 2010.

7. US Department of Health and Human Services. *Child Abuse and Neglect: Critical First Steps in Response to a National Emergency.* Washington, DC: United States Department of Health and Human Services, Office of Human Development Services, United States Advisory Board on Child Abuse and Neglect; 1990.

8. US Department of Health and Human Services. *Child Maltreatment 2011: Reports from the States to the National Child Abuse and Neglect Data Systems.* Washington, DC: United States Department Health and Human Services; 2011.

9. DePanfilis D, Salus MK. *Child Protective Services: A Guide for Caseworkers.* Washington, DC: United States Department of Health and Human Services; 2003.

10. Levine M, Levine L. *Helping Children: A Social History.* New York, NY: Oxford University Press; 1992.

11. United States Department of Health and Human Services. *Child Welfare Outcomes 1998: Annual Report.* Washington, DC: United States Department of Health and Human Services, Administration for Children and Families, Administration on Children, Youth and Families Children's Bureau; 1998.

12. Kempe CH, Silverman FN, Steele BF, Droegemuller W, Silver HK. The battered-child syndrome. *JAMA.* 1962;181(1):17-24.

13. Kempe CH. Sexual abuse, another hidden pediatric problem: the 1977 C. Anderson Aldrich lecture. *Pediatrics.* 1978;62(3):382-389.

14. McCoid AH. The battered child and other assaults upon the family: part I. *Mil Law Rev.* 1965:50:20.

15. Child Abuse Prevention and Treatment Act, 42 USC 510g et seq. Pub L 104-235 (amended 1996).

16. Child Abuse Prevention and Treatment Act (CAPTA), USC 42 §5101-5116 (1996).

17. US Department of Health and Human Services. *Child Maltreatment.* Washington, DC: US Government Printing Office; 2009.

18. Pence D, Wilson C. *Team Investigation of Child Sexual Abuse: The Uneasy Alliance.* Thousand Oaks, CA: Sage Publications, Inc; 1994.

19. Wilson C, Pence D. How should child protective services and law enforcement coordinate the initial assessment and investigation? In: Dubowitz H, DePanfilis, eds. *Handbook for Child Protection Practice*. Thousand Oaks, CA: Sage Publications, Inc; 2000:101-104.

20. Gelles R. Family preservation and reunification: how effective a social policy? In: White S, ed. *Handbook of Youth and Justice*. New York, NY: Kluwer Academic/Plenum Publishers; 2001.

21. Gelles RJ, Welsh J, Welsh R. CAPTA: successes and failures at preventing child abuse and neglect: testimony prepared for United States House of Representatives Committee on Education and the Workforce Subcommittee on Select Education. Committee on Education and the Workforce Web site. http://archives.republicans.edlabor.house.gov/archive/hearings/107th/sed/capta8201/gelles.htm. Accessed March 3, 2003.

22. Smolowe J, Blackman A, Simmons-Washington AM, et al. Case workers: making the tough calls. *TIME*. December 11, 1995.

23. Levi BH, Portwood SG. Reasonable suspicion of child abuse: finding a common language. *J Law Med Ethics*. 2011;39(1):62-68.

24. Dinsmore J. *Joint Investigations of Child Abuse: Report of a Symposium*. Washington, DC: United States Department of Health and Human Services, National Center on Child Abuse and Neglect; 1993.

25. Rowe DS, Leonard MF, Seashore MR, Lewiston NJ, Anderson FP. A hospital program for the detection and registration of abused and neglected children. *N Engl J Med*. 1970;282:950-952.

26. Wilson EP, Hilbert D. A hospital team approach to child abuse. *PA Med*. 1973;69:419-425.

27. National Children's Alliance Web site. http://www.nationalchildrensalliance.org/. Accessed March 3, 2003.

28. National Children's Alliance. Standards for accredited members. National Children's Alliance Web site. http://www.nationalchildrensalliance.org/index.php?s=76. Accessed March 3, 2003.

29. Ells M. Need for a team approach. In: *Forming a Multidisciplinary Team to Investigate Child Abuse*. Washington DC: United States Department of Justice, Office of Justice Programs, Office of Juvenile Justice and Delinquency Prevention; 1998.

30. Wurtele SK, Miller-Perrin CL. *Preventing Child Sexual Abuse: Sharing the Responsibility*. Lincoln, NB: University of Nebraska Press; 1992.

31. Kalichman SC, Craig ME, Follingstad DR. Mental health professionals and suspected cases of child abuse: an investigation of factors influencing reporting. *Community Ment Health J*. 1988;24(1):43-51.

32. Williams HS, Osborne YH, Rappaport NB. Child abuse reporting law: professionals' knowledge and compliance. *South Psychol*. 1987;3:20-24.

33. Drake B. Unraveling "unsubstantiated". *Child Maltreat*. 1996;1(3):261-271.

34. Butz AM, Redman BK, Fry ST, Kolodner K. Ethical conflicts experienced by certified pediatric nurse practitioners in ambulatory settings. *J Pediatr Health Care*. 1998;12(4):176-182.

35. Greipp ME. Ethical decision making and mandatory reporting in cases of suspected child abuse. *J Pediatr Health Care*. 1997;11(6):258-265.

36. Rycraft JR. Redefining child abuse and neglect: narrowing the focus may affect children at risk. *Public Welfare*. 1990;48:14-21.

Chapter 14

Legal Issues

Teresa Scalzo, JD
Kathleen Brown, PhD, RN, NP
Melanie Bragg, JD

Key Points

1. The requirement that protected health information (PHI) "be disclosed for public interest and benefit activities"[1] is important to health care providers because reporting of abuse or neglect and disclosing information regarding victims of abuse, neglect, or domestic violence are considered "public interest and benefit activities."[1] Therefore, some information may be shared in these instances without authorization or permission.
2. When called upon to disclose PHI, a health care professional should speak to his or her legal representative about the parameters of what can be revealed.
3. Criminal court is designed to hold offenders accountable but is not the proper forum for determining issues involving dependency, custody, or other issues impacting a child's welfare. Therefore, it is not uncommon for simultaneous dependency or custody cases to be pending when a crime is prosecuted.
4. The final hearing in a criminal case is a trial before a jury or a judge sitting alone or a plea before a judge. Medical professionals may be called to testify at any of the hearings that occur during a criminal case, either to help the prosecution prove its case or to help the defense defend against allegations. Regardless of which side calls the medical professional as a witness, it is critical for the medical professional to be objective, thorough and truthful.
5. As determined by the landmark United States Supreme Court case *Santosky v Kramer*,[2] the standard of proof required of states seeking to terminate parental rights is "clear and convincing evidence," which is higher than the typical burden of "beyond a preponderance of the evidence" required of civil cases but lower than the burden of "beyond a reasonable doubt" required of a criminal case.[3]
6. The fact that a health care professional performs an examination or makes a report to law enforcement or child protective services (CPS) does not always mean that the person will have to testify in court. A civil or criminal case is not necessarily filed simply because a case was investigated. Even if a case is filed, it may not end up at trial. In fact, most cases never have a formal trial because most cases are criminal cases that are often resolved by plea agreements and most civil cases are resolved by settlements. When a case does go to trial, it is often long after completion of the examination(s) for which the health care provider is expected to provide testimony. The health care provider should always remain in the neutral role of health care provider with his or her first obligation to the patient's health.
7. It is crucial that the health care provider be meticulous and thorough when collecting evidence and recording his or her findings because attorneys try to create doubt by showing inconsistencies, mistakes, and irregularities in these areas.

8. As with any witness, the health care provider may not only be judged by what he or she says, but also by his or her demeanor and appearance. When called as a witness, the health care provider should dress in a neat, clean, professional manner and remember that potential jurors may observe him or her, from the moment of arrival at the courthouse. It is critical to remain calm and polite.
9. A witness who does not understand a question should ask to have it clarified. The witness should not guess or rush to answer questions, but rather, take care to answer all questions thoughtfully and accurately. A witness who does not remember information may ask to refer to his or her records to "refresh his or her recollection."[4] A witness who does not know the answer to a question asked at trial should simply acknowledge that he or she does not know the answer. The witness should always remember that truthfulness and accuracy are critical at all times.

The health care provider evaluating a child for suspected maltreatment will inevitably come into contact with the legal system. Child maltreatment cases may be handled in civil or criminal court, a designation that will subject the matter to vastly different processes. This chapter explains the history and purpose of the CPS system and its relationship with the legal system, gives an overview of mandatory reporting laws, and explains what happens after an initial report of suspected maltreatment is made. This chapter also reviews the Health Insurance Portability and Accountability Act of 1996 (HIPAA) and its impact on child maltreatment cases. Finally, because many health care providers are called upon to testify in cases of suspected child maltreatment, the chapter gives an overview of the various types of related legal proceedings and examines the role of courtroom evidence and testimony.

Child Protective Services

The agency that provides protective services to children is known by different names across the country, including Children and Youth Services and the Department of Family and Youth Services. For the purpose of clarity, this chapter will refer to said agency as child protective services (CPS). An understanding of the history of the state's legal right to intervene in child welfare cases is useful in understanding the legal processes involved in child welfare proceedings. As far back as 1655, criminal courts had jurisdiction over abuse and neglect cases involving children. In or about 1692, states and municipalities determined that local governments and private institutions should bear responsibility for issues concerning children's protection and welfare. The English legal principle of *parens patriae,* which placed "charities, infants, idiots, and lunatics returned to the chancery," under the care of the crown was first used in 1696 and is the statutory basis for the federal and state governments' right to intervene, investigate, and oversee child welfare cases.

It was not until 1825 that states began to enact laws giving social welfare agencies the ability to remove neglected or abused children from their homes or from the streets and place them in orphanages or with other families. In 1835 the Humane Society founded the National Federation of Child Rescue agency to investigate child maltreatment. In the late 1800s private child protection agencies formed to investigate reports of child maltreatment, present cases in court, and lobby for child welfare legislation.

In 1912, the federal Children's Bureau was established to manage federal child welfare efforts. In 1958, amendments to the Social Security Act mandated that states fund child protection efforts. In 1962, C. Henry Kempe and Associates published a paper in the *Journal of the American Medical Association (JAMA)* on the battered child syndrome. The article generated much discussion and public outrage, so much so that 49 states passed child abuse reporting laws by the mid-1960s. By 1974, the federal government passed the Child Abuse Prevention and Treatment Act (CAPTA). CAPTA provided federal funding for a broad range of child abuse and prevention efforts in the United States and mandated that states establish procedures for the investigation of child abuse. In 1980, Congress passed the first comprehensive federal CPS act, the Adoption Assistance and Child Welfare Act of 1980 (Pub L No 96-272), which provided states with economic incentives for reducing the number and length of stay of foster care placements.

Mandatory Reporting Laws

A number of laws mandate the reporting of suspected child abuse. Reports made pursuant to these mandatory reporting laws may bring the health care professional into contact with CPS. The Child Welfare Information Gateway is a very useful Web site for health care providers seeking specific information on the reporting of suspected child abuse. State laws and reporting mechanisms may be accessed through the Child Welfare Information Gateway Web site at www.childwelfare.gov.

While variation between states exists in regard to reporting parameters, such as when a health care professional is mandated to make report and reporting mechanisms, the spirit of the reporting laws, which is to provide a means of encouraging frontline health care providers to report suspected child maltreatment, does not vary. Reporting leads to investigation and should, therefore, provide protection for the child who is in danger of being harmed. Typically, the laws protect health care professionals who report in good faith and establish criminal penalties for those who fail to report suspected abuse. Medical professionals should check with their legal representatives to ensure they understand the specific requirements of reporting.

Barriers to Reporting

Research and clinical experience demonstrates the influence of many factors on the health care provider's decision-making process with regard to reporting suspected child maltreatment. Research asserts that health care providers wish to do the right thing and to protect their patients and the patients' families[5]; however, research also upholds that of the mandated reporters, health care providers report the fewest number of cases. According to the Child Abuse Recognition Experience Study (CARES),[5] three-fourths of injuries thought to be from child abuse are not reported to anyone by providers. According to the Fourth National Incidence Study of Child Abuse and Neglect (NIS-4)[6] conducted by the Department of Health and Human Services in 2010, professional staff in schools recognized and reported the majority of cases involving children who met a harm standard (52%), while reports made by professional staff in hospitals represented only 13% of reported cases. The underreporting of cases of suspected child maltreatment can be attributed to several reasons, a few of which will be explored in the following sections.

Confusion Regarding the Role of Child Protective Services

Health care providers may hold the belief that the sole function of child protective services (CPS) is to remove a child from his or her home; however, this is not the case. Keeping a family together is a high priority for CPS and they only remove a child from his or her home as a last resort. To that end, CPS provides intensive family support, cognitive therapy, and family preservation interventions to avoid removal and assist in the restoration of the family unit.[7] Health care providers may also lack confidence in reporting to CPS and may believe that reports to CPS will be ignored or inappropriately handled. Still, the NIS-4 asserts that a report made to CPS by a hospital is given high priority for investigation.[6]

Additionally, the health care provider may fear becoming involved in the legal system as the result of making a report to CPS. Theodore and Runyan[8] report that 75% of 270 surveyed pediatricians stated their experience of testifying in court in cases of child abuse as having impressed upon them that the court system is harmful or distressing to children. Health care providers may not report suspected abuse if they believe that reporting will not produce what they believe to be a good outcome for the child.[8]

Lack of Ease in Reporting

According to a study in which Feng et al[9] interviewed nurses, physicians, social workers, and teachers, ease of reporting is an important variable related to reporting. Health care providers may be confused about mandatory reporting laws, including to whom and in which cases the report should be made. Time management is a very important issue for health care providers. All providers should have easy access to their local CPS system through which they can report suspected child abuse. By establishing protocols to facilitate reporting, hospitals and clinicians may eliminate confusion regarding reporting laws.

Poor Communication

As specialization increases in nursing and medicine, lines of communication become increasingly difficult to interpret. Health care providers who work with children may not know whom to contact with questions about cases of suspected child abuse and may see the immediate health or safety needs of the child as their only challenge. As such, frontline providers may assume that someone else will deal with the child's nonclinical issues and provide any needed services. Who the other professional might be is often unknown to episodic health care providers.

Health Insurance Portability and Accountability Act

Health care providers may be confused by the role of the Health Insurance Portability and Accountability Act (HIPAA) and may have questions as to how privacy regulations apply to patients and families in cases of suspected abuse. Additionally, hospital-employed attorneys may interpret HIPAA differently from CPS and law enforcement professionals, thereby increasing the confusion. Health care providers with questions about HIPAA should consult their facility guidelines and the rules of their state for additional HIPAA information if questions arise when dealing with a child abuse issue.

Available Resources

Flaherty[10] recommends pediatric health care providers have access to a multidisciplinary team of child abuse specialists to include CPS workers, specialized health care workers, social workers, advocates, prosecutors, and law enforcement. Members of the team should respond to reports of suspected abuse or neglect and meet on a regular basis to develop protocol and procedures for the handling and reporting of suspected cases of child maltreatment. Access to such teams is critical to overcoming a lack of reporting. Such teams serve as a resource for both education and referrals. Unfortunately, easy access to such teams is provided to some, but not all health care providers. In some rural areas of the United States, teams may be located many miles away from where health care providers are working with patients and families. An increase in the number of teams and access to teams via new technologies such as telemedicine is urgently needed.

The importance of interdisciplinary communication and education among professionals who work with children is essential to increasing the reporting of suspected child abuse or neglect via health care. Protection of children in harm's way cannot be achieved without a team effort. Improved lines of communication between health care providers and CPS supported by a dialogue concerning the system and the application of protection mechanisms are critical.

Protected Health Information

Health care professionals recognize the importance of privacy and confidentiality in medical records, the legal particulars of which are represented in HIPPA. Lawmakers, motivated by the fact that an estimated 24% of each health care dollar went to administrative expenses rather than enhanced patient care, moved to enact HIPPA to address rising health care costs. Much of the administrative difficulty and cost could be attributed to the existence of complex coding systems and the lack of sharing of diagnostic or billing methods among providers. As such, experts found the entire health care industry to be unable to move to a single, efficient electronic transaction environment through which administrative effort may be diminished.

Many of the HIPPA rules, such as privacy and confidentiality, were held as standard operating procedure for health care providers long before the legislation was enacted; however, for the first time in history, HIPAA provided federal regulations that further defined and codified the old rules. HIPAA requires: (1) nationwide uniformity, (2) mandatory compliance, and (3) meticulous adherence to the new rules.

HIPAA contains confidentiality provisions and provides that protected health information (PHI) must be disclosed: (1) to individuals who want to have access to or know about any disclosures of their own PHI or (2) to Health and Human Services (HHS) during a compliance investigation or review or enforcement action. PHI is defined as: (1) any oral or recorded information; (2) information on any past, present, and future physical or mental health condition; (3) all health care treatment; and (4) past, present, or future payment for health care. PHI may be disclosed: (1) to the individual who is the subject of the information; (2) for the covered entity's own treatment, payment, and health care operations activities; (3) with informed consent or in circumstances that clearly give the individual the opportunity to agree, acquiesce, or object; (4) incidental use and disclosure to the minimum necessary; (5) for public interest and benefit activities; or (6) for research and other public health purposes with any identifying information removed. Child welfare and other agencies can be considered "covered entities" as long as they are health care providers that transmit PHI in electronic form regarding a transaction covered by HIPAA.

Parents can normally view the medical records of their children except when the parents are not the personal representatives. The 3 exceptions are: (1) when the minor consents to the care and the state law does not require the parent's consent; (2) if the parent agrees that there is a confidential relationship between the minor and the health care provider; and (3) when the minor obtains care at the direction of the court or a person appointed by the court, such as an *ad litem* attorney. If a health care provider, in his or her professional judgment, thinks that a child is in danger or may be a victim of abuse or neglect by the parent, that parent is no longer treated as a personal representative.

Technical definitions aside, the requirement that PHI "be disclosed for public interest and benefit activities"[1] is the detail that is important to health care providers because reporting of abuse or neglect and disclosing information regarding victims of abuse, neglect, or intimate partner violence (IPV) are considered "public interest and benefit activities."[1] Therefore, some information may be shared in these instances without authorization or permission. It protects child health information but allows disclosures with victim consent or when necessary to prevent harm to the victim or others. This detail is important because without it, providers would not be able to comply with the laws that mandate the reporting of child abuse.

HIPAA federal regulations also provide authority for courts to order disclosure of medical records for judicial and administrative proceedings.[1] A covered entity may disclose protected health information in the course of any judicial or administrative proceeding in response to an order of a court or administrative tribunal, provided that the covered entity discloses only the PHI expressly authorized by such order. When called upon to disclose PHI, a health care provider should speak to his or her legal representative about the parameters of what can be revealed.

Overview of Court Systems

"All States have enacted child maltreatment laws that play a significant role in reporting and intervening in cases of child abuse and neglect."[11] When parents are unwilling or unable to provide for the safety and well-being of their children, the state intervenes to enforce these child maltreatment laws.[11] The extent of the state's authority, who responds, and how they respond is governed by state law, which means the response may vary greatly from state to state. Additionally, a child maltreatment case may be heard in in civil court, usually as a dependency or custody case, or it may be heard in criminal court if an offender is prosecuted adding increased variation in case handling.

Civil Court

Dependency Hearings

A dependency hearing is held to determine whether parents are no longer fit to care for their child. Although the process of dependency hearings varies from state-to-state, it is generally CPS that initiates the proceedings by filing a petition with the courts when child abuse is suspected. The report contains the allegations of abuse or neglect as well as a request for the court to determine whether it is in the best of interest of the child that he or she be removed from his or her home or whether the parent's rights should be terminated.[12] The court that hears the case varies by state; however, family or juvenile courts, which have the authority to make decisions about what happens to the child, generally handle the cases. The court analyzes factors such as whether the child is in imminent danger of harm, the child's safety can be assured, and the family is willing to cooperate with keeping the child safe. State statutes determine the standards for decision-making and what factors should be taken into consideration. In severe cases of abuse or neglect, parental rights may be terminated, but termination is a drastic measure that is not undertaken lightly. Hearings for dependency cases are typically closed to the public and may only be attended by those involved in the proceedings.

Various types of hearings are convened throughout the process of a dependency case. An ***emergency hearing*** is called to determine whether immediate intervention is necessary to protect a child who is suspected of having been a victim of abuse or neglect. An ***adjudicatory hearing*** is held to determine the substantive issue of whether the child is in fact a victim of child maltreatment. If the court finds that the child has been abused or neglected, ***dispositional hearings*** are held to determine how to protect the child by considering, among other things, whether a child should be removed from his or her home or if it is sufficient to impose conditions on the parents to keep the child safe. Review hearings later examine whether circumstances have changed and if the continued involvement of the state is necessary.[13]

When medical professionals are required to testify in a dependency hearing, their testimony is generally given at an adjudicatory hearing wherein the court's purpose is to determine if a child has been the victim of abuse or neglect and, if found to be so, what injuries occurred and who caused them. As determined by the landmark United States Supreme Court case *Santosky v Kramer*,[2] the standard of proof required to terminate parental rights is "clear and convincing evidence," which is higher than the typical burden of "beyond a preponderance of the evidence" required of civil cases but lower than the burden of "beyond a reasonable doubt" required of a criminal case.[3] Medical testimony is often presented by the government agency, typically CPS, seeking to prove the child is dependent as a way of meeting its burden and proving the case. For example, if the child was injured or neglected by his or her parent(s), medical testimony can be used to establish the injuries. Therefore, the observations made by the health care provider during an examination can be critical to the outcome of a dependency hearing and may result in their being called to testify.

Custody Cases

The custody case is another type of civil legal proceeding that involves children. Whereas dependency proceedings are initiated by the state, custody proceedings are most often initiated by the filing of a legal pleading requesting a change in custody of the child. A lawyer generally files the pleading on behalf of a parent, guardian, or other person seeking custody of a child; however, it is possible for an individual to file his or her own pleadings without legal representation. It is not uncommon for allegations of child abuse to surface during divorce and custody proceedings. When this happens, a health care provider may be called upon to testify regarding any observations that he or she made during medical examinations of the child or children at the center of the proceedings. Custody cases are generally heard in closed hearings and may take place in front of a master as opposed to a judge. A master is typically an attorney appointed to assist judges with certain types of cases, such as custody cases.

Criminal Court

State law determines which offenses are punishable in criminal court. Crimes of child abuse include homicide, assault, battery, reckless endangerment, rape, and sexual assault among others. Additionally, child neglect and abandonment may be determined to be a crime. It is not uncommon for simultaneous dependency or custody cases to be pending when a crime is prosecuted. Criminal court is designed to hold offenders accountable, but it is not the proper forum for determining issues involving dependency, custody, or other issues impacting a child's welfare.

The multidisciplinary team approach to investigating and prosecuting child abuse cases is viewed by most experts as the optimal response.[14] The multidisciplinary team may include CPS workers, specialized health care workers, social workers, victim advocates, police, and prosecutors, among others. Although the team works together for the benefit of the child, each member has its own role. Specifically, the police are responsible for investigating criminal cases, as a result many police departments employ investigators or detectives with specialized training to handle cases of suspected child maltreatment. Some police departments have specialized units at their disposal. Once a case is investigated, the prosecutor, also called district attorney, state's attorney, or attorney general, is responsible for proving it in court. Like the police, the prosecutor's office may have a special unit that handles child abuse cases. The goal of criminal court is not only to punish the offender for committing a crime but also to protect the public from future misconduct. Additionally, the focus of criminal court is on whether the state can prove the elements of the crime as defined by statute and meet the highest standard of proof under the law of beyond a reasonable doubt.

Criminal cases are initiated in different ways in different states. In some states, an arrest warrant begins the process while in other states, a grand jury indictment is the first step in commencing proceedings. In many states, the first hearing in a criminal case is a public preliminary hearing at which the defendant is present. In other states, the first hearing is an investigation before a grand jury panel composed of citizens where the crime occurred. Unlike the preliminary hearing, the grand jury investigation is closed and the defendant is not present. After a preliminary hearing or grand jury investigation, motions or other pretrial hearings may take place. The final hearing in a criminal case is a trial before a jury or a judge sitting alone. Health care providers may be called to testify at any of these hearings, either to help the prosecution prove its case or to help the defense defend against the allegations. Regardless of which side calls the medical provider as a witness, it is critical for the medical professional to be objective, thorough, and truthful.

Testifying in Court

As previously discussed, a health care provider may be required to testify in court as a result of observations that he or she made while examining a child who is suspected to be the victim of child abuse. The fact that a health care provider performs an examination or makes a report to law enforcement or CPS does not always mean that the person will have to testify in court. A civil or criminal case is not necessarily filed simply because a mandatory reporter filed a report to law enforcement or because a case was investigated. Even if a case is filed, it may not end up at trial. In fact, most cases never have a formal trial because most criminal cases are resolved by plea agreements and most civil cases are resolved by settlements. When a case does go to trial, it is often long after the completion of the examination(s) for which the health care provider is to provide testimony. The length of time it takes for a case to go to trial varies depending on the jurisdiction in which the case if filed; it is not uncommon for cases to take a year or more to get to trial. Health care providers who keep meticulous notes during an examination will be better prepared to testify as the notes will help to refresh their memory when the case finally gets to trial.

It is critical for health care providers to understand the basic tenets of the legal system in order to understand where they fit in the process. Although the structure and rules of the various courts differ in each jurisdiction, some basic concepts remain consistent. Regardless of the court system a health care provider comes into contact with, he or she is expected to be honest, objective, and accurate. The health care provider is not the fact finder, judge, or jury. Instead, the health care provider is a first-line responder who sees a child, often in his or her most critical state of need. Attorneys, police, judges, and CPS expect that the health care provider will conduct thorough exams, write accurate notes, and cooperate with the court process when and if necessary. The health care provider should always remain in the neutral role of health care provider with his or her first obligation to the patient's health.

Few attorneys are willing to call a witness for their case without having had at least one prior conversation with that witness to review what will occur during testimony. By the same token, no health care provider should be willing to testify in a case without meeting with the requesting attorney. Preparation is the key to comfort in the courtroom, and meeting with the attorney before testimony is paramount. At a minimum, advanced preparation with the attorney should allow the witness to know whether or not the health care provider will be testifying as an expert and the general line of questioning.

The process of testifying in court can be a challenging experience for a number of reasons. It is common to be called to testify and then be made to wait for hours because some other situation related to the court process has held up one's testimony. The health care provider often has to clear and rearrange his or her daily schedule to be available for the court time; therefore the health care provider called to testify should be aware that the given schedule might change. Furthermore, the compensation given is usually not comparable to the work time missed.

The health care provider must review all written documentation of the case and be familiar with the details and conclusions of the examination on specific cases. Relying on one's memory of a case can be detrimental to the process. It is the health care provider's responsibility to be clear about the details of the case. Whether expert or fact witness, nervous or calm, remaining professional at all times is the most important component of testifying effectively.

Evidence

It is crucial that the health care provider be meticulous and thorough when collecting evidence and recording his or her findings because attorneys try to create doubt by showing inconsistencies, mistakes, and irregularities in these areas. Medical records must include all pertinent facts and observations. Before testifying, the health care provider should review his or her reports and any evidence he or she collected that may be admitted at the trial.[15]

In court, attorneys call witnesses to give testimony and introduce various types of physical evidence for consideration. Most jurisdictions have formal rules of evidence, although some still follow common law rules, which means that judges determine what is admissible based upon historical practices. There are 2 types of evidence: direct and circumstantial. ***Direct evidence*** is evidence that leads to the point at issue, without the intervention of the proof of any other fact. ***Circumstantial evidence*** is indirect evidence that requires the trier of fact to make an inference or deduction.[16] For example, if a person can testify that he or she looked out the window and saw a person walking across the lawn in the snow, direct evidence exists that a person walked across the lawn in the snow. If instead the person testifies that he or she observed a single set of footprints in the snow on the front lawn, circumstantial evidence exists that someone walked across the lawn. Medical providers will typically provide direct evidence based upon their observations. For example, if a vaginal swab were tested and found to have semen, direct evidence would exist that semen was in the vagina. Circumstantial evidence would exist that a male ejaculated in the child. It is best for medical providers to focus on documenting the facts that would constitute direct evidence; it will be the attorney's job at trial to argue the significance of circumstantial evidence.

Expert Witnesses and Fact Witnesses

Testifying in court can be an intimidating experience. The health care provider will not be required to testify in every case; however, when obligated, he or she may be called upon to serve as a fact witness, expert witness, or both. A ***fact witness*** testifies to what he or she observed. Factual testimony may require the witness to discuss what was collected and how it was collected as well as policies and procedures.[4] An ***expert witness*** is able to testify to opinions or conclusions based upon his or her education, knowledge, and experience when those opinions or conclusions assist the finder of fact in making a decision.[17] Rules governing the testimony of expert witnesses are generally codified in rules of evidence or governed by common law. For example, Federal Rule of Evidence 702 states,[18] "If scientific, technical, or other specialized knowledge will assist the trier of fact to understand the evidence or to determine a fact in issue, a witness qualified as an expert by knowledge, skill, experience, training, or education, may testify thereto in the form of an opinion or otherwise, if (1) the testimony is based upon sufficient facts or data, (2) the testimony is the product of reliable principles and methods, and (3) the witness has applied the principles and methods reliably to the facts of the case."

Before the witness is able to testify as an expert, the judge must be persuaded that the purported expert has knowledge, training, or experience in an area of specialized knowledge that is beyond the abilities of the ordinary juror.[17] Generally, expert testimony begins with the attorney who called the witness asking the witness questions about his or her training, education, and qualifications to show that witness is qualified to testify as an expert. Most states define qualifications broadly and practical experience may qualify an expert to testify. Because education, training, and experience are critical to an expert witness's qualifications, the health care provider who may be called upon to testify as an expert should maintain an up-to-date *curriculum vitae* that details his or her education, including degrees and training programs such as:

— Licenses

— Employment

— Volunteer work in related fields

— Relevant professional experience

— Lectures and training delivered

— Publications

— Awards

— Memberships in professional organizations

— Additional information pertinent to the expert's qualifications[15]

It is helpful when health care professionals have specific training in the medicolegal aspects of evidence collection and documentation of findings that will hold up under courtroom scrutiny. The educational content of SANE training includes addressing the requirements of the legal system. SANE nurses are highly trained in evidence collection, maintaining chain of custody, testifying in court, and issues related to prosecution and plea bargaining.[19] SANE training would benefit all clinicians who evaluate cases of abuse.

Once the witness is established as an expert and recognized by the court as such, the attorney asks the expert's opinion on the issue in question. The opinion portion of the testimony usually consists of the foundation or basis for the opinion followed by the conclusion. An expert may be required to give testimony in the form of an answer to a hypothetical question. The requirements for and format of the questions vary from state-to-state and jurisdiction-to-jurisdiction, so health care providers should try to meet with the attorney before the trial to raise any concerns and correct the attorney if he or she misstates or misinterprets facts or conclusions.[15,20]

Regardless of whether the medical professional is called as a fact witness, expert witness, or both, certain basic principles apply. As with any witness, the health care provider may not only be judged by what he or she says, but also by his or her demeanor and appearance. The witness should dress in a neat, clean, professional manner and remember that potential jurors may observe him or her from the moment of arrival at the courthouse. It is critical to remain calm and polite.[15]

During trial, the attorney calling the witness generally begins by asking open-ended questions as part of the direct examination. Later, the opposing attorney is allowed to cross-examine the witness and will often ask leading questions that suggest the desired response. The health care provider should listen carefully to the question being asked before responding and answer only the question that is asked.[20] Accuracy is critical as a witness may be cross-examined with transcripts from prior testimony. A witness who does not understand a question should ask to have it clarified.[4] The witness should not guess or rush to answer questions, but rather take care to answer all questions thoughtfully and accurately. A witness who does not remember information may ask to refer to his or her records to "refresh his or her recollection."[4] A witness who does not know the answer to a question asked at trial should simply acknowledge that he or she does not know the answer.[15] The witness should always remember that truthfulness and accuracy are critical at all times.

Depositions

A deposition is testimony under oath that is recorded for use in court at a later date. The purpose of a deposition is to obtain information that cannot be learned as readily through written records or general investigation. The lawyer for one side questions a witness on the opposing side. This testimony allows involved attorneys to find out as much as possible about the case, including strengths and weaknesses, and a witness's credibility.

Depositions take place outside the courtroom. Oral testimony is taken under oath, and the proceedings are transcribed. All deposition information is recorded and can be used as official testimony at a later trial. The deposition transcript may be introduced as evidence in court if and when a case proceeds to trial. It is important that the health care provider be as prepared for the deposition as he or she is for an actual court case. Preparation first involves speaking with the attorney to discuss what the expectations of reviewing the case should be. Then the health care provider who is to testify prepares by reviewing the medical record, treatment of the patient, policies and procedures in effect at the time the patient was seen, and scope and standard of nursing practice. Of course, the medical record should not be altered in any way from its original format.

Conclusion

This chapter provided an explanation of the history and purpose of CPS, mandatory reporting laws, and HIPAA. By understanding the role of CPS and the intersection of mandatory reporting laws and HIPAA, the health care provider is better equipped to keep children safe. The chapter also provided an overview of the various types of legal proceedings and where the health care professional fits in those proceedings. Finally, the chapter explained the basic rules of testifying to assist those medical providers called upon to go to court in providing objective and professional testimony.

References

1. 45 CFR §164.512 (e).
2. *Santosky v Kramer*, 455 US 745, 768-69 (1982).
3. Nilson B. Yearning for Zion Ranch raid: lowering the standard of proof for the termination of parental rights. *Brooklyn Law Rev.* 2009;75(1):305-343.
4. Ledray LE, Wolbert Burgess A, Giardino AP. *Medical Response to Adult Sexual Assault: A Resource for Clinicians and Related Professionals.* St. Louis, MO: STM Learning, Inc; 2011.
5. Jones R, Flaherty EG, Binns HJ, et al. Clinician's description of factors influencing their reporting of suspected child abuse: report of the Child Abuse Reporting Experience Study research group. *Pediatrics.* 2008;122(2):259-266.
6. Sedlak AJ, Mettenburg J, Basena M, et al. *Fourth National Incidence Study of Child Abuse and Neglect (NIS-4).* Washington, DC: United States Department of Health and Human Services; 2010.
7. O'Reilly R, Wilkes L, Luck L, Jackson D. The efficacy of family support and family preservation services on reducing child abuse and neglect: what the literature reveals. *J Child Health Care.* 2010:14(1):89-94.

8. Theodore AD, Runyan DK. A survey of pediatricians' attitudes and experiences with court in cases of child maltreatment. *Child Abuse Negl.* 2006;30(12):1353-1363.

9. Feng JY, Fetzer S, Chen YW, Yeh L, Huang MC. Multidisciplinary collaboration reporting child abuse: a grounded theory study. *Int J Nurs Stud.* 2010;47(12):1483-1490.

10. Flaherty EG, Sege RD, Hurley TP, Baker A. Strategies for saving or improving children's lives. *Pediatrics.* 2008;122(suppl 1):S18-S20.

11. Office on Child Abuse and Neglect, Children's Bureau, Goldman J, Salus MK, Wolcott D, Kennedy KY. A coordinated response to child abuse and neglect: the foundation for practice. United States Department of Health and Human Service Administration for Children and Families Web site. http://www.childwelfare.gov/pubs/usermanuals/foundation/foundationh.cfm. Published 2003. Accessed August 17, 2012.

12. Child Welfare Information Gateway. Mandatory reporters of abuse and neglect: summary of state laws. United States Department of Health and Human Services Administration for Children and Families Web site. http://www.childwelfare.gov/systemwide/laws_policies/statutes/manda.cfm. Published 2010. Accessed August 17, 2012.

13. United States Department of Health and Human Services, Child Welfare Information Gateway. Working with the courts in child protection. United States Department of Health and Human Services Administration for Children and Families Web site. http://www.childwelfare.gov/pubs/usermanuals/courts_92/courtsb.cfm. Accessed August 17, 2012.

14. American Prosecutors Research Institute. *Investigation and Prosecution of Child Abuse.* 3rd ed. Thousand Oaks, CA: Sage Publications, Inc; 2004.

15. Scalzo TP. Tips for testifying as an expert witness in a violence against women prosecution. *Voice.* 2006;1(4).

16. Mccormick on Evidence §342, at 308 (6th ed. 2006).

17. Bocchino AJ, Sonenshein DA. *A Practical Guide to Federal Evidence Objections, Responses, Rules, and Practice Commentary.* 9th ed. Louisville, CO: National Institute for Trial Advocacy; 2009.

18. Fed R Evid 702.

19. Logan T, Cole J, Capillo A. Sexual assault nurse examiner program characteristics, barriers, and lessons learned. *J Forensic Nurs.* 2007;3:24-34.

20. Cashman DI, Benak LD. Preparing staff for testimony in sexual assault cases. *J Forensic Nurs.* 2007;3(1):47-49.

Chapter 15

Children in the Violent Home: The Relationship Between Intimate Partner Violence and Child Maltreatment

Judith A. Rosenberg, PhD, MPH, CPNP-PC
Julie A. Nadkarni, MS, ARNP, CPNP
Sandra W. Shulman, BSN, CPNP

Key Points

1. ***Child maltreatment*** is defined as any act or series of acts of commission or omission by a parent or other caregiver that results in harm, potential for harm, or threat of harm to a child.

2. ***Child abuse*** refers explicitly to acts of commission, which may include single or ongoing acts of deliberate or intentional harm to a child.

3. Although male-on-female intimate partner violence (IPV) is more prevalent, female-on-male IPV has a significant incidence. In fact, violence between partners is frequently bidirectional, and individuals involved in bidirectional IPV are more likely to also be involved in other violence with closely related individuals.[1]

4. Higher frequencies of IPV are associated with a greater frequency of physical aggression towards children residing in the same household. Physically aggressive individuals do not tend to specialize with regard to their victim; rather, they are aggressive in their behavior towards everyone.[2] However, it is not always the perpetrator of IPV that perpetrates child maltreatment. In one study, for example, women who were victims of IPV were significantly more likely to have abused or neglected their children.[3] In over two-thirds of households with one or both aggressive parents, both parents engaged in aggression towards their young children.[4]

5. Two stressors in particular that are frequently associated with IPV issues are (1) separation and divorce and (2) substance abuse.

6. Substance abuse cannot be viewed as causative for violence in the home but has been shown in a preponderance of studies to be associated with escalation of all forms of violence within such environments. Alcohol and other inhibition-reducing drugs, such as cocaine, cloud recognition of responsibility and consequences of actions, thereby reducing the barrier to antisocial actions such as violence against one's intimate partner. Alcohol in particular is associated with increased individual proclivity for violent behavior, some of which may be learned as culturally normative behavior.[5]

7. Homes where chronic abuse and neglect is perpetrated by primary attachment figures, such as the parental unit, can have a highly negative impact on the child's ability to develop and maintain friendships, particularly in the school setting.[6] Children who have been subjected to chronic trauma, especially chronic abuse and neglect, are likely to have serious difficulties in becoming successful students.[7]
8. Behavioral regression as a result of trauma deserves further mention. Developmental milestones, including toilet training; cessation of self-soothing behaviors, such as thumb sucking and sleeping alone or with the lights off, can be compromised after a child experiences trauma.[8] Such behavioral regression, seen by some parents as child failures or even intentional, may also increase the risk of abuse and maltreatment by parents.
9. Because of the danger IPV poses for children in the home, pediatric nurses must screen and assess the parents of their patients for IPV, especially if child maltreatment is suspected.
10. Victims of dating violence are at increased risk for injury and are more likely to engage in binge drinking, suicide attempts, physical fights, and sexual activity.[9]

Introduction

Over the past several decades, issues of family violence have shifted from an exclusively private, unspoken matter to an openly discussed and widespread public health problem.[10] According to the National Child Abuse and Neglect Data System[11] (NCANDS), 3.2 million reports of child abuse or neglect involving 5.8 million children were made to state child protection service (CPS) agencies in the United States in 2007. Over a quarter of these reports were subsequently substantiated as incidents of child maltreatment.[11] According to the Centers for Disease Control and Prevention[12] (CDC), 4.8 million intimate partner physical assaults and rapes are perpetrated on women each year, and 2.9 million such assaults are perpetrated on men. In 2005, these assaults resulted in the death of 1510 victims.[13] Given the magnitude of both IPV and child maltreatment and the inferred pain and suffering experienced within the family unit related to both, a relationship between parental IPV and parental maltreatment of children would be expected.[14]

Factors occurring within the family that may infer risk for violence include poverty and other financial stressors, substance use,[5,12] younger adult as the head of the household, cultural background,[15] mental or physical illness in the family, the birth of a child, and separation and divorce.[1,16] Since 2001, military service has become a significant factor as well.[17,18] Children in homes plagued by IPV are at risk of suffering similar maltreatment, either indirectly or directly. Children in homes where one parent is abusing the other or where abuse is mutual between parents, may become involved in that abuse either as passive witnesses or as accidentally or intentionally involved bystanders.[2,16] Children in domestically violent homes may also experience direct abuse either at the hands of the abusive adult partner or the victimized partner.[2,10]

A need remains for health care providers caring for families to protect and advocate for adults and children vulnerable to abuse. This can best be done with comprehensive, universal screening for IPV and child abuse; documentation of forensic findings; and appropriate referrals to victim service organizations and child welfare agencies as indicated.[19]

This chapter assists health care providers caring for families to understand the relationship between IPV and child maltreatment. Following a definition of terminology to be employed, the chapter provides a brief overview of the crimes of IPV and child maltreatment. The chapter goes on to explore different modes of children's involvement in violence within their homes, such as the child as witness to violence and the child as the target of violence. The physical, cognitive, psychosocial, and behavioral responses of children in violent homes will be addressed. Finally, the chapter addresses the health care provider's role in assessing the co-occurrence of IPV and child maltreatment, with emphasis on the assessment and response.

Nomenclature

The terminology used to describe the maltreatment of children has evolved such that different terms may be used in contextually different ways. This chapter, insofar as possible, adheres to the definitions of terms that has been advanced by the CDC.[12,20,21] Wherein the CDC does not provide terminology, nomenclature has been derived from other salient references, which are cited in those definitions. Specific terms that will be employed and their definition as used in this chapter are as follows:

Child maltreatment: Any act or series of acts of commission or omission by a parent or other caregiver that results in harm, potential for harm, or threat of harm to a child. The term maltreatment and abuse are frequently used interchangeably in the literature. However, in this chapter, as in the cited CDC publications, the term ***abuse*** refers explicitly to acts of commission, which may include single or ongoing acts of deliberate or intentional harm to a child.

Intimate partner violence (IPV): Abuse that occurs between 2 people in a close relationship. The term intimate partner includes current and former spouses and dating partners. IPV exists along a continuum from a single episode of violence to ongoing battering. IPV includes 4 types of behavior: (1) ***physical abuse***, (2) ***sexual abuse***, (3) ***threats*** of physical or sexual abuse, and (4) ***emotional abuse***.

Co-occurrence of child and partner maltreatment: Cases where (1) one parent is physically aggressive to the other parent and physically maltreats a child; (2) one parent is aggressive toward the other parent who is physically maltreating a child; or (3) one or both parents are aggressive towards each other and both physically maltreat the child.[10]

Violent home: A household wherein acts of aggression occur repeatedly, promulgated either by isolated individuals or multiple individuals. Household may refer to any living arrangement that represents home to a child. This can include, but is not limited to, traditional single family homes; rotating homes such as shared custody arrangements between separated or divorced parents; or extended family, such as aunts, uncles, grandparents, or foster homes. Aggressive individuals may be parents or guardians but may also be extended relatives and may even be siblings.[22]

Child Maltreatment

According to NCANDS, approximately 3.2 million referrals involving 5.8 million children were reported to CPS organizations. Of these reports, 61.7% were deemed sufficiently credible to warrant an investigation, and 25.2% of these investigations determined at least one child to have been the victim of maltreatment.[11]

If these data from 2007 are inferred to be representative, it may be concluded that there are at least 250 000 new cases of child maltreatment occurring annually in the United States. The perpetrators of maltreatment in 86.5% of cases were the parents or a close relative of the victim. Females (56.5%) were more frequently found to be the perpetrators than males (42.2%). The reporters of child maltreatment were most frequently professionals (57.7%), including teachers, law enforcement officials, social services, and health care workers.[11]

In 2007, child maltreatment resulting in death was estimated to have occurred 1760 times in the United States for an overall child maltreatment death rate of 2.35 per 100 000 children. The true incidence of child abuse fatalities is unknown at least in part because death cases may be inaccurately diagnosed or inadequately investigated.[23] Of all child maltreatment fatalities, 34.1% were attributed to neglect only; 26.4% were attributed to physical abuse only; 35.2% were attributed to multiple maltreatments; and the balance were attributed to other forms of maltreatment, such as sexual abuse or medical neglect. Children aged under 4 years represented 75.7% of the maltreatment fatalities, with the highest rate occurring in males aged under 1 year (18.85 per 100 000 infant males).[11]

While death due to maltreatment is the most extreme outcome, it represents a very small fraction of a quarter of a million annual cases. Unless effective intervention occurs, the victims of child maltreatment are subject to continuing patterns of abuse and neglect. This in turn leads to patterns of immediate and long-term sequelae including[11,24]:

— Impaired brain development leading to cognitive, language, and academic impairment

— Poor overall health

— Poor mental and emotional health such as depression, anxiety, eating disorders, and suicide attempts

— Antisocial traits and violent behavior

— Increased risk of juvenile delinquency, adult criminality, and resultant incarceration

— Increased rates of unemployment and poverty

— Increased rates of Medicaid usage and other channels of social spending

— Increased risk for substance abuse

In addition to the obvious individual costs associated with these short and long-term effects, these sequelae translate directly to societal costs in the form of decreased tax revenue, increased social spending, and increased costs secondary to criminality.[25] Moreover, there is a substantial body of evidence that the victims of maltreatment are at risk of becoming future perpetrators of maltreatment, generally of their own offspring.[25]

Intimate Partner Violence

Public awareness of violence, and particularly IPV, has grown and evolved as a public health and criminal justice concern.[26,27] Between the years 1993 and 1998, IPV victimization occurred in 8 to 10 women per 1000 and in approximately 2 men per 1000. IPV was more prevalent in lower income households (42 per 1000 for incomes below $25 000) than in upper income (23 per 1000 for incomes $25 000 or above) and in households where the heads of house were aged under 25 years (39 per 1000) than in those where the heads of house were aged 25 years or older (22 per 1000). Forty-five percent of female IPV victimization occurred in households where children aged younger than 12 years were present, while only 39% of IPV victimization occurred in households without young children. Only 25% of male IPV victimization occurred in households with young children and 67% occurred in households without children aged younger than 12 years.[28] It must be noted that while male-on-female IPV is more prevalent, female-on-male IPV has a significant incidence. In fact, violence between partners is frequently bidirectional, and individuals involved in bidirectional IPV are more likely to also be involved in other violence with closely related individuals.[1]

IPV is assaultive behavior occurring between partners in marital, dating, and cohabiting relationships. Within IPV relationships, one partner uses various behaviors to exercise power and control over the other. These behaviors may include physical or sexual assault and battery; psychological abuse; financial abuse; or isolation from friends, family members, and coworkers.[5,15,29] IPV crosses racial, social, and economic boundaries; however, socioeconomic factors and factors relating to family dynamic have been identified among risk factors associated with incidence of IPV.[5,15] Additionally, environmental factors have been associated with an elevated risk for IPV (**Table 15-1**).

Fifty percent of female IPV victims and 32% of male IPV victims incurred serious injuries, including gunshot or knife wounds, internal injuries, broken bones, or loss of consciousness as a result of their attacks. Of the IPV victims incurring serious injury, 63% of females and 60% of males did not seek treatment for their injuries. Only 53% of female victims and 46% of male victims reported their attacks to the police.[28] It is the serious underreporting of IPV that may be of greatest concern. **Table 15-2** lists the most frequently cited reasons given among victims of IPV who did not report their attacks to the police.

Table 15-1. Environmental Factors Associated with Elevated Risk Factors for Intimate Partner Violence

— History of poverty with residence in disadvantaged neighborhoods

— Origin dynamics, including poor impulse control and IPV

— Family with history of mental health issues, particularly depression and substance abuse

Data from Tolan P, Gorman-Smith D, Henry D. Family violence. Annu Rev Psychol. *2006;57:557-583.*
Data from Jewkes R. Intimate partner violence: causes and prevention. Lancet. *2002;359(9315):1423-1429.*
Data from Caetano R, Vaeth P, Ramisetty-Mikler S. Intimate partner violence victim and perpetrator characteristics among couples in the United States. J Fam Violence. *2008;23(6):507-518.*
Data from Ehrensaft MK. Intimate partner violence: persistence of myths and implications for intervention. Child Youth Serv Rev. *2008;30(3):276-286.*
Data from Stith SM, McMonigle CL. Risk factors associated with intimate partner violence. In: Whitaker DJ, Lutzker JR, eds. Preventing Partner Violence: Research and Evidence-Based Intervention Strategies. *Washington, DC: American Psychological Association; 2009:67-92.*

Table 15-2. Reasons for Not Reporting Cited by Victims of IPV

— Police couldn't do anything (99.7%).

— Police wouldn't believe report (61.3%).

— It was a minor, one-time incident (37.9%).

— Wanted to protect relationship with attacker or with children (34.8%)

— Didn't want police or court involvement (32.0%)

— Fear of perpetrator (11.7%)

Data from Child Welfare Information Gateway. Child abuse and neglect fatalities 2009: statistics and interventions. United States Department of Health and Human Services Web site. http://www.childwelfare.gov/pubs/factsheets/fatality.cfm. Accessed November 8, 2009.

The Link Between Child Maltreatment and Intimate Partner Violence

The exposure of children to violence on television, in cinema, on the Internet, and even in video games has been postulated to increase violent behavior among American youth.[30] Over recent years, children's exposure to violence within the family, particularly IPV, has been increasingly addressed by health care providers and specifically by nurses.[31-33] Historically, the effect of IPV on children went largely unnoticed, if not completely disregarded, by those caring for IPV victims. Often regarded as extensions of the battered parent, children were rarely viewed as potential victims of abuse and neglect.[34] As health care professionals have approached the family from a broader systems perspective, the physical and psychosocial effects of violence on the marital dyad, on the children, and on future generations have become of increasing concern.[8,35,36]

Children in domestically violent homes are often referred to as the unseen, silent, or secondary victims of violence.[34] Battered women may be unaware of the degree to which their children witness their abuse or fear of losing custody for failing to protect their children in the violent home and, as a result, may minimize the abuse their children have witnessed.[37] The presence of children during episodes of violence may go unnoticed by parents; however, children may directly witness or indirectly overhear violently loud arguments between their parents. Additionally, children, especially younger children, may suffer accidental injuries, either as a result of being struck by objects thrown or while in the arms of the victim parent. Older children may suffer accidental injuries while trying to intervene in parental violence or while trying to protect the parent they perceive as victim during an attack.[4,10] Children may be witnesses to more than one act of violence between their parents, with subsequent acts of violence increasing in intensity, frequency, duration, and potential for lethality over time. Older children may be required to call the police, an ambulance, or both for the victim parent.[4]

Children in homes where IPV occurs may also suffer from direct abuse or neglect inflicted by either parent.[2-4,16] As recently as the mid-1970s, the generally held view was that children residing in homes where interparental violence occurred were no more likely than other children to be the victims of abuse. Improved survey methodology demonstrated that, in fact, such children were victims of physical abuse at a much greater frequency, and by the mid-1990s, it had become clear that IPV and child maltreatment within households were both directly and indirectly linked.[16] Higher frequencies of IPV are associated with greater frequency of physical aggression towards children residing in the same household. Physically aggressive individuals do not tend to specialize with regard to their victim; rather, they are aggressive in their behavior towards everyone.[2] However, it is not always the perpetrator of IPV that perpetrates child maltreatment. In one study, for example, women who were victims of IPV were significantly more likely to have abused or neglected their children.[3] In over two-thirds of households with one or both aggressive parents, both parents engaged in aggression towards their young children.[4]

The Violent Home

The interrelatedness of child maltreatment and IPV that is identified by the preponderance of literature dating from the mid-1970s points to the existence of family dyads that can be defined as violent homes.[1,16] For the purposes of this chapter, the definition of a violent home referenced in the nomenclature section above will be employed, namely that a violent home has one or more individuals who engage in aggressive behavior directed at other individuals in the home on a recurring basis. The violent home may encompass multiple households for a child victim, as is seen in shared custody arrangements between divorced spouses. The perpetrators of violence in the violent home may be any individuals within the household, including parents and those described in the above sections, but

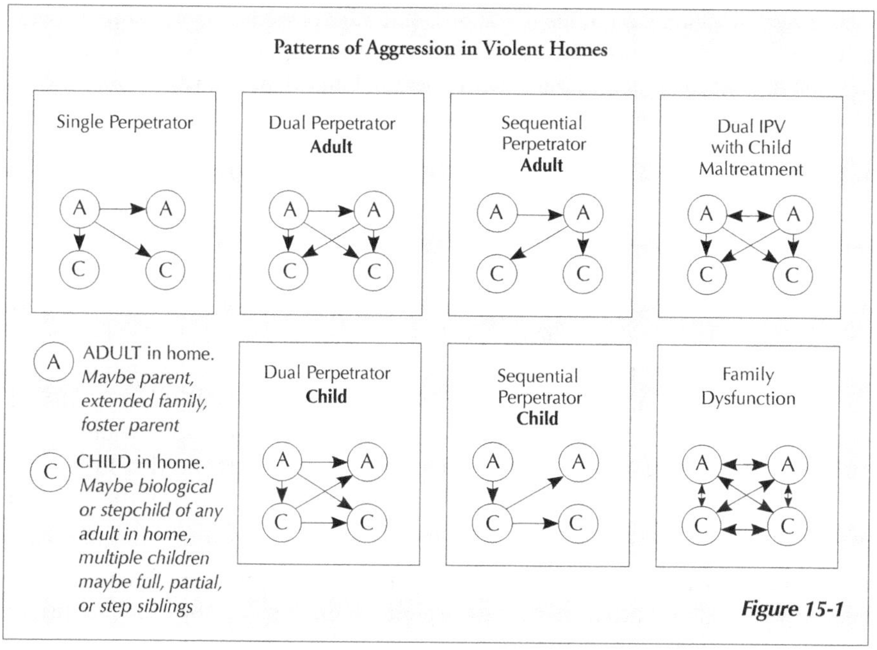

Figure 15-1. *Various patterns of aggression in violent homes.*

may also include extended family or siblings acting aggressively toward each other.[22] Different patterns of aggression in violent homes are shown diagrammatically in **Figure 15-1**. These patterns are an adaptation from models presented by Appel and Taylor[16] but have been extended and modified to reflect the existence of female-on-male, as well as male-on-female IPV,[12] and to reflect the existence of sibling-on-sibling abusive relationships.[22]

In the violent home, resources for coping with commonplace family stressors, such as the birth of a new child, the death of a loved one, new employment, lost employment, or a household emergency such as an automobile accident, are limited.[38] Two stressors in particular are worthy of specific note, inasmuch as they are frequently associated with IPV issues: (1) separation and divorce and (2) substance abuse.

Following separation and divorce, custody and visitation issues can pose problems for individuals who were victims of IPV before the separation. When violent ex-spouses are permitted visitation with their children, they may use visitation as an opportunity to continue harassing and even abusing their former spouse.[39] Following separation of a household wherein IPV was occurring without concomitant maltreatment of children in the home, the violence may escalate to include abuse of the children who serve as surrogates for previously victimized partners. The creation of blended families resulting from a parental death, separation, or divorce may also place a child at risk for exposure to IPV or maltreatment. Children may find themselves as targets of maltreatment by a step-parent, particularly if there is jealousy over their biological parent's previous relationships.[19]

For victims of IPV who must leave their home under duress and seek outside shelter, the situation is frequently very daunting. Shelter space is limited and is even more so for parents who have any number of children who must be sheltered with them. In addition, if one or more of the accompanied children is an adolescent male, then finding a shelter is often impossible as adolescent males may be considered a security risk.

Substance abuse cannot be viewed as causative for violence in the home, but has been shown in a preponderance of studies to be associated with escalation of all forms of violence within such environments.[5,8,40,41] Alcohol and other inhibition-reducing drugs, such as cocaine, cloud recognition of responsibility and consequences of actions, thereby reducing the barrier to antisocial actions such as violence against one's intimate partner. Alcohol in particular is associated with increased individual proclivity for violent behavior, some of which may be learned as culturally normative behavior.[5]

Response Patterns of Children in Violent Homes

Exposure to violence has profound effects on the growth and development of young children such as infants and toddlers. However, most of the literature written about IPV and its impact on children is written about older children. Because the young child may be unable to communicate their feelings verbally, their emotional behavior may be the only indicator of exposure to violence, particularly in the absence of physical findings.[42] Carpenter et al[36] suggest that early traumatic experiences may have devastating effects on growth and development, particularly in establishing behaviors that foster a sense of trust, security, and well-being. Since growth and development progresses rapidly during the first few years of life, it is important for those providing protective services to children to possess knowledge of the social, emotional, and physiological or neurological growth of children exposed to the trauma of IPV from their caregivers.

Early research on infant attachment[43,44] maintained that young children, and particularly infants, will form an attachment to a caregiver by the first year of life. The quality of the mother's bond with her infant is significant in establishing secure attachment relationships. In an optimal situation, a secure attachment relationship will help the infant develop prosocial behaviors that will lend themselves toward social competence and higher cognitive skills. The opposite pattern or lack of attachment is disorganized or disoriented. Infants who were identified as a high-risk group exhibited fear and contradictory behaviors when they needed comfort or protection from their caregivers.[36] A caregiver's lack of response to an infant during a stressful event may result in the infant's inability to comfort or calm him or herself. The effects of adverse environmental exposure on infants and toddlers have been shown to impact the maturation of brain development,[45] which has long-term consequences for cognitive and academic implications. Flaherty et al[8] have shown an association between the overall health of young children and household stressors such as violence.

It is noted in the literature that there is a relationship between IPV and social-, psychological-, and health-related adversities throughout all age groups.[46,47] As health care providers intervene with such families, it is important for them to examine the link between adverse childhood events (ACEs) and the presentation of children in the health care milieu. Nurses in particular may be one of the first to see these children in a variety of health care settings, such as clinics, schools, and childcare centers. "The family is recognized as the most significant socializing agent for children and youths and the locus of important learning both in the normative and deviant domains."[48] Therefore, nurses can play an important role in identifying families at risk of perpetuating IPV over time.

The response of victims after a traumatic event has been described for various crimes, including cases of rape[49] and IPV.[50] With the recognition of posttraumatic stress disorder (PTSD), trauma response patterns have become one of the leading psychiatric diagnoses of this decade. Numerous investigators have addressed the application of traumatic response patterns to children who have been exposed to violence.[45,51-53] Like their adult counterparts, children may also suffer from intrusive thoughts, including nightmares, as a result of experiencing violence or witnessing abuse. They may also display strong avoidance tendencies, especially when an event or location is a reminder of the traumatic event. Emotional numbing or feelings of apathy toward parents, peers, and others may also be noted in children after trauma. Finally, hyperactive startle responses, or responses that are far more dramatic than what the situation calls for, are also characteristic of children who have witnessed or experienced violence. To varying degrees, physical, cognitive, psychosocial, and behavioral responses predictably follow victimization. Additionally, various trauma-specific factors affect the degree to which victims respond. When the victim of a traumatic event is a child, several specific considerations must be weighed in evaluating his or her response. These can include the child's age and developmental level; the frequency, duration, and lethality of the trauma; past trauma history; relationship to the perpetrator; and the individual family characteristics supporting the child.[45,51-53]

The home environment provides a critical foundation on which certain social behaviors are learned and transitions to the school environment are built. Homes where chronic abuse and neglect is perpetrated by primary attachment figures, such as the parental unit, can have a highly negative impact on the child's ability to develop and maintain friendship, particularly in the school setting.[6] Children who have been subjected to chronic trauma, especially chronic abuse and neglect, are likely to have serious difficulties in becoming successful students.[7] Frederick[54] identifies several family factors that are associated with school success, including warmth, expectations of academic success, and consistency. Families where children are treated harshly and abused are likely to foster social maladjustment and dissociative behaviors in the child. Therefore, developing relationships and relating to others may be greatly hindered and lead to considerable social isolation, aggressive behavior, and school failure. Children who are victims of chronic abuse are likely to establish relationships patterned after their unstable home situations which only tend to impede the formation of positive and stable relationships in school. There are reports that maltreated children are disproportionately more likely to have poor academic skills in reading, math, and language. Frederick[54] states that dealing with all aspects of the school environment, including cognitive tasks and behavioral issues, leaves the child at greater risk for failure. Crooks et al[55] report that in understanding the sequelae of child maltreatment for adolescents, the child's family, peers, and school communities are important influences to consider. Family, school, and community relationships have the potential to "either exacerbate, or mitigate early negative experiences"[55] and are identified as protective factors where structure and prosocial role models serve as an important supportive opportunity. For example, a connection to a school with a support system could potentially provide a child with opportunities to excel, achieve academically, and develop prosocial behaviors. However, in a school environment where there is little connectivity (eg, length of stay is limited due to frequent moving), alienation is likely to prevail. Nevertheless, the risk for school-related difficulties is greater for children who reside in violent and abusive homes.

Physical Response

The first step to helping maltreated children is recognizing the signs of abuse and neglect. The first sign generally recognized by the health care provider is the physical response in the form of physical injuries.[56,57] Injuries such as excessive bruising, burns, fractures, or head trauma, especially in the younger child, should raise suspicion for abuse in most pediatric nurses. This is especially true when the explanation given by the parent or caregiver is not consistent with the child's injury or when the explanation is inadequate or developmentally inappropriate for the injury.[58-61] In over 13% of cases, children who are neglected are also victims of abuse[11]; therefore, patterns of neglect, such as malnutrition, lack of necessary medical care, or inadequate supervision resulting in physical harm, should also alert the health care provider to possible abusive maltreatment.

Accidental injuries, which may occur in the course of developing various motor skills, such as walking, running, and riding a bike, may prove difficult to distinguish from those that are intentionally inflicted.[62] Cutaneous injuries are the single most common presentation of physical abuse. Patterned injuries, or injuries with a characteristic size, shape, or texture are likely to be present. Common cutaneous injuries seen with abuse include patterned bruises, burns, bite marks, and ligature marks. The most common characteristics separating abusive from nonabusive cutaneous injuries are location and pattern. Bruising is extremely uncommon in infants and increases in frequency as children become older and more adventurous. A toddler learning to walk may present with a contusion or abrasion on his forehead or chin with a history of a fall. Likewise, his hands and knees may also show the signs of an unsuccessful attempt at walking or running. Accidental bruising in children tends to be located over bony prominences and on the front of the body.[62] Abusive bruising tends to be located away from bony prominences and may involve the head, neck, face, or torso, as well as the extremities. Bruising about the genitalia and inner thighs should raise concern for sexual abuse but may also be the result of toileting issues. Injuries inflicted with an object will often leave bruising or marks reflecting the outline of that object. Bruising sustained from being struck with hands, belts, cords, or paddles may appear linear, looped, or diffuse in pattern. Bruising in different stages of healing is commonly the result of repeated abuse and, if observed, should further raise the health care provider's index of suspicion for abuse. Whether one bruise or multiple bruises, location and pattern must be documented in the child's medical record by health care personnel.[63]

Abusive burns most commonly present as contact burns or immersion burns. Accidental and abusive contact burns can result from hair or clothing irons, space heaters, cigarettes, ovens, or any other hot object. Accidental contact burns usually have indistinct margins and do not occur in multiples. The opposite is true in many cases of abusive contact burns. Accidental scald burns are more likely to be irregular and asymmetrical. Abusive scald or immersion burns commonly result in well-demarcated areas of tissue injury and sparing. Abusive burns include stocking-and-glove patterned burns to the hands and feet, as well as doughnut-shaped burns to the buttocks. Many of these burns are inflicted as a result of toileting issues. In the United States, burns from tap water are the most common form of abusive burns.[59,63]

Cognitive Response

Children who witness IPV and those who are directly abused may experience trauma-related sequelae that affect their cognitive abilities. Hypervigilance and increased arousal and startle responses, symptoms diagnostic of posttraumatic stress response in adults, may be seen in children from violent homes. Avoidance of events and places associated with abuse may also be seen in children. For example, children exposed to violence in the later evening hours may be more avoidant of bedtime rituals because of the association between abuse and nighttime.[45,51-53]

Children of violent homes may have developmental delays that range from mild to severe. Children who reside in violent homes must be focused on survival at the expense of normal developmental activities. Older children may have decreased concentration coupled with difficulty focusing their attention on various tasks and may be easily distracted from daily activities and routines. These symptoms may manifest in school-aged children and adolescents as poor grades and academic skill levels below their expected abilities.[36,45,64] Such a spiral of poor academic performance may in turn lead to increased incidents of abusive discipline at home.

Behavioral Response

Children's behavioral responses to trauma, especially trauma in the form of violence in the home, are often characterized as externalizing or internalizing, or hyperarousal and dissociation respectively.[45] Externalizing behaviors, or behaviors typically expressed outwardly, can be seen in children of all ages. Externalizing behaviors seen in the toddler and school-aged child can begin with periods of increased restlessness and whining and may culminate in crying, yelling, and temper tantrums.[52] Older children who have learned that using violence is an acceptable way to meet their needs may use violence in their everyday lives. They may begin to engage in more delinquent types of behaviors, including lying, stealing, and truancy. Invariably, these types of behaviors result in other deleterious consequences in the home and, possibly, in the criminal justice system.[47,64]

Still, rather than expressing trauma outwardly, some child victims may exhibit internalizing behaviors in response to the trauma. Toddlers and school-aged children may regress behaviorally and seclude themselves from other children.[8] Older children may internalize trauma and act out through sexual promiscuity and early pregnancy. For some teenagers, pregnancy may be seen as a way to disconnect from the family system; ironically, early pregnancy generally serves only to reinforce dependence on the family of origin. In addition to early pregnancy, substance use, isolation, or self-directed violence are also forms of internalization.[65] In severe cases, children may completely dissociate from traumatic events, separating emotional from physical feelings.

Behavioral regression as a result of trauma deserves further mention. Developmental milestones, including toilet training, cessation of self-soothing behaviors such as thumb sucking, and sleeping alone or with the lights off, can be compromised after a child experiences trauma.[8] Such behavioral regression, seen by some parents as child failures or even intentional, may also increase the risk of abuse and maltreatment by parents.

Implications for Nursing Practice

Every nurse, regardless of specialty, will interact with and care for members of a family. Families will present in various stages of development and transition. In recent years, the definition of family has expanded to include more than the traditional 2-parent household. Various family compositions will require care, including the single-parent family, the gay or lesbian family, families in which the primary caregiver is a grandparent or other relative, and adoptive or foster families. Nurses caring for all family types must capitalize on the family's strengths while attempting to minimize or eradicate their weaknesses. This is especially true when working with the violent family. Co-occurrence research emphasizes the need to assess for IPV whenever child maltreatment is present and vice-versa. However, conducting a thorough assessment of child maltreatment in IPV cases is not a universal practice.

Like other health care professionals, pediatric nurses are required to assess for and intervene in cases of suspected child maltreatment; however, their role in caring for adult victims of violence is less well defined. Because of the danger IPV poses for children in the home, pediatric nurses must screen and assess the parents of their patients for IPV, especially if child maltreatment is suspected to be present. Assessing for IPV in a private and nonthreatening manner can allow for greater disclosure by the victim parent. Resources, such as the RADAR card screening tool that is available through the Philadelphia Institute for Safe Families,[66] can assist the pediatric specialty nurse in assessing for the presence of violence in the home and in providing appropriate referral to the victimized parent to seek assistance, or if necessary, safe shelter (**Box 15-1**). It is important to keep in mind that the abused partner or parent may be very reluctant to discuss the violence they have experienced and even more reluctant to take measures to

Box 15-1. RADAR

Routinely screen female patients
Ask direct questions
Document your findings
Assess patient safety
Respond, review options, and refer

Adapted from The Institute for Safe Families; American Academy of Pediatrics, Pennsylvania Chapter. RADAR for pediatrics: a domestic violence intervention. Institute for Safe Families Imagining a Better Future Web site. http://www.instituteforsafefamilies.org/materials/m/radar. Accessed June 18, 2013.

escape the violence.[28] Moreover, caution should be exercised in giving the abused parent printed materials, even hand-written phone numbers, that are associated with support or law enforcement agencies because the individual's safety may be compromised if the abuser finds these in the abused parent's possession.[66]

Pediatric nurses caring for adolescents must begin to screen for dating violence, that is the physical, sexual, or psychological (emotional) violence within a dating relationship.[67] According to the CDC, approximately 1 in 4 teenagers acknowledge some form of physical, sexual, or verbal dating abuse each year, with about 10% incurring a physical injury from a girlfriend or boyfriend.[9] These high rates of dating violence are consistent with the demonstrated increasing risk for IPV with decreasing age.[15] Although both male and female adolescents may equally be victims of abuse (8% of males; 11% of females), they are abusive in different ways. Teenage girls are more likely to yell, threaten to hurt themselves, pinch, slap, scratch, or kick. Teenage boys injure girls more severely and frequently.[67] Youths involved in same-sex dating are just as likely to experience dating violence as youths involved in opposite-sex dating. Victims of dating violence are at increased risk for injury and are more likely to engage in binge drinking, suicide attempts, physical fights, and sexual activity.[9] Signs and symptoms that may be associated with dating violence in an adolescent victim include:

— Poor social skills

— Inability to manage anger and conflict

— Belief that using dating violence is acceptable

— Witnessing violence at home

— Alcohol use

— Having behavior problems in other areas

— Having a friend involved with dating violence

Adolescent patients exhibiting these signs should trigger additional inquiry into the possibility of his or her involvement in dating abuse.

For many of the adolescents who experience dating violence, the lessons learned in early dating may serve as scripts for future relationships. Adolescence has been characterized as a window of opportunity in which an individual may prepare and learn healthy relationship skills such as negation, compromise, and conflict resolution.[68] Whether inpatient or outpatient, the nurse should utilize this window to provide information, discuss situations, and answer any questions the adolescent may have. Nonjudgmental and confidential inquiry into the nature of any sexual activity, including exposure risks for unplanned pregnancy and sexually transmitted infections (STIs), as well as any concurrent drug and alcohol use, is essential. Health care providers must remember that the adolescent may feel more comfortable without the parent or caregiver in the room and should always ask before inquiring about intimate relationships.

Nurses caring for women in family planning, prenatal, obstetric, and postpartum settings should screen for IPV among all patients. An opportune time for female patients to be screened for IPV is at their family planning or yearly gynecologic visits. Additionally, women who present frequently for treatment of STIs, emergency contraception, or unplanned pregnancies should be screened at every clinical encounter because these conditions may be associated with pressured or coerced sex as well as violence. Women receiving prenatal care should be screened a minimum of 3 times during pregnancy for IPV, as current research indicates that domestic violence increases as a pregnancy progresses. Women who frequently miss prenatal appointments or who are screened late in pregnancy should be assessed at every clinical encounter for violence. Positive responses to screening during pregnancy should alert the nurse to the potential for continued abuse of the women and future child maltreatment. Safety planning measures for leaving an abusive relationship should be discussed following a positive response to violence screening, regardless of the woman's immediate intention to leave the relationship. These plans should be reviewed and revised as needed at successive clinical encounters.[66] Positive findings for IPV when there are children in the home should prompt concurrent inquiry into the possibility of child maltreatment.

Conclusion

Children and their families who live in violent homes pose a special challenge for the health care system. Of the 3.2 million reports of suspected child maltreatment that were reported to state agencies in 2007, the majority were made by professionals who, without a personal relationship, just happened to be working with those children.[11] That is, along with school personnel, nurses and other health care personnel represent the front line of defense for children who are the victims of maltreatment. For children who are not yet school-aged, the nurse and his or her health care colleagues stand alone as the front line. Pediatric nurses have a unique position, as they work not only with their primary patient but with that child's primary caregiver and possibly other members of that child's household as well, including siblings and extended family. Because of the propensity for violent behavior to beget additional violent behavior or to produce collateral victims, these nurses must be vigilant in assessing not only for evidence of maltreatment in their primary patients but in the family members that accompany them to the health care visits. The parent who has been successful in protecting his or her child from the violence that has been inflicted on her or himself is unlikely to remain successful forever. It is incumbent on the pediatric practitioner to routinely screen caregivers for abuse; ask questions of the caregivers in the context of discipline and safety, including the safety of the caregiver; document any findings that may indicate abuse; assess the risk to the safety of children and caregiver; and then respond with appropriate follow-up appointments and, where necessary, referrals (RADAR).[66]

There are both real and perceived barriers to the effective implementation of comprehensive screening and intervention programs, that is programs that concomitantly address the entirety of the violent home, namely concomitant IPV and child maltreatment. In some cases, nurses who are primarily trained in pediatrics or in women's health may be reluctant to screen for violence and abuse within families because of inadequate training and lack of experience with high-conflict families. Caring for children who have suffered abuse may make it difficult to provide services for a violent parent who may also have been victimized in the home. Finally, the nurse's own experience with violence in the home must also be recognized as having the potential to affect the care the nurse gives to victims or perpetrators of violence.[69] It is the strong recommendation of these authors that both nurse training programs and nursing continuing education programs provide training in the effective recognition of and intervention into violent homes. An example of this type of program already in place is in the State of Florida, wherein continuing education in IPV is required every third license renewal for all health care providers.

Through routine screening for violent homes, a greater degree of safety can be established for the children and their caregivers who live in those homes. This is because routine screening is itself a form of intervention as it encourages the victims of violence to report their maltreatment in a safe environment. A child may be empowered by the knowledge that someone outside of the home knows of the danger he or she is in and that the individual is available to help seek safety. This in turn may lead to an increase in reporting, and an exodus from such relationships. When children are identified as either being abused or at high risk for experiencing violence, assessment of and mandatory referral to local CPS organizations and law enforcement agencies is indicated to provide immediate relief for the children, and may provide relief for the caregiver victim, as well.

Finally, screening can be a productive intervention when applied to nonviolent families as well. Professional reporting of suspected child maltreatment or IPV is dependent upon interaction of the victims with teachers, health care workers, or other professionals. Screening questions, when asked of individuals who are not in violent homes, increases that individual's awareness and increases the chance that they may recognize violent predilection when it is present in neighbors or friends. Violence thrives when it is hidden from view and is most effectively addressed when it is exposed. The key to increasing the exposure of violence is the awareness and proactive screening activity on the part of all members of the nursing community.

References

1. Tolan P, Gorman-Smith D, Henry D. Family violence. *Annu Rev Psychol.* 2006;57:557-583.
2. Jouriles EN, McDonald R, Slep AM, Heyman RE, Garrido E. Child abuse in the context of domestic violence: prevalence, explanations, and practice implications. *Violence Vict.* 2008;23(2):221-235.
3. Taylor CA, Guterman NB, Lee SJ, Rathouz PJ. Intimate partner violence, maternal stress, nativity, and risk for maternal maltreatment of young children. *Am J Public Health.* 2009;99(1):175-183.
4. Slep AM, O'Leary SG. Parent and partner violence in families with young children: rates, patterns, and connections. *J Consult Clin Psychol.* 2005;73(3):435-444.
5. Jewkes R. Intimate partner violence: causes and prevention. *Lancet.* 2002;359 (9315):1423-1429.
6. Pearlman LA, Courtois CA. Clinical applications of the attachment framework: relational treatment of complex trauma. *J Trauma Stress.* 2005;18(5):449-459.
7. van der Hart O, Nijenhuis ERS, Steele K. Dissociation: an insufficiently recognized major feature of complex posttraumatic stress disorder. *J Trauma Stress.* 2005;18(5):413-423.
8. Flaherty EG, Thompson R, Litrownik AJ, et al. Effect of early childhood adversity on child health. *Arch Pediatr Adolesc Med.* 2006;160(12):1232-1238.

9. Centers for Disease Control and Prevention National Center for Injury Prevention and Control. Understanding teen dating violence fact sheet. Centers for Disease Control and Prevention Web site. http://www.cdc.gov/violenceprevention/pdf/TeenDatingViolence2009-a.pdf. Accessed December 19, 2009.

10. Knickerbocker L, Heyman RE, Smith Slep AM, Jouriles EN, McDonald R. Co-occurrence of child and partner maltreatment: definitions, prevalence, theory, and implications for assessment. *Eur Psychol.* 2007;12(1):36-44.

11. United States Department of Health and Human Services. *Child Maltreatment 2007.* Washington, DC: United States Department of Health and Human Services, Administration on Children, Youth and Families; 2009.

12. Centers for Disease Control and Prevention. Understanding intimate partner violence: fact sheet. Centers for Disease Control and Prevention Web site. http://www.cdc.gov/violenceprevention/pdf/IPV_factsheet-a.pdf. Accessed 2012.

13. Tjaden P, Thoennes N. *Extent, Nature, and Consequences of Intimate Partner Violence: Findings from the National Violence Against Women Survey.* Washington, DC: United States Department of Justice, Office of Justice Programs, National Institute of Justice; 2000.

14. Casanueva C, Martin SL, Runyan DK. Repeated reports for child maltreatment among intimate partner violence victims: findings from the National Survey of Child and Adolescent Well-Being. *Child Abuse Negl.* 2009;33(2):84-93.

15. Caetano R, Vaeth P, Ramisetty-Mikler S. Intimate partner violence victim and perpetrator characteristics among couples in the United States. *J Fam Violence.* 2008;23(6):507-518.

16. Appel AE, Holden GW. The co-occurrence of spouse and physical child abuse: a review and appraisal. *J Fam Psychol.* 1998;12(4):578-599.

17. McFarlane AC. Military deployment: the impact on children and family adjustment and the need for care. *Curr Opin Psychiatry.* 2009;22(4):369-373.

18. Rentz ED, Martin SL, Gibbs DA, Clinton-Sherrod M, Hardison J, Marshall SW. Family Violence in the military: a review of the literature. *Trauma Violence Abuse.* 2006;7(2):93-108.

19. Campbell JC, Lewandowski LA. Mental and physical health effects of intimate partner violence on women and children. *Psychiatr Clin North Am.* 1997;20(2):353-374.

20. Leeb RT, Paulozzi LJ, Melanson C, Simon TR, Arias I. *Child Maltreatment Surveillance: Uniform Definitions for Public Health and Recommended Data Elements.* Version 1.0. Atlanta, GA: Centers for Disease Control and Prevention National Center for Injury Prevention and Control; 2008.

21. Saltzman LE, Fanslow JL, McMahon PM, Shelley GA. *Intimate Partner Violence Surveillance: Uniform Definitions and Recommended Data Elements.* Version 1.0. Atlanta, GA: Centers for Disease Control and Prevention National Center for Injury Prevention and Control; 2002.

22. Phillips DA, Phillips KH, Grupp K, Trigg LJ. Sibling violence silenced: rivalry, competition, wrestling, playing, roughhousing, benign. *ANS Adv Nurs Sci.* 2009;32(2):E1-E16.

23. Crume TL, DiGuiseppi C, Byers T, Sirotnak AP, Garrett CJ. Underascertainment of child maltreatment fatalities by death certificates, 1990-1998. *Pediatrics.* 2002;110(2, pt 1):e18.

24. Zielinski DS. Child maltreatment and adult socioeconomic well-being. *Child Abuse Negl.* 2009;33(10):666-678.

25. Child Welfare Information Gateway. Child abuse and neglect fatalities 2009: statistics and interventions. United States Department of Health and Human Services Web site. http://www.childwelfare.gov/pubs/factsheets/fatality.cfm. Accessed November 8, 2009.

26. Black MC, Breiding MJ; Centers for Disease Control National Center for Injury Prevention and Control. Adverse health conditions and health risk behaviors associated with intimate partner violence—United States, 2005. *MMWR.* 2008;57(05):113-117.

27. Corso PS, Edwards VJ, Fang X, Mercy JA. Health-related quality of life among adults who experienced maltreatment during childhood. *Am J Public Health.* 2008;98(6):1094-1100.

28. Rennison CM, Welchans S. Intimate partner violence. Bureau of Justice Statistics special report: intimate partner violence. Bureau of Justice Statistics Web site. http://www.bjs.gov/content/pub/pdf/ipv.pdf. Published May 2000. Accessed January 9, 2014.

29. Ehrensaft MK. Intimate partner violence: persistence of myths and implications for intervention. *Child Youth Serv Rev.* 2008;30(3):276-286.

30. Strasburger V, Donnerstein E. Children, adolescents, and the media: issues and solutions. *Pediatrics.* 1999;103(1):129-139.

31. Lane WG, Dubowitz H. Primary care pediatricians' experience, comfort and competence in the evaluation and management of child maltreatment: do we need child abuse experts? *Child Abuse Negl.* 2009;33(2):76-83.

32. McDougall T. Safeguarding vulnerable children. *Paediatr Nurs.* 2008;20(3):14-17.

33. Elliott V. Speaking up for children. interview by Catherine Sadler. *Nurs Stand.* 2004;18(19):59.

34. Rhea MH, Chafey KH, Dohner VA, Terragno R. The silent victims of domestic violence—who will speak? *J Child Adolesc Psychiatr Nurs.* 1996;9(3):7-15.

35. Cox CE, Kotch JB, Everson MD. A longitudinal study of modifying influences in the relationship between domestic violence and child maltreatment. *J Fam Violence.* 2003;18(1):5-17.

36. Carpenter GL, Stacks AM. Developmental effects of exposure to intimate partner violence in early childhood: a review of the literature. *Child Youth Services Rev.* 2009;31(8):831-839.

37. Magan RH. In the best interests of battered women: reconceptualizing allegations of failure to protect. *Child Maltreat.* 1999;4(2):127-135.

38. Shipman KL, Rossman BBR, West JC. Co-occurrence of spousal violence and child abuse: conceptual implications. *Child Maltreat.* 1999;4(2):93-102.

39. Shalansky C, Eriksen J, Henderson A. Abused women and child custody: the ongoing exposure to abusive ex-partners. *J Adv Nurs.* 1999;29(2):416-426.

40. Taylor CA, Sorenson SB. Intervention on behalf of children exposed to intimate partner violence: assessment of support in a diverse community-based sample. *Child Abuse Negl.* 2007;31(11-12):1155-1168.

41. Bennett LW. Substance abuse and the domestic assault of women. *Soc Work.* 1995;40(6):760-771.

42. Edleson JL, Ellerton AL, Seagren EA, Kirchberg SL, Schmidt SO, Ambrose AT. Assessing child exposure to adult domestic violence. *Child Youth Services Rev.* 2007;29(7):961-971.

43. Ainsworth MDS, Blehar MC, Waters E, Wall S. *Patterns of Attachment: A Psychological Study of the Strange Situation.* Hillsdale, NJ: Lawrence Erlbaum Associates; 1978.

44. Bowlby J. Attachment and loss: retrospect and prospect. *Am J Orthopsychiatry.* 1982;52(4):664-678.

45. Watts-English T, Fortson BL, Gibler N, Hooper SR, De Bellis MD. The psychobiology of maltreatment in childhood. *J Soc Issues.* 2006;62(4):717-736.

46. Ernst AA, Weiss SJ, Hall J, et al. Adult intimate partner violence perpetrators are significantly more likely to have witnessed intimate partner violence as a child than nonperpetrators. *Am J Emerg Med.* 2009;27(6):641-650.

47. Fang X, Corso PS. Child maltreatment, youth violence, and intimate partner violence: developmental relationships. *Am J Prev Med.* 2007;33(4):281-290.

48. Eisikovits Z, Grauwiler P, Mills LG, Winstok Z. Recent trends in intimate violence: theory and intervention volume II. *Child Youth Services Rev.* 2008;30(6):613-615.

49. Burgess AW, Holmstrom LL. Rape trauma syndrome. *Am J Psychiatry.* 1974;131 (9):981-986.

50. Schwarz ED, Perry BD. The posttraumatic response in children and adolescents. *Psychiatr Clin North Am.* 1994;17(2):311-326.

51. Runyon MK, Faust J, Orvaschel H. Differential symptom pattern of post-traumatic stress disorder (PTSD) in maltreated children with and without concurrent depression. *Child Abuse Negl.* 2002;26(1):39-53.

52. Margolin G, Vickerman KA. Post-traumatic stress in children and adolescents exposed to family violence: I. overview and issues. *Prof Psycho Res Pr.* 2007;38(6):613-619.

53. Putman SE. The monsters in my head: posttraumatic stress disorder and the child survivor of sexual abuse. *J Counseling Dev.* 2009;87(1):80-89.

54. Frederick J, Goddard C. 'School was just a nightmare': childhood abuse and neglect and school experiences. *Child Fam Soc Work.* 2010;15(1):22-30.

55. Crooks CV, Scott KL, Wolfe DA, Chiodo D, Killip S. Understanding the link between childhood maltreatment and violent delinquency: what do schools have to add? *Child Maltreat.* 2007;12(3):269-280.

56. Child Welfare Information Gateway. Recognizing child abuse and neglect: signs and symptoms. United States Department of Health and Human Services Web site. https://www.childwelfare.gov/preventing/overview/recognize.cfm. Accessed January 10, 2014.

57. Botash AS. Child abuse and treatment for medical providers. Child Abuse MD Web site. http://childabusemd.com/. Accessed October 31, 2009.

58. Cheung KK. Identifying and documenting findings of physical child abuse and neglect. *J Pediatr Health Care.* 1999;13(3, pt 1):142-143.

59. Dubowitz H, Bennett S. Physical abuse and neglect of children. *Lancet.* 2007;369(9576):1891-1899.

60. Gilbert R, Kemp A, Thoburn J, et al. Recognizing and responding to child maltreatment. *Lancet.* 2009;373(9658):167-180.

61. Reece RM, Christian CW, eds. *Child Abuse: Medical Diagnosis and Management.* 3rd ed. Elk Grove, IL: American Academy of Pediatrics; 2009.

62. Hymel K, Boos S. Conditions mistaken for child physical abuse. In: Reece RM, Christian CW, eds. *Child Abuse: Medical Diagnosis and Management.* 3rd ed. Elk Grove, IL: American Academy of Pediatrics; 2009:227-256.

63. Jenny C, Reece RM. Cutaneous manifestations of child abuse. In: Reece RM, Christian CW, eds. *Child Abuse: Medical Diagnosis and Management.* 3rd ed. Elk Grove, IL: American Academy of Pediatrics; 2009.

64. Child Welfare Information Gateway. Long-term consequences of child abuse and neglect. United States Department of Health and Human Services Web site. www.childwelfare.gov/pubs/factsheets/long_term_consequences.cfm. Published 2013. Accessed January 10, 2014.

65. Parker B. Abuse of adolescents: what can we learn from pregnant teenagers? *AWHONNS Clin Issues Perinat Women's Health Nurs.* 1993;4(3):363-370.

66. The Institute for Safe Families; American Academy of Pediatrics, Pennsylvania Chapter. RADAR for pediatrics: a domestic violence intervention. Institute for Safe Families Imagining a Better Future Web site. http://www.instituteforsafefamilies.org/materials/m/radar. Accessed June 18, 2013.

67. Herrman JW. There's a fine line...adolescent dating violence and prevention. *Pediatr Nurs.* 2009;35(3):164-170.

68. Wolfe DA, Wekerle C, Scott K, et al. Dating violence prevention with at-risk youth: a controlled outcome evaluation. *J Consult Clin Psychol.* 2003;71(2):279-291.

69. Shea CA, Mahoney M, Lacey JM. Breaking through the barriers to domestic violence intervention. *Am J Nurs.* 1997;97(6):26-33

Chapter 16

Risks to Children in the Digital Age of the Internet and Social Networking*

Elizabeth Dowdell, PhD, MS, RN

Key Points

1. National studies have found that the majority of today's youth are using the Internet as a venue for social interaction, idea sharing, artistic creation, photography, schoolwork, and online journaling or blogging.[1-3]
2. The prolific use of the Internet by youth has also resulted in their exposure to a variety of sexual and violent material, financial scams, cyberbulling, and harassment and placed them at risk for meeting dangerous people or predators.
3. Online risky behavior can be inclusive of more than one behavior. Internet risk behaviors that have been found to cluster together include sharing of personal information (eg, name of school, email address, picture of self); corresponding online with an unknown person or later meeting the person offline; engaging in online-initiated harassment (eg, malicious or offensive jokes); visiting online-initiated sex sites; and overriding Internet filters or blocks.[1,2,4-6]
4. Only 29.4% of the Internet offenders who entered chat rooms used their true identity, over half (58.8%) disguised their identity by name or age, and the remaining 11.8% reported having varied their means of identification.[7]
5. National and local news stations are reporting numerous stories of teens taking nude photos of themselves or others and sharing them by way of texting or posting them online. This practice, now known as *sexting*, refers to "sexual communication with content that includes both pictures and text messages, sent using cell phones and other electronic media."[8] This practice can also include children and teens in the acts of undressing each other, touching each other, or having sex.
5. The media has reported that teens whose inappropriate or lurid photos have been sexted to others have experienced bullying and exclusion by their peer group. As a consequence of this type of shunning, reports suggest these teens have experienced depression and anxiety and have even become suicidal.[9] Additionally, college admissions staff and human resource (HR) departments are increasingly asking for access to personal Web pages to view what the applicant has posted. Sexting-related pictures posted the Internet may reflect poorly on the teen and affect future employment and academic acceptance.

Sections of the following have been adapted, with permission, from the American Journal of Nursing, the monograph *A Multi-Prong Approach to Strengthening Internet Child Safety* from the National Center for Missing and Exploited Children and Chapter 16, *Risks to Children in the Digital Age* by Eileen M. Alexy, RN, MSN.

6. During the history-taking or interview phase of the assessment, questions focused on risky online and offline behaviors can be asked directly. By asking questions about Internet behaviors, health care providers can detect risky Internet behaviors or problems early, much in the way that health care providers screen for other health-risk behaviors, such as smoking and alcohol use.
7. It is essential that the nurse maintain patience with these victims and not blame the child.

Introduction

The advent of the Internet, with its instant worldwide access to information, has transformed daily life and become a primary means of business and personal communication across the world. Over the past decade, Internet use among children and adolescents has shown to be 3 times greater than that of television and 9 times greater than that of radio.[6] More children, adolescents, and young adults are reporting that they use the Internet as their primary mode of communication, social networking, and delivery of personal pictures and information.[1,2,10-12] Adolescents can gain access to the Internet from almost anywhere, including their home computer, a computer at a friend's house, wireless zones, and video game systems. Even cell phones can facilitate electronic communication with anyone else who has a cell phone or email account, 24 hours a day, 7 days a week. With increased access comes increased responsibility on the part of parents, educators, and law enforcement to impose safeguards to protect children from potentially harmful material and potentially risky behavior.

Internet safety and awareness appears to be growing, with many children, adolescents, and parents becoming informed of the potential dangers of the Internet through the media, schools, and even the Internet itself. Adults are generally aware that the Internet is not always safe and understand that children do not perceive the potential threats posed by the Internet. The current generation of high school students take the Internet for granted because they have grown up in a technology-based society wherein the Internet has entirely replaced the full gamut of informational resources upon which earlier generations relied. The dramatic growth in use of, if not reliance on, the Internet has become fully integrated into the current generation of high school students' activities of everyday living.

The world at large has benefitted enormously from the Internet; however, it is becoming increasingly evident that there is a dark side to the Internet. The technology that permits the virtual instant transfer of information to the entire developed world and most of the underdeveloped world is the same technology that can be harnessed as a powerful tool for criminally motivated individuals. Among the many areas of Internet-based criminal activity, the alarming rise in Internet-transmitted child pornography is of global importance. Additionally, there is growing apprehension about the potential for self-exploitation, cyber bullying, harassment, access to pornography, online predators, sexual solicitation, identity theft, and cyberstalking.

When discussing Internet crimes against children, much of the focus of law enforcement, safety programs, and the public has been on identifying and apprehending the offenders. However, a new category consisting of individuals victimized online has emerged. Online victimization often results in offline consequences, specifically sexual victimization, exploitation, and fraud. Health care providers play a pivotal role in providing diagnostic and clinical intervention services to victimized and exploited individuals across the lifespan. The health care provider's biopsychosocial training and presence in facilities where children, adolescents, and families seek services present a unique opportunity to provide intervention, education, and counseling regarding matters of human sexuality and Internet safety. An understanding of the methods used by sex offenders and schemers to exploit and lure children in the context of the Internet is essential for families, law enforcement personnel, nurses, and other health care providers. Knowledge regarding these matters is necessary to develop and provide effective prevention and treatment strategies for child victims and their families in schools, communities, emergency rooms (ERs), and pediatric and psychiatric settings.

Risky Behaviors on the Internet

Risky behavior, a frequent part of an adolescent's growth and development, can increase as the individual ages. Historically, risky behaviors seen in the health arena have included smoking cigarettes, alcohol, and drug use, as well as sexual experimentation. The contemporary health care setting now also sees risk-taking behaviors manifest in the online arena as a result of the increased presence of the Internet in daily life. National studies have found that the majority of today's youth are using the Internet as a venue for social interaction, idea sharing, artistic creations, photography, school work, and online journaling or blogging.[1-3] Still, using the Internet also means that they are at risk for being exposed to a variety of sexual and violent material, financial scams, cyberbullying, harassment, and for meeting dangerous people or predators.[1,2,4,7] Such risk is evidenced by reports made by children and adolescents disclosing exposure to undesired sexual material, explicit pictures, online harassment, and aggressive solicitation.[13] Individual online risky behavior can be inclusive of more than one behavior. Internet risk behaviors that have been found to cluster together include sharing of personal information (eg, name of school, email address, picture of self); corresponding online with an unknown person or later meeting the person offline; engaging in online-initiated harassment (eg, malicious or offensive jokes); visiting online-initiated sex sites; and overriding Internet filters or blocks.[1,2,4-6]

Recent research has found differences regarding online behavior based on age. For example, early adolescents—middle school students (grades 6 through 8, aged 11 through 14 years)—often have different levels of participation when compared to older adolescents that are high school students (grades 9 through 12, aged 15 through 19 years). In one study, middle school students were asked a series of questions about personal information and the Internet.[4,5] As a result, a clustering of Internet risk behaviors was established from the students (20%) who reported posting their pictures on the Internet. The risk behaviors included sharing personal information (eg, name of school, e-mail address, picture of self); corresponding online with an unknown person or later meeting person or developing a relationship; engaging in online-initiated harassment (eg, malicious or offensive jokes); visiting online-initiated sex sites; and overriding Internet filters or blocks. The study found that 20% (81 of the 404 surveyed) of the middle school teen students who posted their picture on the Internet were more likely to post the name of their school and their e-mail address, send their picture to someone online, receive an e-mail or instant message (IM) from an online stranger, and feel more threatened while on the Internet when compared to students who did not post their picture.[4,5]

High school students have also demonstrated a clustering of Internet risk behaviors but reported higher participation rates than middle school students. In one study, 54.4% of the high school student sample reported posting a picture online; that behavior had a significant relationship with the same behaviors as the middle school students, except that the high school students did not post their home address.[7] Instead, high school students were more likely to post their school name and address in lieu of their home address, a finding that may be reflective of their age; use of the Internet; and an outcome of Internet safety programs that now emphasize that an individual should no longer post personal information (eg, home address, phone number) to the Internet. It is important to understand that posting personal information online does not, by itself, appear to be a particularly risky behavior. However, the clustering of several behaviors associated with posting a picture may place the vulnerable youth at risk.[7,14]

There is a growing trend with the youth population wherein personal friends solicit peers online or share personal information with unknown people offline.[5,15] In a 2000 report on the Internet behaviors of children and adolescents, only 3% of the youth interviewed reported that their online friend tried to solicit them. By 2005, 14% of the youth reported their online friends as participating in solicitation or harassment. That there is an increase in the reporting of friends sharing and giving out information is in contrast to the low numbers of youth, only 5%, who have reported any direct sexual solicitation or harassment to law enforcement or to their Internet service providers.[15]

Online Victimization

Children and adolescents may experience any of the following forms of online victimization[13,16]:

— Sexual solicitation by an adult wherein the adult requests the child to participate in sexual activities or a sexual conversation

— Aggressive sexual solicitation, which may involve offline (in-person) contact with the solicitor; potential unwanted exposure to sexual material such as explicit photos

— Online harassment

— Involvement in distressing events where the child finds himself or herself upset or afraid over an online incident

Social Networking Sites

The mid-1970s witnessed the electronic linking of computers to form the basis of computer-mediated scientific collaboration, social interaction, and networking. 2010 witnessed an explosion of social networking sites serving a wide variety of interests and individuals. Indeed, social networks have created a public service that encourages relationships between people and content they wish to share. Not surprisingly, children and adolescents use social networking sites in large numbers. In one study, the majority (88%) of the 2077 high school students in the study reported using social networking sites. Girls reported using social network sites more often than did boys, 91.1% and 84.1% respectively. However, more girls (81.4%) than boys (61.6%) reported using a privacy setting on their social network accounts that made their pages available only to those they granted access.[7] The same study reported that college-age students also use social networking sites, with 91.4% routinely online and Facebook reported as the most popular site used. Female college students (15%) reported visiting a greater variety of Web sites than did their male counterparts (3%).[7] Sex offenders; Internet offenders who self-reported only an Internet-related sexual offense, such as possessing or transmitting child pornography or soliciting a minor over the Internet; and men with a sexual offense that was not Internet-related, including child molesters, rapists, and generic offenders with no known offenses against children who also reported using social networking. In this group, the most popular site among those who reported using a social networking site was Myspace, followed by Facebook. Also, the majority of offenders in this study reported disguising their identities when online in teen or child chat rooms; no reported findings specify if this also applies to their social network profile.[7]

That adolescent and college-age students have been found to have a higher variety of social networking websites than the offender group, including those who lived in the community and may have had unrestricted Internet access depending upon their probation restrictions, which may be reflective of the adolescent's developmental milestones at this age, which include experimenting in order to define self, developing autonomy, and fitting in with peers. That the adult offenders are also using social networking sites supports studies in the published literature that indicate social networks have significant adult use.[1,14,17] Social networking sites such as Myspace and Facebook are currently very popular with both adult offenders and adolescents; however, there are fewer well-known sites that cannot be ignored and must be considered when asking about social networking sites. Tagged™, founded in 2004, gained notoriety in 2012.[18] Tagged enables users to build and customize profiles. Initially targeted at teens in the United States, Tagged was opened to users worldwide aged 13 years and older in October 2006. Tagged implemented several security features to increase online safety for users, including a minimum participation age of 13 years; viewing restrictions to prevent the public from viewing the profiles of 13- and 14-year-old participants; viewing restrictions to prevent the public and users aged 18 years and older from viewing the profiles of 15- and 16-year-old participants; networking restrictions requiring participants to have the e-mail address or surname of the person from whom he or she would like to request friendship; and further networking restrictions requiring the solicited participant to reciprocate any requests for friendship by accepting the solicitor's request. The security measures were not, however, entirely successful. In February 2009, a high school teacher was arrested after having sex with a 14-year-old girl he met on Tagged. It was found that the 32-year-old man had over 100 female friends aged under 17 years. In December 2009, New York Attorney General Andrew Cuomo announced that Tagged and 13 other social networking sites agreed to remove registered sex offenders from among their users as part of the New York Electronic Securing and Targeting of Online Predators Act.[18]

Transparency, not using a privacy setting, is often the standard among adults who create social networking profiles. The majority of adult profiles are open to the general public for viewing and review. Research on social networks has found that most adult Internet users (82%) who maintain an online profile say that their profile is currently visible online, as compared with 77% of online teens.[14] Among the adults who say they have a visible profile, 60% say the profile can be seen by anyone who happens upon it, while 38% say their profile is only accessible to friends.[14] Studies show adolescents tend to make conservative choices with respect to visibility of their profile; 40% said their profile was visible to anyone, and 59% reported that it was restricted to friends only,[1] with high school girls more likely to have and use privacy settings on their social networking Web page than the boys.

Chat Rooms

Internet chat rooms are very popular with children and adolescents.[5,14-16,19] Chat rooms were designed as a place where individuals or groups could share information with another individual or group by way of text. These virtual rooms provide the ability to hold a digital conversation with multiple people and provide a different mode of communication from IM programs that are typically designed for one-to-one communication. The majority of chat room users enter a given room based on a shared interest or other similar connection and use the chat room as a means to discuss topics related to that shared interest. New technology has developed that has enabled the use of file sharing and webcams in the chat room, in addition to the traditional plain text.

For children and adolescents, chat rooms can be a fun place to exchange ideas, experiences, and information on any topic of interest. Many make use of age-appropriate chat rooms, ensuring that the individuals with whom they chat are same-aged peers. Although many children and adolescents use chat rooms without incident, a disturbing finding is emerging from the literature that suggests chat rooms can also be dangerous places. In one recent study, middle school students identified chat rooms as a place to meet, who they believe to be, teenaged strangers online. One-third of the boys and 12.5% of the girls reported accessing open chat rooms with other locations, including game rooms (13.6% of boys) and Web pages (18.8% of girls), with only 9 students indicating that the Web site was monitored by a parent or adult. Of the 59 middle school students who reported chatting with strangers online, 32 met the stranger offline, and 3 reported sexual assault.[4] High school students also reported frequently using chat rooms. When asked about meeting strangers online, high school girls reported that they met the stranger on a specific Web page or site (33.6%), using IM (20%), or in a chat room (6.4%), whereas boys met strangers using IM (24.1%), on a specific Web page or site (12.8%), or in a chatroom (11.3%).[7] Of the high school students who reported meeting offline with a stranger, 22.6% of the boys and 36.9% of the girls reported that "something sexual" happened at the meeting. From this group, 6.8% of the boys and 4.5% of the girls reported being threatened or sexually assaulted as a result of the meeting.[7]

Of importance is the knowledge that adult sex offenders also report accessing teen chat rooms. One study found that 41.7% of the Internet offender sample who were also child molesters reported visiting teen chat rooms, followed by 30% of the Internet-only offenders, and 12.8% of the child-molester-only group.[7] A small percentage of the Internet offenders (29.4%) who entered chat rooms used their true identity, over half (58.8%) disguised their identity by name or age, and the remaining 11.8% reported having varied their means of identification.[7] Offenders were also found to be more likely to introduce the topic of sex into an Internet chat session than middle school or high school students.[7] Internet offenders were most likely to introduce the topic of sex into the first chat session or in the 2nd through 6th session, with the remaining introducing sex in the 7th session.[7] Some differences were noted between the genders in the student populations with boys being more likely to seek out the topic of sex when online than girls.[7] Additionally, high school boys were more likely to report having gone to an inappropriate Web site or chat room, and both early adolescent and adolescent boys were more likely to be exposed to sexual talk than girls.[7]

Self-exploitation Behaviors and Sexting

Self-exploitation, specifically the creating and distributing of explicit or inappropriate pictures of oneself or peers is an emerging high-risk Internet behavior that can have long-term implications. National and local news stations are reporting numerous stories of teens taking nude photos of themselves or others and sharing them by way of texting or posting them online.[9,20] This practice, now known as ***sexting***, refers to "sexual communications with content that includes both pictures and text messages, sent using cell phones and other electronic media."[8] This practice can also include children and teens in the acts of undressing each other, touching each other, or having sex. It is a growing phenomenon as more youth have cell phones capable of sending sexually explicit messages, photos, or videos. A recent study using a national sample of youth aged 12 through 17 years reported that 4% of these adolescents had created and then sent nude, nearly nude, or sexually suggestive images by way of electronic media.[21] Another study asked current high school students about sexting, specifically if they knew about it, had experienced it, or knew of someone who had experienced it. Findings indicated that over 50% of the high school students reported that they knew about sexting, with more girls (56.7%) reporting knowing about sexting than boys (46.9%). Almost one-third of the students (31.3%), again with more girls than boys, knew someone who had engaged in sexting. These numbers changed when the students were asked if they had ever been sexted, with more boys (17.6%) responding that they had been sexted than girls (13.4%).[7]

Sexting images can also be posted on social networking Web sites where they can be downloaded and shared. The potential consequences of such exposure are far-ranging and can include legal charges of child pornography and indecent exposure. In addition, the photos can end up in the hands of child predators.[16] The social implications of sexting can be just as devastating for teens when photos are viewed by members of a team, school, or community. Once something is posted to the Internet, it never goes away; therefore, humiliation and emotional consequences of sexting can be long-term in nature.[16] The media has reported that teens whose inappropriate or lurid photos have been sexted to others have experienced bullying and exclusion by their peer group. As a consequence of this type of shunning, reports suggest these teens have experienced depression and anxiety and have even become suicidal.[9] Additionally, college admissions staff and HR departments are increasingly asking for access to personal Web pages to view what the applicant has posted. Sexting-related pictures posted on the Internet may reflect poorly on the teen and affect future employment and academic acceptance.

Online Relationships

Online relationships are increasing in the adolescent population,[22] and while many can be rewarding, others can be dangerous. Many adolescents choose to enter into a casual online friendship or romantic relationship because the Internet provides easy access to individuals different from their families, schoolmates, and neighbors.[5,22-24] It is not uncommon for children and adolescents to turn to the Internet in order to find some sort of support system or friend. Youth that turn to online relationships for support, affirmation, and affection may do so because of feelings of isolation from their families or peers. Problems identified in the literature that are of concern for the adolescent are frequent parent-child conflicts, a history of psychological distress, low levels of communication ability, and high levels of delinquency.[22] Differences between genders have been identified in the literature, with girls who form close online relationships often having high levels of child-parent conflict, above average levels of depression, a history of a past victimization, and traumatic life events. Boys who form similar relationships tend to be non-Hispanic white and have low communication levels with parents, a history of psychological distress, and high Internet usage.[22]

Youth who form online associations can form unrealistic expectations regarding these relationships. To combat feelings of loneliness and isolation, the adolescent can become fixated on the online relationship, believing that they can depend on these online friends for all social contact and support. For the adolescent whose online relationship is with someone at a distance, troubling feelings may intensify the youth's isolation when the online individual is unable or unwilling to meet offline.[24] Adolescents who form these close online relationships often have associated issues that can put the youth at risk for harassment, bullying, solicitation, and exploitation.

Electronic Aggression

Electronic aggression is a relatively new form of bullying that is increasing in prevalence in the adolescent population. At this time there is no one concrete and widely agreed upon or accepted definition of electronic aggression in the literature. However, Tokunaga[25] has proposed a comprehensive definition that states electronic aggression is "[a]ny behavior performed through electronic or digital media by individuals or groups that repeatedly communicates hostile or aggressive messages intended to inflict harm or discomfort on other." It is a definition that is inclusive of all forms of electronic media and also recognizes that both individuals and groups can perpetrate electronic aggression. Because there is no one definition of or strict criteria governing electronic aggression, there is not a consistent incidence or prevalence rate for electronic aggression; however, reports of cyberbullying and harassment are increasing.[26] Ybarra et al[26] reported from their national cross-sectional online survey of 1588 youths aged 10 through 15 years that 33% experienced online harassment in the past year, with 9% reporting an incident on a social networking site specifically. Another study estimated 9% to 34% of adolescents as victims of electronic aggression, as compared to 4% to 21% of adolescents estimated as perpetrators.[27]

While electronic aggression occurs across the lifespan, the majority of the current literature focuses on the population of children and adolescents. Although much of the current research does not support a relationship between age and electronic aggression, a few researchers have proposed a curvilinear hypothesis wherein electronic aggression occurs with greatest frequency during early adolescence, ages 11 through 13 years. For example, one study supporting this hypothesis involved 3339 youth in grades 5, 8, and 11. The adolescents reported higher rates for verbal and physical bullying than electronic aggression; however, when electronic aggression was looked at independently, it was found to have peaked in middle school and declined in high school. Specifically, electronic aggression had the lowest incidence among 5th graders (4.5%), the highest among 8th graders (12.9%), and had tapered off by 11th grade.[28] Wang et al[29] reported a similar finding, noting that 9th and 10th graders were significantly less involved in electronic aggressions than their younger 6th-grade peers. Interestingly, youths harassed online were significantly more likely to also report 2 or more detentions or suspensions and skipping school in the previous year. Additionally, youth who reported being targeted for Internet harassment were 8 times more likely than all other youth to concurrently report carrying a weapon to school in the past 30 days.[30]

For some students who reported posting their picture online there is a relationship with being vulnerable to online or offline school harassment, also known as electronic aggression.[14] The incidence of being bullied or harassed increased when using IM or having conversations in chat rooms. Although, when these researchers examined school bullying, 64% of youth who were harassed online did not report also being bullied at school.[14] Interestingly, 1 study reported that in the sample, the majority of youth who were targeted by Internet harassment did not appear to be upset by the experience, although almost 2 out of 5 (39%) reported a resulting feeling of emotional distress.[19] The study found that the distressed youths were significantly more likely to be preadolescents as opposed to adolescents and to have less experience with chat room use.[19]

Online Stalking

Stalking refers to harassing or threatening behavior that is engaged in repeatedly and is defined as a course of conduct directed at a specific person that would cause a reasonable person to feel fear.[31] Women are more likely to be the victims, though stalking incidents are reported to the police by men as often as by women, with young adults (most aged under 35 years) composing the majority of the stalking victims.[31] Interestingly, it appears that most victims know their stalker. Nearly 75% of victims in a United States Department of Justice study knew their offender in some capacity, 45% reported that the stalking offenders were acquaintances rather than intimate partners, and 30% of stalking offenders were identified as a current or former spouse or intimate partner.[31]

Technology, specifically the Internet, has become a quick and easy way for stalkers to monitor and harass their victims. This type of electronic harassment has been termed as cyberstalking. In a United States Department of Justice study (sample size: 65 270) more than one in four stalking victims reported that some form of cyberstalking was involved.[31] Victims reported receiving unwanted email (83%) or IMs (35%) from the stalker.[31] The use of electronic monitoring, such as surveillance devices, video, or digital cameras, in conjunction with listening devices or bugs was reported to have been used to stalk 1 in 13 victims who participated in the study.[31] Stalking online or offline may or may not be accompanied by a credible threat of serious harm; however, the potential for psychological damage is high and likely.[32] In the United States, each state has an anti-stalking law of which many adults and adolescents are unaware. As more adolescents go online to blog, network, e-mail, IM, do homework, play games, or shop, the potential for being targeted increases.

The Role of Health Care Providers in the Digital Age

In the diverse and complex health care, child welfare, educational, and juvenile law enforcement settings of the 21st century, professionals are increasingly encountering at-risk and risk-taking children and adolescents. Health care providers can be on the cutting edge of technology advances as learners and educators and impact the online behaviors of children and adolescents. School nurses or those practitioners working with adolescents in the community, inpatient, or outpatient settings are in a unique position to help adolescents and their families develop safe Internet behaviors. By better understanding patterns of Internet use, precursors and correlates of risky Internet behavior, and areas of vulnerability, health care providers can better inform the development of age- and language-appropriate curriculums and literature specifically designed to keep children safer on the Internet. The task, however, is to define the Internet in much the same way as other clearly identified domains of potential risk. The Internet, because it is a powerful force for good as well as a potential hazard, is a far more ambiguous health risk than other more conventional risky behaviors, such as smoking, alcohol use, and substance use. Health care providers care for children and families in a variety of settings and are therefore afforded the opportunity to provide education and counseling.

Awareness and Risk Assessment

Nurses can and do provide education about Internet safety behaviors. Nurses who are in the schools, community, private practice, or outpatient settings can incorporate Internet education into treatment plans when working with children and their families. Educational programs about safe Internet behaviors and risky behaviors in conjunction with resources available to contact for assistance must target parents, health care providers, educators, and other professionals who are in contact with adolescents. Education targeting adolescents about not sharing a friend or family member's Internet contact information must also be included in prevention education. Reinforcing the positive adolescent behavior of sharing both good and bad online experiences with their parents, educators, or clinicians should be encouraged.[23] Families or individuals who have had negative online experiences, must be encouraged by health care providers and other professionals to report inappropriate or dangerous online behaviors to their local police and to the National Center for Missing and Exploited Children (NCMEC), which coordinates the CyberTipline®. The NCMEC website contains links to organizations that have established Internet safety programs that have been used throughout the United States. These programs have used a variety of techniques to educate children and adolescents about Internet safety, such as online learning modules, curriculum-based programs, online games, virtual training, and online or Web-based workshops for adults and parents. Some programs have begun to employ the strategy of peer-to-peer models to promote Internet safety.[23]

During the history-taking or interview phase of the nursing assessment, questions focused on risky online and offline behaviors can be asked directly. By asking questions about Internet behaviors, health care providers can detect risky Internet behaviors or problems early, much in the way that nurses screen for health risk behaviors (eg, smoking, alcohol use). Online risks to children must be discussed in an open forum with developmentally appropriate assessment tools and educational materials. Parents are more often concerned about these issues than are children. Children, especially adolescents, often have a cavalier idea about the Internet,[33] maintaining that exploitation and crime will not happen to them but that they, instead, happen to the "other guy." This attitude is strongly related to their development from children into adolescents and must be factored into all assessments. Online risks to children are a public health concern; therefore, a risk assessment screening should be conducted with both parents and children. Questions that can provide insight into the child's online behaviors and practices include some of the following:

— Does the child surf the Internet alone?

— Does the child go online daily? If so, does he or she spend more than 2 hours per day online?

— Is the computer in a public space at home?

— Is the computer a desktop or a laptop?

— Does the child have a cell phone that has Internet access?

— What types of Internet services does the child use (eg, chat rooms, IM, e-mail)?

— Do the parents have a set of house rules regarding Internet use?

— Do the parents have the child's password(s) for e-mail, cell phone, social networking sites, Web sites, blogs, and other Internet-based applications?

— Does the child have an online profile? Where is this profile posted? Has the parent seen the profile?

— What has the child shared about him or herself online? Where is he or she sharing this information (eg, blog, personal Web site, social networking profile)?

— If the child participates in chat rooms, what types of chat rooms (eg, hobbies, sports, music, gaming)?

— What sites are being visited?

— Who is the child communicating with online?

— What does the child know about the individual(s) he or she is chatting with online? How did he or she meet the individual(s)?

— What types of Web sites does the child access (eg, health information, support groups, hobbies, gaming, music)?

Answers to these questions will indicate whether the child or adolescent is communicating with strangers or participating in other risky online behaviors. Health promotion, plans of care, and Internet safety interventions should be tailored to fit the child or adolescent's stage of development. Information gathered from the nursing assessment and health histories should be analyzed. If the health care provider is alerted to a possible Internet danger, the school hierarchy should convene a staff meeting to determine a plan of intervention. The various community, health, mental health, and educational resources need to be identified, so appropriate referrals may be made.[23]

Parents should be encouraged to surf the Web with their child routinely because it provides an excellent opportunity for the parent to spend quality time with his or her child and allows him or her to gain a better understanding of what the child is being exposed to online. Additionally, spending time online with children gives parents the opportunity to be the teachers. Health care providers should teach that efforts should be made to balance the amount of time children spend online with offline activities. Even though the Internet can be entertaining and educational, children should not become isolated from their real-life peers. In addition, it is beneficial to establish house rules or a contract with children for online safety and to locate computers in a public space, such as a living room, recreation room, classroom, or library. Many Internet safety experts recommend posting the rules next to the computer to avoid the phenomenon of out of sight, out of mind[34,35] (**Table 16-1**).

Table 16-1. Internet Rules for Parents
— Communicate. Talk to your child about sexual victimization and potential online danger.
— Spend time with your children online.
— Have your children teach you about their favorite online destinations.
— Keep the computer in a common room in the house, not in your child's bedroom. It is much more difficult for a computer sex offender to communicate with a child when the computer screen is visible to a parent or another member of the household.
— Use parental controls provided by your service provider, blocking software, or both. While electronic chat can be a great place for children to make new friends and discuss various topics of interest, it is also prowled by computer sex offenders. Use of chat rooms, in particular, should be heavily monitored. While parents should use these mechanisms, they should not totally rely on them.
— Always maintain access to your child's online account and randomly check his or her e-mail. Be aware that your child could be contacted through the Unites States Mail as well.
— Be up front with your child about your access and reasons why.
— Teach your child responsible use of resources online.
— Be aware that there is much more to the online experience than chat rooms.
— Find out what computer safeguards are used by your child's school, the public library, and at the homes of your child's friends. These are all places, outside your normal supervision, where your child could encounter an online predator.
— Understand, even if your child were a willing participant in any form of sexual exploitation, that he or she is not at fault and is the victim.
— Understand that the offender always bears complete responsibility for his or her actions.
(continued)

Table 16-1. Internet Rules for Parents *(continued)*

— Teach your child that they control the technology and that cell phones, laptops, iPads, tablets, and other data devices can be turned off. Encourage children not to sleep with their electronics in bed or near them. Help your child establish routine patterns of technology use during the day and at night.

— Instruct your children:

- — to never arrange a face-to-face meeting with someone they met online
- — to never upload (post) pictures of themselves onto the Internet or online service or to people they do not personally know
- — to never give out identifying information such as their name, home address, school name, or telephone number
- — to never download pictures from an unknown source, as there is a good chance there could be sexually explicit images
- — to never respond to messages or bulletin board postings that are suggestive, obscene, belligerent, or harassing
- — that whatever they are told online may or may not be true

Reprinted from United States Department of Justice; Federal Bureau of Investigation. A parent's guide to Internet safety. The FBI: Federal Bureau of Investigation Web site. http://www.fbi.gov/stats-services/publications/parent-guide/parentsguide.pdf. Accessed June 27, 2013.

Recommendations for parents with young children should include not having online profiles and when early adolescents want a social media page they should be given guidance on what to include in and where to post their profile. An online profile is a list of personal information that Internet service providers let you post online. This information allows other users to know more about you, such as your name, age, sex, address, hobbies, and interests. Children may think having a profile is fun; this is a serious mistake. Online profiles can provide a shopping list of information for sexual predators and can be more harmful than helpful. Knowledge of the types of Internet services children use allows providers to assess risk and to devise individual care plans of education for children, parents, and professionals who work with children. In particular, school nurses and public health nurses are in an excellent position to provide education to children, parents, and teachers regarding the nature of Internet risks.

Handling the Disclosure of Online and Offline Victimization

The most important thing to remember when a child discloses online or offline victimization is to remain calm and nonjudgmental. Often, children who are lured from their homes or schools by someone they encountered online are not completely naive. Frequently, they are curious, troubled, or rebellious adolescents searching for sexual information or companionship.[36] Children who are enticed or duped are usually looking to have their needs for attention and affection met.[36] Regardless of the events, these children have been enticed and manipulated by a shrewd offender, and often they are not fully aware of the consequences of their actions. As Summit[37] found, children who are sexually victimized may recant their stories after disclosure. This frequently occurs because the child or others blame him or her for the interaction. Additionally, the child may become embarrassed and ashamed.[38] It is essential that the health care provider maintain patience with these victims and not blame the child.

The legalities of Internet crimes against children and criminal proceedings brought against offenders differ from state-to-state because of age of consent laws and definitions of sexual assault and statutory rape. For example, if a child victim were 16 years of age and engaged in consensual sexual relations with an offender, in 32 states the 16-year-old would be at or older than the legal age of consent.[39] In these 32 states, offenders can be guilty of crimes such as corrupting the morals of a minor, contributing to the delinquency of a minor, or an equivalent offense because a child or minor is generally considered to be an individual aged under 18 years.[40] Typically, the latter crimes are considered misdemeanors and are not treated as seriously as conventional child sex offenses. However, for those child victims in one of the 18 states where the age of consent is 17 or 18 years, the offender could be charged with more serious criminal sexual offenses.[39,40] It essential for health care providers and nurses to be informed about the applicable statutes in their state of practice. The need for Internet safety and awareness appears to be growing. Many children, adolescents, and parents can be informed of Internet danger through the media, schools, and the Internet itself. If a health care provider suspects a child has been victimized through his or her Internet use, it is essential that the health care provider report it. The NCMEC has instituted a special CyberTipline to report the online victimization of children (**Box 16-1**). In addition to the CyberTipline, NCMEC also provides a variety of free educational materials related to Internet safety for children and adolescents at www.missingkids.com. Further Internet safety information can be downloaded from the Federal Bureau of Investigation at http://www.fbi.gov/stats-services/publications/parent-guide.

Box 16-1. The CyberTipline
The CyberTipline can be accessed by way of the Internet at http://www.cybertipline.com or toll-free at 1-800-843-5678.

Conclusion

The Internet can be a great tool and resource for people of all ages. Using the Internet, however, carries risks despite its potential value. The end result then, for both professionals with children and parents or caregivers, is that use of the Internet requires supervision; it is essential for their safety. If professionals or parents uncover any evidence of illegal activity online or get reports of such activity from children, it is imperative they write down exactly what happened and save the illegal files. Then, they should inform the Internet provider and their local law enforcement. With an appropriate level of caution, children and families will be able to safely access and make full use of the enormous amount of information and communication capabilities available through the Internet.

References

1. Lenhart A, Madden M, Macgill AR, Smith A. Teens and social media: the use of social media gains a greater foothold in teen life as they embrace the conversational nature of interactive online media. Pew/Internet and American Life Project Web site. http://www.pewinternet.org. Accessed May 23, 2008.
2. Mitchell KJ, Wolak J, Finkelhor D. Are blogs putting youth at risk for online sexual solicitation or harassment? *Child Abuse Negl.* 2008;32(2):277-294.

3. Ybarra ML, Diener-West M, Leaf PJ. Examining the overlap in Internet harassment and school bullying: implications for school intervention. *J Adolesc Health.* 2007:41(6)(suppl 1):S42-S50.

4. Dowdell EB. Risky Internet behaviors of middle-school students: communication with online strangers and offline contact. *Comput Inform Nurs.* 2011;29(6):352-359.

5. Dowdell EB, Burgess AW, Cavanaugh D. Clustering of Internet risk behaviors in a middle school student population. *J Sch Health.* 2009;79(11):547-553.

6. Issac D, Cusimano MD, Sherman A, Chipman M. Child safety education and the world wide web: an evaluation of the content and quality of online resources. *Inj Prev.* 2004;10(1):59-61.

7. Dowdell EB, Burgess AW, Flores JR. Original research: social networking patterns of adolescents, young adults, and offenders. *Am J Nurs.* 2011;111(7):28-36.

8. Wolak J, Finkelhor D. Sexting: a typology. University of New Hampshire Web site. http://www.unh.edu/ccrc/pdf/CV231_Sexting%20Typology%20 Bulletin_4-6-11_revised.pdf. Published March 2011. Accessed May 23, 2011.

9. CBS News. "Sexting" shockingly common among teens. CBS News US Web site. http://www.cbsnews.com/stories/2009/01/15/national/main4723161.shtml. Accessed January 15, 2009.

10. Dombrowski SC, Gischlar KL, Durst T. Safeguarding young people from cyber pornography and cyber sexual predation: a major dilemma of the Internet. *Child Abuse Rev.* 2007;16(3):153-170.

11. Lenhart A. Cyberbullying and online teens. Pew/Internet and American Life Project Web site. http://www.pewinternet.org. Accessed May 23, 2008.

12. Mitchell KJ, Wolak J, Finkelhor D. Trends in youth reports of sexual solicitations, harassment and unwanted exposure to pornography on the Internet. *J Adolesc Health.* 2007;40(2):116-126.

13. Wolak J, Mitchell KJ, Finkelhor D. Online victimization of youth: five years later. Alexandria, VA: National Center for Missing and Exploited Children Bulletin; 2006.

14. Madden M, Fox S, Smith A, Vitak J. Digital footprints: online identity management and search in the age of transparency. Pew Internet and American Life Project Web site. http://pewresearch.org/pubs/663/digital-footprints. Accessed May 23, 2008.

15. Wolak J, Mitchell KJ, Finkelhor D. Escaping or connecting? characteristics of youth who form close online relationships. *J Adoles.* 2006;26(1):105-119.

16. National Center for Missing and Exploited Children. What is child pornography? National Center for Missing and Exploited Children Web site. http://www.missingkids.com/missingkids/servlet/PageServlet?LanguageCountry=en_US&PageId=1504. Accessed October 17, 2008.

17. Lenhart A. Social networks grow: friending mom and dad. Pew/Internet and American Life Project Web site. http://pewresearch.org/pubs/1079/social-networks-grow. Accessed on January 16, 2010.

18. WICZ-TV news. Cuomo: social networking sites agree to remove sex offenders from sites. WICZ-TV Web site. http://www.wicz.com/news2005/viewarticle.aspa=11778. Accessed February 6, 2010.

19. Ybarra ML, Mitchell KJ, Wolak J, Finkelhor D. Examining characteristics and associated distress related to Internet harassment: findings from the second youth Internet safety survey. *Pediatrics*. 2006;118(4):e1169-e1177.

20. Golson J. Charges against Clifton girl spark debate about teen's lurid pictures. NJ.com Web site. http://www.nj.com/news/index.ssf/2009/03/nj_joins_others_states_in_crac.html. Published March 29, 2009. Accessed June 15, 2013.

21. Lenhart A. Teens and sexting: how and why minor teens are sending sexually suggestive nude or nearly nude images via text messaging. Pew/Internet and American Life Project Web site. http://www.pewinternet.org/~/media//Files/Reports/2009/PIP_Teens_and_Sexting.pdf. Accessed 2012.

22. Wolak J, Mitchell KJ, Finkelhor D. Close online relationships in a national sample of adolescents. *Adolescence*. 2002;37(147):441-455.

23. Dowdell EB, Bradley PK. Risky Internet behaviors: a case study of online and offline stalking. *J Sch Nurs*. 2010;26(6):436-442.

24. Subrahmanyam K, Lin G. Adolescents on the net: Internet use and well-being. *Adolescence*. 2007;42(168):659-677.

25. Tokunaga RS. Following you home from school: a critical review and synthesis of research on cyber bullying victimization. *Comput Hum Behav*. 2010;26(3):277-287.

26. Ybarra ML, Espelage DL, Mitchell KJ. The co-occurrence of Internet harassment and unwanted sexual solicitation victimization and perpetration: associations with psychosocial indicators. *J Adolesc Health*. 2007;41:S31-S41.

27. David-Ferdon C, Hertz MF. Electronic media, violence, and adolescents: an emerging public health problem. *J Adolesc Health*. 2007;41(6)(suppl 1):S1-S5.

28. Williams KR, Guerra NG. Prevalence and predictors of Internet bullying. *J Adolesc Health*. 2007;14(6)(suppl 1):S14-S21.

29. Wang J, Iannotti RJ, Nansel TR. School bullying among adolescents in the United States: physical, verbal, relational, and cyber. *J Adolesc Health*. 2009;45(4):368-375.

30. Ybarra ML, Mitchell KJ. How risky are social networking sites?: a comparison of places online where youth sexual solicitation and harassment occurs. *Pediatircs*. 2008;121(2):e350-e357.

31. Baum K, Catalano S, Rand M, Rose K. National crime victimization survey: stalking victimization in the United States. *Bureau of Justice Statistics Special Report*. 2009.

32. D'Amico M. Cyberstalking via the net. *Netguide*. 1997;4(2):32.

33. Turow J, Nir L. The Internet and the family 2000: the view from parents, the view from kids. The Annenberg Public Policy Center of the University of Pennsylvania Web site. http://www.appcpenn.org/Internet/family/finalrepor_fam.pdf. Accessed August 7, 2001.

34. Aftab P. *The Parent's Guide to Protecting Your Children in Cyberspace*. New York, NY: McGraw-Hill; 2000.

35. Armagh DS. A safety net for the Internet: protecting our children. *Juvenile Justice*. 1998;5(1):9-15.

36. Lanning KA. Cyber pedophiles: a behavioral perspective. *APSAC Advisor*. 1998;11(4):12-18.

37. Summit RC. The child sexual abuse accommodation syndrome. *Child Abuse Negl.* 1983;7(2):177-193.

38. Crosson-Tower C. *Understanding Child Abuse and Neglect.* 6th ed. Boston, MA: Allyn & Bacon; 2005.

39. Phipps C. Children, adults, sex and the criminal law: in search of reason. *Seton Hall Law J.* 1997;22:1-60.

40. Toth P, McClure K. An overview of selected legal issues involved in computer related child exploitation: many questions, few answers. *APSAC Advisor.* 1998;11(4):19-22

Chapter 17

Prevention of Child Maltreatment

Beverly L. Fortson, PhD*
Joanne B. Martin, DrPH, RN, FAAN
Colby Lokey, MS

Key Points

1. Research has suggested strong perceived social support, a child having a good relationship with at least one parental figure, and a socioeconomic status above the poverty level are associated with a lower risk for child maltreatment.
2. There are 3 types of prevention programs. Universal prevention programs are provided to the general population, regardless of risk, and often aim to educate the general public, all parents, service providers, and others about the scope and consequences of child maltreatment before it ever occurs. Selected prevention programs are targeted to individuals identified as being at-risk or selected, owing to a variety of factors that are often associated with child maltreatment such as poverty, young parental age, parental mental health issues, and parental substance use among others. Indicated prevention programs are designed for families in which child maltreatment has already occurred and for which reports of maltreatment have been substantiated. The goal of such programs is to prevent the recurrence of child maltreatment and minimize its impact on the child and family.[1]
3. Children aged 4 years and younger are at the greatest risk for child-maltreatment-related death, with abusive head trauma (AHT) being a common cause. As noted by Klevens & Leeb,[2] two-thirds of child maltreatment fatalities in children under 5 years of age are caused by AHT.
4. A substantiated CPS report may prevent more serious and even life-threatening child maltreatment from occurring in the future. An unsubstantiated CPS report may also prevent child maltreatment because of the support and additional services that may be provided to families as a result. For example, most states (72.5%) refer both substantiated and unsubstantiated cases to community agencies for services. Without intervention, children who are left in the care of alleged perpetrators are at risk for recurring or new child maltreatment.
5. Nurses working in the emergency room (ER) who see older infants and children admitted for treatment of injuries, ingestions, and acute or chronic conditions are in a key position to assess for suspected child maltreatment or identify the potential for child maltreatment.[5] Moreover, a nurse working in this environment may assess adults admitted for the treatment of injuries resulting from intimate partner violence (IPV) and may assess the risk of child maltreatment for any involved children.

* The findings and conclusions in this chapter are those of the authors and do not necessarily represent the official position of the Centers for Disease Control and Prevention.

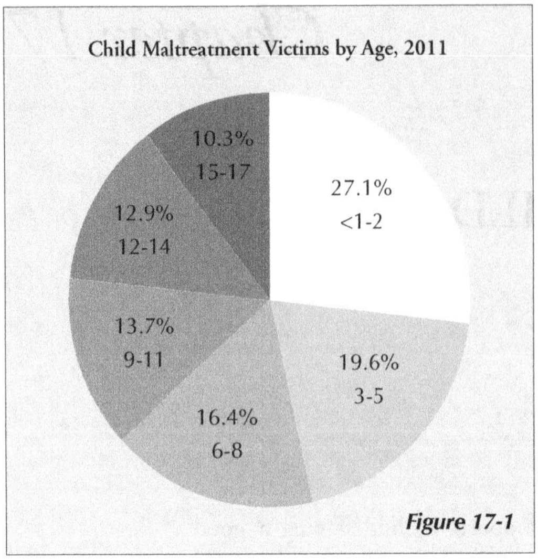

Figure 17-1. *Child maltreatment victims by age, 2011. Data from United States Department of Health and Human Services; Administration for Children and Families; Administration on Children, Youth and Families; Children's Bureau.* Child Maltreatment 2011. *Administration for Children and Families Web site. http://www.acf.hhs.gov/sites/default/files/cb/cm11.pdf. Accessed June 7, 2013.*

While child abuse and neglect was recognized as a major public health problem in the United States in the late 1980s and early 1990s, it was not recognized as a major worldwide public health problem until 1999.[3] The Centers for Disease Control and Prevention (CDC) defines child maltreatment as act(s) of omission or commission committed by a parent or caregiver that results in harm, potential for harm, or threat of harm to a child.[4] Of the 3.4 million referrals for child maltreatment received by child protective services (CPS) in the United States in 2011, 676 569 children were confirmed as victims of abuse or neglect.[5] Although children aged under 3 years are at the highest risk for maltreatment, the risk, in general, decreases with age; children aged birth through 18 years have at least a 1 in 10 chance of being exposed to some form of maltreatment[5] **(Figure 17-1)**. Given that not all incidents of child maltreatment are reported to CPS, this data likely underestimates rates of occurrence. The *Fourth National Incidence Study of Child Abuse and Neglect (NIS-4)* provides a better estimation of child maltreatment and addresses the issue of underreporting by including data from various professionals in a wide range of agencies in representative communities. The NIS-4 estimates 553 330 children experienced abuse and 771 700 children experienced neglect from 2005 through 2006.[6] Recent self-report child-maltreatment-exposure surveys suggest that approximately 20% of children in the United States have a history of child maltreatment, with occurrences varying among the different types of child maltreatment.[7] The types of child maltreatment include physical abuse, sexual abuse, neglect, and psychological abuse (emotional abuse)[4,8] **(Table 17-1)**. In 2011, neglect was the most common cause for a child maltreatment report (78.5%), followed by physical abuse (17.6%), sexual abuse (9.1%), and psychological abuse (9.0%).[5] It should be noted, however, that psychological abuse often occurs in conjunction with many of the other forms of child maltreatment.[5]

Child maltreatment is often associated with negative consequences in both childhood and adulthood. The effects of child maltreatment can range from impaired functioning to death. Research suggests that children with histories of child maltreatment are more likely to engage in bullying behavior and are at a higher risk for victimization by their peers than children without such histories.[9] Additionally, research suggests that children with a history of child maltreatment are at a higher risk for experiencing depressive disorders, negative self-perception (eg, guilt and blame), anxiety disorders, posttraumatic stress disorder (PTSD), and increased aggression than those without such histories.[10-12] As adults, those with histories of child maltreatment may be more likely than those without to struggle with alcoholism, PTSD, drug abuse, anxiety, depression, suicide attempts, and other psychiatric disorders.[13-15] The Adverse Childhood Experiences (ACE) Study documents a strong relationship between abuse exposure or household dysfunction during childhood and several of the risk factors for the major causes of death in adulthood (eg, ischemic heart disease, cancer, chronic lung disease, skeletal fractures, liver disease), such that the more adverse events to which the individual is exposed, the greater the likelihood of negative outcomes.[16] Additionally, researchers have documented an overlap in exposure to child maltreatment and exposure to other types of violence, wherein those individuals who are exposed to child maltreatment are at increased risk of being exposed to other types of violence later in life.[17,18] For example, in a 15-year prospective longitudinal study, Barnes et al[19] found that women with a history of sexual abuse were 2 times as likely to have experienced sexual and physical revictimization than were nonabused comparison females. This chapter reviews the risk and protective factors associated with child maltreatment as well as strategies currently being used to prevent child maltreatment and related negative consequences. This chapter also discusses the role of the nurse in the prevention of child maltreatment.

Table 17-1. Types of Child Maltreatment

Type of Child Maltreatment	Characteristics
Physical abuse	The intentional use of physical force by the caregiver that results in physical injury or risk of physical injury for the child
Sexual abuse	Sexual acts in which there is evidence of oral, anal, or genital penetration; molestation with genital contact; or other unspecified acts that do not necessarily involve genital contact (eg, fondling of breasts or buttocks, exposure to sexual activity)
Neglect	The care required to meet the child's basic needs (eg, physical, emotional, educational) is not provided or the caregiver fails to protect the child from harm or potential harms.
Psychological abuse	Acts that involve torturous restriction of movement (eg, tying or binding); verbal or emotional assault (eg, belittling, scapegoating); or overly punitive, exploitative, or abusive treatment that convey to the child that he or she is "worthless, flawed, unloved, unwanted, endangered, or valued only in meeting another's needs"[4]

Data from Leeb RT, Paulozzi LJ, Melanson C, Simon TR, Arias I. Child Maltreatment Surveillance: Uniform Definitions For Public Health And Recommended Data Elements. *Version 1.0. Atlanta, GA: Centers for Disease Control and Prevention, National Center for Injury Prevention and Control; 2008.*

Risk and Protective Factors Associated With Child Maltreatment

Individual characteristics and environmental factors play a large role in determining whether a child will experience child maltreatment and the negative consequences that can result. A social ecological model composed of 4 levels is often used to understand the individual, relationship, community, and societal factors that either increase the risk for or protect against the victimization or perpetration of child maltreatment, referred to as ***risk factors*** and ***protective factors*** respectively. Cicchetti & Lynch[20] suggested that family-level contextual factors are the most influential in determining child exposure and outcomes. Other factors that might increase the risk for the victimization or perpetration of child maltreatment are as follows:

— Child under 4 years of age

— Low socioeconomic status

— Parental substance abuse or mental health issues

— Familial social isolation

— Child having special needs[5,21-26]

Protective factors, although equally as important as risk factors, have received far less focus in research; however, studies note strong perceived social support, a child having a good relationship with at least one parental figure, and having a socioeconomic status above the poverty level are associated with a lower risk for child maltreatment.[27-29] Other risk and protective factors are included in **Table 17-2**.

Table 17-2. Risk and Protective Factors for the Victimization and Perpetration of Child Maltreatment

RISK FACTORS

— Children younger than 4 years of age

— Special needs of the child that may increase caregiver burden (eg, disabilities, mental retardation)

— Parents' lack of understanding of children's needs and development and lack of parenting skills

— Parents' history of child maltreatment in family of origin

— Substance abuse, mental health issues, or both in the family

— Parental characteristics such as young age, low education, single parenthood, large number of dependent children, and low income

— Nonbiological, transient caregivers in the home (eg, mother's male partner)

— Parental thoughts and emotions that tend to support or justify maltreatment behaviors

— Social isolation

— Family disorganization, dissolution, and violence, including intimate partner violence

— Parenting stress, poor parent-child relationships, and negative interactions

— Community violence

— Concentrated neighborhood disadvantage (eg, high poverty and residential instability, high unemployment rates, and high density of alcohol outlets) and poor social connections

PROTECTIVE FACTORS

— Supportive family environment and social networks

— Nurturing parenting skills*

— Stable family relationships*

— Household rules and child monitoring*

— Parental employment*

— Adequate housing*

— Access to health care and social services*

— Caring adults outside the family who can serve as role models or mentors*

— Communities that support parents and take responsibility for preventing abuse*

**Factors are promising in preventing child maltreatment.*
Data from Centers for Disease Control and Prevention. Child maltreatment: risk and protective factors. Centers for Disease Control and Prevention Web site. http://www.cdc.gov/ViolencePrevention/childmaltreatment/riskprotectivefactprs.html. Updated April 10, 2012. Accessed June 7, 2013.

As noted previously, the environment is one of many factors that influence exposure to and perpetration of child maltreatment. Klein's[30] research supported the importance of the community context in understanding a child's risk for child maltreatment. Neighborhoods with higher rates of child maltreatment referrals were those with inadequate resources for child supervision, more concentrated socioeconomic disadvantage, and greater racial and ethnic diversity. Conversely, Klein[30] found that concentrated affluence in communities was associated with lower rates of child maltreatment. Coulton et al[31] found that neighborhood factors associated with child maltreatment, including socioeconomic disadvantage (eg, income or poverty levels, property values, unemployment, residential instability, and increased child care burden) can contribute to child maltreatment victimization and perpetration; however, the strength of the connection between a child's family and his or her community can serve as protective factors for child maltreatment victimization and perpetration.

Strategies for Preventing Child Maltreatment

Given the rate at which child maltreatment occurs and the associated negative consequences, it is important that the prevention of child maltreatment be a focus for or at least understood by all of those who interact with families and have an opportunity to impact the problem. Child maltreatment prevention programs often fall into 1 of 3 levels based on the target of interest: universal prevention, selected prevention, or indicated prevention. Universal prevention programs are provided to the general population, regardless of risk, and often aim to educate the general public, all parents, service providers, and others about the scope and consequences of child maltreatment before it ever occurs.[1] Selected prevention programs are targeted to individuals identified as being at-risk or selected, owing to a variety of factors that are often associated with child maltreatment, such as poverty, young parental age, parental mental health issues, and parental substance use, among others. Indicated prevention programs are designed for families in which child maltreatment has already occurred and for which reports of maltreatment have been substantiated. The goal is to prevent the recurrence of child maltreatment and minimize its impact on the child and family.[1]

Universal Prevention Programs

Triple P — Positive Parenting Program®

As noted previously, universal interventions to prevent child maltreatment strive to reach all families, not just families at an increased risk for its occurrence. The Triple P — Positive Parenting Program is one example of a universal intervention. Triple P was developed as a population-level system of parenting and familial support and includes 5 intervention levels, each of which aim to enhance parental competence and prevent or change dysfunctional parenting strategies.[32] Level 1 in the Triple P system is the universal level wherein health promotion and social marketing strategies are used to increase parents' access to information on how to deal with common child-rearing issues. Levels 2 through 5 are not universal in their approach as the goal of these levels is to provide parents with information and support that is matched to their needs (**Table 17-3**). In a study of 18 counties in the United States randomly assigned to either the Triple P program or the control group receiving services as usual (ie, services typically offered within the communities without the addition of Triple P), all rates of child maltreatment increased during the study; however, the counties who participated in the Triple P program demonstrated smaller increases in and lower overall rates of substantiated cases. Additionally, the rates at which children were removed from the home and child maltreatment-related injuries occurred decreased from pre- to post-intervention in Triple P counties and were lower than the rates in the control counties where rates increased from pre- to post-intervention.[33]

Table 17-3. Triple P Levels

LEVEL	CHARACTERISTICS
Level 1: *Universal Triple P*	Health promotion and social marketing strategies are used to increase parents' access to information on how to deal with common childrearing issues.
Level 2: *Selected Triple P*	Brief consultations with individual parents or parenting seminars with groups of parents are used with the goal of normalizing parenting interventions.
Level 3: *Primary Care Triple P*	Active skills training occurs for parents who need it to be able to implement the parenting strategies.
Level 4: *Standard and Group Triple P*	Parents are taught to apply skills to a range of target behaviors both at home and in community settings, and the training benefits all children with problems, irrespective of whether the child is diagnosed with a behavioral disorder.
Level 5: *Enhanced Triple P*	Optional addition to Level 4 for families with additional risk factors that can be addressed through skills taught in the intervention (eg, mood management, stress coping).

Data from Sanders MR. Triple P-Positive Parenting Program as a public health approach to strengthening parenting. J Fam Psychol. *2008;22(4):506-517.*

Period of Purple Crying® and Hospital-Based Parent Education Program

Children aged under 4 years are at the greatest risk for child-maltreatment-related death, with AHT being a common cause. As noted by Klevens & Leeb,[2] two-thirds of child maltreatment fatalities in children under 5 years of age are caused by AHT. Two universal prevention programs have been developed to prevent AHT[34,35] by providing information regarding AHT to all parents of newborns before hospital discharge. One such program, the Period of Purple Crying, aims to acknowledge that infant crying can be frustrating, but there are ways to handle the crying aside from shaking the infant.[34] Mothers who participated in the Period of Purple Crying program reported increased knowledge about AHT and infant crying and were more likely to report having shared information about the dangers of shaking and the importance of walking away if frustrated.[34] Dias et al[35] reported on an AHT prevention program that was implemented in hospitals in an 8-county region in New York. Nurses used a brochure and an 11-minute video to present parents with information on AHT and then asked parents to sign a commitment statement verifying they received and understood the materials. During the period of intervention, rates of AHT declined by 47% when compared to the previous 6-year control period.[35] Randomized CDC-funded clinical trials of both AHT programs are currently underway. This research seeks to provide more comprehensive information about the impact of these programs on population rates of AHT.

Adults and Children Together Against Violence Parents Raising Safe Kids Program (ACT Program)

Another universal program designed for early prevention of child maltreatment is the Adults and Children Together Against Violence Parents Raising Safe Kids program (ACT program).[36,37] As a universal prevention program, the ACT program aims to educate communities and families to create safe, healthy environments that protect children and youth from violence. This program focuses on teaching parents about child development, both the causes and consequences of violence, anger management skills, problem-solving skills, and discipline techniques not involving physical punishment.[36] In one of the first evaluations of the program,[37] an attempt was made to ensure that the programs from which parents were recruited did not target individuals who had already engaged in child maltreatment. Instead, parents were recruited from a comprehensive social service agency and parent programming sites. In their evaluation, Portwood et al[37] found that participation in the ACT program resulted in a reduction in the use of harsh verbal and physical discipline and an increase in nurturing behavior at posttreatment and at a 3-month follow-up. In another study that examined the impact of the program in a community sample, Knox et al[36] found that parents who participated in the ACT program demonstrated significantly lower instances of hitting children with objects and spanking when compared to a comparison sample that did not receive the training. In addition, the ACT program parents showed a significant improvement in parenting skills and violence prevention–related knowledge, behaviors, and beliefs when compared to baseline.[36] While many of the other programs described herein focus mainly on positive parenting skills, which are essential in reducing frustration, violence, and the use of physical punishment, this program explicitly focuses on educating parents about violence and teaching them ways to reduce violence and the use of physical punishment. Although the potential exists for some parents and educators to shy away from a program that explicitly teaches alternatives to corporal punishment, this program shows promise as the research demonstrates that many of the parents who have participated in the program benefitted from the teaching and implemented the skills and techniques in their parenting practices.

Child Sexual Abuse Prevention Programs

Child sexual abuse prevention programs are typically school-based and aim to educate children, families, teachers, and other members of the community about child sexual abuse.[38] In general, such programs teach children skills aimed at reducing the risk of becoming a victim of child sexual abuse, including how to call for help and identify dangerous or risky situations, personal boundaries, and undesired forms of touching.[38-40] In addition to teaching children these skills, school-based programs also encourage disclosure and open communication, try to decrease self-blame in children who have been abused, and aim to empower bystanders or witnesses to prevent or report inappropriate sexual behaviors. Research has demonstrated that children who participate in school-based education programs aimed at preventing child sexual abuse are 6 to 7 times more likely to use the protective skills taught in simulated dangerous or risky situations when compared to children who did not participate in such programs.[40] It is unclear, however, whether child sexual abuse prevention programs actually reduce child sexual abuse.[41] Moreover, it may be unrealistic to expect children to fend off adult predators; therefore, many child sexual abuse prevention programs, such as Darkness to Light, now focus the responsibility of preventing child sexual abuse on adults. Still, more work is needed to further develop and evaluate programs focused on the prevention of perpetration to determine whether they reduce the risk of child sexual abuse.

Prevention Programs for Selected and Indicated Populations

Safe Environment for Every Kid (SEEK)

The Safe Environment for Every Kid (SEEK) program is a model of pediatric primary care aimed at reducing child maltreatment for selected populations such as those at risk of child maltreatment. SEEK trains primary care providers to identify and address the risk factors for child maltreatment, including maternal depression, history of or current substance abuse, use of harsh punishment, and extreme stressors.[42] A study examining the effectiveness of the SEEK model compared families who participated in the SEEK program to those who completed services as usual and found that families who participated in the SEEK program had fewer CPS reports than families who completed services as usual (13.3% and 19.2% respectively), reported fewer occurrences of severe physical assault, and were more likely to adhere to medical care and ensure their children had timely immunizations.[42]

Home Visiting Programs

Like the SEEK program, home visiting programs are typically provided to selected populations, which most often include low-income pregnant women or new mothers who are at risk for child maltreatment. In randomized trials conducted in the United States, the evidence of effectiveness for home visiting programs is mixed, with some models showing few or no effects and others showing strong effects.[43,44] The mixed effects are likely the result of 2 factors: (1) home visitation is only the mechanism by which content is delivered to participating families; and (2) variation of content included in home visiting models.

Healthy Families America® (HFA)

Healthy Families America (HFA) is the most widely implemented model of home visiting and is based on 12 critical elements that fall under 3 broad domains: service initiation, service delivery, and staff characteristics **(Table 17-4).** HFA home visiting typically begins in the first 3 months after birth and continues until the child is aged 3 through 5 years. Approximately three-fourths of the HFA professionals trained to conduct home visits have either graduated from college (37%) or have some college education (39%) beyond high school, and a large percentage (67%) have received instruction at the college level in the helping professions such as social work and early childhood education.[45,46] Randomized evaluations of the HFA program have yielded mixed results or, in many cases, no evidence for its effectiveness in preventing child maltreatment.[47] Healthy Families New York is an example of an HFA program that has shown some promise in decreasing risk factors associated with child maltreatment such as harsh parenting and decreases in self-reported serious abuse; however, these results were found only in a subsample of families (eg, first-time mothers who enrolled in home visiting during pregnancy).[48,49]

Nurse Family Partnership® (NFP)

Nurse Family Partnership (NFP) is another widely implemented home visiting program. NFP enrollment is typically limited to low-income, first-time mothers and their infants because they are at an increased risk for adverse outcomes, including child maltreatment.[50] NFP home visiting always begins during pregnancy, usually in the first or second trimester, and can continue until the child's second birthday. NFP home visitors are registered nurses, with almost all holding baccalaureate degrees. The nurses, following a detailed guide, address a number of factors with participating families, including child maltreatment; dietary intake; signs of illness in children; creating safe households; reducing cigarette, alcohol, and illegal drug use; and other topics. Rigorous research on NFP suggests the program is effective at preventing child maltreatment in

Table 17-4. HFA Critical Elements

SERVICE INITIATION

— Services begin prenatally or at birth.

— A standardized assessment tool is used to identify families most in need of services.

— Families can voluntarily participate in services.

SERVICE CONTENT

— Intensive services are provided and a plan is made to increase or decrease the frequency of services.

— Culturally competent services are provided.

— The focus of services is on support to the parent, parent-child interactions, and child development.

— Families should be linked to a medical provider to assure optimal health and development, with links to additional service providers as needed.

— Home visitor caseloads should be such that home visitors have enough time to spend with each family to meet their needs and plan for future activities.

STAFF CHARACTERISTICS

— Home visitors should have good interpersonal skills and display a willingness to work in or with culturally diverse communities.

— Home visitors should be prepared to handle the situations to which they might be exposed when working with at-risk families.

— Home visitors should receive intensive training specific to their role to understand the essential components of family assessment and home visitation.

— Home visitors should receive ongoing, effective supervision.

Data from Healthy Families America. About us: critical elements. Healthy Families America Web site http://www.healthyfamiliesamerica.org/about_us/critical_elements.shtml. Accessed June 7, 2013.

low-income, first-time mothers, and the results persist over time.[51,52] The NFP program has also been shown to reduce the number of subsequent pregnancies, use of welfare, and criminal behavior in women who participated in the home visiting program when compared to women in the comparison group.[52,53]

Behavioral Parent Training Programs (BPT)

In recent years, empirical support for behavioral parent training (BPT) programs aimed at preventing physical abuse and neglect and its recurrence has grown substantially, with support for the use of BPT to systematically address and prevent child maltreatment growing as well.[54-56] While most BPT programs were initially developed as a way to help parents address child behavior problems, the programs have been shown to be successful in preventing recidivism for abuse in families with substantiated cases of child maltreatment and in reducing child maltreatment risk factors in high-risk families.[54,55,57,58] When implemented as a measure to prevent child maltreatment, BPT programs most often focus on selected and indicated populations.

Highly trained professionals typically deliver BPTs, successful examples of which include Project SafeCare, Parent Child Interaction Therapy (PCIT), and The Incredible Years®, to one family at a time over the course of several sessions. BPT programs, which are based on social learning theories and principles, often teach parents behavior management techniques and positive interaction skills to decrease parental and child frustration, as well as externalizing behaviors in the child that may cause an escalation in parental behavior and result in the implementation of harsh parental discipline.[59,60] Therefore, it is reasonable to assume that BPT programs may be effective in the prevention of child maltreatment, specifically physical abuse,[61,62] which is often related to harsh parental discipline, negative parent-child interaction styles, and high levels of parenting stress.[63,64] BPT programs have also demonstrated positive effects in families with a history of neglect and involvement in the child welfare system, some with severe and chronic histories of involvement with child welfare.[55,58]

SafeCare®

SafeCare is a highly structured in-home parent training program that focuses on parent-child interactions, home safety, and health skills in families with children aged birth through 5 years of age.[57] A study conducted with parents reported to CPS for physical abuse or neglect found that parents who completed the SafeCare program were less likely to have a re-report of physical abuse or neglect than families who completed services as usual at a 36-month follow-up; recidivism rates were 15% and 46% respectively.[57] In a randomized clinical trial of SafeCare in a high-risk population, the event survival trend for the amount of time between referral and re-report of child maltreatment was 103 days for the standard home-based mental health services group and 200.5 days for the SafeCare participants.[65] These differences were not statistically significant, but the trend favored SafeCare participants.

Parent Child Interaction Therapy (PCIT)

PCIT is a parent training program designed for families with children aged 2 through 7 years of age with behavior problems.[60] PCIT consists of 2 phases: (1) child-directed interaction (CDI) and (2) parent-directed interaction (PDI). The CDI phase is often referred to as the ***relationship enhancement phase*** where parents are taught skills that decrease coercive parent-child interactions, while the PDI phase is referred to as the ***discipline phase***, and parents are taught behavior management and discipline skills. A study examining the effectiveness of PCIT in a group of physically abusive parents in the child welfare system found that parents who participated in PCIT had significantly fewer subsequent reports of physical abuse (19%) than parents who participated in services as usual (49%).[54] In a study of families with chronic and severe histories of neglect or physical abuse, PCIT plus a motivational enhancement was effective at reducing future child welfare reports, with a stronger effect observed when children were returned to the home sooner rather than later.[55]

The Incredible Years®

The Incredible Years is a BPT program that focuses on families with children aged 2 through 12 years who are at risk for or currently exhibiting conduct problems or attention-related disorders.[66] Separate programs also exist for teachers and children; reviews are currently underway to evaluate a parenting program for children aged birth through 3 years. Like other BPTs, The Incredible Years is effective at reducing harsh parenting and conduct problems and at increasing positive discipline and nurturing parenting.[66] In evaluations of The Incredible Years with at-risk samples, parents demonstrated lower negative and higher positive parenting scores after participating in the program than those parents who did not participate.[67] Additionally, it was found that parents who participated in the program made significant positive changes in parenting behaviors, irrespective of whether or not they had a previous history of involvement with CPS.[67] In a study consisting primarily of families with a history of neglect, Linares et al[68] found that positive parenting skills increased in parents and foster parents who participated in The Incredible Years program when compared to controls, and the improvements were greatest when parents attended 6 or more program sessions.

The Role of Nurses in Preventing Child Maltreatment

Education about the scope and consequences of child maltreatment and prevention programming related to child maltreatment begins in training programs. Nurses, like other professionals, are expected to engage in continuing education programs throughout their career; information related to child maltreatment can be obtained during the trainings. All nurses should understand their role in reporting suspected child maltreatment and should know the policies and procedures for reporting suspected child maltreatment that govern the hospital, clinic, school, or agency in which they work before the need arises (see *Chapter 13, Child Protective Services and Child Abuse*). A nurse is not expected to determine if child maltreatment has occurred; rather, CPS is responsible for determining if a report is substantiated or unsubstantiated. If there is reason to suspect child maltreatment, a formal report should be made to CPS in accordance with the policy of the employer and laws of the state where the incident occurred. Nurses should never assume a report has already been made to CPS. Although nurses and other mandated reporters may wonder whether making a report to CPS is worthwhile given that not all reports to CPS are investigated, it should be acknowledged that multiple reports from different sources may mean that CPS is more likely to investigate or substantiate a referral.[69] Approximately 10% to 15% of unsubstantiated reports are substantiated when re-reported.[70] In addition, referrals from professionals are more likely to be substantiated than referrals from family, friends, and neighbors.[69]

A CPS report that is substantiated may prevent more serious and even life-threatening child maltreatment from occurring in the future. A CPS report that is unsubstantiated may also prevent child maltreatment because of the support and additional services that may be provided to families as a result. For example, most states (72.5%) refer both substantiated and unsubstantiated cases to community agencies for services.[71] Without intervention, children who are left in the care of alleged perpetrators are at risk for recurring or new child maltreatment.[69]

The roles of nurses vary greatly within the profession. As a result, nurses are often employed in a number of settings, providing them with a number of opportunities to participate in the prevention of child maltreatment. For example, nurses employed in primary care settings, hospitals, schools, and community agencies have contact with children and families. Information on the way in which nurses can assist in preventing child maltreatment in each of these settings is provided in the following sections.

Hospital Settings

Maternity Units

Nurses who work in maternity units have opportunities to prevent child maltreatment because of their contact with a mother after the birth of her child. Most efforts to prevent child maltreatment in this situation are provided to all mothers, including those at an increased risk for child maltreatment. For example, in many hospitals, before each mother and infant is discharged home, maternity nurses conduct interventions to prevent AHT, as previously described. In addition, nurses ensure that infants are safely transported home in a properly installed car seat and provide instructions for safe sleep. To compensate for early discharge, some hospitals offer home visits to all families within 1 to 3 days after discharge.[72,73] During a home visit, a nurse assesses the mother's postpartum health status and conducts a newborn inspection. Since the nurse is actually in the home, he or she is able to assess the safety and appropriateness of the home environment. This opportunity allows the nurse, when necessary, to make appropriate referrals to community resources, including home visiting programs that are designed to prevent child maltreatment.

Neonatal Intensive Care Unit (NICU)

Infants admitted to the neonatal intensive care unit (NICU) are at increased risk of child maltreatment as a result of their age and medical condition(s).[74] Nurses in the NICU are in a prime position to prevent child maltreatment because they have opportunities to observe the parents and other primary caregivers during the extended period of time the infants are in the NICU. For example, nurses may observe that parents rarely visit, interact inappropriately verbally or physically, or self-report intimate partner violence. NICU nurses are responsible for teaching primary caregivers, usually parents, how to care for their infant and for ensuring the parent is capable of providing competent care before the infant is discharged home. If parents cannot demonstrate they can perform necessary procedures, provide 24-hour care, and appropriately assess the need for medical intervention, NICU nurses cannot recommend discharge.

Emergency Room (ER)

Nurses working in the emergency department (ER) who see older infants and children admitted for treatment of injuries, ingestions, and acute or chronic conditions are in a key position to assess for suspected child maltreatment or identify the potential for child maltreatment. Moreover, a nurse working in this environment may assess adults admitted for the treatment of injuries resulting from IPV and assess the risk of child maltreatment for any involved children. If child maltreatment is suspected, the nurse should follow the procedures of the employer and the laws of the state in reporting the incident, as described earlier. Some hospitals have child abuse teams that work in the ER and include nurses specializing in the assessment of child maltreatment; these nurses have expertise and training that allows them to assess for and recognize the signs of child maltreatment and, if available, should be consulted in cases where child maltreatment is suspected (see *Chapter 13, Child Protective Services and Child Abuse*).

Primary Care

Prenatal care and well-child care should include routine screening for a wide range of problems in the home and family, including maternal mood disorders, substance abuse, and IPV, all of which are risk factors for child maltreatment. In their roles in the primary care setting, nurses may administer screening tools or ask specific questions of the child or family and may probe further about specific issues occurring in the home. Based on information provided by the child or family, nurses may make referrals to appropriate community resources, or they may educate the family on a potential topic to prevent current or future problems. For example, using a developmental framework, nurses can discuss home safety and what is expected of children during different developmental periods to prevent injuries and ingestions. Education about child development and appropriate expectations of children at different ages may also lessen parental frustration and harsh punishment that can be associated with normal infant crying and other issues of childhood, such as toilet training.

School Settings

School nurses deal with a wide range of child maltreatment-related behaviors, from child sexual abuse (eg, rape of a child by an older cousin) to neglect (eg, persistent lice). Because school nurses operate in a non–health care setting, they practice good clinical judgment and understand how to apply CPS reporting policies. School nurses may assist counselors and teachers in providing universal prevention programs for child sexual abuse. Teachers may be the first ones to identify students who exhibit signs and symptoms of potential child maltreatment and often consult with the school nurse or refer children to the nurse when such issues arise. Given that the signs and symptoms of child maltreatment can be confused with other health problems, proper diagnosis and treatment is essential. On campuses with school-based or school-linked clinics, the nurse can not only refer the student for evaluation, but he or she can more easily convey the reason for the referral, ensure the appointment is kept, and facilitate appropriate follow-through.

Other Settings

Nurses can be an effective voice in preventing child maltreatment in other settings. For example, nurses can educate decision-makers and influential community leaders at the local, state, or national level about health-promoting policies that would contribute to reduced child maltreatment, such as improved access to health care, safe adequate housing, enhanced food and nutrition supplements at home and school, and quality affordable child care. Nurses can also provide credible testimony before Congress using personal experience to illustrate the consequences of existing public policies. Additionally, nurses can develop and disseminate effective interventions and programs to reduce child maltreatment. Nurses developed 2 of the evidence-based programs described in this chapter. Harriet Kitzman, a public health nurse educator in Boston was instrumental in developing the internationally renowned NFP model of home visitation. Additionally, Kimberly Monarch, Chief Operating Officer (COO) of the NFP National Service Office and former Chief Executive Officer (CEO) of Sigma Theta Tau, spearheads dissemination efforts to ensure fidelity to the NFP model and sustainability over time. Carolyn Webster-Stratton, professor of nursing at the University of Washington, is a licensed clinical psychologist and nurse practitioner (NP) and is responsible for the development of The Incredible Years. Many other nurses make major contributions to preventing child maltreatment through research, education, and practice.

Conclusion

Child maltreatment is a serious public health problem that affects the lives of millions of children across the United States. While efforts to recognize the prevalence of child maltreatment and how it affects the lives of children have come a long way, much work still needs to be done to prevent child maltreatment. It is imperative for adults to assume the responsibility for ensuring the safety of children. All adults, including nurses and other health care professionals, must also collaborate if child maltreatment is truly going to be prevented. It is the responsibility of adults and communities to understand and learn about the various types of abuse, recognize the warning signs, and make reports as needed. Additional work is needed to ensure programs not only target individuals and families but also other adults in the community and society at large in order to affirm their role in protecting children and preventing child maltreatment.

References

1. O'Connell ME, Boat T, Warner KE, eds. *Preventing Mental, Emotional, and Behavioral Disorders Among Young People: Progress and Possibilities.* Washington, DC: National Academies Press; 2009.

2. Klevens J, Leeb RT. Child maltreatment fatalities in children under 5: findings from the National Violence Death Reporting System. *Child Abuse Negl.* 2010;34(4):262-266.

3. World Health Organization. WHO recognizes child abuse as a major public health problem. World Health Organization Web site. http://www.who.int/inf-pr-1999/en/pr99-20.html. Published April 8, 1999. Accessed June 7, 2013.

4. Leeb RT, Paulozzi LJ, Melanson C, Simon TR, Arias I. *Child Maltreatment Surveillance: Uniform Definitions For Public Health And Recommended Data Elements.* Version 1.0. Atlanta, GA: Centers for Disease Control and Prevention, National Center for Injury Prevention and Control; 2008.

5. United States Department of Health and Human Services, Administration for Children and Families, Administration on Children, Youth and Families Children's Bureau. Child maltreatment 2011. Administration for Children and Families Web site. http://www.acf.hhs.gov/sites/default/files/cb/cm11.pdf. Accessed June 7, 2013.

6. Sedlak AJ, Mettenburg J, Basena M, et al. Fourth National Incidence Study of Child Abuse and Neglect (NIS–4). Washington, DC: United States Department of Health and Human Services, Administration for Children and Families; 2010.

7. Finkelhor D, Turner H, Ormrod R, Hamby SL. Violence, abuse, and crime exposure in a national sample of children and youth. *Pediatrics.* 2009;124(5):1411-1423.

8. Miller-Perrin CL, Perrin RD. Child Maltreatment: An Introduction. 2nd ed. Thousand Oaks, CA: Sage Publications; 2007.

9. Shields A, Cicchetti D. Parental maltreatment and emotion dysregulation as risk factors for bullying and victimization in middle childhood. *J Clin Child Psychol.* 2001;30(3):349-363.

10. Briere J, Jordan CE. Childhood maltreatment, intervening variables, and adult psychological difficulties in women: an overview. *Trauma Violence Abuse.* 2009;10(4):375-388.

11. Dubner AE, Motta RW. Sexually and physically abused foster care children and posttraumatic stress disorder. *J Consult Clin Psychol.* 1999;67(3):367-373.

12. Kaplow JB, Widom CS. Age of onset of child maltreatment predicts long-term mental health outcomes. *J Abnorm Psychol.* 2007;116(1):176-187.

13. Hankin BL. Childhood maltreatment and psychopathology: prospective tests of attachment, cognitive vulnerability, and stress as mediating processes. *Cognitive Ther Res.* 2005;29(6):645-671.

14. Lo CC, Cheng TC. The impact of childhood maltreatment on young adults' substance abuse. *Am J Drug Alcohol Abuse.* 2007;33(1):139-146.

15. MacMillan HL, Fleming JE, Streiner DL, et al. Childhood abuse and lifetime psychopathology in a community sample. *Am J Psychiatry.* 2001;158(11):1878-1883.

16. Felitti VJ, Anda RF, Nordenberg D, et al. Relationship of childhood abuse and household dysfunction to many of the leading causes of death in adults: the Adverse Childhood Experiences (ACE) study. *AM J Prev Med.* 1998;14(4),245-258.

17. Holt S, Buckley H, Whelan S. The impact of exposure to domestic violence on children and young people: a review of the literature. *Child Abuse Negl.* 2008;32(8):797-810.

18. Renner LM, Slack KS. Intimate partner violence and child maltreatment: understanding intra- and intergenerational connections. *Child Abuse Negl.* 2006;30(6):599-617.

19. Barnes JE, Noll JG, Putnam FW, Trickett PK. Sexual and physical revictimization among victims of severe childhood sexual abuse. *Child Abuse Negl.* 2009;33(7):412-420.

20. Cicchetti D, Lynch M. Toward an ecological/transactional model of community violence and child maltreatment: consequences for children's development. *Psychiatry.* 1993;56(1):96-118.

21. Ammerman RT, Kolko DJ, Kirisci L, Blackson TC, Dawes MA. Child abuse potential in parents with histories of substance use disorder. *Child Abuse Negl.* 1999;23(12):1225-1238.

22. Berger LM. Income, family structure, and child maltreatment risk. *Child Youth Serv Rev.* 2004;26(8):725-748.

23. Hibbard RA, Desch LW; the Committee on Child Abuse and Neglect and Council on Children with Disabilities. Maltreatment of children with disabilities. *Pediatrics.* 2007:119(5):1018-1025.

24. Hussey JM, Chang JJ, Kotch JB. Child maltreatment in the United States: prevalence, risk factors, and adolescent health consequences. *Pediatrics.* 2006;118(3):933-942.

25. Sidebotham P, Heron J; the Avon Longitudinal Study of Pregnancy and Childhood Study Team. Child maltreatment in the "children of the nineties": a cohort study of risk factors. *Child Abuse Negl.* 2006;30(5):497-522.

26. Wu SS, Ma CX, Carter RL, et al. Risk factors for infant maltreatment: a population-based study. *Child Abuse Negl.* 2004;28(12):1253-1264.

27. Freisthler B, Bruce E, Needell B. Understanding the geospatial relationship of neighborhood characteristics and rates of maltreatment for black, Hispanic, and white children. *Soc Work.* 2007;52(1):7-16.

28. Thomas D, Leicht C, Hughes C, Madigan A, Dowell K. Emerging practices in the prevention of child abuse and neglect. United States Department of Health and Human Services Web site. http://www.childwelfare.gov/preventing/programs/whatworks/report. Accessed June 7, 2013.

29. Muller RT, Goebel-Fabbri AE, Diamond T, Dinklage D. Social support and the relationship between family and community violence exposure and psychopathology among high risk adolescents. *Child Abuse Negl.* 2000;24(4):449-464.

30. Klein S. The availability of neighborhood early care and education resources and the maltreatment of young children. *Child Maltreat.* 2011;16(4):300-311.

31. Coulton CJ, Crampton DS, Irwin M, Spilsbury JC, Korbin JE. How neighborhoods influence child maltreatment: a review of the literature and alternative pathways. *Child Abuse Negl.* 2007;31(11-12):1117-1142.

32. Sanders MR. Triple P-Positive Parenting Program as a public health approach to strengthening parenting. *J Fam Psychol.* 2008;22(4):506-517.

33. Prinz RJ, Sanders MR, Shapiro CJ, Whitaker DJ, Lutzker JR. Population-based prevention of child maltreatment: the U.S. Triple P system population trial. *Prev Sci.* 2009;10(1):1-12.

34. Barr RG, Rivara FP, Barr M, et al. Effectiveness of educational materials designed to change knowledge and behaviors regarding crying and shaken-baby syndrome in mothers of newborns: a randomized controlled trial. *Pediatrics.* 2009;123(3):972-980.

35. Dias MS, Smith K, DeGuehery K, et al. Preventing abusive head trauma among infants and young children: a hospital-based, parent education program. *Pediatrics.* 2005;115(4):e470-e477.

36. Knox MS, Burkhart K, Hunter KE. ACT Against Violence Parents Raising Safe Kids program: effects on maltreatment-related parenting behaviors and beliefs. *J Fam Issues.* 2010;32(1):55-74.

37. Portwood SG, Lambert RG, Abrams LP, Nelson EB. An evaluation of the Adults and Children Together (ACT) Against Violence Parents Raising Safe Kids program. *J Prim Prev.* 2011;32(3-4):147-160.

38. Finkelhor D. The prevention of childhood sexual abuse. *Future Child.* 2009;19(2):169-194.

39. Davis MK, Gidycz CA. Child sexual abuse prevention programs: a meta-analysis. *J Clin Child Adolesc.* 2000;29(2):257-265.

40. Zwi KJ, Woolfenden SR, Wheeler DM, et al. School-based education programmes for the prevention of child sexual abuse. *Cochrane Database Syst Rev.* 2007;18(3):1-36.

41. Mikton C, Butchart A. Child maltreatment prevention: a systematic review of reviews. *B World Health Organ.* 2009;87(5):353-361.

42. Dubowitz H, Feigelman S, Lane W, Kim J. Pediatric primary care to help prevent child maltreatment: The Safe Environment for Every Kid (SEEK) model. *Pediatrics.* 2009;123(3):858-864.

43. Gonzalez A, MacMillan HL. Preventing child maltreatment: an evidence-based update. *J Postgrad Med.* 2008;54(4):280-286.

44. Sweet MA, Appelbaum MI. Is home visiting an effective strategy? A meta-analytic review of home visiting programs for families with young children. *Child Dev.* 2004;75(5):1435-1456.

45. Diaz J, Oshana D, Harding K. Healthy Families America: 2003 annual profile of program sites. Chicago, IL: Prevent Child Abuse America; 2004. Working paper number 123104.1.

46. Healthy Families America. Characteristics of effective home visitors. Healthy Families America Web site. http://www.healthyfamiliesamerica.org/downloads/home_visitors.pdf. Accessed June 7, 2013.

47. Harding K, Galano J, Martin J, Huntington L, Schellenbach CJ. Healthy Families America effectiveness: a comprehensive review of outcomes. *J Prev Interv Community.* 2007;34(1):149-179.

48. DuMont K, Mitchell-Herzfeld S, Greene R, et al. Healthy Families New York (HFNY) randomized trial: effects on early child abuse and neglect. *Child Abuse Negl.* 2008;32(3):295-315.

49. Rodriguez ML, DuMont K, Mitchell-Hersfeld SD, Walden NJ, Greene R. Effects of Healthy Families New York on the promotion of maternal parenting competencies and the prevention of harsh parenting. *Child Abuse Negl.* 2010; 34(10):711-723.

50. Nurse-Family Partnership. Evidence-based public policy. Nurse-Family Partnership Web site. http://www.nursefamilypartnership.org/public-policy. Accessed June 7, 2013.

51. Eckenrode J, Ganzel B, Henderson CR Jr, et al. Preventing child abuse and neglect with a program of nurse home visitation. *JAMA*. 2000;284(11):1385-1391.

52. Olds DL, Eckenrode J, Henderson CR Jr. Long-term effects of home visitation on maternal life course and child abuse and neglect: fifteen-year follow-up of a randomized trial. *JAMA*. 1997;278(8):637-643.

53. Olds DL, Kitzman H, Hanks C, et al. Effects of nurse home visiting on maternal and child functioning: age-9 follow-up of a randomized trial. *Pediatrics*. 2007;120(4):e832-e845.

54. Chaffin M, Silovsky JF, Funderburk B, et al. Parent-child interaction therapy with physically abusive parents: efficacy for reducing future abuse reports. *J Consult Clin Psychol*. 2004; 72(3):500-510.

55. Chaffin M, Funderburk B, Bard D, Valle LA, Gurwitch R. A combined motivation and parent-child interaction therapy package reduces child welfare recidivism in a randomized dismantling field trial. *J Consult Clin Psychol*. 2011;79(1): 84-95.

56. Whitaker DJ, Lutzker JR, Shelley GA. Child maltreatment prevention priorities at the Centers for Disease Control and Prevention. *Child Maltreat*. 2005;10(3): 245-259.

57. Gershater-Molko RM, Lutzker JR, Wesch D. Using recidivism data to evaluate project SafeCare: teaching bonding, safety, and health care skills to parents. *Child Maltreat*. 2002;7(3):277-285.

58. Letarte MJ, Normandeau S, Allard, J. Effectiveness of a parent training program "Incredible Years" in a child protection service. *Child Abuse Negl*. 2010;34(4):253-261.

59. Eisenstadt TH, Eyberg SM, Bodiford McNeil C, Newcomb K, Funderburk B. Parent-child interaction therapy with behavior problem children: relative effectiveness of two stages and overall treatment outcome. *J Clin Child Psychol*. 1992;22(1),42–51.

60. Hembree-Kigin TL, Bodiford McNeil C. Parent-Child Interaction Therapy. New York, NY: Springer Science+Business Media, LLC; 1995.

61. Urquiza AJ, Bodiford McNeil C. Parent-child interaction therapy: an intensive dyadic intervention for physically abusive families. *Child Maltreat*. 1996;1(2):134-144.

62. Ware LM, Fortson BL, McNeil CB. Parent-child interaction therapy: a promising intervention for abusive families. *Behav Analyst Today*. 2003;3(4):375-382.

63. Black DA, Heyman RE, Smith Slep AM. Risk factors for child physical abuse. *Aggress Violent Beh*. 2001;6(2-3):121-188.

64. Milner JS. Social information processing in high-risk and physically abusive parents. *Child Abuse Negl*. 2003;27(1):7-20.

65. Silovsky JF, Bard D, Chaffin M, et al. Prevention of child maltreatment in high-risk rural families: a randomized clinical trial with child welfare outcomes. *Child Youth Serv Rev*. 2011;33(8):1435-1444.

66. Webster-Stratton C, Reid M. Adapting The Incredible Years, an evidence-based parenting program, for families involved in the child welfare system. *J Child Serv*. 2010;5(1):25-42.

67. Webster-Stratton C, Reid MJ, Hammond M. Preventing conduct problems, promoting social competence: a parent and teacher training partnership in head start. *J Clin Child Psychol*. 2001;30(3):283-302.

68. Linares LO, Montalto D, Li M, Oza VS. A promising parenting intervention in foster care. *J Consult Clin Psychol.* 2006;74(1):32-41.

69. Child Welfare Information Gateway. Decision-making in unsubstantiated child protective services cases: synthesis of recent research. United States Department of Health & Human Services Web site. http://www.childwelfare.gov/pubs/focus/decisionmaking/decisionmaking.pdf. Published June 2003. Accessed June 7, 2013.

70. Way I, Chung S, Jonson-Reid M, Drake B. Maltreatment perpetrators: a 54-month analysis of recidivism. *Child Abuse Negl.* 2001;25(8):1093–1108.

71. United States Department of Health and Human Services, Office of the Assistant Secretary for Planning and Evaluation, Administration for Children and Families, Administration on Children, Youth and Families Children's Bureau. Investigation. In: National study of child protective services systems and reform efforts: review of state CPS policy. Assistant Secretary for Planning and Evaluation Web site. http://aspe.hhs.gov/hsp/cps-status03/state-policy03/. Published April 2003. Accessed June 7, 2013.

72. Escobar GJ, Braveman PA, Ackerson L, et al. A randomized comparison of home visits and hospital-based group follow-up visits after early postpartum discharge. *Pediatrics.* 2001;108(3):719-727.

73. Frank-Hanssen M, Hanson KS, Anderson MA. Postpartum home visits: infant outcomes. *J Community Health Nurs.* 1999;16(1):17-28.

74. Bugental DB, Beaulieu DA, Silbert-Geiger A. Increases in parental investment and child health as a result of an early intervention. *J Exp Child Psychol.* 2010;106(1):30-40.

Chapter 18

Human Trafficking: A Health Care Perspective

Reena Isaac, MD
Karen C. Harpold, JD
Angelo Giardino, MD, PhD

Key Points

1. While traditional slavery may have been quite apparent in its time and sanctioned by national governments, human trafficking (HT) persists and thrives today in secrecy because it has become a highly profitable criminal business.
2. Once an HT victim has been identified, the health care system has the opportunity to provide essential health care assessments to determine the physical and psychological needs of the victims and set in motion interventions that may rescue victims from their criminal victimization.
   a. One out of every 3 teens living on the street in the United States will be lured into prostitution within 48 hours of leaving home. Such numbers defy the belief that such activity only occurs in other countries. The average age of entry into sex trafficking is 12 or 13 years old.
3. Homeless youth; runaway or "throwaway" children; children with past sexual or physical abuse; children with learning or physical disabilities; and children with low self-esteem are all among those most vulnerable to domestic human trafficking.
4. If the health care provider suspects that the patient may be a potential victim of HT, he or she should isolate the patient from any accompanying individual; doing so will allow the health care provider to safely ask the patient direct questions and facilitate a discussion about his or her situation.
5. If the interview and resulting answers suggest that the patient may be an HT victim, the health care provider practicing in the United States should make use of the federal Department of Health and Human Services hotline for further assistance (1-888-3737-888).
6. Kellogg & Sugarek's[1] TEAMSTAT approach is one of the approaches that health care providers may use when evaluating and interacting with potential victims of human trafficking and abuse.

   Tell them your agenda
   Express concern
   Assure normalcy of feelings
   Medical issues
   Safety issues
   Test and treat presumptively
   Access appropriate psychological and legal assistance
   Timely follow-up

7. While HT victims may not fully disclose their histories of exploitation, the health care provider may still be able to obtain and document important information regarding the victim's experience and chronicling of his or her health. Such interactions will allow for a continuing opportunity to build trust and rapport with the child victim, with the mutual goal of safeguarding the health of the patient.

8. Once a government's activity in combating HT is assessed, countries are ranked as Tier 1, Tier 2, or Tier 3. Countries that are fully compliant with the Trafficking Victims Protection Reauthorization Act (TVPRA) minimum standards receive Tier 1 status; nations that do not meet TVPRA standards receive a Tier 3 status. Tier 3 countries may be subject to nonhumanitarian sanctions and opposition on the part of the United States to other benefits from organizations such as the World Bank. In 2010, the United States included itself in the rankings, based on the same standards to which other countries are held.

9. Perhaps the most significant challenge the health care provider faces when evaluating a victim of HT is meeting his or her need for a safe house, or a place of shelter, and protection if he or she is a victim of forced prostitution. Recovery can be a long and difficult process, and an ideal safe house can offer education, job training, life-skills training, individual and group therapy, recreational activities, and other long-term support services.

Human slavery, despite the world's collective, progressive views and struggles for human rights over the centuries, continues in the modern era in the form of HT. While traditional slavery may have been quite apparent in its time and sanctioned by national governments, HT persists and thrives today in secrecy because it has become a highly profitable criminal business. Within the last 2 decades, the collective awareness of this vast expanding global industry has increased as the global community has seen more and more of the faces of trafficking victims who are tricked or coerced into forced labor and sexual exploitation. The International Labor Organization estimates human trafficking to be a $32 billion per year industry.[2] This criminal industry is driven by political unrest, economic inequities, high demands for cheap labor and the sex trade, vulnerable and desperate populations seeking a better life, and the perceived low risk for prosecution.[3] HT is the fastest growing criminal industry in the world and is currently the second largest source of income for organized crime, second only to the illegal drug industry.[4]

Nurses and other related health care providers have a role to play in stemming this tide. Nurses on the front line of clinical care can help detect HT victims as one of the few professionals likely to interface with trafficked victims during their captive experience.[5,6] The Family Violence Prevention Fund states that 28% of victims of trafficking reported contact with the health care system at least once during their captive period.[7]

Health care professionals, including nurses, therefore, hold a unique and pivotal position as important stakeholders in confronting the challenge of HT. Unlike a more traditional health care problem, however, HT is a multifaceted criminal activity that requires nurses to look beyond the information available in the health care arena and possess knowledge regarding how to interface with the social services and legal communities. Once an HT victim has been identified, the health care system has the opportunity to provide essential health care assessments to determine the physical and psychological needs of the victims and set in motion interventions that may rescue victims from their criminal victimization.[8,9]

Nurses should look beyond common health care issues and familiarize themselves with the legal issues surrounding HT that may affect both international and domestic victims.

Table 18-1. Needs of Victims of Human Trafficking

	International		Domestic
	Adults	Children	Children
Emergency			
Safety	X	X	X
Housing	X	X	X
Food or clothing	X	X	X
Translation	X	X	
Legal guardianship		X	X
Short- or Long-term			
Transitional housing	X		X
Long-term housing	X		X
Permanency placement		X	
Legal assistance	X	X	X
Advocacy	X	X	X
Translation	X	X	X
Medical care	X	X	X
Mental health or counseling	X	X	X
Substance abuse treatment			X*
Transportation	X		X
Life skills	X	X	X
Education	X	X	X
Financial assistance or management	X		X
Job training or employment	X	X	X
Child care	X		X
Reunification or repatriation	X	X	X

**While substance abuse treatment may be a need for international victims, providers contacted by this study only identified a need for domestic child victims.*

Reprinted from Clawson HJ, Dutch NM, Salomon A, Goldblatt GL. Study of HHS programs serving human trafficking victims. Office of the Assistant Secretary for Planning and Evaluation Web site. http://aspe.hhs.gov/hsp/07/humantrafficking/Final/index.shtml. Published December 2009. Accessed June 10, 2013.

Additionally, health care providers should be aware of the social services available to victims of trafficking.[10] **Table 18-1** lists the needs of children, adolescents, and adults who may be international or domestic victims of HT. In order to help victims of HT, health care providers should know how to refer and access services and supports to meet their needs.

This chapter describes the scope of the HT problem both from an international and a domestic United States perspective and will focus primarily on the role health care providers can play in dealing with this problem. After reviewing the health care issues that may arise for child, adolescent, and adult victims of HT, the chapter explores specific clinical approaches to the health care encounter based on Kellogg & Sugarek's[1] TEAMSTAT model. Additionally, an overview of the legal issues related to human trafficking is provided, looking at both international and domestic aspects. Finally, the chapter summarizes details of a national community needs assessment conducted in the United States in an effort provide health care providers with the tools needed to activate community services and supports necessary to serve HT victims.

Human Trafficking: A Multifaceted Problem

HT is a multidimensional problem. When considering HT in the United States, it is important to keep in mind several different aspects of the problem. First, HT consists of both international and domestic dimensions. Second, HT is typically divided into 2 major forms that may overlap, namely (1) forced labor and (2) commercial sexual exploitation. Third and finally, HT impacts all ages, claiming child, adolescent, and adult victims. Each aspect has a fundamental impact on efforts directed at identifying and responding to HT since supports and services designed for foreign adult nationals who are victims of forced labor look very different from those designed for domestic minors who are victims of sexual exploitation. In short, HT is a messy problem that manifests itself in a complicated way. Since this is a relatively new area for research and advocacy, some of the available literature comprehensively addresses all of these dimensions, while others are more limited in focus. It is important for the health care provider to use the available literature to inform his or her care, realizing that the literature itself may be messy like the problem it addresses and may at times address international adult victims, at times international child victims, at other times domestic child or adolescent victims, and still at other times adult victims. The demonstrated state of the available literature on human trafficking is the reality of an evolving field.

Scope of the Problem

A criminal activity such as HT wherein perpetrators seek to avoid being discovered is likely to be difficult to adequately quantify. Consequently, it is hard to come by accurate numbers related to the scope of the problem of HT. It is estimated, however, that at least 12.3 million people in the world are estimated to be living as slaves at any given time; 56 % of these victims are women and girls.[11] It is further estimated that approximately 17 500 foreign nationals are trafficked into the United States annually.[12] In addition, despite the United States' position as a prominent developed nation, American homeless children and adolescents find themselves at risk for a number of problems, including sexual exploitation and sex for survival. Estimates for the number of child victims of domestic HT vary, but it is estimated that approximately 200 000 American children are at a high risk of being lured into the sex industry annually.[13]

Domestic child and adolescent victims of HT within the United States have different profiles than international victims. Most minor domestic victims are exploited in the commercial sex industry.[14] One out of every 3 teens on the street will be lured into prostitution within 48 hours of leaving home.[14] Entry into sex trafficking may occur as early as 12 or 13 years of age.[13]

Homeless children and adolescents, teens and young adults for whom it is not possible to live in a safe environment with a relative and who have no other safe alternative living arrangement[4,15] find themselves at risk for a number of problems, including HT. The National Coalition for the Homeless notes that there are 3 interrelated causes for homeless youth, namely family problems, economic pressures, and residential instability. Homeless youth find themselves in high risk situations in which exploitation is common and risk for physical and sexual assaults is high. These youths may experience physical and mental health problems, have no consistent way to attain necessary health care, and typically have difficulty continuing in school and supporting themselves financially.[15]

Related Health Problems

The various forms of HT have a profound impact on the health of an individual. The experiences of abuse, rape, social manipulation, and economic exploitation can result in a range of consequences on the mental, physical, and reproductive health of child victims and place them at risk for drug and alcohol abuse. It is important to understand the various stages traversed by most victims and how such sentinel episodes may result in the presenting manifestations of clinical signs and symptoms in order to successfully appreciate the clinical picture of victims of HT, identify such victims, and address their unique health care needs.[6]

Human Trafficking: Risk Factors

Common factors exist that may make certain individuals and populations more vulnerable to exploitation. Poverty, interpersonal violence, war, and economic hardships can be contributing factors that drive individuals to either seek out or be enticed by promises of a better and fruitful life elsewhere.[6,16] Such are the environments of most internationally trafficked victims. Individuals who are already disenfranchised from society or their families are at higher risk of being victimized. At-risk populations include:

— Homeless youth

— Runaway or "throwaway" children

— Children with past sexual or physical abuse

— Children with learning or physical disabilities

— Children with low self-esteem

Still, some youth come into contact with potential human traffickers in public places, such as movie theaters, schools, bus stops, and shopping malls.[17]

Displacement from Known and Familiar Surroundings

Human traffickers use force, intimidation, or enticement to lure victims. Physical removal may be subtle or brisk in its criminal implementation, but the result in the same in that the victim is placed in an unfamiliar situation and environment. The international victim may also be confronted with new languages, customs, and unknown persons. Physical assaults, unpredictable and unforeseen dangers, and unsafe travel conditions, such as lack of food and shelter or protection from the elements, may further add to the mental and physical stress of these victims.

Potentially Hazardous Nature of Expected Service

Persons involved in forced labor services may be expected to operate under extreme working conditions, such as working very long or unusual hours while enduring physical and psychological stress. Those working in the sex trade industry are at risk for sexually transmitted infections (STIs), pregnancy, and sexual and physical assaults.[18] An inability to control the number of clients and forced unprotected sex are possible abuses victims of forced prostitution may endure. Squalid living conditions, deprivation of food and human contact, and threats of violence and sexual assaults may also persist.

In an effort to maintain control of captive victims, perpetrators may force the victims to live or work in a location with high security measures, such as bars on windows, barbed wire, or security cameras. Other forms of control may include debt bondage; control of the victim's money, passports, or other important identifying documents; and threats of deportation or retaliation towards family members. Further isolation, alienation, and disorientation of child victims occur as communication with their family is prohibited. Mechanisms such as beatings, sexual assaults, and psychological anguish are used in the subordination of victims. Additionally, social isolation and distrust of legitimate authority figures (eg, law enforcement, protective agencies) are fostered in these environments. Many victims may develop traumatic bonding with the perpetrator in which a paradoxical cognitive distortion of the relationship and reciprocal positive feelings between the captor and hostage exist. For example, the child or adolescent victim may believe he or she is in love with his or her pimp or trafficker and may defend the pimp's actions, protect his or her identity, or both. Victims may dually show fear, distrust, and anger toward authority figures. Such a reaction is considered to be a form of human survival that allows the victim to cope in a stressful captive scenario and abusive situation.[4,19]

The exploitation that is a hallmark of the HT victim's experience can result in various medical consequences and health risks that may be detected in the health care setting by a health care provider who is aware of the signs and symptoms for which he or she is looking. While the health risks associated with HT have not been well recognized or documented, research and utilization of the medical literature on refugees, sex workers, and victims of interpersonal violence can allow for certain extrapolation and parallels of health consequences for trafficked victims.[18,20,21]

What sets HT apart from other traumatic events that may occur as a single event, such as stranger rape or physical assault, is the repetitive and continuous nature of the abuse. A victim may present with one or a combination of the previously described adverse health conditions.[8] When HT victimizing events occur over time and in combination, this pattern of inflicted traumas may result in a multiplicity of symptoms as noted in other types of chronic abuse (eg, childhood trauma, intimate partner violence [IPV], or torture).[22,23]

Specific Physical Health Issues

Any form of extreme physical stress can result in bodily injury, whether by forced manual labor or by direct violence. Physical abuse, confinement, and torture may result in unexplained injuries or signs of chronic abuse. Ligature marks created by ropes, cuffs, or chains are possible notable physical findings that may manifest in the victims of HT and may be indicative of efforts on the part of the perpetrator to detain or confine the victim. Cigarette burns, scratches and contusions are also possible notable physical findings that may be indicative of torture and abuse. Such methods further maintain control of the captive victim. Furthermore, tattooing may be used to further de-identify and dehumanize the victim as well as act as a branding tool for the trafficker and pimp. Hepatitis or other blood-borne infections may be of concern if unhygienic techniques were used when placing the tattoos. Poor living and working conditions may result in various respiratory or other related infections, such as tuberculosis (TB) and parasitic infections. Deprivation of sleep, food, light, and basic necessities may further contribute to the poor health and well-being of victims. Fatigue, exhaustion, and malnutrition may manifest in the HT victim as a result. Since seeking medical care for victims is a low priority for perpetrators, many medical and dental concerns may be ignored, thereby resulting in exacerbated preexisting conditions by the time medical attention is ultimately sought. Such actions may lead to disability or even death. It is crucial for the health care provider to realize that any physical finding that is inconsistent with the history provided must elicit concern and suspicion of abuse.

Reproductive and Gynecological Health

Minors and adults who are used as sex trade workers are at high risk of contracting STIs, including human immunodeficiency virus (HIV) and other blood-borne viruses.[24] Additionally, adolescent and adult HT victims face potential unwanted and unexpected pregnancies and gynecological complications stemming from unsafe abortions.[6,8]

Sexual violence perpetrated by men against women may involve both physical force or nonphysical coercion (eg, bribes, trickery, threats) to compel victims to have sex against their will. Traffickers may enforce a practice in which a sex worker must block her menstrual cycle by inserting foreign materials, such as sponges and mattress stuffing, into the vaginal vault. Complications stemming from this practice, as cited from a study in Brazil, especially when these items are maintained in the vagina for prolonged periods of time, include pain during intercourse, abnormal vaginal discharge, chronic infections, pelvic inflammatory disease (PID), and septic shock.[25] Chronic pain and foul odor associated with this practice may continue even after the victim has been removed from the trade.

Mental Health

Trauma has associated affective, behavioral, and cognitive consequences in minors and adults. Acute anxiety and stress disorder, conduct disorders, and personality disorders are well recognized in children living in victimizing circumstances.[24,25] Continued belittlement, humiliation, or intimidation; economic restrictions or confiscations of earnings; and other controlling behaviors further diminish victims and their ability to cope. Victims of HT may also suffer from low self-esteem, suicidal thoughts, and poor socialization and interpersonal relationships.[18,24] Victims of HT are likely to have suffered from abuse, stress, and depression similar to victims of other forms of violence.[18,22] Drug and alcohol abuse is also seen.[6,26]

Neglected Health Care Needs

The criminals who perpetrate HT against minors and adults are engaged in a criminal commercial enterprise; therefore, a constant and productive group of victims is the ultimate goal for these perpetrators. Given this expectation and the knowledge of the illegal nature of the activity, many traffickers do not allow for proper and timely pursuits of medical needs of their victims, regardless of age, child, adolescent, or adult, or status, international or domestic. The victims may be unclear as to when his or her last medical visit was. Thus, many afflictions harbored by the victims may be at advanced stages when finally presented to a health care setting due to the delay in seeking proper medical care.

Screening and Identification of Potential Victims

As stated previously, HT victims, either minor or adult, domestic or international, who appear in a health care setting are likely to be suspicious of most authority figures and reluctant to reveal too much personal information for fear of retaliation by their captors or, in the case of an international victim, possible deportation. Interacting with such victims requires sensitivity, compassion, and a nonjudgmental approach. As victims are unlikely to quickly reveal themselves as victims, if they recognize themselves as such, health care providers must be aware of subtle and nonverbal clues that may indicate abuse. It is important to realize that while many victims may not fully disclose abusive or concerning circumstances during a single interaction, it is prudent to obtain as much information as possible for their health and safety and begin developing a rapport and environment of trust for future encounters to the health care setting.[27]

Certain signs or red flags may be noted during the evaluation and should trigger concerns that the identification of a victim may be at hand. The signs or red flags discussed in the following sections must be considered; however, it must be noted that the list is not exclusive to HT victims since traumatic experiences that include exposure to violence or threats would likely manifest in a similar fashion.[4]

Such signs should be interpreted within the context of the clinical setting and the specific patient being evaluated. This is not a complete list but should be considered a clinical guide for critical clinical thinking and consideration.

History and Interview

- The patient is not allowed or able to speak for him or herself; patient is accompanied by an overly controlling and verbal speaker who insists on being present or interpreting for the patient.
- Patient is unable to provide a current address or claims to be just visiting.
- Patient does not know the city in which he or she resides.
- Patient reports that he or she cannot come and go as he or she wishes.
- Patient reports working excessively long or unusual hours; patient appears anxious to return quickly to work.
- Patient reports living in a home or environment with high security measures (eg, bars on windows, barbed wires, security cameras).
- Patient is evasive or untruthful in regard to age or identification.
- Patient is not in control of his or her own identification documents.

Physical Exam

- Patient is in general poor health, malnourished.
- Patient appears anxious, depressed, or submissive or displays nervous or paranoid behavior.
- Patient demonstrates poor eye contact.
- Patient is discovered to have evidence of brandings (eg, tattoo with symbol or name of trafficker) on his or her skin.
- Patient reacts apprehensively at references to law enforcement.
- Patient demonstrates flat affect.
- Patient presents with chronic infection that could have easily been treated medically if he or she had sought routine medical care.
- Patient demonstrates an addiction to drugs or alcohol.
- Patient exhibits unexplained injuries or signs of prolonged or untreated illness/disease
- Patient presents with bodily injuries (eg, signs of physical or sexual abuse, physical restraint, or torture); of particular concern are injuries that cannot be explained or whose explanation is inconsistent with the history provided.

The health care provider should first assess and then attend to the medical needs and resulting required treatments for the patient. If the health care provider suspects that the patient may be a potential victim of HT, he or she should isolate the patient from any accompanying individual; doing so will allow the health care provider to ask the patient direct questions and facilitate a discussion about his or her situation. The health care provider should be aware of those around when conducting the interview and providing resources to the victim. When interviewing a potential HT victim, it is important for the health care provider to be aware that many victims may have been coached as to how to answer certain questions and may have been provided a sort of cover story suggesting that he or she is a visiting student or tourist.[4]

The United States Department of Health and Human Services' (USDHHS) Campaign to Rescue and Restore Human Trafficking Victims suggests several questions that health care professionals can ask when screening potential victims of HT, including the following[28]:

— Can you leave your job or situation if you want?

— Can you come and go as you please?

— Have you been threatened if you try to leave?

— Have you been physically harmed in any way?

— What are your working or living conditions like?

— Where do you sleep and eat?

— Do you sleep in a bed, or on a cot, or on the floor?

— Have you ever been deprived of food, water, sleep or medical care?

— Do you have to ask permission to eat, sleep, or go to the bathroom?

— Are there locks on your doors and windows so you cannot get out?

— Has anyone threatened your family?

— Has your identification or documentation been taken from you?

— Is anyone forcing you to do anything that you do not want to do?

If the interview and resulting answers suggest that the patient may be an HT victim, the health care provider practicing in the United States should make use of the federal Department of Health and Human Services hotline for further assistance (1-888-3737-888).

TEAMSTAT Approach to Evaluation

Kellogg & Sugarek's[1] TEAMSTAT approach, as detailed in the following section, is one of the approaches that health care providers may use when evaluating and interacting with potential victims of human trafficking and abuse. TEAMSTAT is a mneumonic acronym representing the different aspects of the evaluation process as follows:

— **T**ell them your agenda.

— **E**xpress concern.

— **A**ssure normalcy of feelings.

— **M**edical issues

— **S**afety issues

— **T**est and treat presumptively.

— **A**ccess appropriate psychological and legal assistance.

— **T**imely follow-up

Tell Them Your Agenda

The health care professional should begin the evaluation and interview by informing the patient about the types of questions that he or she will be asking and the purpose of these questions. In order to foster trust and open communication, the health care provider should progress in a clear, direct, and nonjudgmental manner. The health provider may begin the interview by stating, "I'm going to ask you some questions about your body and health and about any possible harmful situations that may have happened to you. Some questions might be uncomfortable, but I am asking these questions to figure out what I need to look and test for, so I can help you for your safety and health." It is important to discuss the limitations of confidentiality at the beginning of the interview. For example, health care providers are obligated by law to report suspected cases of child abuse. In like turn, the health care provider is obligated to make a report if the patient intimates that he or she intends to harm him or herself or other persons.

Express Concern

Blending concern with the presenting medical complaint is an effective technique. For example, the health care provider may state, "I am concerned about your symptoms. Have you ever been checked for sexual infections?" This method, executed in a nonjudgmental, patient-focused manner, dually reduces stress in the patient and enhances trust and informational exchange.

Assure Normalcy of Feelings

During the interview, the child or adolescent may express feelings of guilt, fear, or anxiety surrounding potential situations of abuse, risky behaviors and lifestyles, and victimization. The clinician must acknowledge the sensitive nature of these disclosures and react to such admissions in a nonjudgmental, sensitive manner by restating the purpose for the interview questions as they relate to the child's health, welfare, and safety. The professional may validate the child's feelings by acknowledging that these feelings are normal or expected among children who have been through the same challenges and may say, "I know this is really hard for you to talk about, but I talk with many other kids in your situation, and it's not unusual to have the feelings that you do. Remember, I am asking these question to help me decide on how best to help you in your examination."

Medical Issues

A full medical history, including past medical history, hospitalizations, gynecological histories and problems, injuries, behavioral or psychiatric treatment, drug or alcohol use, pregnancy, and menstrual history should be obtained. The results of tests, pregnancy or otherwise health related, and details of the patient's sexual history should be obtained in order to understand potential risks and past concerns. While the patient may forget or misrepresent his or her medical history, it is important for the health care provider to obtain as much of the history as possible.

The health care professional should open this portion of the interview with nonleading, nonthreatening questions and may state, "I usually talk to teens whenever they may have been hurt or touched in a way that made them uncomfortable or scared. Has anything like this ever happened to you?" Some victims of prostitution and pornography may not consider their victimization as frightening or hurtful. More poignant questions may be required when the patient responds with no to this question such as, "Has anyone ever touched you on your private parts with any parts of their body that might be considered inappropriate?"

Physical abuse or victimization may be elicited by asking, "Have you ever been with anyone who hit or hurt you," or directed questions regarding violence by adults who initiate the victim's participation in prostitution or pornography.

Safety Issues

It is important to establish the victim's safety and anticipate the plan for discharge before leaving the health care setting. When discussing their own physical or sexual victimization or drug addiction, teenagers or children may reveal substance use and violence among family members. If the child is a victim of prostitution, pornography, physical abuse, or sexual abuse and is accompanied by a parent, the parent's belief of and support for the child should be clearly established before the child is discharged. The health care provider should inquire of the child's thoughts on or tendencies for running away, including his or her reasons, frequency, and final outcomes.

Test and Treat Presumptively

Medical management of child or adolescent victims of pornography or prostitution should include testing for STIs, pregnancy, and HIV. When appropriate, prophylactic treatment regimens for STI and pregnancy should be offered.

Access Appropriate Psychological and Legal Assistance

Crisis intervention services should be provided to the adolescent or child victim at the time of his or her medical evaluation when indicated. A clinical social worker can provide valuable assistance in locating community recourses and financial assistance. The health care professional is obligated to report suspected child abuse as determined by the laws of each state.

Timely Follow-up

Continuity of medical care is important in the assessment of healing injuries resulting from both physical and sexual abuses, management and treatment of STIs, and education of birth control and barrier methods. Monitoring of and counseling for drug and alcohol abuse and addictions may also be pursued by following drug levels, if necessary.

Documentation

While HT victims may not fully disclose their histories of exploitation, the clinician may still be able to obtain and document important information regarding the victim's experience and chronicling of his or her health. Such interactions will allow for a continuing opportunity to build trust and rapport with the child victim with the mutual goal of safeguarding the health of the patient. When information and a history are obtained from the patient regarding abuses, such information should be properly documented. The interview should be conducted, as mentioned previously, in a nonleading and open-ended format to allow the patient to report his or her experiences. The patient's responses to the clinician's inquiries should be recorded in addition to the patient's appearance and affect as they provide visual cues to the circumstances and experiences of the patient. Findings from the physical examination, including photo documentation as appropriate, should be recorded clearly and properly (see *Chapter 4, The Physical Examination in the Evaluation of Suspected Child Maltreatment: Physical Abuse and Sexual Abuse Examinations*).

Practical Action

The health care provider may find himself or herself feeling overwhelmed by the task of handling a case where HT is suspected as a result of the significant and broad nature of the victim's comprehensive needs. Realizing that numerous social agencies exist in the community to provide protection and disperse services to both domestic and international victims is the first step in providing these children with the help they need. When the health care provider suspects that a child has been the victim of abuse, he or she should make a report to law enforcement or child protective services (CPS) as required by law. The clinician should explain his or her duty to report such crimes of abuse to the patient. Additionally, the federal hotline number (1-888-3737-888) is available as a resource to provide further assistance for HT-related inquiries and cases.

Legal Response to Human Trafficking: Overview for Health Care Providers

Since HT is at its core a criminal activity that harms victims, it is important for nurses and other health care providers to have a basic familiarity with the legal landscape that impacts victims. In an effort to combat criminal networks that defy borders, the United Nations (UN) ratified The Convention Against Transnational Organized Crime and the Protocols Thereto (the Convention) in 2004.[2] The UN established the Convention to present a united front against the transnational criminal problems facing the world's citizens, especially HT. The Convention promulgated a set of guidelines aimed at severely undermining HT networks, protecting the victims of this heinous trade, and punishing those who seek to exploit others. It was ratified as the Protocol to Prevent, Suppress and Punish Trafficking in Persons, Especially Women and Children (the Protocol). Because there is no international law enforcement body that can prosecute trafficking, the authors of the Protocol sought to erect a unified framework that all nations could try to build within their respective countries to better confront global trafficking and other forms of organized crime.[29] There are currently 117 signatories to the Protocol, including the United States.

Prevention

The Protocol urges signatories to enter into programs, studies, and human aid projects to better understand how trafficking networks develop and fester and how to prevent these networks from forming by reducing poverty worldwide. Countries are encouraged to engage in bilateral and multilateral efforts in the form of economic, cultural, social and educational development projects targeted at promoting the well-being of at-risk segments of the population, particularly women and children. Additionally, because trafficking is an international trade with no respect for national borders, the Protocol asserts the necessity of nations to cooperate in law enforcement endeavors and effective border control while treating the victims of trafficking with dignity and respect.

Protection

In keeping with the United Nation's mission of global respect for human rights, the Protocol proposes that signatories develop a legal framework aimed at not only ensuring the protection of trafficked persons but also providing them with housing, counseling, medical care, and training and opportunities for work. Furthermore, special education and health care programs for youths may need to be implemented since many exploited persons are minors. The Protocol urges signatories to criminalize any attempt to traffic persons, including prosecuting accomplices and others who are involved in organizing or directing trafficking. The United States, which signed the Protocol on December 13, 2000, enacted the Trafficking Victims Protection Act (TVPA) in 2000 and the Trafficking Victims Protection Reauthorization Act (TVPRA) in 2008.[30] Under TVPA, the State Department is responsible for publishing the Trafficking in Persons (TIP) Report annually. The 2009 TIP Report highlights some of the innovative programs being used around the world to provide protection for victims of trafficking. For example, an Uzbek organization called Istiqbolli Avlod operates in the United Arab Emirates, a major destination for trafficked Uzbek women.[12] Between September 2008 and February 2009, Istiqbolli Avlod successfully used cultural and language outreach to repatriate most of the 41 Uzbek women found to be incarcerated in jails in the United

Arab Emirates. Similarly, the Jordanian ministry of labor has created a fund to provide humanitarian assistance to trafficking victims and even to pay for the legal costs of civil and criminal suits against traffickers.

Criminalization

The TVPRA asks foreign governments to supply information related to trafficking investigations, convictions, prosecutions, and sentences to the United States government. For instance, in 2008 reports submitted to the United States recorded a total of 5212 prosecutions and 2983 convictions worldwide. The TIP Report includes a tier ranking system that is categorized into the 3 focus areas of trafficking prevention: prosecution, protection, and prevention. Once a government's activity in combating HT is assessed, countries are ranked as Tier 1, Tier 2, or Tier 3. Countries that are fully compliant with TVPA minimum standards receive Tier 1 status; nations that do not meet TVPA minimum standards and have taken no steps toward achieving those standards are ranked as Tier 3. Tier 3 countries may be subject to nonhumanitarian sanctions and opposition on the part of the United States to other benefits from organizations such as the World Bank. In 2010, the United States included itself in the rankings, based on the same standards to which other countries are held.[11,31]

In between these tiers, there are Tier 2 and Tier 2 watch list nations. Tier 2 countries do not fully comply with TVPA minimum standards but are making significant efforts to bring themselves into compliance. Nations are placed on the Tier 2 watch list when the absolute number of trafficking victims reported is very significant or is significantly increasing or the country fails to provide evidence that it is increasing its efforts to combat HT from the previous year. Evidence of efforts to combat trafficking, includes increased investigations, prosecutions, convictions of trafficking crimes, and efforts to provide greater assistance to victims. It also includes efforts to decrease complicity by government officials in HT.

Trafficking Victims Protection Act

The TVPA focuses on 3 aspects to combat human trafficking: prevention of the crime, prosecution of the trafficker, and protection for victims. Under this law, the USDHHS can certify international HT victims as trafficked persons. Once certified, victims are eligible for physical and mental health services, housing, food stamps, and educational and vocational programs as well as legal services and translation services. Victims of the more severe forms of international trafficking may also be granted a T-visa, which allows them to remain in the United States for 3 years and offers them protection under the law. After 3 years, the victim may apply to adjust his or her status to become a lawful permanent resident. Domestic trafficking, on the other hand, lacks the same comprehensive system that the TVPA provides to victims of international trafficking.

International Victims

In order to be granted T-visa nonimmigrant status, the applicant must prove that he or she (1) has been a victim of a severe form of human trafficking; (2) is physically present in the United States or certain territories of the Unites States because of that trafficking; (3) is either under 15 years of age or has complied with any reasonable request for assistance in the investigation or prosecution of the trafficker; and (4) would suffer extreme hardship if removed from the country.[30] An immigrant is ineligible for a T-visa if he or she participated in trafficking others.

Based on those requirements, a trafficking victim who is aged 15 years or older must assist law enforcement in the investigation or prosecution of the trafficker and show extreme hardship if deported. HT victims often require medical attention, risk societal stigmatization, or face potential harm at the hand's of their trafficker's associates, circumstances which fulfill the extreme hardship criterion of the T-visa.

Despite the fact that the United States is authorized to grant 5000 T-visas annually, it granted only 247 T-visas to trafficking victims and 171 T-visas to derivative family members in fiscal year 2008. The Department of Justice (DOJ) has acknowledged a disparity between estimates of trafficking victims in the United States and those victims that have been located and assisted. Helga Konrad, Special Representative on Combating Trafficking in Human Beings for the Organization for Security and Cooperation in Europe, noted that the United States T-visa levels were remarkably low in 2003, with 328 granted, and that these levels fell further in the year 2004 to 136. Additionally, she criticized the United States government's requirement that trafficking victims assist law enforcement agencies in prosecuting traffickers as "benign coercion." Therefore, while the United States is taking decisive legislative and enforcement measures to prevent and curb trafficking, more efforts could be made to find, protect, and rehabilitate victims.

HT victims are often hidden from public view and difficult to locate, which could be a contributing factor to the United States' T-visa level. This is especially true in the context of labor trafficking, which may involve one person performing domestic labor in a private home or a few hundred people working under what appears to be legitimate circumstances in a factory. In addition, victims may not view themselves as victims, instead believing that they are obligated to pay off a debt regardless of the circumstances or feeling guilty that they are in the United States illegally. Victims may also have become so psychologically abused that they are dependent on their traffickers, who often train the victims to give certain answers to police and tell them they will be deported to their home counties in shame if they report their situations to authorities.[30]

Additionally, law enforcement officers who encounter HT victims may lack sympathy for the situation as a result of a lack of cooperation on the part of the victim or a lack of training regarding how to identify victims.

Domestic Victims

Currently, there is no assistance available for domestic victims under TVPA. However, on December 23, 2008, TVPA was reauthorized as the Trafficking Victims Protection Reauthorization Act (TVPRA). Even though the reauthorization still does not provide assistance for domestic victims, it includes a few provisions that make prosecution of trafficking offenders easier for domestic victims and others. TVRPA now includes a new trafficking-specific conspiracy statute that prohibits peonage, enticement into slavery, forced labor, trafficking, sex trafficking, and domestic servitude. TVPRA also includes a new provision penalizing those who knowingly benefit from participating in a venture that engages in trafficking. Previously, only the sex trafficking statute contained such a provision. TVPRA also strengthens the crime of sex trafficking of a minor by eliminating the knowledge-of-age requirement in certain instances. Previously, proof was required to identify the victim as a minor. In the past, the government was required to prove that the defendant actually knew that force, fraud, or coercion would be used to cause a person to engage in a commercial sex act. New language in the statute requires only that the defendant acted in reckless disregard of the fact that such means would be used.

Providers

The majority of providers that come in contact with HT victims do so incidentally. Often their meeting occurs through centers that provide legal or immigration services, such as Catholic charities, ethnically specific service centers, such as Boat People SOS Immigration Service Center in Houston, and nonprofit or faith-based centers.[32]

Victims are sometimes referred to service providers by law enforcement, if the law enforcement agency has a policy of recognizing minor trafficking victims as such instead of as delinquents. Police anti-trafficking task forces accomplish a majority of initial contact with HT victims. A number of coalitions that include collaboration between law enforcement agencies and nongovernmental agencies, such as the Human Trafficking Rescue Alliance (HTRA), have formed in numerous cities across the United States.[33] HTRA includes the FBI's Innocence Lost task force, which centers its investigations on domestic minor sex trafficking. HTRA works to ensure that the needs of both the international and domestic populations of victims are being addressed.

Perhaps the most significant challenge the health care provider faces when evaluating a victim of HT is meeting his or her need for a safe house, or a place of shelter, and protection if he or she is a victim of forced prostitution. Recovery can be a long and difficult process, and an ideal safe house can offer education, job training, life-skills training, individual and group therapy, recreational activities, and other long-term support services.

The Safe House NOW task force is a model program that has brought together representatives from the FBI, local law enforcement, courts, United States and district attorneys, child protective service (CPS) and juvenile probation, women's groups, and nonprofit and faith organizations to develop a plan to provide therapeutic, medical, educational, and housing resources to children caught up in sex trafficking. In the summer of 2010, Arrow Child & Family Ministries[34] was contacted by the task force and Children At Risk regarding the need for a safe house for domestic victims of child sex trafficking in Texas.[7] It is the goal of this coalition to open Freedom Place in late 2011 and to provide a rehabilitative haven for up to 24 female victims of HT.

There are a number of successful organizations currently providing a safe environment to rescued victims of trafficking who serve as an example of best practices for others wishing to emulate their model. Standing Against Global Exploitation (SAGE) is a San Francisco nonprofit organization committed to bringing an end to the commercial sexual exploitation of children and adults. SAGE offers many services to survivors, including in-custody crisis counseling, assessment, traditional services for young women detained at San Francisco's Juvenile Justice Center, mental health services, transgender and men's programs, and a John's school.[35] The San Francisco area appears to be better situated to address the needs of HT victims than most other metropolitan areas in the United States.

Angela's House, which is located in Atlanta, GA and owned by the Juvenile Justice Fund, is a safe house and residential group home for child and adolescent victims of commercial sexual exploitation.[36] This facility, combined with various shelters for the homeless and victims of domestic abuse, forms a network of organizations that provide services to victims of HT. Angela's House is a group home in an undisclosed location outside of Atlanta that houses 6 girls at a time. Normally, girls complete treatment in 4 to 6 months, but if a girl needs more time to complete her treatment, she can stay longer. Seventy-five percent of the girls in Angela's House come to the group home from the juvenile court or the Department of Juvenile Justice. The other 25% are placed in Angela's House through recommendations from the Division of Family and Children Services (DFCS), concerned citizens, parents, or other agencies. Education and counseling services are provided to all girls staying in Angela's House. As is the case in other metropolitan areas, Atlanta has a need for more facilities for male victims of commercial sexual exploitation.

Girls Educational and Mentoring Services (GEMS) is a shelter in New York City that provides direct services and shelter to female trafficking victims aged 12 through 21 years.[37] Rachel Lloyd, a survivor of commercial sexual exploitation herself, founded the organization 30 years ago. Because GEMS has functioned successfully since its creation in 1999, the service providers have gained a great deal of expertise in the area of providing services to girls who have been in prostitution. Therefore, they are also able to provide training to other organizations interested in GEMS and thereby secure additional income programming.

Covenant House, an organization founded to provide services to homeless and runaway youth and young adults, has 20 facilities throughout the country, as well as facilities internationally.[38] Its New York location deals with international, domestic male, and female victims. This organization provides counseling, referrals, educational and vocational programs, medical services, legal services, youth leadership opportunities, and outreach services to homeless youth, including trafficking victims. Covenant House helps over 70 000 children every year through its residential and nonresidential programs and includes a program for victims of HT. Youth are allowed shelter at the Covenant House facility so long as they fit within the organization's age range and are not a potential risk to anyone else.

Children of the Night is one of the most successful programs dealing with child victims of commercial sexual exploitation in the country.[39] Children of the Night is located in Van Nuys, a suburb of Los Angeles. The program has been helping victims of child prostitution for nearly 30 years.[5] This organization focuses solely on minors who are victims of sex trafficking and reaches out to victims through several avenues. The facility can accommodate 24 victims; however, Children of the Night also provides services to victims who do not reside at the shelter. Furthermore, through their hotline, they are able to help between 10 000 and 13 000 people a year.

At their residential shelter, children can arrive as young as 11 years of age and are allowed to stay until they are 18 years of age. In case of necessity, some children are allowed to stay up to age 18½ years. The duration of stay for trafficking victims varies widely, from as little as a few months to up to 4 years.

Children of the Night provides comprehensive care for its residents. Education is provided to the children through an on-site private school.[39] Like GEMS in New York City, Children of the Night uses poetry as a creative outlet for the victims in their shelter. One of the most noteworthy aspects of Children of the Night is that it is one of the few programs nationwide that caters to victims of sexual exploitation, regardless of the sex of the victim.[6] In fact, 40% of Children of the Night's clients are boys under the age of 18 years. The lack of care for transgender and male victims of sexual exploitation is frequently identified by experts in the field as being one of the biggest gaps in direct services.

Responding When No Services Exist: National Community Needs Assessment

An informed and responsive community is necessary to serve both the international and domestic victims of HT. As with most effective community development projects, a needs assessment that inventories the services and supports that are available and the ones that need to be built in the future is a typical starting point for coordinated action. Nurses and other health care providers who seek to activate their communities and further develop the health, social services, and legal supports and services needed by victims of HT can use this needs assessment as a starting point for such advocacy.

The National Institute of Justice commissioned the National Needs Assessment of Service Providers and Trafficking Victims, guided by the following specific questions related to service provision[40]:

— What services currently exist for trafficking victims?

— How responsive are these services to victims?

— What are the barriers to providing services to trafficking victims?

— What assistance or support do service providers need to effectively serve trafficking victims?

The national needs assessment consisted primarily of a telephone interview of a national sample of service providing agencies, supplemented with a focus group interview of such agencies and a focus group of HT victims. The telephone interview was offered to 159 agencies; 98 completed the interview for a response rate of 62%. The interviews were conducted between October 2002 and January 2003; the focus groups were conducted in February 2003. The types of agencies that participated are listed in **Figure 18-1**. The service providing agencies that completed the telephone interviews tended to serve a variety of vulnerable populations and nearly one-third served only trafficking victims. **Figure 18-2** lists the types of clients served. Specifically examining the types of HT victims who were served by the responding agencies, nearly two-thirds of the victims were dealing with forced prostitution. **Figure 18-3** displays the various other forms of forced labor and sex trade–related activities. As might be expected, the types of needs that the HT victims had were broad in nature and large in number. The needs spanned immediate needs for housing, medical care, and legal services as well as long-term needs such as job training and drug treatment services (**Figure 18-4**). Finally, and not surprisingly, the respondents that reported being hindered in their ability to serve HT victims identified a number of barriers. **Figure 18-5** shows the common barriers; high on the list are inadequate resources, training, and coordination among agencies and professionals dealing with these victims. The national needs assessment concluded with a number of recommendations, including a recommendation for enhanced training among all professionals who might come in contact with HT victims and, therefore, be in the position to identify and refer these victims for services.

Conclusion

Victims of HT carry a unique set of health care needs; addressing those needs is one of the first steps in drawing them back into society and out from under their veiled existences. Assessing and treating their various physical ailments, the resultant sequelae and complications of their industries and living conditions, and addressing their mental health needs allows for the treatment of the individual and his or her basic human needs. The health care professional has a unique and vital role to play in both the identification of these victims and the possible continued treatment of their present and ongoing health needs. Various local and regional agencies and organizations may coordinate to address the other social and legal needs of the victim that further draw the individual out of the shadow of secrecy and shame. Being as health care professionals are recognized as potential catalysts for the identification of these victims, it is vital that providers are trained and educated in the recognition of the signs of human trafficking and are aware of the next steps involved in rescuing the victims.

As a first step, if the nurse and health care team's assessment suggests that the patient may be a victim of trafficking, the nurse should contact the National Human Trafficking Resource Center (NHTRC) hotline (1-888-3737-888) for further assistance. Trained

Figure 18-1. *Type of agencies and organizations represented in the sample. Reprinted from Clawson HJ, Small KV, Go ES, Bradley WM. Needs assessment for service providers and trafficking victims. United States Department of Justice Web site. http://www.ncjrs.gov/pdffiles1/nij/grants/202469.pdf. Updated 2003. Accessed February 13, 2011.*

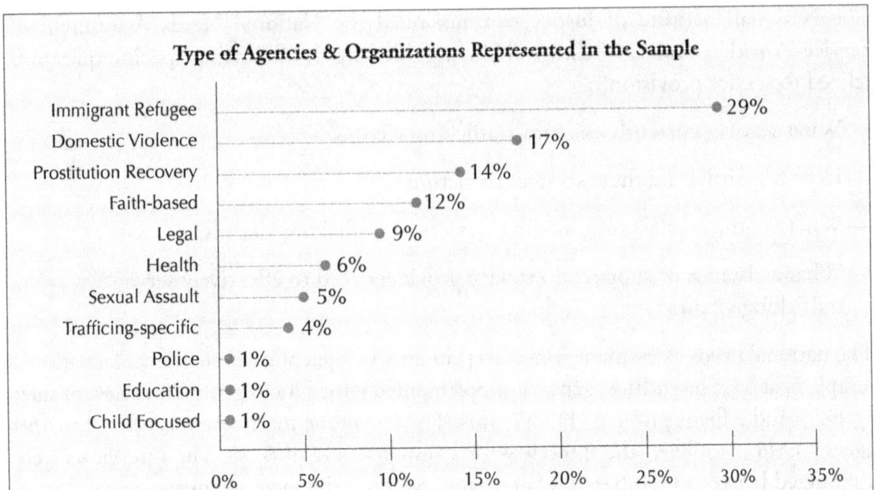

Figure 18-1

Figure 18-2. *General type of patients served. Reprinted from Clawson HJ, Small KV, Go ES, Bradley WM. Needs assessment for service providers and trafficking victims. United States Department of Justice Web site. http://www.ncjrs.gov/pdffiles1/nij/grants/202469.pdf. Updated 2003. Accessed February 13, 2011.*

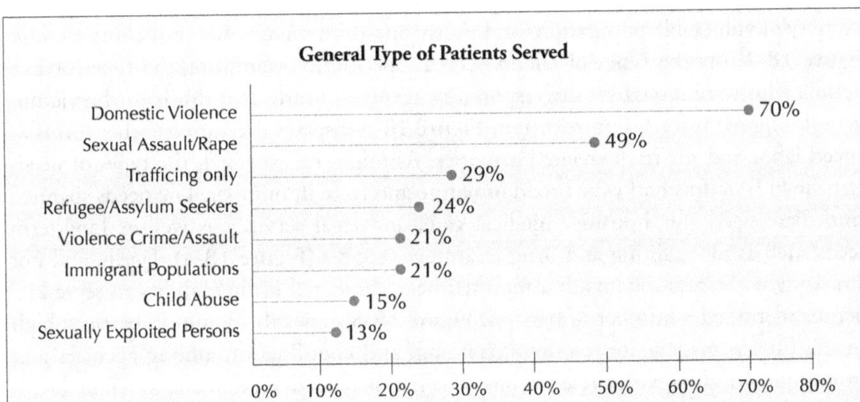

Figure 18-2

Figure 18-3. *Types of trafficking victims. Reprinted from Clawson HJ, Small KV, Go ES, Bradley WM. Needs assessment for service providers and trafficking victims. United States Department of Justice Web site. http://www.ncjrs.gov/pdffiles1/nij/grants/202469.pdf. Updated 2003. Accessed February 13, 2011.*

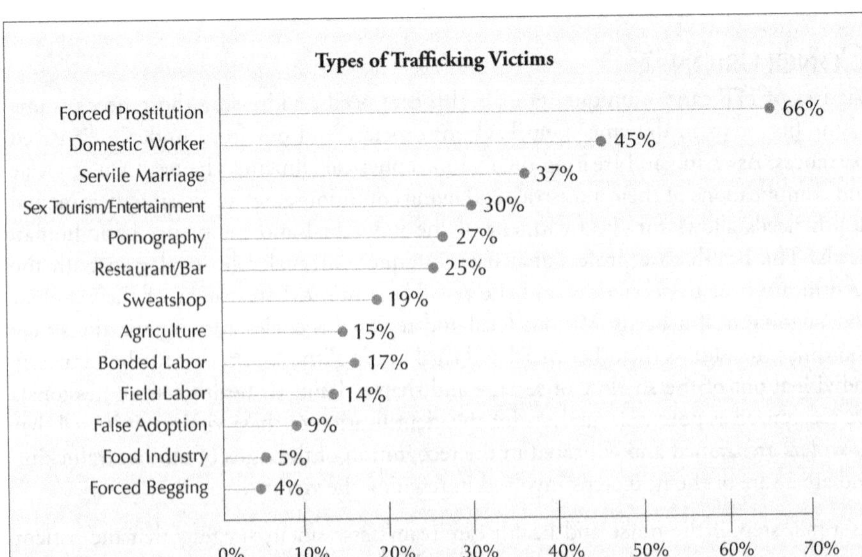

Figure 18-3

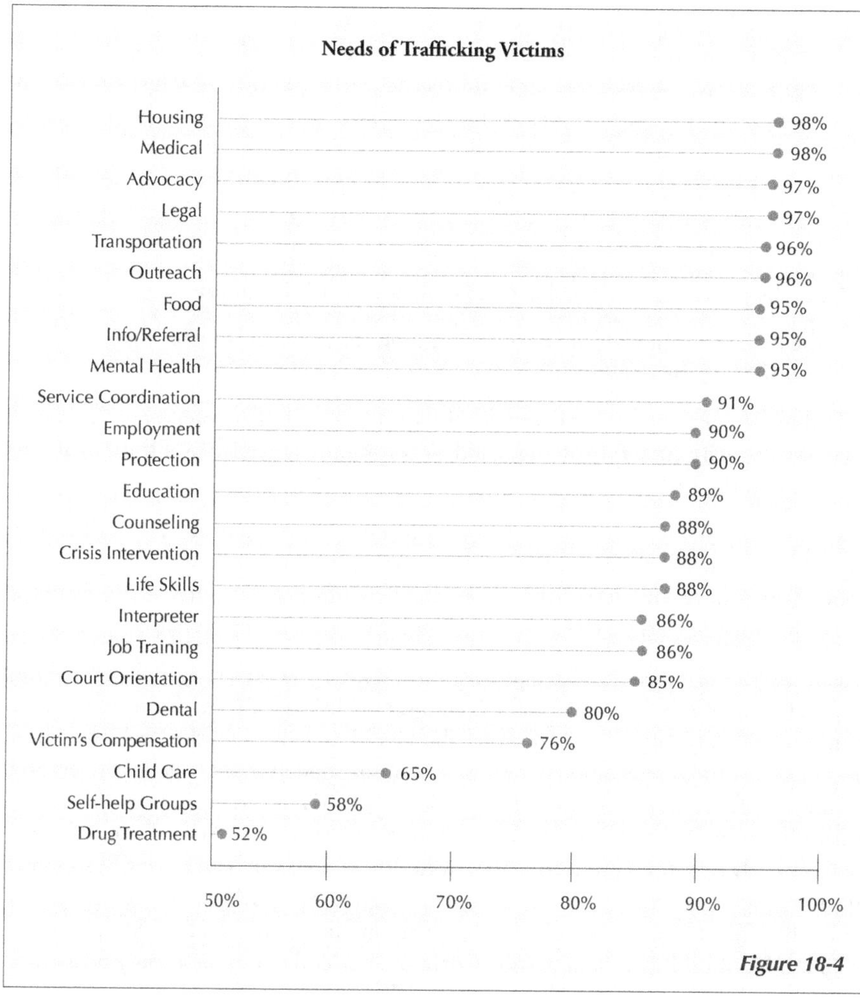

Figure 18-4. *Needs of trafficking victims. Reprinted from Clawson HJ, Small KV, Go ES, Bradley WM. Needs assessment for service providers and trafficking victims. United States Department of Justice Web site. http://www.ncjrs.gov/pdffiles1/nij/grants/202469.pdf. Updated 2003. Accessed February 13, 2011.*

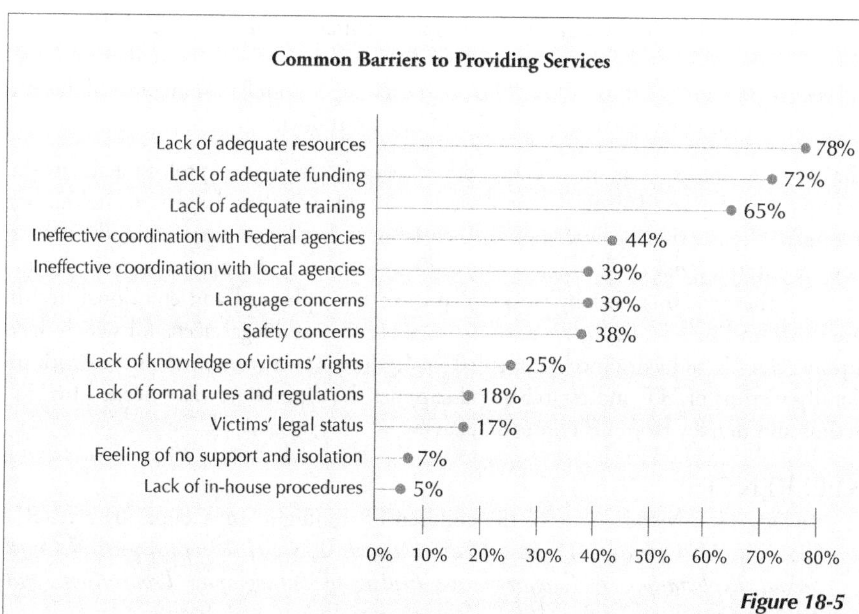

Figure 18-5. *Common barriers to providing services. Reprinted from Clawson HJ, Small KV, Go ES, Bradley WM. Needs assessment for service providers and trafficking victims. United States Department of Justice Web site. http://www.ncjrs.gov/pdffiles1/nij/grants/202469.pdf. Updated 2003. Accessed February 13, 2011.*

personnel will help determine whether the person is truly a victim of trafficking and may connect the victim to local resources in the community. The hotline can help determine the appropriate next steps and referrals for the victim. The hotline may further assist in assessing the level of danger to the victim. The following points should be considered when evaluating a patient who is suspected of having been the victim of HT:

— Is the trafficker present with the victim?

— What will happen if the patient does not return to the trafficker?

— Does the patient believe he, she, or a family member is in danger?

— Is the patient a minor? If the victim is a minor, the provider is under legal obligation to contact CPS.

A child is defined as an individual under the age of 18 and, therefore, cannot properly consent to sexual activity; therefore, child prostitution is included as a form of severe trafficking in the TVPA.

Law enforcement may need to be involved to ensure the safety of the victim. It is important to provide all resources directly to the patient and only when the patient is alone. If the patient is not receptive to accepting such information at that time, encourage him or her to call at a time when he or she needs help or someone to talk to.

The development of health-related prevention and intervention strategies for trafficking may be based on existing models of prevention established for other forms of violence against women (eg, IPV, rape, and sexual abuse) and models established for integration of immigrants and reintegration of returnees.[6] Future models could include gender- and culture-specific strategies developed for various potential areas, such as medical care, social service practices, health education, and public awareness. Several organizations have currently developed guidelines on how health workers can better identify, support, and refer victims of various forms of violence and control. Many of these programs primarily offer information and knowledge about the plight of HT. One particular program, Houston Rescue and Restore Coalition, currently in its pilot study phase, not only provides the knowledge and awareness of HT to health professionals but also builds on the skills of identification and referral of a potential victim of human trafficking.[31] This program aims to raise awareness and instill a basic skill set on how to identify, refer, and report potential victims of HT. The program's target population includes all health professionals who may encounter a victim of human trafficking.

The bottom line is clear, nurses and other related health care professionals are in a unique position to identify potential victims of HT, whether the victims be minors or adults, whether they be exploited for their labor or for sexual purposes, and whether they are international or domestic victims. Once detected, the nurse can assist in the rescue of these victims, first by working to meet their physical and emotional health care needs and then by being aware of the social service and legal needs for which they require referrals and assistance. Informed professionals and communities can work to identify victims of HT and establish and support the types of services needed by HT victims and thereby stop this criminal behavior.

References

1. Kellogg ND. Medical care of the children of the night. In: Cooper S, Estes RJ, Giardino AP, Kellogg ND, eds. *Medical, Legal, & Social Science Aspects of Child Sexual Exploitation: A Comprehensive Review of Pornography, Prostitution, and Internet Crimes.* St. Louis, MO: STM Learning, Inc; 2005:350-368.

2. Feingold DA. Human trafficking. *Foreign Policy.* 2005(150):26-32.
3. Watts C, Zimmerman C. Violence against women: global scope and magnitude. *Lancet.* 2002;359(9313):1232-1237.
4. United States Department of Health and Human Services, Administration on Children, Youth and Families. The campaign to rescue and restore victims of human trafficking: identifying and interacting with victims of human trafficking. Administration on Children, Youth and Families Web site. http://www.acf.hhs.gov/trafficking/campaign_kits/tool_kit_health/identify_victims.html. Updated 2010. Accessed August 2010.
5. Miller E, Decker MR, Silverman JG, Raj A. Migration, sexual exploitation, and women's health: a case report from a community health center. *Violence Against Women.* 2007;13(5):486-497.
6. Zimmerman C, Yun K, Watts C, et al. *The Health Risks and Consequences of Trafficking in Women and Adolescents: Findings From a European Study.* London, UK: London School of Hygiene & Tropical Medicine; 2003.
7. Family Violence Protection Fund: World Childhood Foundation. *Turning Pain Into Power: Trafficking Survivors' Perspectives on Early Intervention Strategies.* San Francisco, CA: Family Violence Protection Fund; 2005.
8. Barrows J, Finger R. Human trafficking and the healthcare professional. *South Med J.* 2008;101(5):521-524.
9. Dovydaitis T. Human trafficking: The role of the health care provider. *J Midwifery Women's Health.* 2010;55(5):462-467.
10. Clawson HJ, Dutch NM, Salomon A, Goldblatt GL. Study of HHS programs serving human trafficking victims. Office of the Assistant Secretary for Planning and Evaluation Web site. http://aspe.hhs.gov/hsp/07/humantrafficking/Final/index.shtml. Published December 2009. Accessed June 10, 2013.
11. United States Department of State Office to Monitor and Combat Trafficking in Persons. Major forms of trafficking in persons: trafficking in persons report 2010. United States Department of State Web site. http://www.state.gov/g/tip/rls/tiprpt/2010. Updated 2010. Accessed May 18, 2011.
12. United States Department of State Office to Monitor and Combat Trafficking in Persons. Major forms of trafficking in persons: trafficking in persons report 2009. http://www.state.gov/g/tip/rls/tiprpt/2009/123126.htm. Updated 2009. Accessed October 2010.
13. Polaris Project. What is human trafficking? Polaris Project Web site. http://www.polarisproject.org/human-trafficking/human-trafficking-faqs#What is human trafficking? Accessed August 2010.
14. Hammer J, Finkelhor D, Sedlak AJ. Runaway/thrownaway children: national estimates and characteristics. *NISMART Bulletin Series.* 2002. NCJ196469.
15. National Coalition for the Homeless. Education of homeless children and youth. National Coalition for the Homeless Web site. http://www.nationalhomeless.org/factsheets/education.html. Updated 2009. Accessed 2011.
16. Watts C, Zimmerman C. Violence against women: global scope and magnitude. *The Lancet.* 2002;359(9313):1232-1237.

17. Boxill NA, Richardson DJ. Ending sex trafficking of children in Atlanta. *Affilia.* 2007;22(2):138-149.

18. Jeal N, Salisbury C, Turner K. The multiplicity and interdependency of factors influencing the health of street-based sex workers: a qualitative study. *Sex Transm Infect.* 2008;84(5):381-385.

19. de Fabrique N, Roman SJ, Vecchi GM, Van Hasslet VB. Understanding stockholm syndrome. *FBI Law Enforcement Bull.* 2007;76(7):10-15.

20. Carswell K, Blackburn P, Barker C. The relationship between trauma, post-migration problems and the psychological well-being of refugees and asylum seekers. *Int J Soc Psychiatry.* 2011;57(2):107-119.

21. Hossain M, Zimmerman C, Abas M, Light M, Watts C. The relationship of trauma to mental disorders among trafficked and sexually exploited girls and women. *Am J Public Health.* 2010;100(12):2442-2449.

22. Dube SR, Anda RF, Felitti VJ, et al. Childhood abuse, household dysfunction, and the risk of attempted suicide throughout the life span: Findings from the adverse childhood experiences study. *JAMA.* 2001;286(24):3089-3096.

23. Thomsen AB, Eriksen J, Smidt-Nielsen K. Chronic pain in torture survivors. *Forensic Sci Int.* 2000;108(3):155-163.

24. Cohen JA, Mannarino AP. Trauma-focused cognitive behavioural therapy for children and parents. *J Child Adolesc Ment Health.* 2008;13(4):158-162.

25. Cutajar MC, Mullen PE, Ogloff JRP, Thomas SD, Wells DL, Spataro J. Psychopathology in a large cohort of sexually abused children followed up to 43 years. *Child Abuse Negl.* 2010;34(11):813-822.

26. Raymond JG, Hughes DG. *Sex Trafficking of Women in the United States: International and Domestic Trends.* Washington, DC: Coalition Against Trafficking Women; 2001.

27. Sabella D. The Role of the Nurse in Combating Human Trafficking. *AM J Nurs.* 2011;111(2):28-37.

28. United States Department of Health and Human Services, Rescue and Restore Victims of Human Trafficking. Resources: screening tool for victims of human trafficking. Administration for Children and Families Web site. http://www.acf.hhs.gov/sites/default/files/orr/screening_questions_to_assess_whether_a_person_is_a_trafficking_victim.pdf. Accessed June 10, 2013.

29. United Nations Office on Drug and Crimes. *United Nations Convention Against Transnational Organized Crime and the Protocols Thereto.* New York: United Nations;2004.

30. Victims of Trafficking and Violence Protection Act of 2000, HR 3244, 106th Cong (2000).

31. Moore AJ. *An Intervention Mapping Approach: Identification of Human Trafficking Victims by Health Professionals* [dissertation]. Houston, TX: University of Texas School of Public Health; 2010.

32. Boat People SOS. Where we work: US branches. Boat People SOS Web site. http://www.bpsos.org/mainsite/where-we-work/us-branches/34-houston.html. Accessed June 10, 2013.

33. Harris County Sheriff's Office. Human Trafficking Rescue Alliance (HTRA). Harris County Sheriff's Office Web site. http://webservices.hcso.hctx.net/HumanTrafficking/default.asp. Accessed June 10, 2013.

34. Arrow Child and Family Resources. Overview. Arrow Child and Family Ministries Web site. http://www.arrow.org/family/Freedom-Place.html. Accessed June 10, 2013.

35. The Sage Project. Home. The Sage Project Web site. http://sagesf.org. Accessed June 10, 2013.

36. Youth Spark. Angela's House. Youth Spark Web site. http://www.youth-spark.org/learn/our-programs/legacy-programs/angelas-house. June 10, 2013.

37. Girls Educational and Mentoring Services. GEMS Web site. http://www.gems-girls.org. Accessed June 10, 2013.

38. Covenant House. CHNY. Covenant House Web site. http://covenanthouseny.org. Accessed June 10, 2013.

39. Children of the Night. Children of the Night Web site. http://www.childrenofthe night.org. Accessed June 10, 2013.

40. Clawson HJ, Small KV, Go ES, Bradley WM. Needs assessment for service providers and trafficking victims. United States Department of Justice Web site. http://www.ncjrs.gov/pdffiles1/nij/grants/202469.pdf. Updated 2003. Accessed February 13, 2011.

Chapter 19

Substance Dependence and Child Maltreatment

Hillary Mowbray, MD
Rebecca Girardet, MD
Angelo P. Giardino, MD, PhD

Key Points

1. Children living in homes with a substance user are at risk for neglect or abuse resulting from household dysfunction and changes in adult behavior that can occur with chemical addiction.
2. A recent analysis of data from a national survey of child well-being found that child protective service (CPS) workers' perceptions of parental substance dependence is associated with a greater likelihood of case substantiation and child removal, irrespective of the presence of other risk factors for child maltreatment.[1]
3. The *Diagnostic and Statistical Manual of Mental Disorders-IV-TR (DSM-IV-TR)*[1] defines chemical dependence as "a pattern of substance use leading to significant impairment in functioning" with coexisting problems at work, school, or home; use in situations that are hazardous; legal problems; or continued use despite significant problems.
4. The children of substance users may suffer from adjustment problems, impaired emotional development, increased level of anxiety and depression, low self-esteem, lack of control over the environment, and increased risk for substance abuse problems later in life.
5. Johnson and Leff[2] found that predictive factors of child resilience include the caregiver's ability to provide for the basic needs of the child, the child's coping skills, the age of the child at the onset of the addiction or relapse, and family support.
6. Efforts to decrease chemical dependency may reduce the prevalence of child maltreatment and improve overall adult health outcomes.
7. Caring for children can be stressful in the absence of substance abuse or other stressors. Potential triggers for child abuse may occur at any time and include an infant's inconsolable crying, feeding difficulties, failed toilet training, or unrealistic expectations. For a parent or caregiver who is impaired, the ability to effectively deal with the potential triggers is decreased.
8. The nursing assessment should include both formal questioning conducted in a nonjudgmental manner and physical observations.
9. Addiction to drugs or alcohol is considered a chronic medical condition, and treatment is neither easier nor more complicated than treating diabetes, hypertension, or asthma.

Introduction

Substance dependence is an immense public health problem in the United States. According to data collected in a recent national survey, just over 9% of Americans aged

12 years or older admitted to having used an illicit drug during the previous month, and 2.6% reported nonmedical use of prescription psychotherapeutic agents. In the same survey, 6.5% of Americans disclosed heavy drinking, defined as having 5 or more drinks on each of 5 or more consecutive days, within the previous 30 days.[3] Substance dependence is not only harmful to the user but also to his or her family and community. The family members of the substance user, particularly the dependent children, may suffer repercussions. The risk for all types of child abuse and neglect, including physical abuse, sexual abuse, nutritional neglect, medical neglect, and educational neglect, is increased in the setting of substance abuse. Health care providers play an important role in assessing both child abuse and substance abuse and should be aware of the current research relating to each. Given the pervasive nature of substance dependence, children of substance users will be part of the health care system, though most of these children go unrecognized and experience medical evaluations wherein their unique needs are not identified. Nurses are uniquely positioned to identify children exposed to substance abuse as well as youth actively using or abusing drugs or alcohol. This chapter discusses the children whose caregiver(s) exhibits substance dependence, provides resources to screen for and recognize clues to identify the child and family dealing with substance dependence issues, discusses commonly abused drugs, and addresses strategies for relieving the problem.

Scope

In 2012, an estimated 23.9 million people reported using illicit drugs in the United States.[3] According to data collected from 2002 to 2007 by the United States Department of Health and Human Services (USDHHS), 8.3 million children aged 18 years and under (11.9%) lived with at least 1 parent who was dependent on or abused alcohol or an illicit drug during the previous year. Of these children, almost 7.3 million (10.3%) lived with a parent who was dependent on or abused alcohol and about 2.1 million (3%) lived with a parent who was dependent on or abused illicit drugs (**Figure 19-1**). More children were found to be living with affected fathers than mothers (5.4 million versus 3.4 million).[4] **Figure 19-2** shows the percentage of children living with substance abuse by their age.

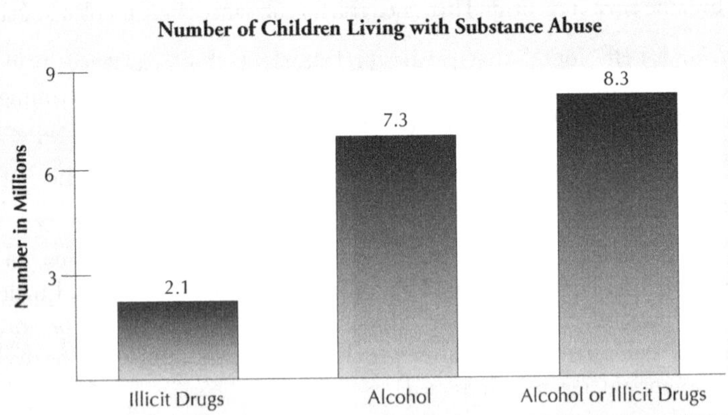

**Includes biological, step-, adoptive, or foster children. Children under 18 years of age who were not living with one or more parents were excluded from this analysis. Approximately 4.0 percent of children under age 15 were not living with one or more parents.*
Source: 2002 to 2007 SAMHSA National Surveys on Drug Use and Health (NSDUHs). **Figure 19-1**

Figure 19-1. Estimated numbers of children aged 18 years and under living with one or more parents with past year substance dependence or abuse (2002 to 2007). Reprinted from Office of Applied Studies, Substance Abuse and Mental Health Services Administration. Children living with substance-dependent or substance-abusing parents: 2002 to 2007. Substance Abuse and Mental Health Services Administration Web site. http://www.samhsa.gov/data/2k9/SAparents/SAparents.pdf. Published April 16, 2009. Accessed June 5, 2013.

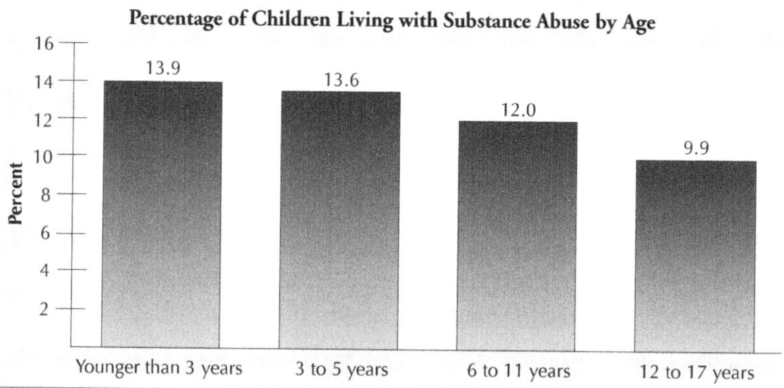

Figure 19-2

**Includes biological, step-, adoptive, or foster children. Children under 18 years of age who were not living with one or more parents were excluded from this analysis. Approximately 4.0 percent of children under age 15 were not living with one or more parents.*
Source: 2002 to 2007 SAMHSA National Surveys on Drug Use and Health (NSDUHs).

Figure 19-2. *Percentages of children under 18 years of age living with one or more parents with past year substance dependence or abuse, by child's age (2002 to 2007). Reprinted from Office of Applied Studies, Substance Abuse and Mental Health Services Administration. Children living with substance dependent or substance-abusing parents: 2002 to 2007. Substance Abuse and Mental Health Services Administration Web site. http://www.samhsa.gov/data/2k9/SAparents/SAparents.pdf. Published April 16, 2009. Accessed June 5, 2013.*

Children living in homes with a substance user are at risk for neglect or abuse resulting from household dysfunction and changes in adult behavior that can occur with chemical addiction. It is estimated that between one-third and two-thirds of children involved with Child Protective Services (CPS) have parental substance abuse as a contributing factor to their maltreatment.[5] The true number of affected children may be higher; however, research in this area is plagued by difficulties, the most notable of which is a lack of a standard methodology for reporting data on the part of CPS and substance abuse treatment programs. Efforts toward establishing a standard methodology, such as using standard definitions, have not been successful at increasing the reliability of collected data. Furthermore, self-reporting, a common methodology used in data collection, has known limitations, including deception and inaccurate recollection.

Limited data provide insight into the extent of the problem. A report from New York City found that 77% of the city's 1994 foster care expenditures were related to parental drug and alcohol addiction.[6] In a 1997 nationwide survey of 915 professionals working in the child welfare system, The National Center on Addiction and Substance Abuse (CASA) reported nearly 80% of professionals felt that substance abuse contributed to at least half of all cases of child maltreatment and approximately 40% thought that substance abuse was a factor in over three-quarters of cases.[6] Based on summative data, CASA estimated that substance abuse caused or contributed to 7 of every 10 cases of child maltreatment.[6] The high numbers of substance-exposed children in child welfare systems may be at least partially the result of repeated drug offenses by their caregivers. Smith and Test[7] noted that while the likelihood of subsequent allegations of maltreatment is high among families reported to CPS for a substance-exposed infant, the increased risk stems almost entirely from subsequent drug-related allegations. Parents involved with CPS were separated into 2 groups (drug-related and control); parents in the drug-related group were not more likely to incur other types of maltreatment allegations than parents in a nondrug control group.[7] Likewise, a recent analysis of data from a national survey of child well-being found that CPS workers' perceptions of parental substance dependence is associated with a greater likelihood of case substantiation and child removal, irrespective of the presence of other risk factors for child maltreatment.[8]

However, other investigations have found substance abuse to be strongly predictive for both physical abuse and neglect irrespective of social and demographic variables.[9]

Chemical Dependence

While no universally accepted definition of substance abuse exists, a person is generally thought to have a substance abuse problem when addiction to substances ingested to produce a high or alter body function interferes with his or her life. The *Diagnostic and Statistical Manual of Mental Disorders-IV-TR (DSM-IV-TR)*[1] defines chemical dependence as "a pattern of substance use leading to significant impairment in functioning" with coexisting problems at work, school or home; use in situations that are hazardous; legal problems; or continued use despite significant problems.

The morbidity and consequences of chemical dependence have been well studied and documented and include the following:

— Work problems

— Illness

— Marital strain

— Financial problems

— Unemployment

— School problems

— Decreased parental monitoring or lack of parenting

— Poor home management

— Lack of family communication skills

— Decreased family cohesion

— Increased family conflict

— Frequent family moves

— Crimes

— Intimate partner violence (IPV) and child abuse

The substance user may suffer from comorbid psychiatric illnesses such as depression, anxiety, posttraumatic stress disorder (PTSD), bipolar disorder, and attention deficit hyperactivity disorder (ADHD). The children of substance users may suffer from adjustment problems, impaired emotional development, increased level of anxiety and depression, low self-esteem, lack of control over the environment, and increased risk for substance abuse problems later in life.[2,6,10,11]

Chemical dependency is a familial problem stemming from both genetic factors and environmental settings that may cross generations. Efforts are underway to understand and identify genes contributing to addiction. The term "reward deficiency syndrome" has been coined to describe individuals who may lack the genes involved in the processing of neurotransmitters that are important to the brain's regulation of addictive, impulsive, and compulsive behaviors. The environment an individual is exposed to during growth and development plays an important role in such aspects as coping skills and socialized behaviors. Substance users may not recognize the degree to which drugs or alcohol contribute to their problems due to biologic changes in brain functions and maladaptive behaviors.

Intergenerational factors are not only relevant to substance abuse, but also to child abuse. Children who grow up with the challenge of living with an addicted caregiver are at risk because the same genetic and environmental risk factors are transmitted to the child.[12] Conners et al[13] studied 4084 children affected by maternal addiction wherein the majority of mothers studied had a history of having been abused by their parents (57.4%) or by another person (73.6%), and more than three-quarters reported family members as having been involved in drug-related activities. The women also had high rates of physical and mental health problems, and many were involved in the criminal justice system. The children in the study also had high rates of poverty (91.3%) and child welfare involvement (56.6%), relatively high rates of physical health complaints, and nearly a quarter had been the subject of a school complaint of bad behavior.[13]

Children of Substance Users

The child of a parent who uses substances is affected by his or her caregiver's addiction(s). The child's parents might make every effort to conceal the problems; however, children are inherently wise to their surrounding environment and possess an almost universal ability to adapt to different situations. A child may exhibit different behaviors based on unique expectations set by various caregivers tasked with his or her care. For example, when a child visits his or her grandparents, a negative behavior, such as whining, may disappear because the child knows that grandma does not tolerate whining. No one may have ever explicitly told the child not to whine, but the child learned that the reaction elicited from his or her grandmother differed from that elicited from his or her mother or father. Learned behaviors are apparent in interactions with the impaired caregiver. The child may learn to be very quiet and stay out of the way when a parent is under the influence.

Chemical dependence is a family disease and affects every member of the family, though the degree to which children are affected varies widely even within the same family and depends upon many factors. While some children of substance abusers may appear to be unaffected, productive members of society, some children never overcome the effects and may suffer with their own addictions to an even greater extent than their parents. Johnson and Leff[2] found that predictive factors of child resilience include the caregiver's ability to provide for the basic needs of children, the child's coping skills, the age of the child at the onset of the addiction or relapse, and family support.

Chemical dependency is often associated with other household stressors, making it difficult to attribute child outcomes to caregiver addiction alone. For instance, poverty is common among households that include chemically dependent individuals as the addiction is typically expensive and impairs the caregiver's ability to seek optimal employment. Additionally, low education is often a consequence of substance addiction and may further limit caregiver employment prospects. Substance-using parents may also suffer from mental illnesses and impaired relationships. Symptoms found among children living in households with a substance-dependent caregiver are listed in **Table 19-1**.

The prevalence of household stressors and the recognition of chemical dependency as a medical condition complicate decisions regarding child protection. Children living in poverty are at risk for maltreatment, but poverty alone is not generally considered cause for CPS intervention. Likewise, physical or mental impairment of the caregiver is not typically used as grounds for intervention, unless severe. As previously noted, the presence of a chemically dependent individual in the home often appears to influence CPS decisions. No clear process exists to determine which substance abuse cases constitute child maltreatment, although the collaboration of both substance abuse and child abuse professionals greatly enhance the safety of children living in homes where there is substance abuse.[11]

Table 19-1. Symptoms Resulting From Growing Up With Substance Abuse

Category of Problems	Symptoms or Problems
Emotional	— Anxiety — Depression — PTSD — Poor self-esteem — Lack of empathy — Inability to form friendships — Social stigma — Substance abuse
Academic	— Educational neglect — Delinquency — Learning problems — Concentration problems — Lack of parental support
Developmental	— Lack of bonding — Developmental delay — Behavior problems
Neglect	— Lack of food and resources — Lack of supervision — Children parenting other children

Data from United States Department of Health and Human Services, Administration for Children and Families, Administration on Children, Youth, and Families Children's Bureau. Child maltreatment 2009. Administration for Children and Families Web site. http://www.acf.hhs.gov/programs/cb/pubs/cm09/cm09.pdf. Published December 31, 2009. Accessed June 5, 2013.

Child Maltreatment

Child maltreatment can have long-lasting effects on brain structure, mental and psychological states, behaviors affecting health and safety, social functioning, life expectancy, and overall health care costs.[14] The Adverse Childhood Experiences (ACE) studies evaluated the long-term impact of events occurring in the first 18 years of life with a complete health assessment correlating risk and disease among adult patients at a large health maintenance organization (HMO). Questions directed at participants elicited responses indicating exposure to abuse, neglect, household dysfunction, substance abuse, mental illness, criminal behavior, and IPV. The studies found a graded relationship between the number of ACEs experienced and negative adult health and well-being, including risk of depression and suicide attempts, multiple sexual partners, sexually transmitted infections (STIs), smoking, alcoholism, and sleep disturbances.[15,16] In a study examining the relationship of adverse experiences to later drug use, Dube et al[17] reported that the most significant factors leading to early and severe drug abuse were exposures to ACEs. In particular, the results suggested that two-thirds of parenteral drug use is attributable to abusive or traumatic childhood experiences.[17] Wu et al[18] also described a similar graded relationship of poor adult health outcomes and negative childhood experiences among adults with comorbid substance use disorders and mental health problems. The proportion of adults in this group who reported histories of multiple negative childhood stressors, including child maltreatment, was greater than among the HMO population of the ACE studies.[18] The findings of these investigations indicate that efforts to decrease chemical dependency may reduce the prevalence of child maltreatment and improve overall adult health outcomes. Additionally, using family treatment drug courts has demonstrated improvement in the desired outcomes of decreased substance abuse and family reunification.[19]

Caring for children can be stressful in the absence of substance abuse or other stressors. Potential triggers for child abuse may occur at any time and include an infant's inconsolable crying, feeding difficulties, failed toilet training, or unrealistic expectations.[20] For a parent or caregiver who is impaired, the ability to effectively deal with the potential trigger is decreased. Children are at increased risk for maltreatment when the timing of potential triggers coincide with critical events in substance abuse periods such as a methadone addict's high which increases violent behaviors, an opioid addict's withdrawal period, or any addict's sleep deprivation.

Children thrive in an environment that is consistent and secure and thereby conducive to the development of behavioral and emotional self-regulation. Families provide the environment and framework for the development of the child. By establishing routines and rules, children develop expectations that form the basis of support systems. These support systems are disrupted or dysfunctional in families with substance abuse. Chemically dependent parents lack the ability to provide structure or discipline in family life but often expect their children to be competent at a wide variety of tasks earlier than do non–substance-abusing parents. The unrealistic expectations experienced by children in these households leads to increased risks for child maltreatment.

Common Characteristics and Confounders

Substance abuse does not usually occur in isolation nor does child maltreatment. Determining a single causative factor is challenging in an environment layered with risks; however, substance abuse has been proven to be an independent risk factor for abuse and neglect. Pelham[21] studied the effects of deviant child behavior and found that alcohol and drug abuse alone may cause or contribute to neglect or violent behavior toward children. Additionally, Conners et al[13] studied mothers enrolled in a chemical dependency program and found that a child's risk of exposure to violence was positively correlated with the severity of their mothers' substance use. Other investigators have identified maternal depression, anger, and difficulties regulating emotions as important potential risks for child abuse.[22] Interestingly, Testa and Smith[23] have discussed the inherent overlap of substance abuse and child maltreatment and postulated that the other risk factors of parental depression, social isolation, homelessness, or IPV may be more directly responsible for maltreatment than substance abuse.

Societal Costs

Given the extent of the problem of child maltreatment stemming from substance abuse, the costs to society are profound; however, determining a dollar amount is difficult because of the nature of such costs. Different forms of societal costs include quantifiable indices such as increased burden on CPS, increased health care costs, crime, loss of productivity, as well as unquantifiable indices such as lost potential of effected children. The economic cost of illicit drug use in the United States in 2002 was estimated to be $180.9 billion dollars[24] with the total costs of alcoholism in 1998 estimated to be $185 billion.[25]

CASA estimated that substance abuse accounted for approximately $10 billion (70%) of federal, state, and local government spending on child welfare systems in 1999.[6] The annual costs related to just one of the medical complications of substance abuse with a preventable outcome in the United States is staggering. In 2002, fetal alcohol syndrome (FAS) was estimated to cost more than $4 billion.[26] Smith and Smith[27] attempted to quantify the costs stemming from childhood psychological problems, reporting long-term economic damages of $300 000 in lost family income and a total lifetime cost for all those affected of $2.1 trillion[27] (**Figure 19-3**).

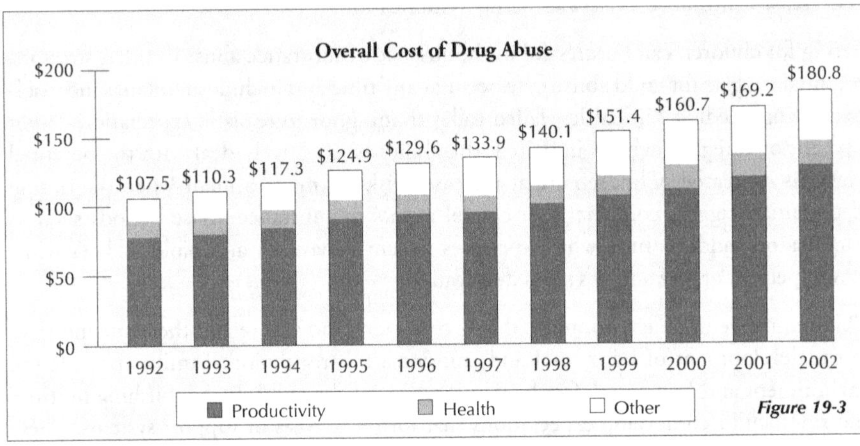

Figure 19-3. *Overall cost of drug abuse, 1992 to 1998 (in billions of dollars). Reprinted from Agency for Healthcare Research and Quality. Five major steps to intervention (The "5 As"). Agency for Healthcare Research and Quality Web site. http://www.ahrq.gov/professionals/clinicians-providers/guidelines-recommendations/tobacco/5steps.html . Published December 2012. Accessed August 20, 2013.*

Obtaining a History of Substance Abuse

The most important, and often most elusive, step in helping a family deal with chemical dependency is to identify the problem. The discussion of dependency can be complicated by several factors, including denial, conflict of interests, and negative perception and must, therefore, be addressed knowledgeably. Denial, as seen with other chronic illnesses, such as persistent poor eating habits in the face of obesity or continued cigarette use despite a diagnosis of asthma, is an important aspect of chemical dependency, as many users minimize the extent of their substance use. An inherent conflict of interest exists for the patient when he or she is asked to provide a history of his or her drug or alcohol use to the health care provider, because the patient knows drugs are illegal and consuming alcohol daily is not healthy. Additionally, substance abuse is associated with shame and rejection. Because of the adverse feelings associated with substance abuse, many health care providers simply avoid discussions involving the use of drugs and alcohol despite widespread prevalence of addiction.[28] The health care professional must be comfortable with addressing the problem of dependency so the patient or family can feel comfortable revealing the problem. A substance user will not likely reveal a problem if a perceived concern for the patient is lacking and he or she does not identify a benefit in making such an admission. Some health care professionals have difficulty dealing with their own personal biases or experiences and, as a result, are not comfortable addressing the behaviors of others. Asking questions in an open and nonjudgmental manner will put the interviewee at ease and facilitate a conversation.

Assessing Substance Abuse

The assessment should include both formal questioning in a nonjudgmental manner and physical observations. The American Academy of Pediatrics (AAP) Committee

Table 19-2. Screening Tools for Alcohol and Drug Use*

Alcohol Consumption Screening Tools	Description
CAGE/Family CAGE	Relatively quick and easy to use; CAGE is an acronym with each letter representing a question from the screening tool.
T-ACE	Screens for prenatal use; T-ACE is an acronym representing the categories of questions (tolerance, annoyance, cut down, eye opener).
CRAFFT	Useful with adolescents; CRAFFT is an mnemonic acronym representing important words in the various questions.
Rapid Alcohol Problems Screen — Quantity Frequency (RAPS4-QF)	6-item questionnaire; found to be more sensitive than CAGE.[29]
AUDIT	10-item questionnaire
Drug Use Screening Tools	Description
The National Institute on Drug Abuse (NIDA) Quick Screen and Modified ASSIST	Four-item questionnaire with follow-up questions for positive responses; also screens for drug use.
Substance Abuse Subtle Screening Inventory (SASSI)	Psychological screens for substance use disorders

**Additional screening tools available through the Web-based search engine for screening instruments hosted by the Alcohol and Drug Abuse Institute at the University of Washington at http://lib.adai.uw.edu/instruments/.*

on Substance Abuse endorses screening for substance use as a part of routine health care and ongoing anticipatory guidance starting with the prenatal visit.[29] A number of assessment tools are available to the health care provider, as outlined in **Table 19-2**. Despite the number of available formal screening tools, systematic reviews have failed to demonstrate effective reduction in substance use, improved health outcomes among adults screened in primary care settings, or reduced risk of maltreatment for children of substance-dependent parents.[30,31]

Rarely do caregivers or adolescents openly ask for help with addiction, so the health care provider must look for clues to an underlying problem. The assessment should include both the child and his or her caregiver(s) and should take into account the child's developmental stage. The health care provider should assess both the child's and the caregiver's appearance, taking care to note if either the child or the caregiver is dirty or disheveled; smells of body odor; or smells strongly of cologne, the application of which may indicate an effort to mask the smell of marijuana or crack. The health care provider should also assess the interactions between the child and caregivers, noting if the child is out of control, demonstrates behavior that is inappropriate for his or her age, or appears withdrawn or timid. Additionally, the health care provider should be aware of the answers provided to standard history questions, noting if the caregiver demonstrates an inappropriate, rude, or defensive tone; appears fidgety; lacks interest in the child or knowledge about the child's condition; or reveals discrepancies in his or her answers or behaviors, such as reports of being unemployed while having an abundance of expensive items. The clinician should also assess for any physical clues that may be indicative of neglect, such as an excessively thin or overweight child, or abuse, such as marks or injuries, as with any examination.

Despite an excellent assessment, the signs of substance abuse often remain hidden. After all, the caregiver is likely skilled at hiding his or her substance abuse from others. Some children and adults will, nonetheless, answer straight-forward questions, such as:

— Do either of your parents use alcohol or drugs?

— What happens when they drink or use drugs?

— Do you use alcohol or drugs?

The complete clinical picture based on all aspects of interaction can provide valuable clues to an underlying problem of substance abuse if the health care provider is knowledgeable and alert to the signs and symptoms. A stepwise approach to tie the assessment to action is the National Institute of Drug Abuse intervention steps, the 5 As, demonstrated in **Table 19-3**.

Table 19-3. The 5 As

Question	Information
Ask	Ask direct questions to determine if substance abuse is a problem in the home.
Advise	Discuss the problem in a nonjudgmental manner. Educate the family.
Assess	Determine risk to child and if appropriate notify CPS.
Assist	Refer to appropriate resources and support.
Arrange	Ensure follow up is provided.

Adapted from Agency for Healthcare Research and Quality. Five major steps to intervention (The "5 As"). Agency for Healthcare Research and Quality Web site. http://www.ahrq.gov/professionals/clinicians-providers/guidelines-recommendations/tobacco/5steps.html. Published December 2012. Accessed August 20, 2013.

Physical Effects

Chemical dependency has long been a focus of medical research and continues as such today. Researchers have explored the possibility of a genetic link to chemical dependency in familial, adoption, and twin studies while focusing much of their investigative attention on the neurologic systems affected by chemical substances. Neurotransmitters such as dopamine, the primary neurotransmitter effecting brain function and pathways and a factor in addiction; serotonin; norepinephrine; and gamma-aminobutyric acid (GABA); opioid; and cannabinoid receptors have all been studied in light of addiction. Additionally, researchers have investigated the genetic differences apparent in the way in which substances are metabolized by the liver. **Table 19-4** identifies several classes of drugs and the physical effects experienced as a result of consumption.

Table 19-4. Chemical Substances and Related Informations

Drug Class	Epidemiology	Physical Effects	Drug Testing	Other Related Information
Depressants: alcohol, barbiturates, benzodiazepines, flunitrazepam (Rohypnol), gamma-hydroxybutyrate (GHB), methaqualone	Approximately 23% of the population in the United States reports binge drinking (5 or more drinks on one occasion) and 6.5 % reports heavy drinking (5 or more drinks on 5 or more days in the previous month).[3]	— Low doses reduce anxiety, provide relaxation or induce drowsiness, and lower inhibitions. — Higher doses cause slurred speech, emotional volatility, nausea, loss of coordination, visual distortions, impaired memory, sexual dysfunction, loss of consciousness, respiratory depression. — Chronic use can cause depression, neurologic deficits, hypertension, liver and heart disease. — Overdoses can be deadly.	— Blood or breathalyzer used for alcohol. — Screening immunoassays used for benzodiazepines, barbiturates, and a wide variety of drugs allowing for cross-reactivity. — Flunitrazepam is cross-reactive with benzodiazepines; therefore, confirmatory testing should be performed if the drug is suspected. GHB is rapidly cleared from the urine and may only be detected through gas chromatography mass spectroscopy (GC-MS).	The combination of alcohol and cocaine is more toxic than either substance alone due to liver metabolism of cocaethylene.

(continued)

Table 19-4. Chemical Substances and Related Informations *(continued)*

Drug Class	Epidemiology	Physical Effects	Drug Testing	Other Related Information
Psychoactive drugs: marijuana, ketamine, phencyclidine (PCP), lysergic acid diethylamide (LSD), mescaline, psilocybin, dextromethorphan	Marijuana was the most commonly used (7.3% of the population aged 12 or older) illicit drug in the United States.[3]	— Impairs motor function (all drugs in class), increases heart rate and blood pressure. — Marijuana produces euphoria, slowed thinking and reaction time, confusion, and long-term use may result in impaired memory and anxiety. — Ketamine produces delirium, depression, and respiratory depression at high doses. — Hallmarks of PCP ingestion are panic and aggression. — Psilocybin causes nervousness and paranoid effects. — When taken in high doses, dextromethorphan has euphoric, psychedelic, and dissociative properties.	— Screening immunoassays for marijuana and PCP — False-positive results for marijuana are uncommon, though marinol (prescribed for nausea related to chemotherapy patients and to stimulate appetite in AIDS patients) will also cause a positive screen. — Passive exposure to marijuana smoke and use of herbal products (eg, hemp) will not cause a positive screen except in extreme cases. — Marijuana mimics (eg, K2, Spice) are not detected by current immunoassays. — Dextromethorphan can cause a false-positive immunoassay result for PCP (even at therapeutic doses).	Dextromethorphan is found in many over-the-counter cough medications.

(continued)

Table 19-4. Chemical Substances and Related Informations *(continued)*

Drug Class	Epidemiology	Physical Effects	Drug Testing	Other Related Information
Stimulants: amphetamine, cocaine, ±3,4-methylenedioxymethamphetamine (MDMA, ecstasy), methamphetamine, methylphenidate	0.6% of the population in the United States uses cocaine and 0.2% of the population use methamphetamine.[3]	— Stimulants may result in increased heart rate and blood pressure, feelings of exhilaration, increased mental alertness, decreased appetite, weight loss, nervousness, insomnia, tremors, loss of coordination, irritability, anxiety, delirium, panic, impulsive behavior, aggressiveness, psychosis, heart failure. — Cocaine may elevate body temperature and cause chest pain and strokes. — MDMA produces hyperthermia, and cardiac, liver, and kidney toxicity.	— Screening immunoassay used for methamphetamine. — Some Parkinson's medications may cause a positive drug test for amphetamines.	— In 2005, federal regulations limiting the purchase of ingredients used to manufacture methamphetamine decreased use; much of the drug currently used in the United States is imported from Mexico. — Cocaine is sometimes used for its vasoconstrictive effects in dental or otolaryngologic procedures. — Amphetamines are found in some diet agents and cold products, though their availability in the United States has been curtailed.

(continued)

Table 19-4. Chemical Substances and Related Informations *(continued)*

Drug Class	Epidemiology	Physical Effects	Drug Testing	Other Related Information
Opiates: codeine, fentanyl, heroin, morphine, opium, oxycodone, hydrocodone	Nearly 3% of the population in the United States uses prescription psychotherapeutic drugs (primarily pain relievers) nonmedically.[3]	— Most opiates can result in pain relief, euphoria, drowsiness, constipation, confusion, respiratory depression, and nausea. — Heroin can produce a staggering gait.	— Codeine ingestion can result in a positive immunoassay result for both codeine and morphine. — Oxycodone and methadone require assays specific to these drugs. — Fentanyl is not detectable on standard screening tests, but only with GC/MS.	Seen among teenaged population, "pharm parties" involve mixing various prescription drugs together to create "trail mix" for consumption. The dangerous game is complicated by drug-drug interactions, as is the concomitant use of alcohol.
Inhalants: paint thinners, gasoline, glue, air fresheners, body sprays	Unknown	May result in loss of inhibition, headache, slurred speech, wheezing, memory impairment, weight loss, unconsciousness, sudden death.	No routine screening test available.	

Data from Department of Health and Human Services, Substance Abuse and Mental Health Services Administration, Office of Applied Studies. Results from the 2007 National Survey on Drug Use and Health: national findings. Health Services Administration Web site. http://www.samhsa.gov/data/nsduh/2k7nsduh/2k7Results.htm. Accessed 2012.

Substance use leaves an imprint on the health of the family, despite efforts on the part of the substance user to protect his or her loved ones. Unpredictable daily routines and parenting can lead to suboptimal development and learning in infants and toddlers who need consistency in order to feel confident about exploring the surrounding environment and making connections with people. Infants exposed to substances prenatally can exhibit increased crying, difficulty soothing, and disturbances of sleeping and eating. Young children living with a substance-dependent parent are at increased risk of accidental ingestion or even purposeful ingestion by caregivers desiring to produce a sedative effect, as seen when a caregiver gives alcohol to a child to help them sleep. Older children may experience attachment disorders, depression, anxiety, aggression, PTSD, ADHD, conduct disorders, and learning disabilities. Older children are also at increased risk for developing unhealthy behaviors, such as heightened sexual activity and experimentation with drugs or alcohol.

Intrauterine Drug Exposure

Data collected by the Substance Abuse and Mental Health Services Administration (SAMHSA) suggests that rates of chemical use among substance-dependent women decline during pregnancy.[32] Rates of alcohol consumption, binge drinking, and marijuana use declined from 19% during the first trimester to 6.2% in the third trimester for women who were pregnant during the period 2002 to 2007. A high proportion of women resumed use of these substances following pregnancy,[32] which demonstrates the need for targeted assistance in the pediatric and postpartum settings.

The effects of substance use on the fetus depend upon many factors. The gestational age at time of ingestion, substance(s) used, method of ingestion, dose, and frequency of use determine whether damage occurs. Individual differences in metabolism in both mother and the fetus may also play a role.

Alcohol is the only known addictive substance to have the potential to produce a recognized malformation syndrome. Alcohol readily crosses the placenta and causes its most deleterious effects during the first trimester, a period when many women are unaware of the growing fetus. FAS is characterized by craniofacial abnormalities, low birth weight, failure to thrive (FTT), developmental delay, abnormalities of muscle tone, and learning and behavior problems. FAS and alcohol-related neurodevelopmental disorders are characterized by less severe involvement of organ systems. A safe dose of alcohol to prevent the spectrum of alcohol-related disorders in the fetus has not been determined because the amount of alcohol consumed may or may not correlate with the severity of symptoms.

While potentially harmful during the fetal and perinatal periods, substances other than alcohol have not been conclusively found to result in permanent negative outcomes. In a study of 717 newborns exposed prenatally to cocaine, exposed infants were approximately 500 grams lighter and half an inch shorter than nonexposed peers at the time of delivery and were born 1.2 weeks earlier, but no morphological pattern was found. Exposed infants were more likely to be jittery, have autonomic instability, and have a high-pitched cry during the early newborn period. By 2 years of age, however, there was no demonstrable difference in IQ between the groups.[33] Likewise, while infants prenatally exposed to opiates may experience a well-defined pattern of withdrawal symptoms, such as jitteriness, irritability, loose stools, respiratory distress, and possible seizures shortly after birth, a permanent syndrome related to opiate exposure in utero has not been described. Cocaine, tobacco, and methamphetamine use during pregnancy may increase the risk of miscarriage and premature delivery related to the vasoconstrictive effects of each drug. Like cocaine, neither tobacco nor methamphetamine is associated with known permanent effects on prenatally exposed infants; however, tobacco use during and following pregnancy has been linked to an increased risk of sudden infant death syndrome (SIDS).[33]

Attempts to ascribe infant health outcomes to particular substances are complicated by the intertwined social and physical stressors experienced by substance-dependent women. In a study of cocaine-exposed infants, Bauer et al[34] found that mothers using cocaine during pregnancy were more likely than control subjects to smoke cigarettes and marijuana and drink alcohol. The infants of the mothers who used cocaine were more likely to enter into to protective custody and to be put up for adoption and were less likely to be breastfed than infants born to other mothers.[34] Similarly, in a sample of pregnant women using methamphetamine, 25% smoked tobacco, 6% used marijuana, and approximately 23% drank alcohol. These women were also more likely to be single, were less educated, received less prenatal care, and were more likely to receive public financial assistance than women in a control group.[35] Given the complex interplay of adverse factors experienced by pregnant women with addiction problems, the American College of Obstetricians and Gynecologists (ACOG) Committee on Ethics issued an opinion discouraging legal interventions in cases of maternal substance use stating that this approach unjustly singles out the most vulnerable women and creates the potential for criminalization of otherwise legal behaviors, such as smoking tobacco and drinking alcohol. The ACOG further pointed out that legal approaches might have the unintended consequence of reducing rates of prenatal care for these high-risk pregnancies. Additional unintended consequences might include a hindrance of chemical dependency treatment, which is shown to be more effective during pregnancy than at other times in a woman's life because pregnant women tend to be particularly motivated.[36]

Drug Testing

The most dependable method for determining whether an individual is using chemical substances is to test for the presence of commonly used substances using the various appropriate testing methods. Drug testing of federal employees in their place of employment was introduced by Ronald Reagan in 1986 and resulted in federal standards of drug testing as regulated by SAMHSA. The guidelines indicate the process of drug testing should include proper collection of a specimen, initiation of chain of custody, and appropriate analysis of the specimen by a certified laboratory. The health care provider should be aware of the limits of drug testing when making decisions regarding interventions, such as contacting law enforcement or CPS based on test results. (For further information, review *Chapter 5, Laboratory Findings, Diagnostic Testing, and Forensic Specimens in Cases of Child Sexual Abuse.*) The metabolites of abused substances differ in rate of absorption, distribution, metabolism, and excretion, all of which may affect test results. Additionally, the way in which a drug is consumed can determine how long the drug may be detected by a given test. The possibility of sample adulteration should also be considered whenever specimen collection is unobserved.

Laboratory investigation of drug use includes both screening testing and confirmatory testing. A positive test result is determined by detecting the substance at a specific threshold. Screen threshold levels are designed to differentiate between exposure and active use of a substance and are set at nationwide standards by SAMHSA. Screening tests are designed for maximum sensitivity, in an effort to reduce the possibility of missing positive specimens; therefore, it is possible for a person who did not consume a given substance but was exposed to it in one way or another to test positive for the substance. The health care provider should be aware that a positive test cannot determine which type of drug within a drug class was detected due to limits of the testing technique. For example, the immunoassay for benzodiazepines is designed to cross-react to any metabolite in the drug class. Also, natural products and dietary supplements have known cross-reactivity with some illicit drugs (eg, dextromethorphan, a common nonprescription cough suppressant, may cause a false positive drug test result for opiates). Furthermore, a study of Internet-obtained dietary supplements showed that almost half of the products studied were contaminated with illegal drugs; most of the products manufactured in the United States were not found to be contaminated.[37] With any drug screen, the chain of custody should be maintained to prevent contamination, substitution, or dilution.

If a screening test is positive for a particular drug or if the suspected drug is not available on the screening test, further testing may be required. Gas chromatography mass spectroscopy (GC-MS) or high-performance liquid chromatography can be performed in specialized laboratories to confirm the presence of a given drug; however, higher cost and longer processing times associated with confirmatory testing may prove problematic.

Neonatal drug testing is controversial. According to the ACOG Ethics Committee Opinion on drug and alcohol abuse, universal screening combined with intervention and referral to treatment is recommended for routine prenatal care. This policy does not share universal support. A study by Roberts[38] of a high-risk population demonstrated decreased prenatal care as the unintended result of prenatal drug testing. Women were "mistrustful of providers' often inconspicuous efforts to discover drug use." Due to potential risks to the fetus associated with prenatal exposure to substances, allegations of child abuse may be raised. Criminal charges against chemically dependent pregnant women on the grounds of child abuse have not resulted in widespread support; rather, the focus has shifted to substance abuse education and opening treatment opportunities for women with families. Additionally, criminal charges on grounds of child abuse are considered by some to be unjust since treatment is often not available.[39]

Urine

Urine drug testing uses an immunoassay that screens for multiple drugs at one time. The tests are rapid, fairly inexpensive, and readily available. Different brands vary in the range of compounds detected while sensitivity varies depending on the drug concentration in the urine and the cutoff concentration of the immunoassay. The cut-off concentration is set to the lowest drug concentration that can be reliably detected. These levels are based on consumption of the drug, along with individual variability. Detection time for most drugs is 1 to 3 days from the time of consumption based on dose, route of administration, metabolism, urine volume, and urine pH. Lipid soluble drugs, such as marijuana, diazepam, and phencyclidine (PCP), can be detected at longer intervals in long-term users.

Hair

Human hair, which typically grows 1 cm per month, can retain evidence of substance use. The concentration of retained drug metabolites can be affected by bleaching or other cosmetic treatments as well as by individual characteristics, such as hair structure, porosity, growth, and melanin content. Testing hair for evidence of substance use affords the greatest length of time for detection, typically a minimum of 1 week up to several months from the time of consumption, depending on individual hair growth. Due to the variability of metabolite presence in each hair follicle, reliability can be called into question when low levels of drug concentration are revealed. Proper specimen handling and washing in the laboratory can help differentiate between drug use and drug exposure.[37]

Other Testing Modalities

Serum testing is the ideal method for determining if an individual has consumed alcohol; however, most other drugs are eliminated from the blood within minutes to hours of consumption, narrowing the focus of this type of testing. The presence of alcohol may also be determined with breathalyzers, devices that measure the mass of alcohol per volume of breath. Sweat testing is useful for monitoring drug use over a several-week period and is most often used by government agencies or treatment programs. The reliability of sweat-test results has come under question because the ability to manipulate test results is higher than with other forms of testing. Saliva testing provides the quickest results, but wide spread use is limited by cost, required supervision time to ensure a 10-minute to 30-minute period of fasting before collection, and accuracy. In addition, maternal drug use over the several months before delivery may be determined by testing the newborn's meconium.

Treatment of Substance Abuse

Treating substance abuse is as complex a problem as the reasons that an individual becomes an addict. Substance abuse involves many aspects of an individual's life, with each aspect requiring careful attention for successful treatment. The needs of women entering treatment programs who are involved with CPS, for instance, are notably different from other patients. Women with chemical dependency problems and child welfare issues typically have more children and financial difficulties and are more likely to have histories of physical abuse than other women entering treatment.[40]

The benefits of abstinence from substance use include improved parenting ability, a regaining of relationships, an ability to become a productive member of society, and increased resources for constructive endeavors. Unfortunately, treatment is not available to a majority of substance abusers in the United States. In 2012, 9.2% (an estimated 23.9 million persons) of the population aged 12 years or older was classified with substance dependence or abuse in the past year. Among those who sought treatment but did not receive it, 48.3% cited the cost of care or insufficient medical insurance as the primary explanation, 26.3% stated that they were not ready to stop using, and 8.2% said that they lacked adequate transportation or that treatment options were not convenient.[3] **Figure 19-4** lists the substances for which treatment was received in 2012 among people aged 12 years and older.

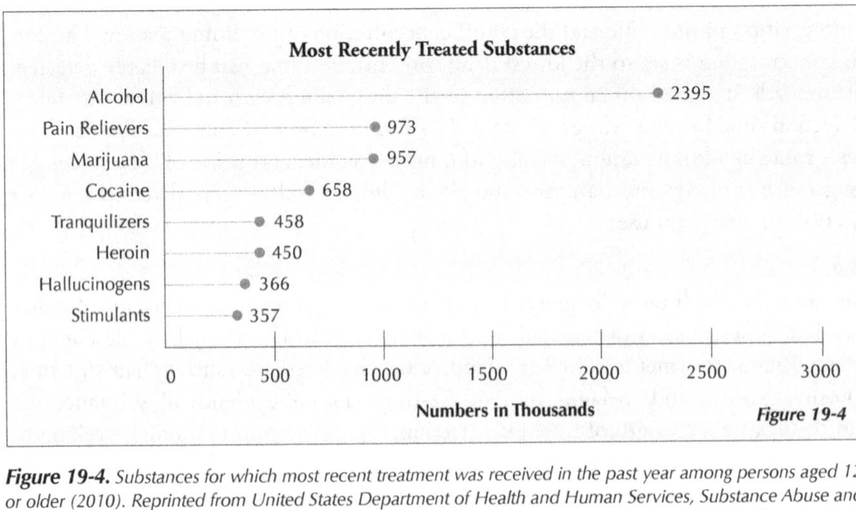

Figure 19-4. *Substances for which most recent treatment was received in the past year among persons aged 12 or older (2010). Reprinted from United States Department of Health and Human Services, Substance Abuse and Mental Health Services Administration, Center for Behavioral Health Statistics and Quality. Results from the 2012 National Survey on Drug Use and Health: summary of national findings. Substance Abuse and Mental Health Services Administration (SAMHSA) Web site. http://www.samhsa.gov/data/NSDUH/2012SummNatFindDetTables/NationalFindings/NSDUHresults2012. Published September 2013. Accessed June 25, 2014.*

Table 19-5. Adults and Teens Who Relapsed After Drug and Alcohol Treatment

	Adults (N=160)	Adolescents (N=188)
Gender (% male)	90	45
Years of Age (SD)	44.8 (8.0)	15.9 (1.2)
Ethnicity (%)		
Caucasian	64	74
Hispanic	11	18
African-American	21	3
Other	5	5
Comorbid Psychopathology (%)		
ASPD (adults)/Conduct Disorder (teens)	16.9	86.0
Panic Disorder	3.8	4.6
Obsessive Compulsive Disorder (OCD)	5.0	23.7
Post-Traumatic Stress Disorder (PTSD)	28.1	N/A
Generalized Anxiety Disorder (GAD)	1.9	16.0
Schizophrenia	5.0	N/A
Major Depression/Dysthymia	18.1	62.6
Bipolar Disorder	6.3	19.8
Attentive Deficit Hyperactivity Disorder (ADHD)	N/A	34.4

Adults = current; Adolescents = primary

Copyright © American Psychological Association. Reproduced with permission from Ramo DE, Brown SA. Classes of substance abuse relapse situations: a comparison of adolescents and adults. Psychol Addict Behav. *2008;22(3):372-379.*

Principles of substance abuse treatment have been established through research. The guidelines can be applied to best suit individual needs and form the basis for most treatment programs. Treatment is a long process of initial detoxification followed by ongoing therapies and relapse prevention. Complications and setbacks occur at each phase of the process and should be expected. Many programs incorporate medication and behavioral therapy to assist with difficulties.

Much like any chronic illness requiring long-term treatment, individuals have varying success at compliance with avoiding harmful behaviors. Addiction to drugs or alcohol is considered a chronic medical condition, and treatment is neither easier nor more complicated than treating diabetes, hypertension, or asthma.[41] Treatment of comorbid conditions with access to health care and mental health providers is essential to maintaining sustained recovery. **Table 19-5** lists results of 18-month relapse rates by comorbidity and ethnicity from a study of adults and adolescents completed in 2008.

Treatment types and styles are vast and varied. Programs can be administered inpatient or outpatient with private or public funding. Participation can be voluntary or mandatory. Mandatory programs, which are often administered by law enforcement, judicial systems, child welfare systems, or while incarcerated, are associated with higher success rates. A pilot study comparing family drug court with intensive case management services found improved results for the drug court based on parameters of positive child welfare disposition, substance use, mental health, parenting, and family functioning.[42] Green et al[43] also found improved outcomes with family drug courts in the form of shorter wait times for entering treatment, higher incidences of completed treatment episodes, and longer treatment duration. Green at al[43] also found that the children of parents involved with family drug courts experienced decreased wait times for permanent placement and increased rates of reunification. Further research has continued to support these conclusions and show earlier exit of the child welfare system.[19]

McLellan et al[41] conducted a literature review comparing adherence and relapse rates for drug dependence with chronic condition management for type 2 diabetes, hypertension, and asthma and concluded that adherence and relapse rates among adults were similar across all conditions. **Figure 19-5** reflects this comparison.

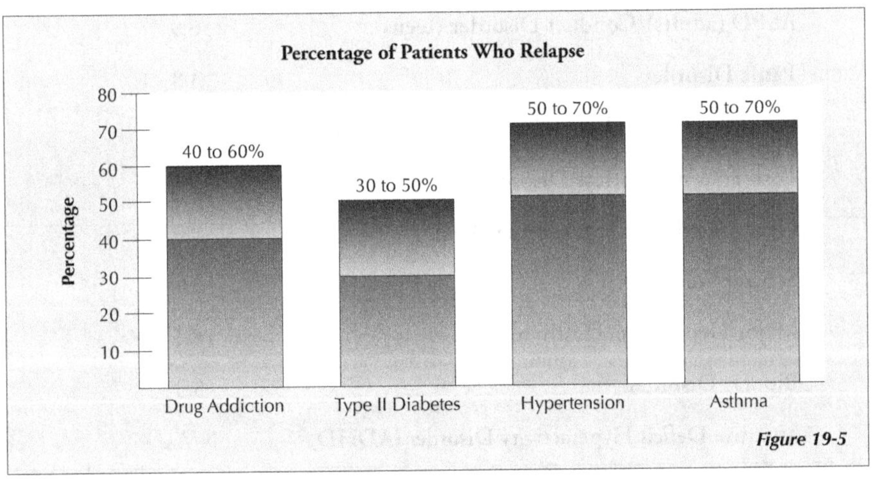

Figure 19-5. *Relapse rates are similar for drug addiction & other chronic illnesses. Adapted from McLellan AT, Lewis DC, O'Brien CP, Kleber HD[41]; Graham AW, Schultz TK, Wilford BB, eds; American Society of Addiction Medicine[44]; Dekker FW, Dieleman FE, Kaptein AA, Mulder JD[45]; Gerstein DR, Harwood HJ, eds; Committee for the Substance Abuse Coverage Study Division of Health Care Services[46]; Graber AL, Davidson P, Brown AW, McRae JR, Woolridge K[47]; Kurtz SMS[48]; Lowinson JH, Ruiz P, Millman RB, eds.[49]; O'Brien CP, McLellan AT[50]; McLellan AT, Metzger DS, Alterman AI, Woody GE, Durrell J, O'Brien CP[51]; McLellan AT, Alterman AI, Metzger DC, et al[52]; Moos RH, Finney JW, Cronkite RC[53]; Schaub AF, Steiner A, Vetter W[54]; Sinnock P[55]; Clark LT[56]; National Institute on Drug Abuse.[57]*

Research has demonstrated differences in the brain functioning of chemically dependent users and non–substance users. Medications restore brain function and prevent relapse for opioid, tobacco, and alcohol addiction. These medications block the typical response of the substance and allow the user to develop alternative patterns of behavior. The FDA has approved 3 medications for treating alcohol dependence: naltrexone, acamprosate, and disulfiram. Naltrexone, an opioid receptor blocker, is effective in reducing the desire to drink in some individuals; still, others are resistant to its effects, thereby limiting its widespread use. Naltrexone is also sometimes used to reduce the side effects of opiate dependence, though its usefulness is limited. Acamprosate helps to reduce symptoms of protracted withdrawal, such as insomnia, anxiety, restlessness, and, in patients with severe dependence, dysphoria. Disulfiram, which blocks the normal metabolism of alcohol, causes an uncomfortable reaction of flushing and nausea upon consumption of alcohol. Many programs administer disulfiram under surveillance because noncompliance is common. Methadone and buprenorphine are effective medications for the treatment of opiate addiction that suppress withdrawal symptoms and relieve cravings by targeting opioid receptors. Research and development of additional therapies is ongoing and include drug-specific vaccines to prevent drugs from reaching the brain.[58]

Once recovery is sustained, supportive measures are put in place. Peer-based support groups include Alcoholic Anonymous (AA), Narcotics Anonymous (NA), and Oxford House. The latter are "democratically run, self-supporting, drug free homes"[59] and can be found in various municipalities throughout the country. The Arkansas Center for Addictions Research Education and Services started a treatment program for pregnant and postpartum women with dual diagnosis in response to a need for alternative treatment programs that included childcare. The program includes outpatient substance abuse treatment, safe residential living to include women and their children under age 5 years, children's programs and services, integrated mental health treatment, and medical care. The program has experienced challenges and successes but may serve as a model for similar programs.[60]

Research has demonstrated that chemically dependent adults who participate in residential drug maintenance programs for at least 6 months demonstrate fewer instances of substance use at their 2-year follow-up and better outcomes in terms of employment and self-regulation than those who participate for less than 6 months.[61] The prolonged recovery period that is typically required to make drug treatment successful has implications for families involved with child welfare systems since agencies are required to achieve permanency for children within limited timeframes. The Adoption and Safe Families Act of 1997, aiming to limit emotional trauma to children, requires that agencies move to terminate parental rights once a child has been in foster care for 15 of the previous 22 months unless there is a compelling reason not to do so. Unfortunately, treatment facilities that accommodate parents with children are not available in many communities, and lack of medical insurance and other financial difficulties may limit patient access even where services exist. The goals of successful parent treatment and family reunification may also be hindered by ineffective communication links between treatment providers and welfare agencies.[62]

Treatment Challenges

Treatment difficulties are multifaceted and frequently encountered. Substance abuse treatment workers and child welfare workers have different priorities, timelines, and definitions of success, and a lack of coordination between the 2 groups is common. Additionally, most programs suffer from a lack of funding and adequate staffing. A lack of trust or negative perception is present with most governmental involvement, particularly with CPS.

In a revealing study of drug user's attitudes toward parenting, Rhodes et al[63] showed consistent attempts on the part of the substance user to minimize the damage to the involved children. The substance users attempted to keep the drug use secret from their children and to keep the family as normal as possible. A primary reason given for not seeking treatment was the fear of having the children taken into protective custody; however, the children were also given as a primary reason for enabling the users to continue any effort of recovery.[63]

Despite these inherent challenges, substance abuse treatment is a wise cultural endeavor. Studies have proven that treatment for substance abuse is a worthwhile and cost-effective investment. The annual cost of drug and alcohol treatment was estimated to be $21 billion in 2003; however, recent cost-benefit analyses of treatment programs demonstrate an average cost-benefit ratio of 7:1 meaning that every $1 spent in treatment generates $7 in increased savings as a result of decreased criminal activity, decreased health care costs, and increased wages.[64]

The Future of Treatment

Additional research on the connections between substance abuse and child maltreatment consisting of clear definitions for congruent data collections across disciplines, methodological soundness, and tracking of long-term outcomes is imperative. Coordination between CPS and substance abuse specialists is essential in order to address the different needs of and services for chemically dependent individuals and their families. Evidence-based practice is essential to the validity and continued development of this field of knowledge.

Conclusion

Substance abuse is a very common problem that increases a child's risk for maltreatment. Open, supportive dialogue between nurses and patients and their families is vital to finding solutions to these overlapping harms. Awareness of the different drugs of abuse and understanding the complexities of treatment will assist and improve the quality of nursing care. After reading this chapter, nurses can begin to integrate the information provided into daily practice to improve the lives of individuals affected by substance abuse. Resources are provided to remain abreast of the most recent innovations in identifying and treating this chronic illness.

Appendix 19-1: Additional Resources

Appendix 19-1. Additional Resources

Organization	Information
Al-Anon Family Groups	http://www.alanon.com
Alcoholics Anonymous (AA)	http://www.aa.org
Centers for Disease Control and Prevention (CDC) Youth Risk Behavior Surveillance System (YRBSS)	http://www.cdc.gov/nccdphp/dash/yrbs
Families Anonymous	http://familiesanonymous.org
Monitoring the Future	http://www.monitoringthefuture.org
National Association for Children Advocates (NACA)	http://www.nacoa.org/aboutnacoa.htm
National Council on Alcoholism and Drug Dependence, Inc. (NCADD)	217 Broadway, Ste 712 New York, NY 10007 Phone: (212) 269–7797 Fax: (212) 269–7510 E-mail: national@ncadd.org HOPE LINE (24-hour affiliate referral): 800-NCA–CALL (800-622-2255) http://www.ncadd.org
National Institute on Alcohol Abuse and Alcoholism (NIAAA)	http://www.niaaa.nih.gov

(continued)

Appendix 19-1. Additional Resources *(continued)*

Organization	Information
National Institute on Drug Abuse (NIDA)	http://www.drugabuse.gov
National Organization on Fetal Alcohol Syndrome	1200 Eton Court, NW Third Floor Washington, DC 20007 Toll-free Phone: 800-66–NOFAS Fax: (202) 466–6456 http://www.nofas.org
Shoutinginside.com	http://www.shoutinginside.com
United States Department of Health Substance Abuse and Mental Health Services Administration (SAMHSA)	http://www.samhsa.gov **Treatment Facility Locator:** Phone: 800-662–HELP http://www.findtreatment.samhsa.gov
United States Department of Health and Human Services SAMHSA Office of Applied Studies	http://oas.samhsa.gov/nhsda.htm
United States Department of Health and Human Services Assistant Secretary for Planning and Evaluation	Blending Perspectives and Building Common Ground: *A Report to Congress on Substance Abuse and Child Protection April 1999* http://aspe.hhs.gov/hsp/subabuse99/chap1.htm
The White House, President Barack Obama Office of National Drug Control Policy	www.whitehousedrugpolicy.gov/streetterms/default.asp

References

1. American Psychaitric Association. *Diagnostic and Statistical Manual of Mental Disorders*. 4th ed. Text revision. Arlington, VA: American Psychiatric Association; 2000.
2. Johnson JL, Leff M. Children of substance abusers: overview of research findings. *Pediatrics*. 1999;103(5, pt 2):1085-1099.
3. United States Department of Health and Human Services, Substance Abuse and Mental Health Services Administration, Center for Behavioral Health Statistics and Quality. Results from the 2012 National Survey on Drug Use and Health: summary of national findings. Substance Abuse and Mental Health Services Administration (SAMHSA) Web site. http://www.samhsa.gov/data/NSDUH/2012SummNatFindDetTables/NationalFindings/NSDUHresults2012. Published September 2013. Accessed June 25, 2014.
4. Office of Applied Studies, Substance Abuse and Metal Health Services Administration. Children living with substance-dependent or substance-abusing parents: 2002 to 2007. Substance Abuse and Mental Health Services Administration Web site. http://www.samhsa.gov/data/2k9/SAparents/SAparents.pdf. Published April 16, 2009. Accessed June 5, 2013.

5. United States Department of Health and Human Services, Administration for Children and Families, Administration on Children, Youth, and Families Children's Bureau. Child maltreatment 2009. Administration for Children and Families Web site. http://www.acf.hhs.gov/programs/cb/pubs/cm09/cm09.pdf. Published December 31, 2009. Accessed June 5, 2013.

6. The National Center on Addiction and Substance Abuse at Columbia University. No safe haven: children of substance-abusing parents. The National Center on Addiction and Substance Abuse at Columbia University Web site. http://www.casacolumbia.org/articlefiles/379-No%20Safe%20Haven.pdf. Published January 1999. Accessed June 5, 2013.

7. Smith BD, Test MF. The risk of subsequent maltreatment allegations in families with substance-exposed infants. *Child Abuse Negl.* 2002;26(1):97-114.

8. Berger LM, Slack KS, Waldfogel J, Bruch SK. Caseworker-perceived caregiver substance abuse and child protective services outcomes. *Child Maltreat.* 2010;15(3):199-210.

9. Chaffin M, Kelleher K, Hollenberg J. Onset of physical abuse and neglect: psychiatric, substance abuse, and social risk factors from prospective community data. *Child Abuse Negl.* 1996;20(3):191-203.

10. National Institute on Drug Abuse. Drugs, brains and behavior: the science of addiction. National Institute on Drug Abuse Web site. http://www.drugabuse.gov/publications/science-addiction. Revised August 2010. Accessed June 5, 2013.

11. Young NK, Nakashian M, Yeh S, Amatetti S. *Screening and Assessment for Family Engagement, Retention, and Recovery (SAFERR).* Rockville, MD: Substance Abuse and Mental Health Services Administration; 2006.

12. Diamond-Berry KP. The consequences of intergenerational chemical addiction on infants, toddlers, and families. *Zero to Three.* 2007;27(4):5-10.

13. Conners NA, Bradley RH, Mansell LW, et al. Children of mothers with serious substance abuse problems: an accumulation of risks. *Am J Drug Alcohol Abuse.* 2004;30(1):85-100.

14. Mikton C, Butchart A. Child maltreatment prevention: a systematic review of reviews. *Bull World Health Organ.* 2009;87(5):353-361.

15. Dube SR, Felitti VJ, Dong M, Giles WH, Anda RF. The impact of adverse childhood experiences on health problems: evidence from four birth cohorts dating back to 1900. *Prev Med.* 2003;37(3):268-277.

16. Chapman DP, Wheaton AG, Anda RF, et al. Adverse childhood experiences and sleep disturbances in adults. *Sleep Med.* 2011;12(8):773-779.

17. Dube SR, Felitti VJ, Dong M, Chapman DP, Giles WH, Anda RF. Childhood abuse, neglect, and household dysfunction and the risk of illicit drug use: the adverse childhood experiences study. *Pediatrics.* 2003;111(3):564-572.

18. Wu NS, Schairer LC, Dellor E, Grella C. Childhood trauma and health outcomes in adults with comorbid substance abuse and mental health disorders. *Addict Behav.* 2010;35(1):68-71.

19. Bruns EJ, Pullmann MD, Weather ES, Wirschem ML, Murphy JK. How effects of a multidisciplinary family treatment drug court on child and family outcomes: results of a quasi-experimental study. *Child Maltreat.* 2012;17(3):218-230.

20. Belsky, J. Etiology of child maltreatment: a developmental-ecological analysis. *Psychol Bull.* 1993;114(3):413-434.

21. Pelham WE, Lang AR, Atkeson B, et al. Effects of deviant child behavior on parental distress and alcohol consumption in laboratory interactions. *J Abnorm Child Psychol.* 1997; 25(5):413-424.

22. Hien D, Cohen LR, Caldeira NA, Flom P, Wasserman G. Depression and anger as risk factors underlying the relationship between maternal substance involvement and child abuse potential. *Child Abuse Negl.* 2010; 34(2):105-113.

23. Testa MF, Smith B. Prevention and drug treatment. *Future Child.* 2009;19(2):147-168.

24. Executive Office of the President, Office of National Drug Control Policy. The economic costs of drug abuse in the United States 1992-2002. https://www.ncjrs.gov/ondcppubs/publications/pdf/economic_costs.pdf. Published December 2004. Accessed June 5, 2013.

25. Harwood HJ. Updating Estimates of the Economic Costs of Alcohol Abuse in the United States: Estimates, Update Methods, and Data. National Institute on Drug Abuse and the National Institute on Alcohol Abuse and Alcoholism, National Institutes of Health, Department of Health and Human Services Web site. http://pubs.niaaa.nih.gov/publications/economic-2000/. Published 2000. Accessed January 8, 2013.

26. Lupton C, Burd L, Harwood R. Cost of fetal alcohol spectrum disorders. *Am J Med Genet C Semin Med Genet.* 2004;127C(1):42-50.

27. Smith JP, Smith GC. Long-term economic costs of psychological problems during childhood. *Soc Sci Med.* 2010;71(1):110-115.

28. Werner MJ, Joffe A, Graham AV. Screening, early identification, and office-based intervention with children and youth living in substance-abusing families. *Pediatrics.* 1999; 103(5, pt 2):1099-1112.

29. Kulig J; The American Academy of Pediatrics Committee on Substance Abuse. Tobacco, alcohol, and other drugs: the role of the pediatrician in prevention, identification, and management of substance abuse. *Pediatrics.* 2005;115(3):816-821.

30. Nygren P, Nelson HD, Klein J. Screening children for family violence: a review of the evidence for the US Preventative Services Task Force. *Ann Fam Med.* 2004;2(2):161-169.

31. Polen MR, Whitlock EP, Wisdom JP, Nygren P, Bougatsos C. *Screening in Primary Care Settings for Illicit Drug Use: Staged Systematic Review for the United States Preventive Services Task Force.* Rockville, MD: Agency for Healthcare Research and Quality (US); 2008. Report No. 08-05108-EF-1.

32. Office of Applied Studies, Substance Abuse and Mental Health Services Administration. Substance use during pregnancy: 2002 and 2003 update. Substance Abuse and Mental Health Services Administration Web site. http://www.samhsa.gov/data/2k5/pregnancy/pregnancy.htm. Updated May 12, 2008. Accessed October 10, 2011.

33. Mitchell EA, Milerad J. Smoking and Sudden Infant Death Syndrome. World Health Organization Background Paper, Available at http://www.who.int/tobacco/media/en/mitchell.pdf. Accessed June 25, 2014.

34. Bauer CR, Langer JC, Shankaran S, et al. Acute neonatal effects of cocaine exposure during pregnancy. *Arch Pediatr Adolesc Med.* 2005;159:824-834.

35. Arria AM, Derauf C, Lagasse LL, et al. Methamphetamine and other substance use during pregnancy: preliminiary estimates from the Infant Development, Environment, and Lifestyle (IDEAL) study. *Matern Child Health J.* 2006;10(3):293-302.

36. American College of Obstetrics and Gynecology Committee on Ethics. ACOG committee opinion no. 321: maternal decision making, ethics, and the law. *Obstet Gynecol.* 2005;106(5, pt 1):1127-1137.

37. Dasgupta A. *A Health Educator's Guide to Understanding Drugs of Abuse Testing.* Sudbury, MA: Jones & Bartlett Publishers; 2010.

38. Roberts SC, Nuru-Jeter A. Women's perspectives on screening for alcohol and drug use in prenatal care. *Women's Health Issues.* 2010; 20(3):193-200.

39. American College of Obstetrics and Gynecology. ACOG committee opinion no. 422: at-risk drinking and illicit drug use: ethical issues for obstetric and gynecologic practice. *Obstet Gynecol.* 2008;112(6):1449-1460.

40. Grella CE, Hser YI, Huang YC. Mothers in substance abuse treatment: differences in characteristics based on involvement with child welfare services. *Child Abuse Negl.* 2006;30(1):55-73.

41. McLellan AT, Lewis DC, O'Brien CP, Kleber HD. Drug dependence, a chronic medical illness: implications for treatment, insurance, and outcomes evaluation. *JAMA.* 2000;284(13):1689-1695.

42. Dakof GA, Cohen JB, Henderson CE, et al. A randomized pilot study of the Engaging Moms Program for family drug court. *J Subst Abuse Treat.* 2010;38(3):263-274.

43. Green BL, Furrer C, Worcel S, Burrus S, Finigan MW. How effective are family treatment drug courts?: outcomes from a four-site national study. *Child Maltreat.* 2007;12:43-59.

44. Graham AW, Schultz TK, Wilford BB, eds; American Society of Addiction Medicine. *Principles of Addiction Medicine.* 2nd ed. New York, NY: Harcourt Brace Press; 1998.

45. Dekker FW, Dieleman FE, Kaptein AA, Mulder JD. Compliance with pulmonary medication in general practice. *Eur Respir J.* 1993;6(6):886-890.

46. Gerstein DR, Harwood HJ, eds; Committee for the Substance Abuse Coverage Study Division of Health Care Services. *Treating Drug Problems: A Study of the Evolution, Effectiveness, and Financing of Public and Private Drug Treatment Systems. Vol I.* Washington, DC: National Academy Press; 1990.

47. Graber AL, Davidson P, Brown AW, McRae JR, Woolridge K. Dropout and relapse during diabetes care. *Diabetes Care.* 1992;15(11):1477-1483.

48. Kurtz SMS. Adherence to diabetic regimens: empirical status and clinical applications. *Diabetes Educator.* 1990;16(1):50-56.

49. Lowinson JH, Ruiz P, Millman RB, eds. *Substance Abuse: A Comprehensive Textbook.* 2nd ed. Baltimore, MD: Williams & Wilkins; 1992:56-59.

50. O'Brien CP, McLellan AT. Myths about the treatment of addiction. *Lancet.* 1996;347(8996):237-240.

51. McLellan AT, Metzger DS, Alterman AI, Woody GE, Durrell J, O'Brien CP. Is addiction treatment "worth it"? public health expectations, policy-based comparisons. In: Fox JS, ed. *Proceedings of Josiah Macy Conference on Medical education.* New York, NY: Josiah Macy Foundation; 1995:165-212.

52. McLellan AT, Alterman AI, Metzger DC, et al. Similarity of outcome predictors across opiate, cocaine, and alcohol treatments: role of treatment services. *J Consult Clin Psychol.* 1994;62(6):1141-1158.

53. Moos RH, Finney JW, Cronkite RC. *Alcoholism Treatment: Context, Process, and Outcome.* New York, NY: Oxford University Press; 1990.

54. Schaub AF, Steiner A, Vetter W. Compliance to treatment. *Clin Exp Hypertens.* 1993;15(6):1121-1130.

55. Sinnock P. Hospital utilization for diabetes. In: National Diabetes Data Group. *Diabetes in America: Diabetes Data Compiled 1984.* NIH publication no. 85-1468. Bethesda, MD: United States Department of Health and Human Services, Public Health Service, National Institutes of Health, National Institute of Arthritis, Diabetes, and Digestive and Kidney Disease; 1985.

56. Clark LT. Improving compliance and increasing control of hypertension: needs of special hypertensive populations. *Am Heart J.* 1991;121(2, Pt 2):664-669.

57. National Institute on Drug Abuse. *Principles of Drug Addiction Treatment: A Research Based Guide.* 2nd ed. Bethesda, MD: National Institutes of Health; 1999.

58. Kinsey BM, Jackson DC, Orson FM. Anti-drug vaccines to treat substance abuse. *Immunol Cell Biol.* 2009;87:309-314.

59. Oxford House. The purpose and structure of Oxford House. Oxford House Web site. http://www.oxfordhouse.org/userfiles/file/purpose_and_structure.php. Accessed April 16, 2012.

60. Worley LL, Connors NA, Crone CC, Williams VL, Bokony PA. Building a residential treatment program for dually diagnosed women with their children. *Arch Women's Ment Health.* 2005;8(2):105-111.

61. Jason LA, Olson BD, Ferrari JR, et al. An examination of main and interactive effects of substance abuse recovery housing on multiple indicators of adjustment. *Addiction.* 2007;102(7):1114-1121.

62. Administration for Children and Families, Substance Abuse and Mental Health Services Administration, Office of the Assistant Secretary for Planning and Evaluation. Blending perspectives and building common ground: a report to Congress on substance abuse and child protection. Assistant Secretary for Planning and Evaluation Web site. http://aspe.hhs.gov/hsp/subabuse99/subabuse.htm#ack. Published April 1999. Accessed June 5, 2013.

63. Rhodes T, Bernays S, Houmoller K. Parents who use drugs: accounting for damage and its limitation. *Soc Sci Med.* 2010;71(8):1489-1497.

64. McCarty D. Policy brief: substance abuse policy research program. Substance Abuse Policy Research Program Web site. http://www.saprp.org/knowledgeassets/knowledge_brief.cfm?KAID=1. Accessed June 5, 2013.

Chapter 20

Forensic Nursing

Kathy Bell, MS, RN, SANE-A, SANE-P

Key Points

1. The term *forensic nursing* applies to both the living and the deceased. Forensic nurses encounter patients who have experienced intentionally or accidentally inflicted physical trauma.
2. Forensic Nursing had been defined as "The application of forensic aspects of health care combined with the biological, psychological, social, and spiritual education of the registered nurse in the scientific investigation and treatment of trauma and death" of victims, perpetrators of violence, criminal activity, and traumatic accidents.[1]
3. Primary prevention on the part of the forensic nurse requires the implementation of strategies to stop violence before it occurs. Implemented strategies should aim to decrease the factors that put people at risk for experiencing violence and increase the factors that protect people or buffer them from risk.[2]
4. Secondary and tertiary prevention take place after violence has occurred. The goal of secondary prevention is to identify and eliminate risk factors or problems, while the goal of tertiary prevention is to develop interventions to minimize the impact of the violence and restore health, wellness, and safety as soon as possible.[3]
5. A forensic nurse should be proficient in identifying injuries, understanding mechanisms of injury, piecing together patterns of injury, and identifying patterned injuries, all of which culminate in a suspicious awareness of that which lies beyond the obvious.
6. A nurse with forensic knowledge should know the difference between several key and frequently confused terms, including ***patterned injury, patterns of injury, sharp force injury,*** and ***blunt force injury.*** This detail of injury type may seem insignificant in most cases, but for the forensic case, could be a deciding factor in associating a weapon found at a crime scene with a patient's injuries.

Introduction

Violence and trauma is pandemic. Still, until recently, a significant disconnect existed between the health care and judicial system in the United States with regard to the victims of violent crimes. Among the factors that contributed to the gap were differences in language among professionals. The language used by the professionals in the health care system was foreign to the professionals in the judicial system and vice versa, which lead to instances of miscommunication. Additionally, actions taken in one or the other system were taken without regard to the implications of said actions on the processes or procedures of the other system. Fortunately, forensic nursing now exists as a conduit through which these 2 very different systems might be linked.

History of Forensic Nursing

Historically, images of morgues and thoughts of pathology have been conjured by the term forensic; however, the term forensic nursing applies to both the living and the deceased. Forensic nurses encounter patients who have experienced intentionally or accidentally inflicted physical trauma. For the living patient, such trauma may include covert emotional trauma in addition to overt physical trauma. Because the effects of violence and trauma are far-reaching, forensic nurses may also interact directly with the victim's family, friends, and community groups during the course of the victim's care or through education and prevention activities.

Although relatively new to the United States, living forensics has been practiced in the United Kingdom, Australia, and Canada for over 200 years and, until recently, was practiced in a secure psychiatric setting.[4] Still deeper roots of forensic practice can be traced to *Hsi Duan Yu* (The Washing Away of Wrongs), a Chinese publication dating back to 1248 AD. *Hsi Duan Yu* describes how to distinguish drowning from strangulation, thereby establishing itself as the first recorded application of medical knowledge in the solving of a crime.[4] Additionally, the process on which the foundation of forensic nursing was laid and the evolution of modern nursing in general can be found in various 20th century writings about victims of war and abuse and the mentally ill.[5] For example, Nutting & Dock's 1907 publication, *A History of Nursing: the Evolution of Nursing Systems From the Earliest Times to the Foundation of the First English and American Training Schools For Nurses*, describes the traits and customs of nursing as applied to the condition of humankind.

Forensic nursing attained the global designation of specialty practice in the 1990s, bringing with it qualified clinicians uniquely equipped to blend biomedical knowledge with an understanding of the basic principles of law and human behavior.[1] In 1991, forensic nursing was defined as "the application of forensic aspects of health care combined with the biological, psychological, social, and spiritual education of the registered nurse in the scientific investigation and treatment of trauma and death" of victims, perpetrators of violence, criminal activity, and traumatic accidents.[1] As such, the forensic nurse provides direct services to individual patients and consultation services to agencies representing nursing, medical, and legal professionals. For example, the forensic nurse may be called as an expert witness to provide testimony regarding a particular investigative death process, such as time, manner, or cause of death, or to offer specialized diagnoses of specific conditions. Within forensic nursing, there are more specialized, population-focused areas of practice as well, such as forensic nurse death investigators, sexual assault nurse examiners (SANEs), legal nurse consultants, and forensic geriatric and pediatric nurse clinicians.[1]

In *Forensic Nursing*,[6] one of the first texts devoted to this specialty practice, Lynch states as follows:

> [The] forensic nurse is viewed as an integral member of the multidisciplinary investigative team consisting of health care professionals, law enforcement agencies, social science advocates, and forensic scientists. The effectiveness of the forensic nurse is based in part on the nurse's ability to interact with other professionals and to view the victim or offender in the humanitarian nursing perspective, a unique kind of nursing. As health is viewed on a continuum, it is essential to provide patients with interventions and resources that will help them to reestablish a sense of balance. The forensic nurse examiner strives to facilitate optimum functioning, which begins with objectively assessing the problem, applying the nursing process to achieve mutually established goals, and providing a humane, caring interaction.

Because of the pioneering efforts of interested and motivated nursing professionals, new professional roles and educational programs for the forensic nursing fields are being continuously identified and developed based on Lynch's definition of the field of and concept of the multidisciplinary team.

In 2008, the International Association of Forensic Nursing (IAFN) readdressed the definition of forensic nursing. To include the efforts of members in all countries, the organization simplified the definition to "the practice of nursing globally when health and legal systems intersect."[7] Although there are other organizations that support and promote the practice of forensic nursing, the IAFN plays an important role in the advancement of the profession. According to the IAFN,[7] the organization:

> [C]ame into existence during the summer of 1992, when 74 nurses, primarily sexual assault nurse examiners, came together and formed the organization. The vision of this founding group was to develop an organization that would encompass a wide and diverse body of those who practice nursing within the arena of the law. Nurses that apply concepts and strategies to provide interventions to victims of violent crime or perpetrators of criminal acts were included in this field of practice. This included nurses as diverse as death investigators, correctional nurse specialists, forensic psychiatric nurses, legal nurse consultants, forensic geriatric specialists, nurse attorneys, forensic clinical specialists, forensic gynecology nurses, and other nursing roles defined as forensic practice as they evolve. One year later, the organization had more than tripled in members and held its first Scientific Assembly, with some 160 members in attendance. On the organizations 10th anniversary there were 2000 members. The membership is now over 3000 and represents 24 countries.

Since the beginning, IAFN has promoted quality forensic nursing care and created standards that provide a flexible framework intended to fit within the practice of different countries. These include *Forensic Nursing: Scope and Standards of Practice*; standards of practice for intimate partner violence and SANEs; and education guidelines for adult and pediatric SANEs, forensic nurse death investigators, and forensic nurses working in the realm of IPV.

The most recent publication of *Forensic Nursing: Scope and Standards of Practice* was a cooperative effort of the American Nurses Association (ANA) and the IAFN. It provides the forensic nurse with guidance to practice competently. Although published in the United States, it offers an international perspective for a global network of forensic nurses; the scope of practice includes the history and evolution of forensic nursing and a discussion of practice characteristics and skills. Goals, trends, and issues within forensic nursing as they apply to education, research, populations, genetics, and genomics are also discussed. The scope of practice provides a description of educational preparation and certification and a description of the levels of forensic nursing practice. The standards of forensic nursing practice can be categorized as practices or performance[8]:

— Standards of Practice

  — Assessment

  — Diagnosis

  — Outcomes identification

  — Planning

  — Implementation

  — Evaluation

— Standards of performance
  — Quality of practice
  — Education
  — Professional practice
  — Evaluation,
  — Collegiality
  — Collaboration
  — Ethics
  — Research
  — Resource utilization
  — Leadership

Nurses have always worked with forensic patients; however, a lack of focus existed as to how such patients intersected with the law or legal proceedings once the patient was outside of the health care system. This uncertainty created a gap that was subject to any number of interpretations based on setting (eg, emergency room [ER], correctional facility, psychiatric facility, or patient setting) or vantage point (eg, victim, offender, or community). The forensic nursing specialty developed in response to this gap and has lead to, among other things, an increase in forensic knowledge among nursing professionals that has allowed for better preservation of evidence and a reduction in the number of instances in which the integrity of bullet holes is compromised, bags of clothing are thrown away or remanded to the perpetrator, or evidence is washed away. Forensic nursing applies the nursing process and provides compassionate care and promotion of health while at the same time assuring that sound forensic principles are applied during care.

Events that led to and have supported the development of forensic nursing involve both nursing and non-nursing organizations.[8,9]

— 1948: Article V in the Universal Declaration of Human Rights declares, "No one shall be subjected to torture or to cruel, inhuman or degrading treatment or punishment."

— 1984: The United States Surgeon General identifies violence as a public health issue and health care providers as key agents in ameliorating the effects of violence in our communities.

— 1991: Virginia Lynch conceptualizes the forensic nurse in her master thesis.

— 1991: ANA publishes a position statement on violence as a nursing practice issue.

— 1992: The Joint Commission puts standards in place for the identification and treatment of forensic patients.

— 1995: Forensic Nursing is officially recognized by the ANA as a specialty of nursing.

— 1997: The ANA and IAFN cooperatively publish the Scope and Standards of Forensic Nursing.

— 2000: Healthy People 2010 is developed; action objectives are set, including several that are forensic in nature[10]:

  — Reduce firearm-related deaths.

  — Extend state-level child fatality review of deaths due to external causes for children aged 14 years and younger.

  — Reduce nonfatal poisonings.

  — Reduce deaths caused by suffocation.

  — Reduce homicides.

  — Reduce maltreatment and maltreatment fatalities of children.

  — Reduce the rate of physical assault by current or former intimate partners.

  — Reduce intentional injuries resulting from alcohol- and illicit drug-related violence.

  — Reduce the annual rate of rape or attempted rape.

  — Reduce sexual assault other than rape.

  — Reduce physical fighting among adolescents.

  — Reduce weapon carrying by adolescents on school property.

  — Reduce work-related assaults.

Scope of Violence

In 2002, the World Health Organization (WHO) published its first ever document on violence in the world examining a broad spectrum of violence, including child abuse and neglect by caregivers, youth violence, violence by intimate partners, sexual violence, elder abuse, suicide, and collective violence.[11] The report asserts:

— 1 in 4 women will experience sexual violence by an intimate partner in her lifetime.

— One-third of adolescent girls' first-time intercourse will be forced.

— 20% of women and 5% to 10% of men report child sexual abuse.

— 6% of the elderly report abuse.

— Violence kills 1.6 million people every year.

  — 1424 deaths per day are the result of homicide.

  — 2160 deaths per day, 1 death every 40 seconds, are the result of suicide

  — 840 deaths per day, 35 deaths per hour, are the result of armed conflict.

    — Of the 191 million deaths attributed to armed conflict throughout the 20th century, half were civilians.

In addition to each person killed, there are 20 to 40 more that are injured, resulting in millions over the course of the year. There is no way to accurately measure the cost of an individual's suffering. It is possible, however, to measure the cost of violence in terms of health care dollars. Individuals that have experienced violence and abuse access health care 2 to 2.5 times more frequently than those who have not experienced such trauma.[12] In 2003, the Center for Disease Control (CDC) estimated the health-related costs of rape, physical assault, stalking, and homicide against women by an intimate partner to exceed $5.8 billion annually. In 2005, the CDC estimated that more than 51 000 people in the United States died as a result of violence. The costs of those deaths totaled $47.2 billion, with costs related to lost work accounting for $47 billion and expenses related to medical treatment costs accounting for $215 million.[13] In 2008, the Academy on Violence and Abuse placed the incremental cost of violence and abuse to the health care system at somewhere between $333 billion and $750 billion annually.[13] As such, the incidence of injuries and death from violence has been identified as a major public health issue.

Roles

The health determinants set by Healthy People 2020 include providing service to patients and communities in addressing violence among the duties of the forensic nurse, a role fulfilled alongside public health nurses. In this public health approach, the forensic nurse serves as content expert, clinician advisor, or clinical manager of care facilities that may contribute to a community response to injury prevention.[5]

Prevention

Primary Prevention

Primary prevention on the part of the forensic nurse requires the implementation of strategies to stop violence before it occurs. Implemented strategies should aim to decrease factors that put people at risk for experiencing violence and increase the factors that protect people, or buffer them, from risk.[2] Forensic nurses can participate in primary prevention efforts by participating in a community stance against violence and ensuring that elected officials and media outlets consider nonviolence a priority by supporting public programs providing education about violence, ways for victims of violence to get help, and ways in which third parties may intervene in cases of suspected violence. Primary prevention can also include teaching parenting skills to first-time parents, particularly teenage parents, or those whose children have special needs in a community setting as a means to educate and provide resources in building on protective factors.

Secondary and Tertiary Prevention

Secondary and tertiary prevention take place after violence has occurred. The goal of secondary prevention is to identify and eliminate risk factors or problems while the goal of tertiary prevention is to develop interventions to minimize the impact of the violence and restore health, wellness, and safety as soon as possible.[3] For example, a forensic nurse may participate in screening patients for violence, secondary prevention, and referring them to community organizations for further assistance, tertiary prevention.[5]

Women who reported having been the victim of IPV incurred 17% more primary care visits, 14% more specialist visits, and 27% more prescription refills than women who had not been abused. The women who reported having been the victim of IPV were also more likely to use services in the areas of mental health, substance abuse, hospital outpatient care, ER care, and acute inpatient care during and after periods of IPV.[14] Additionally, IPV is noted to be a leading cause of traumatic death among new and expectant mothers.[15] The consequences of IPV indicate why utilization of prevention activities at all levels by nurses is of the utmost importance in minimizing the effects of violence on children and families.

Skills

A forensic nurse brings several important skills to every patient encounter no matter the setting or patient set, not the least of which is caring. Hammer, Moynihan and Pagliaro[16] state that caring has always been a "hallmark of professional nursing" and that caring should be curious and questioning. Patton[5] further expands on the subject by asserting that caring must not be only for patients, but also for oneself and that "a sense of self worth must be cultivated and nurtured to the degree that caring is conscious, objective, and demanding of the truth." Additionally, a forensic nurse should be proficient in identifying injuries, understanding mechanisms of injury, piecing together patterns of injury, and identifying patterned injuries, all of which culminate in an awareness of that which lies beyond the obvious. For example, the forensic nurse presented with a family recently admitted for injuries sustained as the result of a severe automobile accident might question whether the accident was indeed an accident or perhaps an attempt on the part of an IPV offender to intentionally annihilate the family. The forensic nurse presented with a female child admitted with genital bleeding or discharge might question if the symptoms are the result of sexual abuse, urethral prolapse, or viral condition. Similarly, the forensic nurse presented with a child with behavioral problems might question whether the child is disobedient or if the child is experiencing or witnessing abuse at home. Once presented with a patient, the nurse must apply the forensic nursing process to provide appropriate care to the patient. *Forensic Nursing: Scope and Standards of Practice*[8] addresses the nursing process in detail and outlines the duties a forensic nurse is expected to competently perform (**Table 20-1** and **Table 20-2**).

Table 20-1. Standards of Practice

Duty	Description	Example
Assessment	Collect data pertinent to the patient's health or the situation.	Conduct patient interviews or evidence collection.
Diagnosis	Develop a diagnosis based on the assessment data.	Determine if the injury was intentionally inflicted or accidental.
Outcomes identification	Individualize expected outcomes.	Coordinate a team review of a suspected physical child abuse to determine a safe environment for that child.
Planning	Develop a plan to achieve expected outcomes.	Address wound care, basic safety planning, education, and referrals for the patient who has experienced IPV.
Implementation	Implement the plan.	Provide referrals to professionals outside of the health care system and possibly coordinate care and health teaching. The advanced practice registered nurse (APRN) may provide consultations and exercise prescriptive authority.
Evaluation	Appraise performance.	Administer patient satisfaction questionnaires.

Data from American Nurses Association, International Association of Forensic Nurses. Forensic Nursing: Scope and Standards of Practice. *Silver Spring, MD: American Nurses Association; 2009.*

Table 20-2. Scope of Practice

Duty	Description	Example
Quality of practice	Enhance the quality and effectiveness of practice.	Objectively and factually document all care provided.
Education	Obtain knowledge required of professionals in the field.	Participate in continuing education.
Professional practice evaluation	Applies evidence-based principles	Participate in peer review.
Collegiality	Interact with colleagues appropriately.	Deliver educational presentations to peers.
Collaboration	Work in partnership with others.	Participate in a task force.

Data from American Nurses Association, International Association of Forensic Nurses. Forensic Nursing: Scope and Standards of Practice. *Silver Spring, MD: American Nurses Association; 2009.*

Education

Education is paramount to the forensic nurse's ability to adhere to and apply the scope and standards of practice. Since the early 1990s, education institutions have experienced an explosion of programs designed to provide field-specific education to the forensic nurse. These programs touch every part of the forensic nurse's education path, including entry-level nursing programs, doctorate programs, and continuing education. Forensic nurses may participate in these programs in a variety of settings, such as the traditional classroom, online, or a combination of the two.[5] Core concepts are currently being developed, though debate exists regarding which should be included in forensic nursing educational programs.[5] In 2010, the IAFN Board of Directors designated a forensic nursing core curriculum committee. The committee met over the course of a year and ultimately submitted an outline for an education course for entry into forensic nursing practice.

In addition to education, specific certifications may need to be obtained by the forensic nurse in order to practice in this specialized field. For example, the Forensic Nursing Certification Board introduced the first sexual assault nurse examiner adult/adolescent certification (SANE-A) in 2002. Four years later, the board began offering the first sexual assault nurse examiner pediatric/adolescent certification (SANE-P). Other organizations offer certifications that have a specialty area of focus, such as death investigation and legal nurse consultants. Nurses should check with their state board of nursing to determine specific certification and practice requirements.

Forensic patient care facilities include, but are not limited to, hospitals, schools, correctional facilities, medical examiner offices, homes, and nursing homes. Nearly every patient encounter has the potential for need of forensic nursing knowledge. Forensic nurses may see victims of sexual assault, IPV, child abuse, child sexual abuse, and food and drug tampering. Additionally, forensic nurses may encounter patients who have come into contact with environmental hazards, experienced epidemiological issues, or suffered fatal injury or trauma.

Knowledge of Injuries and Trauma

An understanding of injuries and trauma is important in most specialty areas of forensic nursing. A nurse with forensic knowledge should know the difference between several key and frequently confused terms, including patterned injury and patterns of injury and sharp force injury and blunt force injury. A patterned injury is a wound that exhibits the appearance or characteristics of the object with which it was inflicted. A pattern of injury is a combination or distribution of external or internal injuries that suggest a causative mechanism or sequence of events. Sharp force injuries that are inflicted with a very sharp knife are often incorrectly documented as lacerations. Sharp force injuries include cuts, or incisions, and stab wounds. Cuts or incisions are injuries made when a sharp object comes in contact with the skin with sufficient pressure to divide it. Blunt force injury has common subdivisions that are designated as abrasions, contusions, lacerations, and fractures and are caused by a tearing, shearing, or scraping motion. An example that includes both sharp force and blunt force trauma is when a surgeon takes a scalpel and makes an incision, sharp force, in the abdomen of a patient that has experienced a liver laceration, blunt force, as a result of steering wheel impact. This detail of injury type may seem insignificant in many cases, but for the forensic case, could be a deciding factor in associating a weapon found at a crime scene with a patient's injuries.

The forensic nurse should also be aware of the complicated nature of bruising. Recent literature has shown that it is nearly impossible to accurately date a bruise based on appearance.[17] Bruise age-dating charts should not be used in order to avoid confounding an already complicated forensic situation. For example, using a dating chart, a yellow bruise may be documented as an old bruise; however, research shows that a variety of variables, such as the patient's age, lighting in the room, and number of researchers observing the wound, impact the accuracy of dating the age of a bruise.[17] In the area of child maltreatment, such a determination could impact the decision of law enforcement as to who to charge with a crime based on who was with the child when an injury occurred. It is imperative that health care professionals have an understanding of the nature of bruising as well as the required associated documentation (see *Chapter 4, The Physical Examination in the Evaluation of Suspected Child Maltreatment: Physical Abuse and Sexual Abuse Examinations*).

Recognizing Emotional Trauma

Physical and emotional trauma often occur concurrently; therefore, forensic nurses may interact with patients that exhibit no outward signs of trauma. Where physical injury exists there also exists emotional trauma, the impact of which can be devastating. Research conducted as a part of the CDC's Adverse Childhood Experiences (ACE) Study[18] examined the impact of 10 common childhood experiences on an individual's life expectancy and quality of life **(Table 20-3)**.

Documentation

Accurate and objective documentation of injuries, evidence, and care is an essential element of the forensic medical examination. It is important for the forensic nurse to record the victim's words exactly as he or she says them and to use quotation marks to identify the patient's words. Often, what seems to be insignificant matters; therefore, everything should be recorded. Documentation should be neat and legible, using proper spelling and grammar. Failure to provide this level of detail gives the appearance of a lack of professionalism. It is advised that the nurse review his or her documentation for thoroughness and errors and correct any mistaken information or omissions before completing the examination. Additionally, the nurse should use landmarks that cannot

Table 20-3. Common Childhood Experiences That Impact Life Expectancy and Quality of Life

— Recurrent physical abuse
— Recurrent severe emotional abuse
— Contact sexual abuse
— Incarcerated family member
— Violence against mother
— Household substance abuse
— Chronic depression, mental illness, suicidal
— One parent lost during childhood
— Physical neglect
— Emotional neglect

Data from Centers for Disease Control and Prevention. Adverse Childhood Experiences (ACE) Study. Centers for Disease Control and Prevention Web site. http://www.cdc.gov/ace/index.htm. Updated June 1, 2012. Accessed September 2012.

be easily challenged. Since a number of professionals from different fields may be required to review a given record, the forensic nurse should avoid using abbreviations and jargon in order to avoid confusion. The forensic nurse should not include or imply his or her own personal opinion in the documentation (see *Chapter 9, Documenting the Evaluation of Suspected Child Maltreatment Cases*).

Forensic Photography

Photography is another form of forensic documentation. Forensic photography should provide visual evidence as to the location, size, and detail of a patient's injuries. Each injury should be photographed a minimum of 3 times and in such a manner that disallows any individual viewing the photograph to question the location, size, or nature of the injury. As a rule, it is nearly impossible to take too many photographs; however, it is very possible to take too few. When compiling sets of injury photographs for documentation, the nurse must identify the set by either including a photograph of the individual or his or her medical face sheet (see *Chapter 9, Documenting the Evaluation of Suspected Child Maltreatment Cases*).

Evidence Collection

The Forensic Nursing Scope and Standard of Practice clearly includes evidence collection as one of the roles of the forensic nurse.[8,19] The forensic evidence collection portion of an examination involves linking a victim to a suspect, the victim to the crime scene, and the suspect to the crime scene. The nurse should take care to note that victims are not parts of crime scenes and should not be objectified as such while still respecting the fact that the victim has been in a crime scene. As such, the forensic nurse should handle the patient carefully to ensure effective evidence collection while simultaneously promoting good patient care.

Physical evidence encompasses any and all objects that can establish that a crime has been committed or can provide a link between a crime and its victim or a crime and its perpetrator. This link is guided by Locard's exchange principle, which states that when 2 surfaces come together, there is likely a transfer of material from one to the other.[20]

Whether it is body fluids, dirt and plant materials, fingerprints, or hair and fibers, a possibility of transfer exits.

Some general guidelines for evidence collection include:

— Photography first

— Handle as little as possible.

— Never use plastic bags to collect evidence, instead use previously unused brown paper bags or boxes.

— Store one item per bag.

— Air-dry wet material when possible.

— Use bindles inside envelopes.

— Adhere to chain of custody.

A systematic approach to evidence collection begins with photography. The very basic process of evidence collection involves observing, photographing, and then collecting. By beginning evidence collection with photography, the nurse is able to provide an accurate representation of what he or she observed at the onset of the process before the process itself changed anything. Once the collection process commences, the nurse should handle evidence minimally to prevent loss and destruction. Chain of custody requires authenticating and carefully documenting every location to which the evidence travelled, every person who handled the evidence, and every action performed concerning the evidence. Strict adherence to chain of custody will eliminate questioning as to the integrity of the evidence when submitted in the courtroom (see *Chapter 9, Documenting the Evaluation of Suspected Child Maltreatment Cases*).

Expert Witness

Providing testimony is another key role of the forensic nurse. Court proceedings are not normally taught in nursing school; however, forensic nursing programs include testimony as a part of the curriculum. As potential expert witnesses, all nurses should have an up-to-date resume and curriculum vitae on hand outlining current and past nursing practice and educational activities **(Table 20-4)**.

When giving testimony, nurses should understand that he or she is not there to make or break a case but rather to offer information that is important and relevant for the court to hear. The nurse may be called as an expert or a fact witness. As an expert witness, the court recognizes that he or she possesses experience, training, or knowledge and has authority to provide specific explanations to the court. The forensic nurse witness must be careful not to exceed the limits of the field of professional nursing practice. For

Table 20-4. Tips for Providing Testimony
— Be prepared.
— Be familiar with your documentation.
— Be aware of your policies and procedures.
— Dress professionally.
— Tell the truth.
— Avoid jargon and speak in terms that can be understood.

example, although a nurse may be familiar with various aspects of an investigation of child sexual abuse, it is important that the nurse stays within the bounds of his or her individual education and experience when testifying.

Conclusion

Forensic nursing continues to evolve as a profession. Forensic nursing offers patients compassion, safety, and high regard during a vulnerable time while simultaneously offering objective documentation, properly handled evidence, and impartial testimony to the legal community. Still, the forward development of the profession hinges on continued research. Any research article is only as good as its use enhancing forensic practice, guiding theory, and leading to additional research questions.[21] Peer-reviewed journals, such as the Journal of Forensic Nursing and many other supportive journals provide forensic practitioners with evidence on which to base their practice and with which to provide comprehensive care.

References

1. Lynch VA. Forensic nursing sciences. In: Hammer R, Moynihan B, Pagliaro EM, eds. *Forensic Nursing: A Handbook for Practice*. Sudbury, MA: Jones & Bartlett Publishers; 2006.
2. Center for Disease Control and Prevention. Principles of prevention. Veto Violence Web site. http://www.vetoviolence.org/pop/education-training.html. Accessed September 2012.
3. Chamberlain L. A Prevention primer for domestic violence: terminology, tools, and the public health approach. VAWnet Web site. http://www.vawnet.org/applied-research-papers/print-document.php?doc_id=1313. Published 2008. Accessed September 2012.
4. Barber Duval JS, Dougherty CM, Sullivan MK. Forensic nursing. In: James SH, Nordby JJ, eds. *Forensic Sciences: An Introduction to Scientific and Investigative Techniques*. 3rd ed. Boca Raton, FL: CRC Press, Inc; 2005.
5. Patton S. Forensic nursing in the community. In: Stanhope M, ed. *Public Health Nursing: Population-Centered Health Care in the Community*. 8th ed. Maryland Heights, MO: Elsevier; 2012.
6. Lynch VA. *Forensic Nursing*. St. Louis, MO: Mosby Inc; 2006.
7. International Association of Forensic Nurses. History of IAFN. International Association of Forensic Nurses Web site. http://www.iafn.org/displaycommon.cfm?an=1&subarticlenbr=149. Published 2006. Accessed September 2012.
8. American Nurses Association, International Association of Forensic Nurses. *Forensic Nursing: Scope and Standards of Practice*. Silver Spring, MD: American Nurses Association; 2009.
9. Burgess AW, Berger AD, Boersma RR. Forensic nursing: investigating the career potential in this emerging graduate specialty. *Am J Nurs*. 2004;104(3):58-64.
10. Healthy people 2020. Healthy People 2020 Web site. Healthypeople.gov/2020/. Updated August 20, 2012. Accessed September 2012.
11. World Health Organization. World report on violence and health. World Health Organization Web site. http://www.who.int/violence_injury_prevention/violence/world_report/outline/en/. Published October 3, 2002. Accessed September 2012.

12. Dolezal T, McCollum D, Callahan M. *Hidden Costs in Health Care: The Economic Impact of Violence and Abuse.* Eden Prairie, MN: Academy on Violence and Abuse; 2009.

13. Center for Disease Control and Prevention. Cost of violent deaths in the United States. Center for Disease Control and Prevention Web site. http://www.cdc.gov/violenceprevention/violentdeaths/. Updated February 24, 2011. Accessed September 2012.

14. Center for Disease Control and Prevention. Costs of intimate partner violence against women in the United States. Center for Disease Control and Prevention Web site. http://www.cdc.gov/ncipc/pub-res/ipv_cost/ipv.htm. Updated October 16, 2009. Accessed September 2012.

15. Clements PT, Holt KE, Hasson CM, Fay-Hiller T. Enhancing assessment of interpersonal violence (IPV) pregnancy-related homicide risk within nursing curricula. *J Forensic Nurs.* 2011;7(4):195-202.

16. Hammer R, Moynihan B, Pagliaro EM, eds. *Forensic Nursing: A Handbook for Practice.* Sudbury, MA: Jones & Bartlett Publishers; 2006.

17. Nash KR, Sheridan DJ. Can one accurately date a bruise?: state of the science. *J Forensic Nurs.* 2009;5(1):31-37.

18. Center for Disease Control and Prevention. Adverse childhood experiences (ACE) study. Center for Disease Control Web site. http://www.cdc.gov/ace/index.htm. Updated June 1, 2012. Accessed September 2012.

19. Burgess AW, Piatelli MJ, Pasqualone G. Criminalistics and the forensic nursing process. *J Forensic Nurs.* 2011;7(2): 97-104.

20. Saferstein R. *Criminalistics: An Introduction to Forensic Science.* 5th ed. Englewood Cliffs, NJ: Prentice Hall, Inc; 1995.

21. Amar AF, Clements PT. Toto's guide to reading and using research manuscripts for forensic nursing practice. *J Forensic Nurs.* 2008;4(1):49-51.

Index

A

Appendices, boxes, figures and tables are indicated by a, b, f, and t respectively

B

C

D

E

F

I

J

K

L

M

N

O

P

R

S

T

U

V

W

Y

CPSIA information can be obtained at www.ICGtesting.com
Printed in the USA
LVOW05s0902280115

424662LV00002B/2/P